Handbook of Pediatric Imaging

Handbook of Pediatric Imaging

Edited by

Lori L. Barr, M.D.

Assistant Professor
Departments of Radiology and Pediatrics
University of Cincinnati College of Medicine
Staff Radiologist
Department of Radiology
Children's Hospital Medical Center
Cincinnati, Ohio

Churchill Livingstone
New York, Edinburgh, London, Melbourne, Tokyo

Library of Congress Cataloging-in-Publication Data
Handbook of pediatric imaging / edited by Lori L. Barr.
p. cm.
Includes bibliographical references and index.
ISBN 0-443-08697-4
1. Pediatric radiography. 2. Pediatric diagnostic imaging.
I. Barr, Lori L.
[DNLM: 1. Diagnostic Imaging—in infancy & childhood. WN200
H236]
RJ51.R3H36 1991
618.92'00757—dc20
DNLM/DLC
for Library of Congress 91-15899
CIP

Distributed in the United Kingdom by Churchill Livingstone, Robert Stevenson House, 1–3 Baxter's Place, Leith Walk, Edinburgh EH1 3AF, and by associated companies, branches, and representatives throughout the world.

Accurate indications, adverse reactions, and dosage schedules for drugs are provided in this book, but it is possible that they may change. The reader is urged to review the package information data of the manufacturers of the medications mentioned.

The Publishers have made every effort to trace the copyright holders for borrowed material. If they have inadvertently overlooked any, they will be pleased to make the necessary arrangements at the first opportunity.

Acquisitions Editor: *Robert A. Hurley*
Production Designer: *Jill Little*
Production Supervisor: *Christina Hippeli*

Printed in the United States of America

First published in 1991 7 6 5 4 3 2 1

To the best, Lu and Lee Barr, and Steve Dent

Contributors

Lori L. Barr, M.D.
Assistant Professor, Departments of Radiology and Pediatrics, University of Cincinnati College of Medicine; Staff Radiologist, Department of Radiology, Children's Hospital Medical Center, Cincinnati, Ohio

Susan D. Stansberry, M.D.
Assistant Professor, Department of Radiology, University of Texas Medical Branch at Galveston; Staff Radiologist, Department of Radiology, Child Health Center, Galveston, Texas

Janet L. Strife, M.D.
Professor, Departments of Radiology and Pediatrics, University of Cincinnati College of Medicine; Staff Radiologist, Department of Radiology, Children's Hospital Medical Center, Cincinnati, Ohio

Leonard E. Swischuk, M.D.
Professor of Radiology and Pediatrics, and Director, Division of Pediatric Radiology, Department of Radiology, University of Texas Medical Branch at Galveston, Galveston, Texas

Preface

The *Handbook of Pediatric Imaging* guides the general radiologist through a thought-provoking review of pediatric radiology. It is written from the perspective of one who enjoys being immersed in the uniqueness of pediatric radiology but who has not forgotten the frustration encountered when faced with volumes of information before board examinations. The handbook reviews, in a concise fashion, what other authors have adequately covered and details areas omitted from other works.

The contents have been organized to provide the reader with the easiest method of committing imaging approaches and diagnoses to memory. In some instances, organ systems are considered as a whole; in other cases an anatomic region is discussed. The interpretation skills emphasized by Dr. Swischuk in Chapter 1 resound throughout the remaining chapters. This design reinforces a logical method of pediatric image evaluation and deductive reasoning that reflects how we were taught pediatric radiology and how we choose to teach our future colleagues.

Pediatric radiology has been revolutionized by recent imaging modalities that use nonionizing radiation. Ultrasonography and magnetic resonance imaging are no longer examinations added to the radiologic work-up but are often the first steps in a child's diagnosis. The effective combination of fluoroscopic skills, which have changed little over the past two generations, and technical expertise bordering on science fiction is especially gratifying in pediatric radiology. What other radiologic subspecialist, after performing such technologic wizardry, is rewarded with the richness of a child's smile?

Lori L. Barr, M.D.

Acknowledgments

The actual writing of this book took far less time than did the preparation of the manuscripts and illustrations by countless people at Children's Hospital Medical Center, the University of Cincinnati College of Medicine, the University of Texas Medical Branch at Galveston, and Churchill Livingstone. Very little of the material in this handbook is the author's own work. I am indebted to the many unnamed investigators on whose work this book is based. The suggested readings are not exhaustive and contain only a small percentage of the references consulted; many of the suggested readings contain extensive references as well.

Special thanks to my mentors and colleagues, Drs. Ronald L. Eisenberg, Donald R. Kirks, and Leonard E. Swischuk, who continue to encourage and support me in my efforts as author and academician. Drs. Susan D. Stansberry and Janet L. Strife generously contributed their professional expertise, sacrificing a significant amount of personal time. They deserve my sincere thanks.

I appreciate the permission granted by several writers and publishers to reproduce illustrations from various works. Special thanks to Dr. Depak Bedi for his contributions.

I thank Drs. William S. Ball, Jr., George S. Bisset III, Erin C. Prenger, and Sanford A. Rubin for their careful review of the text, which resulted in valuable criticisms and suggestions.

I deeply appreciate the long hours of typing done by Ms. Carol Amundsen, Ms. Carmen Floeck, Ms. Toni Hanson, Ms. Juanita Hunter, Ms. Brenda Moore, Ms. Thelma Sanchez, Ms. Marlena Tyre, and Ms. Margaret Walden. However, the combined efforts of these highly skilled secretaries does not match the selfless contributions of dexterity, enthusiasm, and time by Ms. Sallie Kroeger. She serves as a shining example of flexibility because she single-handedly typed seventy percent of the text with no prior knowledge of medical terminology.

The photographs and artwork were rapidly and beautifully produced by Medical Center Information and Communications at the University of Cincinnati College of Medicine. I especially thank Mr. Carl Jones and Ms. Meredith Flerlage for their assistance. The editorial skills of Mr. Robert Hurley and Ms. Bridgett Dickinson at Churchill Livingstone were especially useful. I deeply appreciate the patience and understanding both editors exhibited throughout this process.

The book is dedicated to my husband, Mr. Steven R. Dent, who has given the most time to this effort. Considering that the book evolved during our engagement and marriage, he was extremely understanding and helpful. The rapport he developed with our file room clerks while helping me select illustrations continues to benefit me. My parents were also extremely supportive during this time. I thank them for their love, motivation, and assistance. I dedicate this book to them for the love and encouragement they have given me since birth.

I thank God for providing me with the opportunity to apply myself to this project and hope that it reflects the richness of my chosen profession.

Lori L. Barr, M.D.

Contents

1

Image Interpretation

Leonard E. Swischuk

The general principles of image interpretation in pediatric patients are the same as those used in adults. There are, of course, adjustments for the size of the patient and frequently, a different list of differential diagnostic possibilities for any given constellation of findings is required. Otherwise one begins the assessment of a pediatric radiograph much the same as with an adult radiograph. In this regard, one first should determine how many abnormal findings are present, and begin to construct a differential diagnosis for each abnormal finding. It is best to avoid the trap of trying to construct the differential diagnosis for the entire complex of findings too soon. It is true that this is easier to accomplish with experience but it is still better to provide a differential diagnosis for each finding, and dovetail these differential diagnostic lists to come up with a final list of the most likely possibilities.

Using the above approach, the initial review of a chest x-ray such as in Figure 1–1 yields two rather obvious findings: smallness and increased density of the right hemithorax (Fig. 1–1A). The general causes for the finding of a small hemithorax are hypoplasia (congenital or acquired) or atelectasis. There are many causes of atelectasis but at this point it probably is not worthwhile to delineate them, as atelectasis might not be the problem. If it is, etiologic possibilities will need consideration later.

The next finding, increased density of the small lung, simply implies that the lung contains less air than normal. This can occur with atelectasis, pulmonary hypoplasia, or agenesis. A congenitally hypoplastic lung is radiolucent and shows diminished blood flow because of associated pulmonary artery hypoplasia, or even absence. Agenesis of a lung, on the other hand, produces increased density of the small hemithorax. With complete agenesis the hemithorax is totally opaque but with partial agenesis opacity is less pronounced. Therefore, in our case, partial agenesis would be more likely than complete agenesis, while simple hypoplasia of the lung can be excluded. On lateral view, it becomes apparent that the increased density of the small hemithorax is due to increased density of the upper and middle lobes. The lower lobe is aerated and, in fact, overdistended (Fig. 1–1B); therefore it would seem that the increased density of the hemithorax noted on the frontal view of the chest either is due to atelectasis or agenesis of the right upper and middle lobes.

At this point, familiarity with the so-called hypogenetic right lung syndrome would be helpful. Although this entity can occur on the left, it almost exclusively occurs on the right and is comprised of agenesis of the upper and middle lobes. The radiographic findings are precisely those seen in Figure 1–1 and the condition is associated with other abnor-

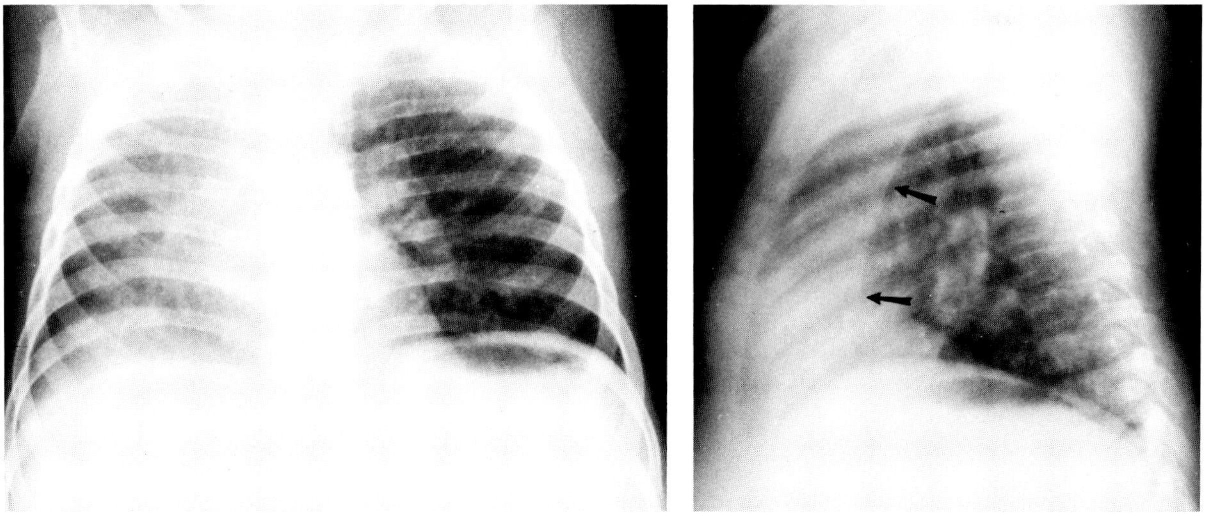

A B

Fig. 1–1 Problem of uneven aeration of the chest. **(A)** The right hemithorax is small and semiopaque. The left lung is radiolucent and shows normal or exaggerated blood flow. The abnormality is on the right. **(B)** Lateral view demonstrating a retrosternal density (*arrows*), an important clue to the diagnosis of this case.

malities such as the scimitar syndrome and accessory diaphragm. The hypogenetic right lung syndrome, therefore, is a very likely possibility but atelectasis of the right upper and middle lobes cannot be excluded. Only further studies or review of old films will determine which of these diagnoses is correct. In this patient the problem was the hypogenetic right lung syndrome and the patient was asymptomatic.

The foregoing case demonstrates the value of assessing each abnormal finding separately. In other instances the differential diagnosis for each abnormal finding is so similar that considering the findings separately is less rewarding. This frequently occurs with bone lesions because bone can only respond to a noxious insult in so many ways and, in fact, bone destruction is simply due to increased osteoclastic activity. This is a nonspecific response on the part of the bone and can be seen with any number of pathologic entities. In such cases, periosteal new bone deposition also often occurs but the differential diagnosis for it and for bone destruction is essentially the same. Therefore, crisscrossing lists of differential diagnostic possibilities for each study is relatively nonproductive and it is best to turn to broad categories of disease and determine whether the findings noted could be produced by these disease categories (i.e., congenital, inflammatory, metabolic, neoplastic, etc.).

For example, in Figure 1–2 the radiograph shows a destructive lesion of the femur in a 5-year-old boy that also shows associated periosteal new bone deposition. Clearly some relatively rapid disease process is present but yet because the periosteal bone is not layered, an extremely aggressive lesion is less likely. Congenital problems producing the findings in Figure 1–2 and presenting at 5 years of age are unlikely, but infection is a good possibility. On the other hand, if one immediately makes note of the fact that most bone infections (osteomyelitis) occur in the metaphyses of long bones, the diaphyseal location of the lesion seen in Figure 1–2 would mitigate against the diagnosis. In other words, even though the radiographic findings are quite compatible with osteomyelitis, the location is not particularly good. By the same token, hematologic diseases (leukemia, sickle cell anemia, etc.) also usually produce metaphyseal lesions and thus the diaphyseal location of the lesion in our case would mitigate against a hematologic disorder.

Next, one might consider metabolic or endocrinologic abnormalities and of these about the only possi-

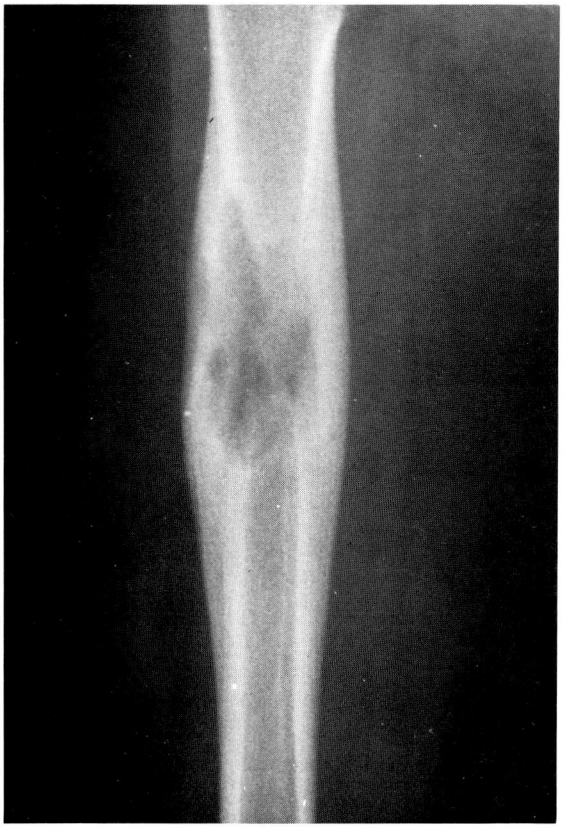

Fig. 1–2 Note the moderately aggressive, mid-diaphyseal destructive lesion in the femur. There is abundant periosteal new bone deposition however, that, is rather mature and solid-appearing.

ble lesion is the brown tumor of hyperparathyroidism. However, if one also notes that the bone, in general, is not demineralized, a brown tumor would not be a good possibility. Traumatic lesions or physical insults to the bone need not be considered as they do not result in the type of bone destruction seen in Figure 1–2. Neoplasms, on the other hand, are a distinct possibility and in fact should be high on one's list. Bone neoplasms can be either primary or secondary and it is well known that most metastases occur in the metaphyseal region of a long bone. A diaphyseal location is not out of the question but is much less likely. The two primary bone tumors most often seen during childhood are osteosarcoma and Ewing's sarcoma. The patient is a little young for both and furthermore, osteosarcomas almost invariably occur in the metaphyses of the long bones; therefore the location of our lesion strongly precludes this possibility. Ewing's tumor, on the other hand, since it commonly occurs in the diaphysis, remains a viable possibility, even though the patient is a little young. However, because Ewing's tumor usually produces delicate, layered periosteal new bone deposition, absence of such new bone greatly weakens the case for Ewing's sarcoma.

Finally, in children, and indeed in young adults, one always must consider the group of diseases known as the reticuloendothelioses (histiocytosis X). This group of diseases can produce a variety of bony lesions and although most often they have a very benign appearance, in children (especially in the midshaft of the femur and humerus) destruction often is so profound that periosteal new bone deposition (usually more solid than layered) is seen, and a malignant disease process is at first suggested. When all of this is considered, histiocytosis X becomes a very strong possibility in our patient and indeed should be the number one choice. This patient did, in fact, have histiocytosis X and no other bony lesions.

If the analysis of any image is approached in one of the two methods just outlined, or if the two methods are combined, seldom will one not be able to offer the referring clinician a well-constructed and pertinent differential diagnosis.[1,2] In many cases and certainly as experience grows, one can even suggest the most likely possibility. Occasionally even a specific diagnosis can be suggested, but it should be remembered that the job of the radiologist is not so much to pinpoint the diagnosis in every case as to analyze the findings individually, and produce an appropriately weighted list of differential diagnostic possibilities.

SUGGESTED READINGS

1. Reuter MB, Felson B: Gamuts in Radiology: Comprehensive List of Roentgen Differential Diagnosis. Audiovisual Radiology of Cincinnati, Cincinnati, 1975
2. Swischuk LE: Differential Diagnosis in Pediatric Radiology, Williams & Wilkins, Baltimore, 1984

2

Face and Neck

Lori L. Barr

RADIOGRAPHIC TECHNIQUES

Plain radiographic analysis of the face may be indicated for a variety of conditions including nasal stuffiness, epistaxis, fever of unknown origin, trauma, or localized asymmetry. Three standard views often obtained are the Waters view, Caldwell's view and a lateral view. When the patient is well-positioned for a Waters view, the petrous pyramids are seen at the floor of the maxillary sinuses. This is achieved by having the central ray perpendicular to the radiograph and acute angulation above the orbitomeatal line (Fig. 2–1). The amount of angulation varies with the head size of the child and may be anywhere from 10 to 37 degrees. This view provides excellent visualization of the maxillary sinuses, nasal septum, hard palate, and coronoid process of the mandible. Caldwell's view is obtained by angling the central ray approximately 15 degrees cranial to the orbitomeatal line (Fig. 2–2). The ideal radiograph has the petrous pyramids projected at the level of the posterior floor of the orbit. This provides excellent visualization of the frontal and ethmoid sinuses, orbital rims, sphenoid wings, and the nasal septum. The lateral view is obtained with the patient in the direct lateral position and the central ray perpendicular to the radiograph (Fig. 2–3). This provides excellent visualization of the sphenoid sinus, hard palate, nasopharynx, frontal sinus, and the velum. Specialized views such as nasal views, the submentovertex view, and orbital views may be used when clinically indicated.

PARANASAL SINUS GROWTH

The maxillary sinuses are aerated at birth, the lateral margin is underneath the infraorbital canal by 2 years of age and lateral to the infraorbital canal by 5 years of age. The sinus continues to expand until the age of 9. The ostia of the maxillary sinuses are located high on the lateral nasal walls and drain into the hiatus semilunaris. Even in premature infants aerated maxillary sinuses are easily identified on the Waters view. The maxillary sinuses are the most likely of the paranasal sinuses to be diseased.

At birth, the ethmoid sinuses are usually aerated and very little growth occurs thereafter. Because each sinus is made up of numerous air cells lying one in front of the other, their overlap may be radiographically projected as septal blurring even when fully aerated. The anterior ethmoid air cells empty into the hiatus semilunaris, the middle into the middle meatus, and the posterior cells into the superior meatus.

Even though the sphenoid sinuses become aerated before 2 years of age, the central location within the calvaria makes evaluation difficult on both frontal and lateral radiographs. The sphenoid sinus ostia are located along the anterior walls of the sinus draining into the sphenoethmoidal recesses.

The frontal sinuses are the last to become aerated

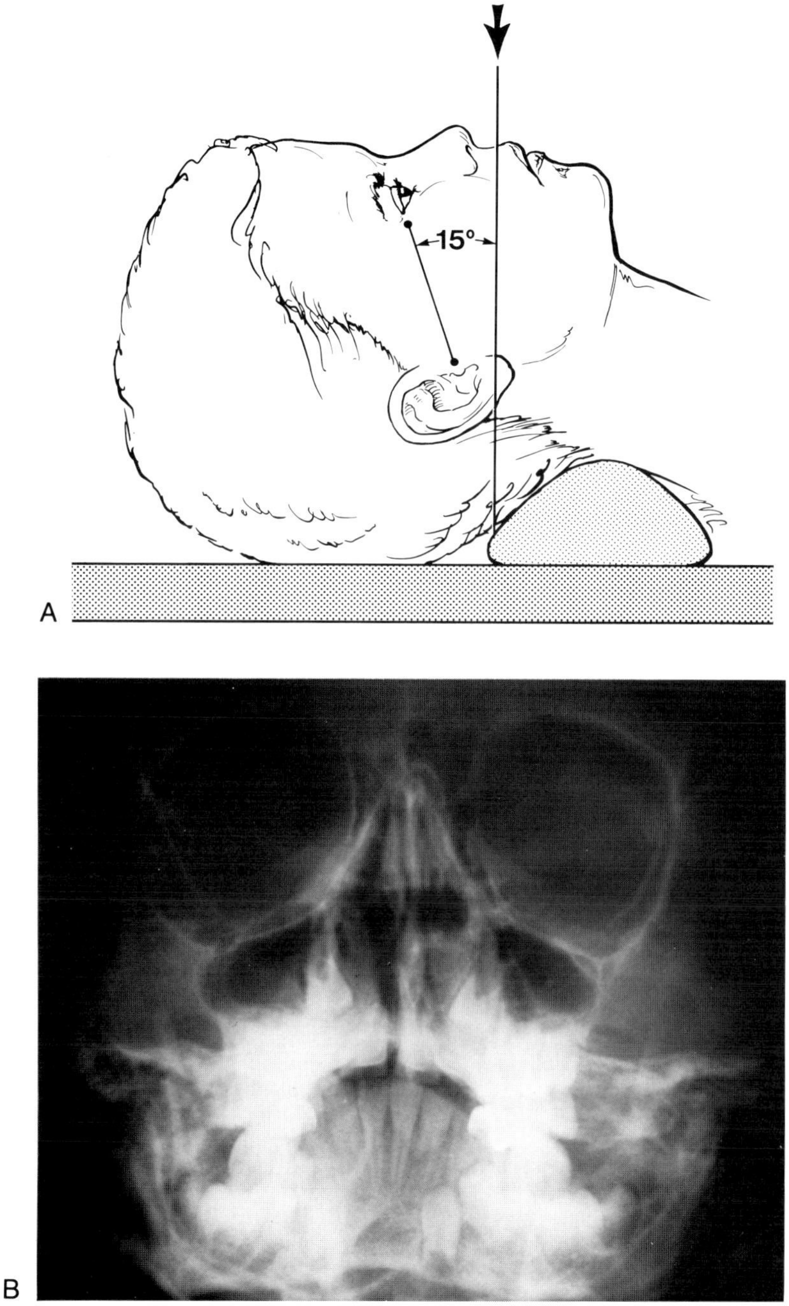

Fig. 2–1 Waters view. **(A)** Note the head positioning, useful in infants for a reverse Waters view. The amount of orbitomeatal line angulation may vary between 10 to 37 degrees dependig on head size. **(B)** Although the angulation of the tube was excellent for this Waters view, note the malalignment of the nasal septum with the front teeth. The result is pseudothickening of the lateral wall of the right maxillary sinus; improper positioning is the most common cause of opacification of a child's sinus.

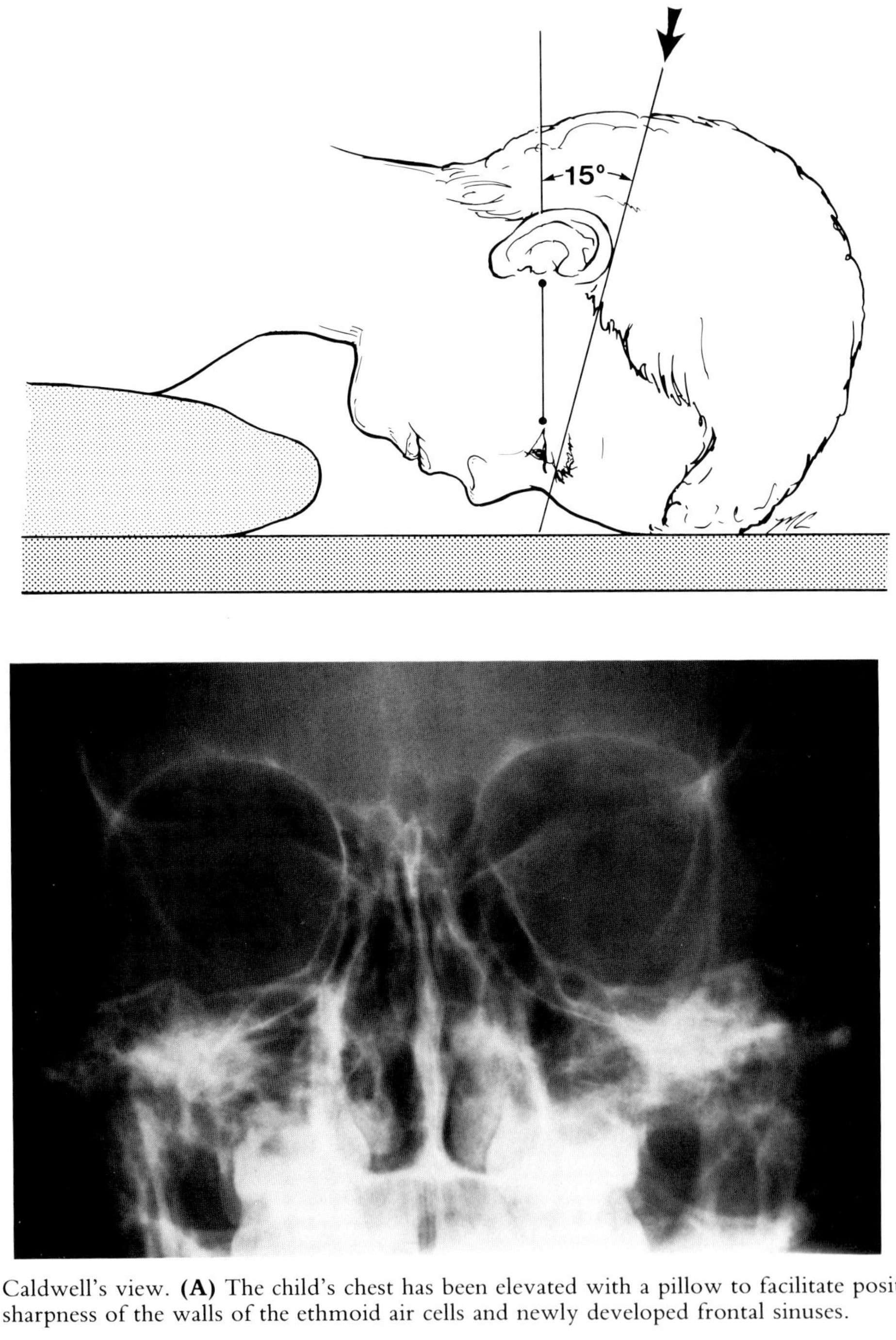

A

B

Fig. 2–2 Caldwell's view. **(A)** The child's chest has been elevated with a pillow to facilitate positioning. **(B)** Note the sharpness of the walls of the ethmoid air cells and newly developed frontal sinuses.

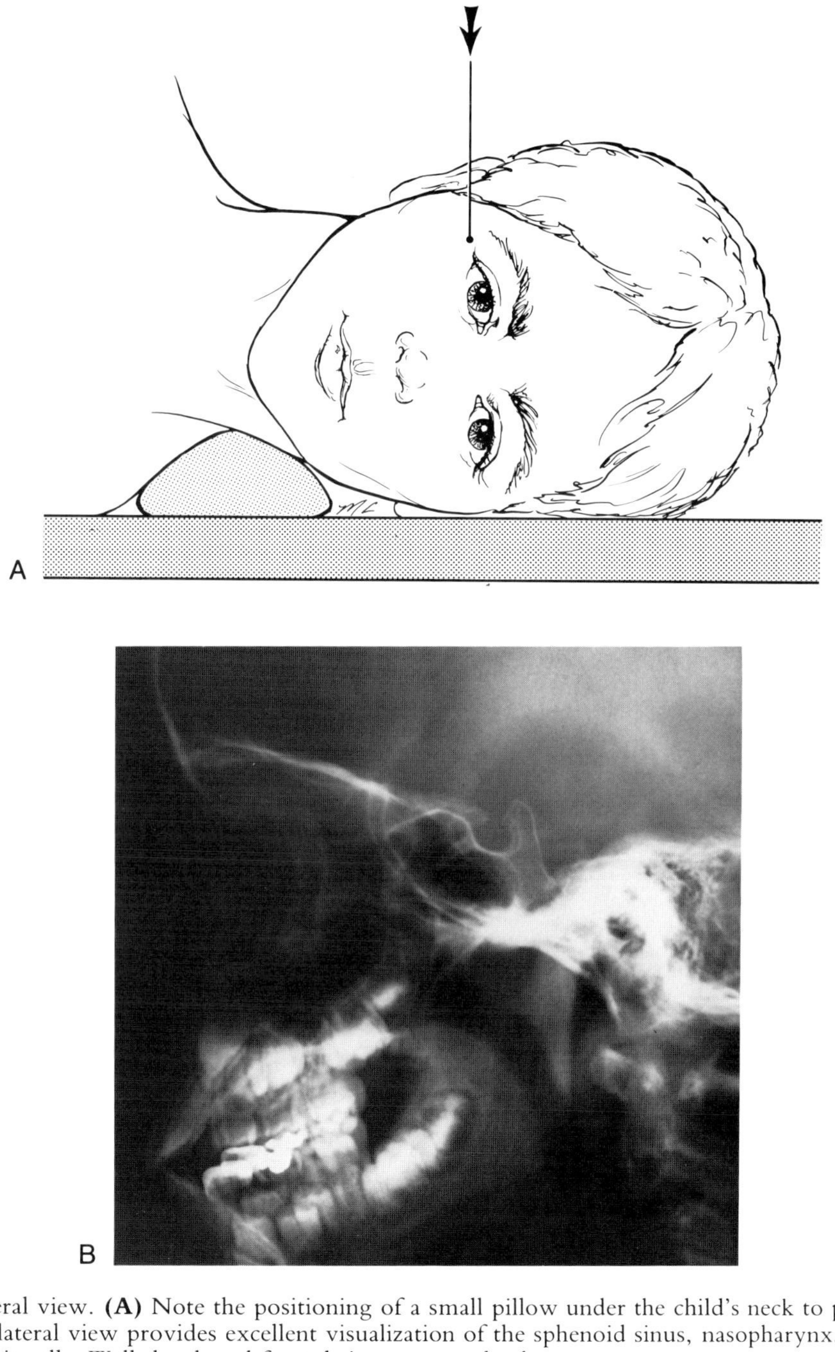

Fig. 2–3 Lateral view. **(A)** Note the positioning of a small pillow under the child's neck to prevent head tilt. **(B)** The lateral view provides excellent visualization of the sphenoid sinus, nasopharynx, hypopharynx, and mastoid air cells. Well-developed frontal sinuses may also be seen.

and usually extend above the superior orbital rim by 10 years of age. The frontal sinus drains via the frontonasal duct or into the anterior ethmoid air cells.

Both the paranasal sinuses and the nasopharynx are lined with the same type of mucoperiosteum. Many of the pathologic processes affecting the paranasal sinuses involve the nasopharynx as well. If surgery is planned, evaluation of the nasopharynx and the paranasal sinuses is best achieved by coronal 5-mm computed tomography (CT) scans obtained at 5-mm increments. In children, use of intravenous (IV) contrast material is uncommon. If there is a question concerning whether a sinus is hypoplastic or obliterated by a mass, magnetic resonance imaging (MRI) may differentiate fatty bone marrow in the underpneumatized sinus from other soft tissue masses (Fig. 2–4). In complex facial anomalies requiring reconstruction either the multi-imaging planes provided by MRI or three-dimensional reconstruction with CT help in preoperative planning (Fig. 2–5). In either case, small children must be sedated and sometimes require general anesthesia for cross-sectional imaging.

NASOPHARYNX AND PARANASAL SINUS OPACIFICATION

Normal

When one encounters apparent pathology on any image, it is important to ask whether there are variations of normal or technical factors that could mimic disease. With opacification of the nasopharynx or paranasal sinuses, both conditions apply. In young patients, positioning is difficult due to the small size of the head and may result in overlap of the maxilla and unerupted tooth buds over the maxillary sinuses. It is important to keep in mind the ages at which the sinuses become aerated since a lack of aeration in the frontal sinus, for example, may be secondary to the patient's age rather than to a pathologic process. In the posterior aspect of the nasopharynx, the most common cause of a mass is hypertrophy of normal lymphoidal tissue (Fig. 2–6). This may result in hypernasal speech requiring audio-enhanced videofluoroscopic evaluation. Depending on the size of

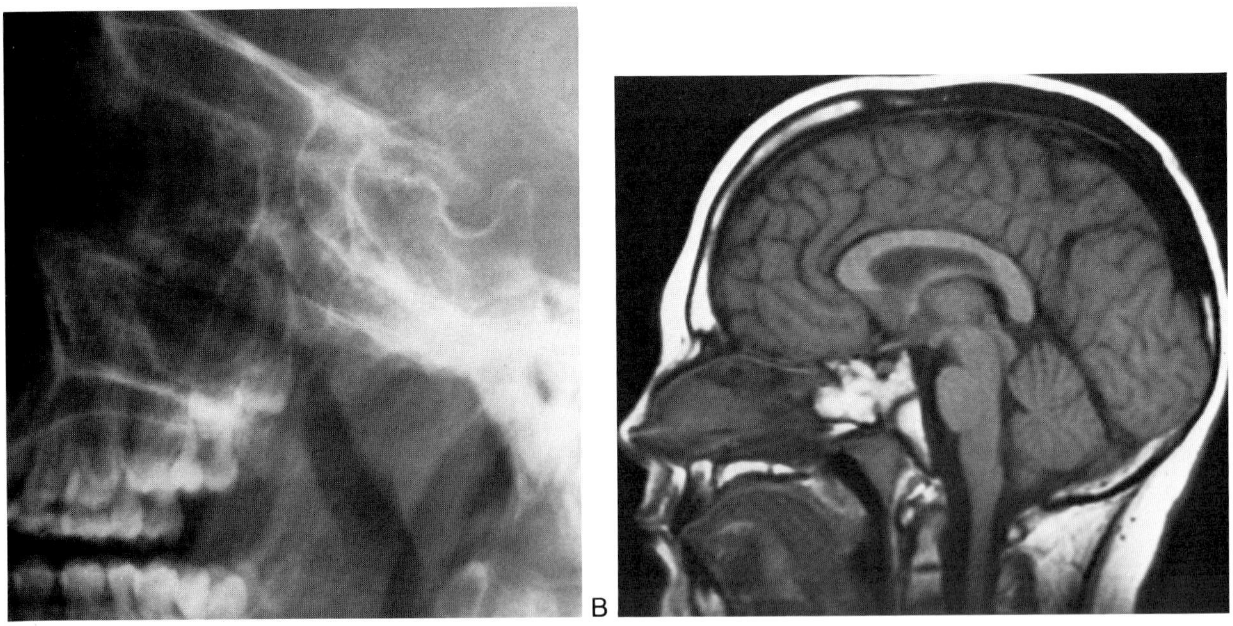

A B

Fig. 2–4 Hypoplastic sphenoid sinus. **(A)** Lateral view demonstrates absence of aeration in the region of the sphenoid sinus in this 10-year-old patient. **(B)** T_1-weighted sagittal MRI slice demonstrates fat within bone marrow filling the usual site of the sphenoid sinus, which has not developed yet in this patient. The fat is high in signal intensity.

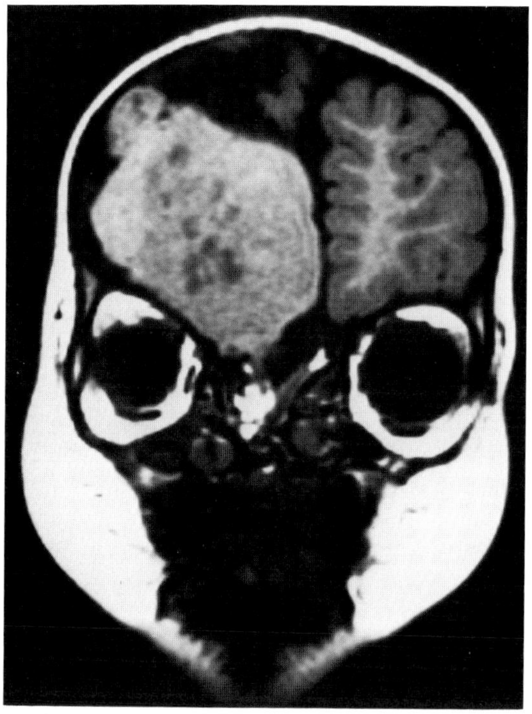

A

Fig. 2–5 Facial anomalies. **(A)** Coronal T_1-weighted MRI demonstrates profound hypertelorism in this patient with a large right frontal teratoma that has extended into the nasal cavity and widened the bones. **(B)** Another child with Apert's syndrome demonstrates a hypoplastic maxilla and severe frontal bossing on the lateral projection of the three-dimensional CT scan. **(C)** Frontal projection demonstrates ridging along the synostotic coronal sutures bilaterally and an enlarged metopic suture compensating for the early closure of the other sutures.

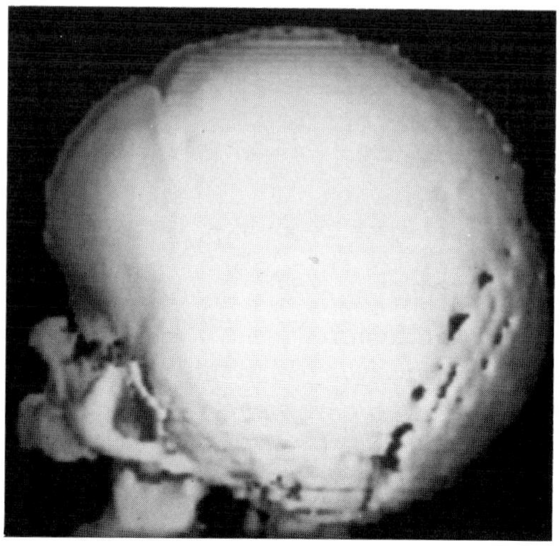

B

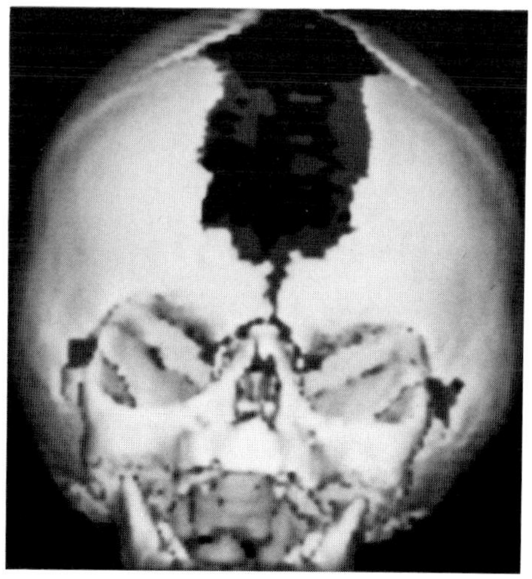

C

NASOPHARYNGEAL/PARANASAL SINUS OPACIFICATION

Normal
- Poor patient positioning
- Age-related underaeration
- Lymphoid hypertrophy

Congenital
- Inclusion cysts
- Hypoplasia/aplasia
- Cystic fibrosis
- Choanal atresia
- Nasal meningocele/encephalocele
- Nasal dermoid
- Tornwalt's cyst

Inflammation
- Infection (bacteria, virus, fungus)
- Osteomyelitis
- Granulomatous disease (Wegener's, sarcoidosis)
- Allergic sinusitis
- Adenomatous/inflammatory polyps
- Antrochoanal polyp
- Mucus retention cysts
- Mucocele

Neoplasm
- Osteoma
- Epithelial papilloma
- Juvenile angiofibroma
- Rhabdomyosarcoma
- Lymphoma
- Lymphoepithelioma
- Meningioma
- Hemangioma
- Schwannoma
- Sarcoma

Systemic/generalized
- Eosinophilic granuloma
- Fibrous dysplasia
- Hemolytic anemias
- Von Willebrand's disease

Trauma
- Fracture
- Foreign body
- Barotrauma

Iatrogenic
- Postoperative
- Antral lavage
- Postirradiation

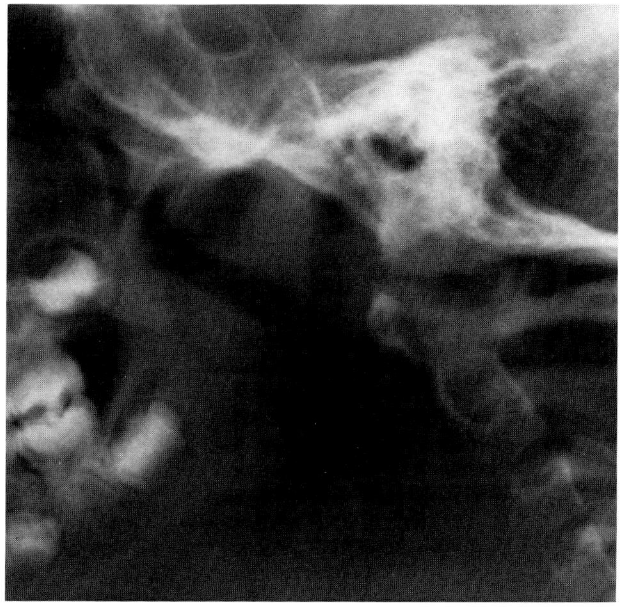

Fig. 2–6 Normal lymphoid hypertrophy. Note the fullness in the superior posterior portion of the nasopharynx of this patient with hypernasal speech.

the velopharyngeal portal, the hypertrophied lymphoid tissue may play an important role in approximation of the velum with the posterior pharyngeal wall. Removal of the lymphoidal tissue may worsen the patient's speech instead of improve it.

Congenital

The development of the nose stems from fusion of lateral and medial nasal processes. Midline facial defects such as cleft palate, cleft lip, bifid nose, and hypertelorism involve the floor of the nose and prevent implantation of the nasal septum. Occasionally, midline defects will result in nasal encephaloceles, meningoceles, inclusion cysts, or nasal dermoids. The frontal sinus is most likely to demonstrate variable degrees of unilateral hypoplasia or even aplasia. When bilateral aplasia of the frontal sinuses is seen, predisposing conditions such as mucoviscidosis (cystic fibrosis) and thalassemia major should be considered. In the remainder of the paranasal sinuses, asymmetry between the two sides is more likely to be due to a pathologic process than hypoplasia. Maxillary hypoplasia may be recognized by an increased downward slanting of the maxillary sinus roof. The sinus walls continue to be sharply outlined despite the size discrepancy. Not only is mucoviscidosis associated with

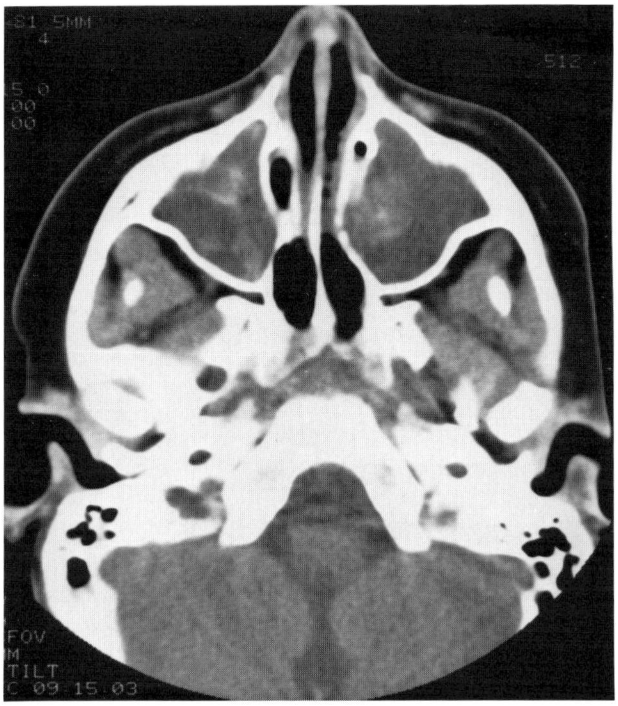

Fig. 2–7 Cystic fibrosis. Note the thickened mucoperiosteum lining the walls of both totally opacified maxillary sinuses. Contrast material has not been given. The high density material in the center of the sinuses represents inspissated mucus.

A

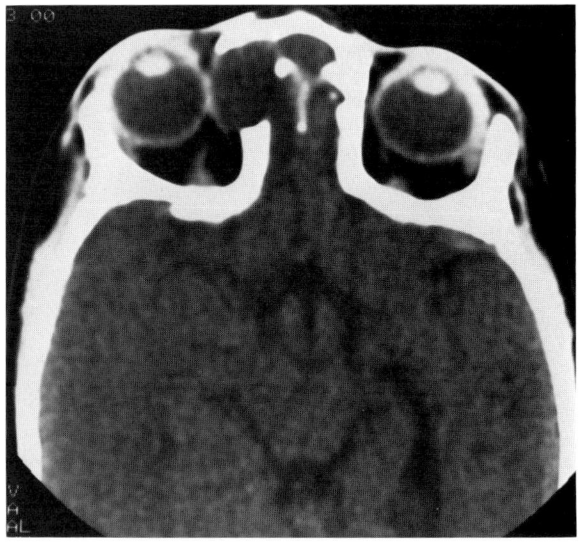

Fig. 2–8 Basal cephalocele. **(A)** Axial CT scan demonstrates a mass of cerebrospinal fluid density interrupting the medial wall of the right orbit. (*Figure continues.*)

sinus aplasia, it may result in the formation of hypertrophic nodular mucosa throughout the nasopharynx and the paranasal sinuses. Radiographically this appears as symmetric mucoperiosteal thickening of all of the sinuses. The thick tenacious mucus may totally opacify the paranasal sinuses and the nasopharynx. With CT, the mucus has an increased attenuation when compared to thickened mucoperiosteum (Fig. 2–7). Although the appearance is classic for cystic fibrosis with inspissated mucus, other conditions, such as fungal sinusitis, may have the same appearance. Because the problem is chronic, the sinuses often are generous in size and demonstrate outward bowing of the walls.

Choanal atresia, unless bilateral, is a relatively innocuous congenital cause of nasal obstruction diagnosed clinically by the inability to pass a small catheter through the nasopharynx. CT provides the surgeon with the exact level of obstruction and presence of bony obstruction prior to surgical intervention.

Encountering a midline nasal or nasopharyngeal mass in the neonatal period should alert one to the possibility of abnormal closure of the anterior neuropore during intrauterine life, which leads to the formation of cephaloceles. Although most cephaloceles are located in the occipital region, basal cephaloceles are not uncommon (Fig. 2–8). The presence of brain within the cephalocele alters the surgical approach. Small amounts of brain tissue may be missed if CT is the only imaging modality used. MRI, subarachnoid injection of metrizamide followed by CT, or subarachnoid injection of ^{99m}Tc-DTPA establishes the presence of communication prior to surgery.

Inclusions of primitive totipotential cells lead to formation of cysts, dermoids, and teratomas. Congenital inclusion cysts are likely to form at fissure sites. The globulomaxillary cyst is a rare inclusion cyst arising between the roots of the lateral maxillary incisor and canine teeth. It appears as a soft tissue mass of the maxillary sinus.

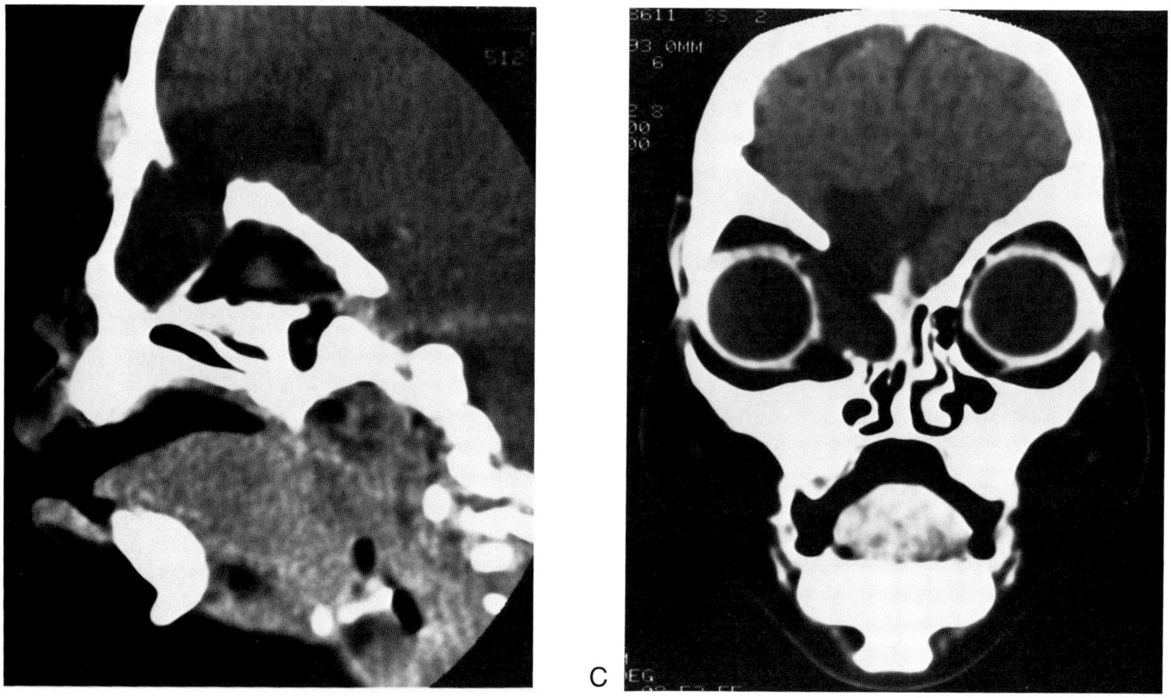

B C

Fig. 2–8 (*Continued*). **(B)** Sagittal CT scan demonstrates bony interruption of the anterior cranial fossa. The density of the mass is equal to that of the cerebrospinal fluid in the extra-axial spaces. **(C)** Coronal CT scan demonstrates lateral displacement of the right globe, obliteration of the right ethmoid air cells, and left nasal septal deviation because of the basal cephalocele. A repeat study was performed after contrast material injection into the subarachnoid space. The cephalocele did not communicate.

Inflammation

Inflammation or infection may cause a variety of plain radiographic findings, including paranasal sinus opacification, mucoperiosteal thickening, air/fluid levels, and rounded soft tissue masses. It is of utmost importance to correlate radiographic images with the clinical history of the patient. While air/fluid levels are the most reliable radiographic sign of acute sinusitis in children, a differential diagnosis of blood, transudate, and iatrogenic fluid must be considered when the clinical history is not available. The most common cause of acute sinusitis in children is viral upper respiratory tract infection (Fig. 2–9). It is only when the sinus ostia become occluded that bacterial or fungal overgrowth leads to sinusitis requiring medical intervention. In the normal host, bacterial sinusitis presents as an acute febrile illness with nasal stuffiness and a nighttime cough. The clinician may choose to treat the patient with antibiotics and no radiographic correlation. However, if the child is still symptomatic after an adequate course of antibiotic therapy, radiographs should be obtained and a referral made to an otorhinolaryngologist. If endoscopy or surgical intervention is planned, CT is indicated. The findings of bacterial sinusitis on CT include total opacification of the sinuses or air/fluid levels (Fig. 2–10). In chronic sinusitis (more likely to occur in the immunocompromised host), sinus wall expansion may be seen (Fig. 2–11). Often circumferential mucoperiosteal thickening is present and there is increased attenuation of the material located centrally, which opacifies the sinuses. This material may represent sterile inspissated mucus, fungus (aspergillosis, candidiasis, actinomycosis), or other unclassified organisms (mucormycosis). CT is extremely helpful in diagnosing complications related to sinusitis, including periorbital cellulitis, osteomyelitis, cavernous sinus thrombosis, subperiosteal abscesses, and epidural abscesses. The earliest radiographic finding of osteomyelitis is loss of the mucoperiosteal line identifying the sinus wall. In chronic indolent osteomyelitis,

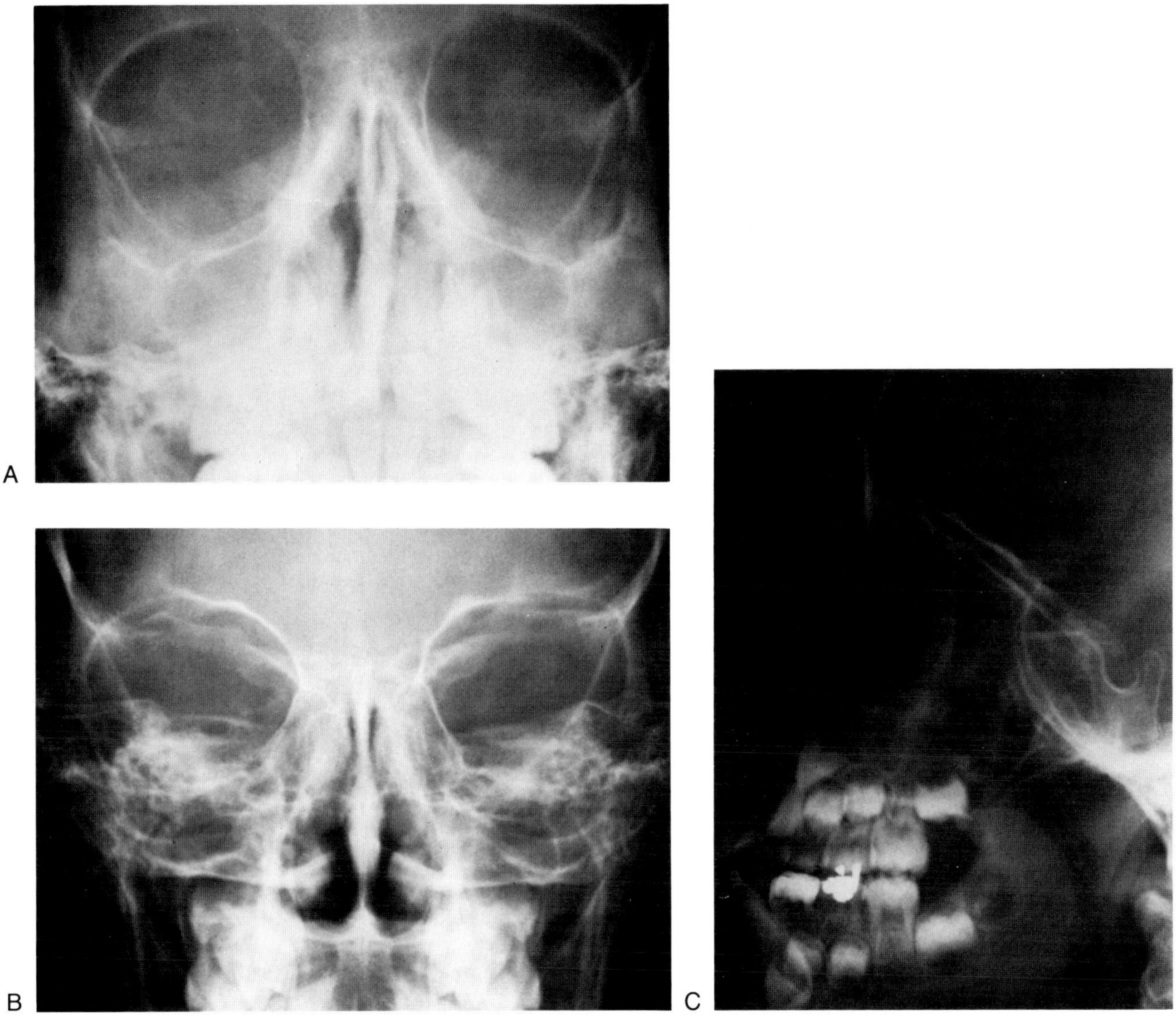

Fig. 2–9 Acute sinusitis. **(A)** Waters view demonstrates total opacification of both maxillary sinuses. **(B)** Caldwell's view demonstrates total opacification of the ethmoid air cells but normal nasal mucosa. **(C)** Lateral view demonstrates total opacification of sphenoid sinus. The patient complained of headaches but was afebrile. The pansinusitus cleared without antibiotic therapy. For comparison, note the normal appearance of the same child in Figs. 2–1B, 2–2B, and 2–3B.

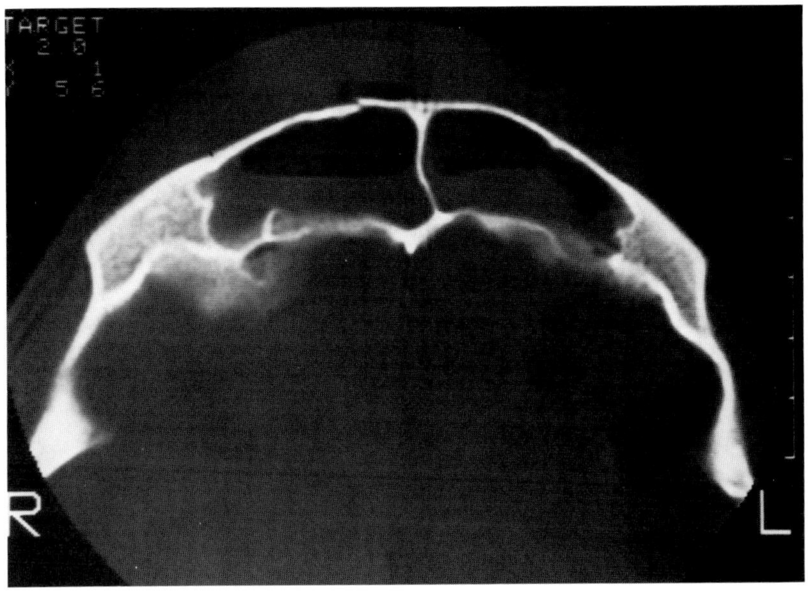

Fig. 2–10 Acute sinusitis. Note the air/fluid levels in both frontal sinuses consistent with acute sinusitis. The prefrontal soft tissue swelling and subcutaneous air suggest the development of Pott's puffy tumor and bony dehiscence. These complications of frontal sinusitis were not accompanied by intracranial extension.

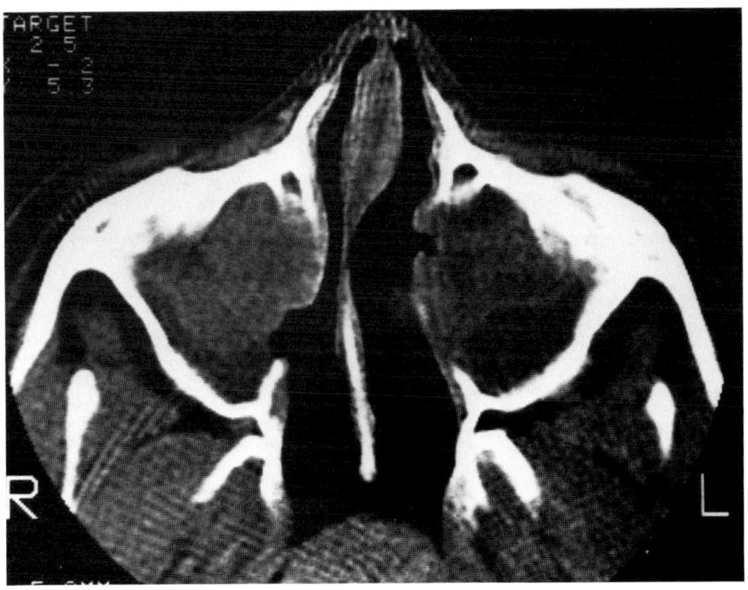

Fig. 2–11 Sinus wall expansion. Note the bulging of the medial walls of the maxillary sinuses inward toward the nasal passages. Both sinuses are totally opacified due to inspissated mucus and chronic sinusitis.

changes include sclerosis of the sinus walls and occasionally sequestrum formation. The incidence of intracranial complications of sinusitis is approximately 3 percent.[21]

Granulomatous disease begins in the nasal cavity with secondary spread into the paranasal sinuses. Tuberculosis, Wegener's granulomatosis, sarcoidosis, and midline granuloma (rare in children) may all present as focal or widespread mucoperiosteal thickening of the nasal cavity and sinuses (Fig. 2–12). Bilateral involvement is the rule and sinus wall expansion is associated. The most common finding seen in children is circumferential mucoperiosteal thickening of the maxillary sinuses. However, with chronic longstanding disease localized cartilage or bone destruction may occur. Wegener's granulomatosis is the most common granulomatous disease of childhood and consists of a triad of upper respiratory tract granulomas, pulmonary disease, and glomerulonephritis. Pathologically, both vasculitis and necrotizing granulomas are identified. Cyclophosphamide is the treatment of choice.

Children with allergies, asthma, or cystic fibrosis may develop uniform circumferential mucoperiosteal thickening involving the majority of the sinuses and the nasal cavity. The inflammatory adenomatous polyp is thought to be the most common new growth in the nasopharynx of children, although it is rarely considered a neoplasm. While polyps less than 1 cm in size often are not radiographically distinguished, nasal polyposis is the most common cause of expansion of the nasal cavity. On noncontrast CT scans, both inflammatory and allergic polyps have a similar density (10 to 18 HU). With injection of IV contrast material, the inflammatory polyp will enhance. However, because treatment is similar in both conditions, contrast enhanced CT scans are usually not performed. A specific form of adenomatous polyp formation is the antrochoanal polyp, which arises from the floor of one of the maxillary sinuses. Five percent of adenomatous polyps are antrochoanal. The polyp grows, opacifies the sinus, extends through the sinus ostium, and dangles into the nasopharynx. Patients usually present with nasal stuffiness or with hypernasal speech. Radiographic examination reveals a nasopharyngeal mass and an opacified maxillary sinus (Fig. 2–13). The treatment of choice is complete surgical excision. Recurrence is rare with treatment. However, if the polyp is snared instead of resected, recurrence rates are high.

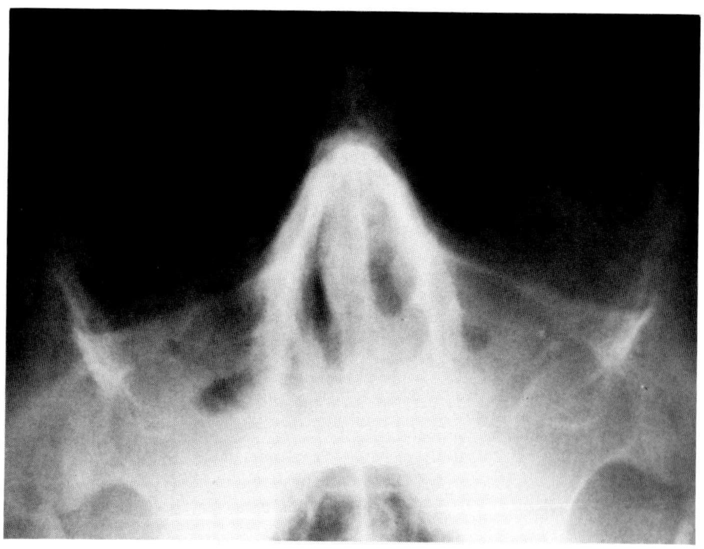

Fig. 2–12 Wegener's granulomatosis. Note the circumferential mucoperiosteal thickening involving both maxillary sinuses and nasal passages in the Waters view of this patient.

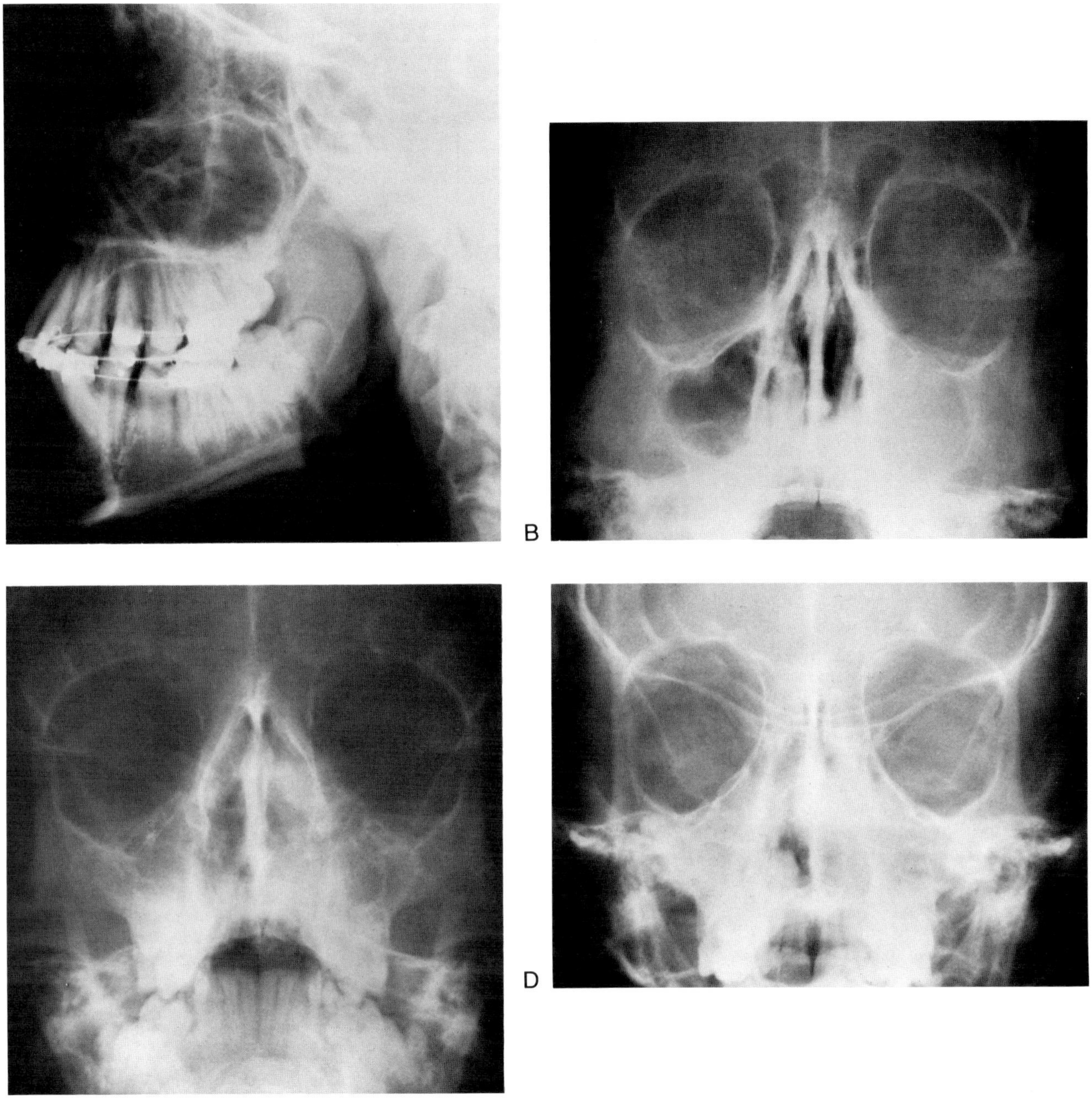

A B C D

Fig. 2–13 Antrochoanal polyp versus inflammatory polyposis. **(A)** The lateral view of this patient with nasal stuffiness reveals a large soft tissue mass extending below the level of the soft palate. The nasopharyngeal air space is obliterated. **(B)** Waters view demonstrates total opacification of the left maxillary sinus consistent with the diagnosis of an antrochoanal polyp extending out of the left maxillary sinus and dangling into the nasopharynx. **(C)** By contrast, Waters view of this child with cystic fibrosis demonstrates total opacification of both maxillary sinuses and a suggestion of a mass in the left nasal passage. These findings are suspicious for inflammatory polyposis. **(D)** Caldwell's view of the same patient demonstrates a left nasopharyngeal mass that proved to be an inflammatory polyp. Note the total opacification of the ethmoid air cells consistent with polyposis.

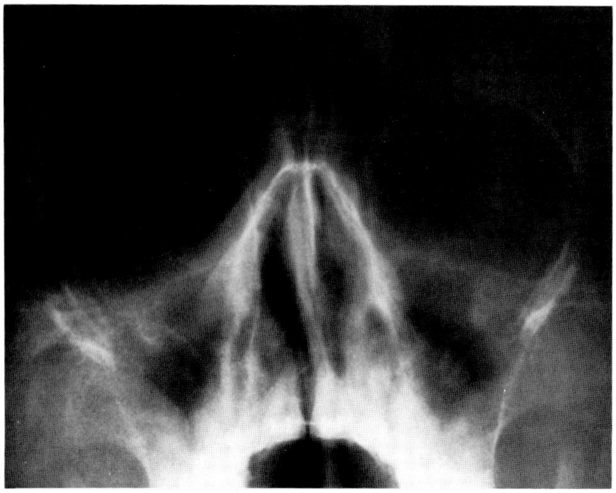

Fig. 2–14 Mucus retention cyst. Note the circumferential mucoperiosteal thickening present in both maxillary sinuses. The rounded soft tissue density arising from the floor of the left maxillary sinus represents a mucus retention cyst.

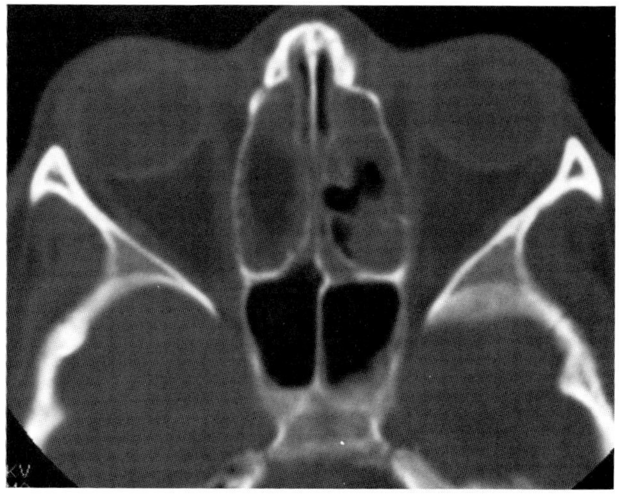

Fig. 2–15 Mucocele. Note the expansion of the walls of the ethmoid air cells medially and laterally. On the right, no aeration is demonstrated. A rim of soft tissue density surrounds a fluid collection. These findings are consistent with early mucocele formation.

Another cause of a rounded soft tissue mass in one of the paranasal sinuses is the mucus retention cyst (Fig. 2–14). This most commonly occurs in the floor of the maxillary sinus following an episode of chronic sinusitis. While most retention cysts occur as an incidental finding on facial radiographs or cross-sectional imaging studies of the brain, a small number may increase in size expanding the sinus wall and causing erosion.

The most common cause of sinus wall expansion is mucocele formation, which usually occurs in the frontal sinuses. The ethmoids and maxillary sinuses may also be involved. On plain radiographs, an opacified sinus is seen with a smooth wall instead of normal scalloping. The density of the mucocele never exceeds that of the adjacent facial bones (Fig. 2–15).

Neoplasm

Neoplasms arising in the paranasal sinuses/nasal cavity often cause symptoms of nasopharyngeal obstruction. These include hypernasal speech, nasal stuffiness, diplopia, and recurrent ear infections from obstruction of the eustachian tubes.

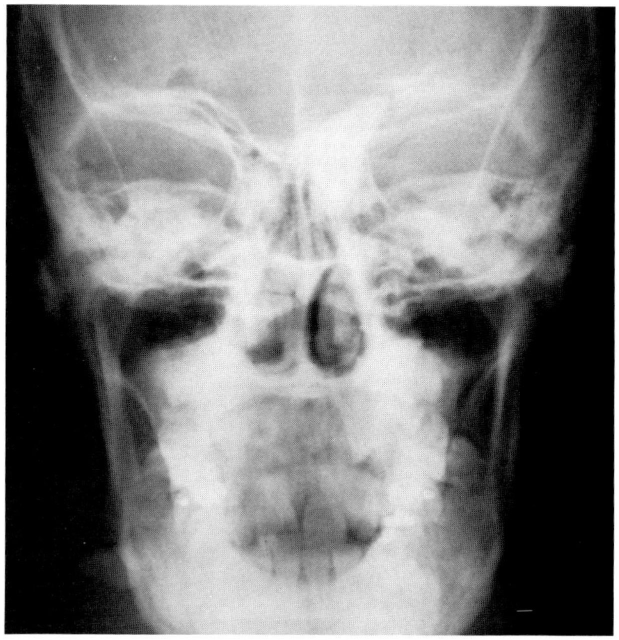

Fig. 2–16 Multiple osteomas. Sharply demarcated bone density masses arise in the left frontal sinus and in the ethmoid air cells bilaterally. Note the similar lesions arising from both sides of the mandible. This patient had Gardner's syndrome.

The most common benign tumor of the paranasal sinuses is the osteoma (Fig. 2–16). The frontal sinus is the usual site of growth followed by the ethmoid and maxillary sinuses. Although the majority of osteomas are densely calcified, noncalcified osteomas may rarely occur and are difficult to differentiate from polyps and retention cysts. Osteomas are slow-growing and will expand the involved sinus wall. When multiple facial osteomas are seen the diagnosis of Gardner's syndrome should be recognized. This syndrome includes multiple osteomas associated with colonic polyps and pigmented mucous membrane lesions. Since the intestinal polyps are adenomatous, the referring physician and family should be informed of the increased incidence of adenocarcinoma. Other rare, benign tumors of the sinuses include epithelial papillomas, hemangiomas, schwannomas, neurofibromas, and meningiomas.

The most common benign nasopharyngeal tumor of childhood is the juvenile angiofibroma. The tumor occurs most frequently in pubescent males presenting with epistaxis and nasal obstruction. Although the tumor is histologically benign, it is aggressive, expanding the pharyngeal structures and growing through the surrounding foramina. On the lateral plain view, anterior bowing of the posterior wall of the maxillary antrum may be noted (Fig. 2–17). Either enhanced CT or MRI is useful for demonstration of tumor vascularity and infratemporal fossa extension that may alter the surgical approach. Cross-sectional imaging is also useful in monitoring response to hormonal therapy prior to surgery. Angiography may define the origins of feeding vessels, embolization may decrease intraoperative blood loss.

Malignant nasopharyngeal and paranasal sinus tumors in children are quite rare. Although squamous cell carcinoma is the most common cell type in adults, lymphoepithelioma is the most common in children. Other cell types include rhabdomyosarcoma and lymphoma. Most malignant tumors in the nasopharynx demonstrate a soft tissue mass with evidence of bone destruction. Cross-sectional imaging will identify infiltration into the infratemporal fossa or parapharyngeal space. The nasopharynx and paranasal sinuses are an important site for metastatic disease in children, especially secondary to neuroblastoma.

Systemic Diseases

Several generalized conditions may obliterate the paranasal sinuses, including severe hemolytic anemias, such as sickle cell disease and thalassemia major, eosinophilic granuloma, and fibrous dysplasia. Von Willebrand's disease has a peculiar predilection for bleeding into the paranasal sinuses and should be considered in the differential diagnosis of multiple air/fluid levels. The hemolytic anemias cause thinning of the cortex and widening of the medullary spaces. The maxillary sinuses may be obliterated by expansion of the maxilla (Fig. 2–18). Fibrous dysplasia causes increased density of the involved bone with expansion of the medullary space by fibrous material with scattered calcific components. If fibrous dysplasia is monostotic, it may be difficult to differentiate from benign bone tumors such as osteoblastoma or ossifying fibroma (both rare in children). Eosinophilic granuloma causes focal destruction and may involve any portion of the face or calvaria.

Trauma

When air/fluid levels are encountered in the paranasal sinuses, trauma must be suspected. Facial fractures are usually accompanied by soft tissue swelling. However, the presence of a foreign body, if small, may have a more indolent clinical course causing localized sinusitis due to an obstructed ostium. Barotrauma is secondary to rapid compression of the air-filled spaces creating a vortex that draws blood into the paranasal sinuses or middle ear from surrounding vessels. This may occur during scuba diving or airline travel, especially if sinus or middle ear disease is present. Air/fluid levels occur in the affected air spaces.

When a child sustains a blow to the face, facial radiographs are often obtained during the emergency room visit. The full extent of facial fractures is best delineated by CT. The most common fractures involving a single bone include the mandible, nasal bones, zygomatic arches, and inferior orbital floor (blowout fracture). The mandible is best evaluated by panoramic views, although most fractures may be detected with the combination of mandibular views and a Towne or submentovertex view. The Towne

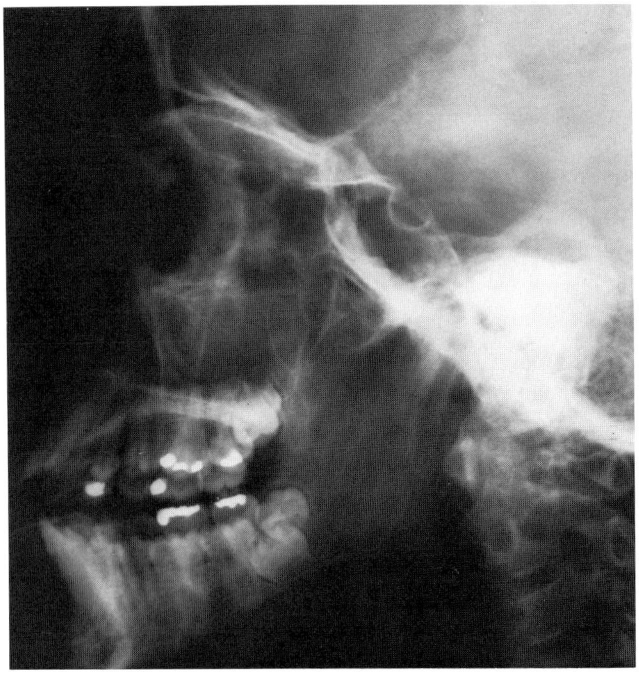

A

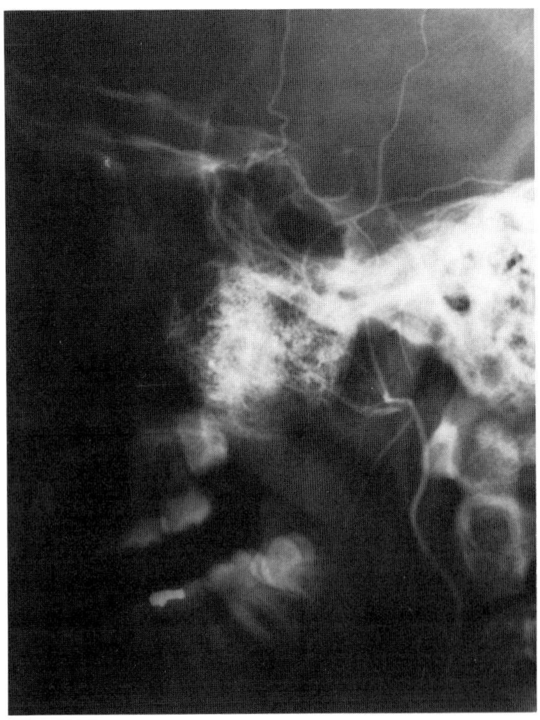

B

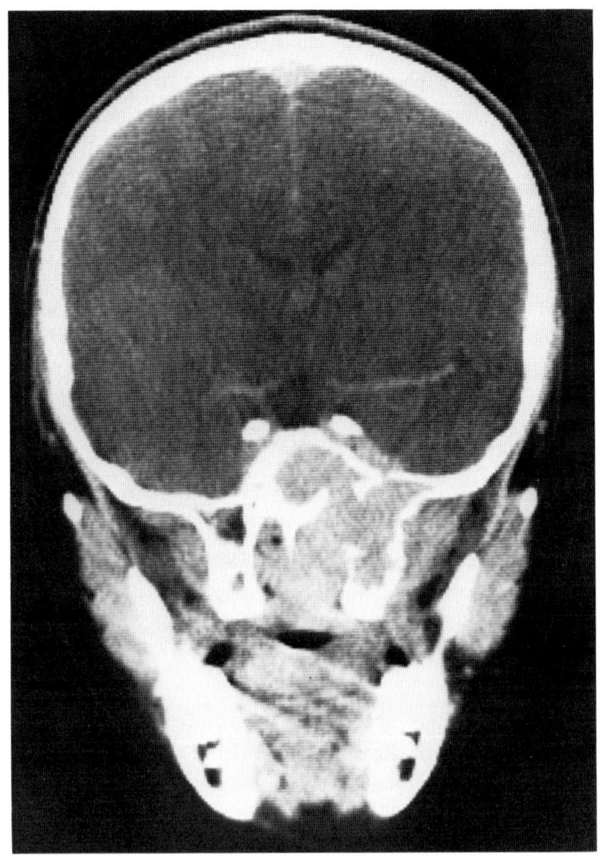

C

Fig. 2–17 Juvenile angiofibroma. **(A)** Lateral view of a patient presenting with epistaxis. Note the obliteration of the nasopharyngeal air space and anterior bowing of the posterior wall of one of the maxillary sinuses suspicious for a juvenile angiofibroma. **(B)** Injection of contrast material into the left external carotid artery of another patient demonstrates dense enhancement of a large juvenile angiofibroma that was subsequently embolized. **(C)** Enhanced coronal CT scan demonstrates enlargement of the nasopharynx with bony destruction by an enhancing juvenile angiofibroma. The tumor had invaded the left middle cranial fossa.

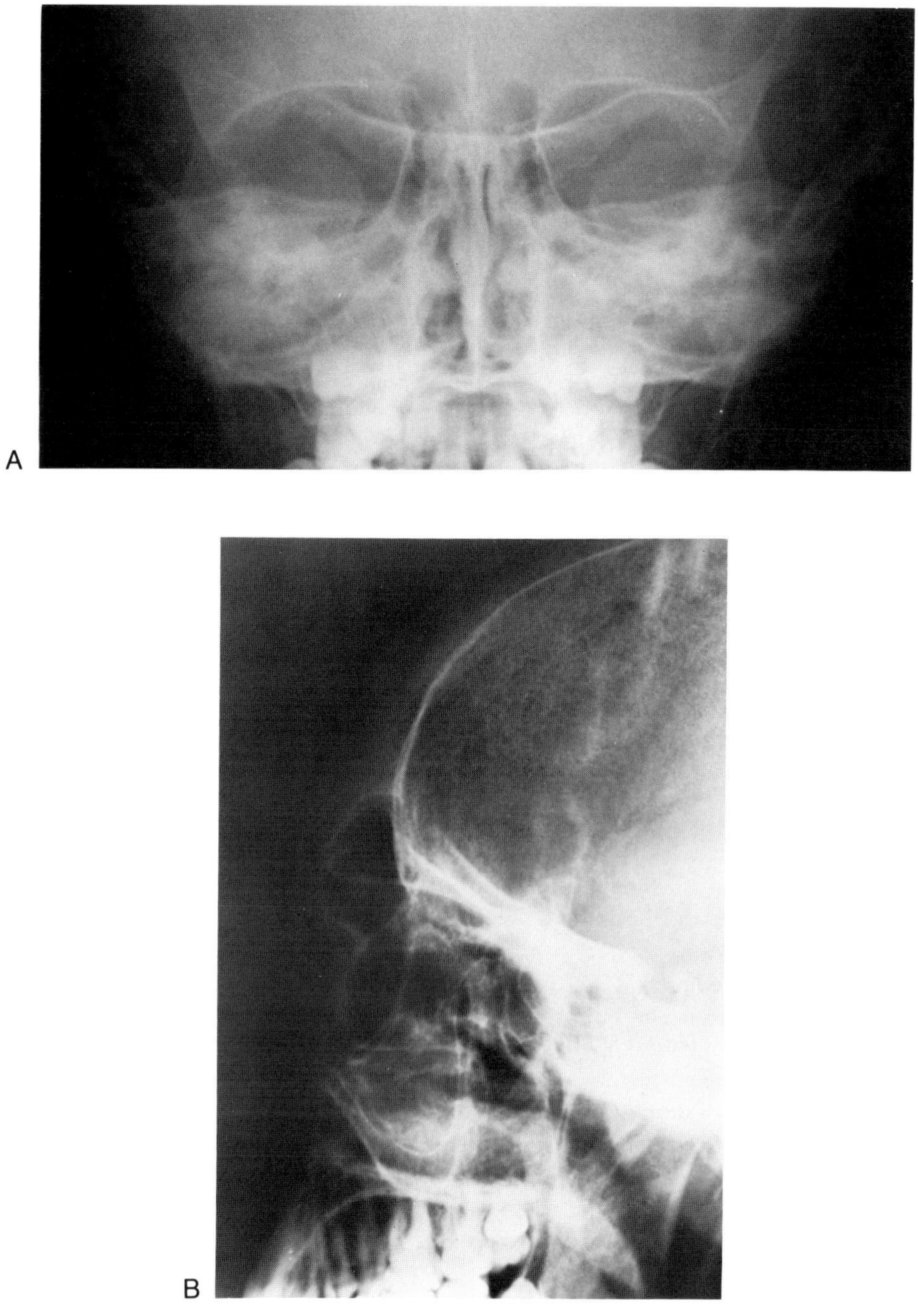

Fig. 2–18 Thalassemia. **(A)** Frontal view of a child with thalassemia demonstrates prominence of the maxilla and obliteration of the maxillary sinuses. Note preservation of the ethmoid air cells and nasal passages. **(B)** Lateral view of the face 11 years later demonstrates severe thickening of the diploë and total obliteration of the maxillary sinuses. The frontal and sphenoid sinuses are preserved.

view is also useful in identification of zygomatic arch fractures (Fig. 2–19). The orbital rim fracture is sustained by a direct blow to the orbit with pressure directed inward. The weakest wall is inferior, resulting in the classic "teardrop" herniation of fat and/or inferior rectus muscle through the roof of the maxillary sinus. Clinically, the patient develops impaired upward gaze, diplopia, and sometimes enophthalmos. Both CT and MRI demonstrate the herniated muscle into the maxillary sinus as well as information about possible optic nerve compromise (Fig. 2–20).

Complex facial fractures are less common in children but include naso-orbital fractures, the Le Fort fractures, and tripod fractures. There is a high association of cerebrospinal fluid leak with naso-orbital fractures. This is secondary to interruption of the fovea ethmoidalis and cribriform plate where the dura attaches. Coronal computed tomograms provide the most information about the integrity of anterior cranial fossa.

Le Fort fractures may be the result of direct facial trauma or may be induced during reconstructive facial surgery. The Le Fort I is a transverse maxillary fracture at the level of the hard palate. The Le Fort II is a pyramidal midfacial fracture separating the maxilla, frontal, and zygomatic bones at the suture lines. The medial and inferior orbital walls are disrupted. The Le Forte III fracture is also termed *craniofacial disjunction*. The medial and inferior orbital walls are separated, as well as the posterior orbital floors, to the level of the inferior orbital fissures. Fractures continue through the maxillary antra to the level of the pterygoid plates and up through the lateral orbital walls. Healing complex facial fractures may result in asymmetry of the paranasal sinuses due to calcified callus formation about the fracture site (Fig. 2–21).

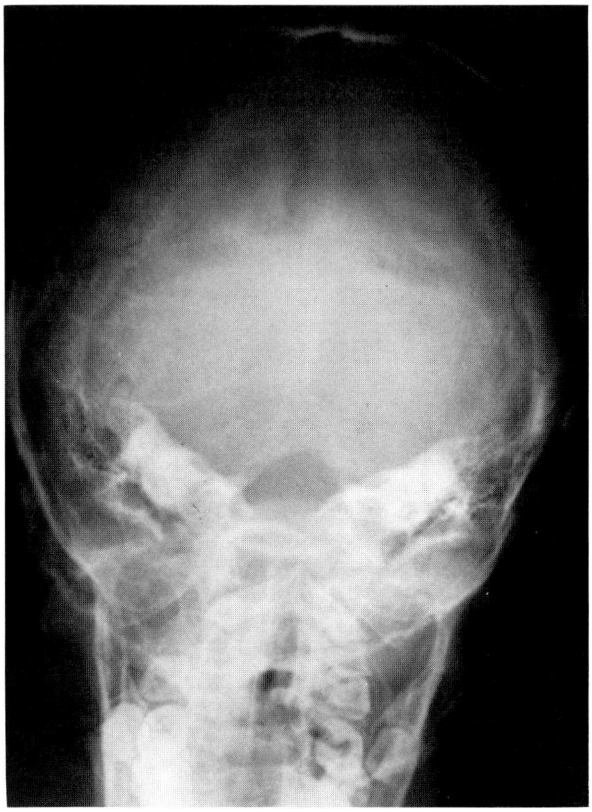

Fig. 2–19 Right zygomatic arch fracture. The Towne view exaggerates the length of both the mandible and the zygomatic arches. The fracture lines through the right zygoma are easily identified in this projection.

Iatrogenic

Indications for nasopharyngeal and paranasal sinus surgery include congenital deformities, recurrent sinusitis unresponsive to medical therapy, benign or malignant neoplasms and internal reduction of facial fractures. CT is the best method of postoperative evaluation. It is imperative to obtain a baseline scan within 8 weeks following surgery for resection of malignant neoplasms. Any soft tissue mass occurring in the postoperative sinus should be clinically evaluated to rule out the presence of tumor.

Antral lavage is the second most common cause of air/fluid levels in the paranasal sinuses. If saline is used to rinse the paranasal sinuses, air/fluid levels may persist for 4 days. Delaying the radiographic examination 1 week will prevent confusion.

Focal sclerosis of the facial bones, which may occur if a child undergoes radiation therapy, is difficult to differentiate from osteomyelitis. A child with a history of radiation therapy to the face requires scrutiny of the sinus radiographs to detect radiation-induced sarcomas, which occur rarely after a variable latent period.

A

B

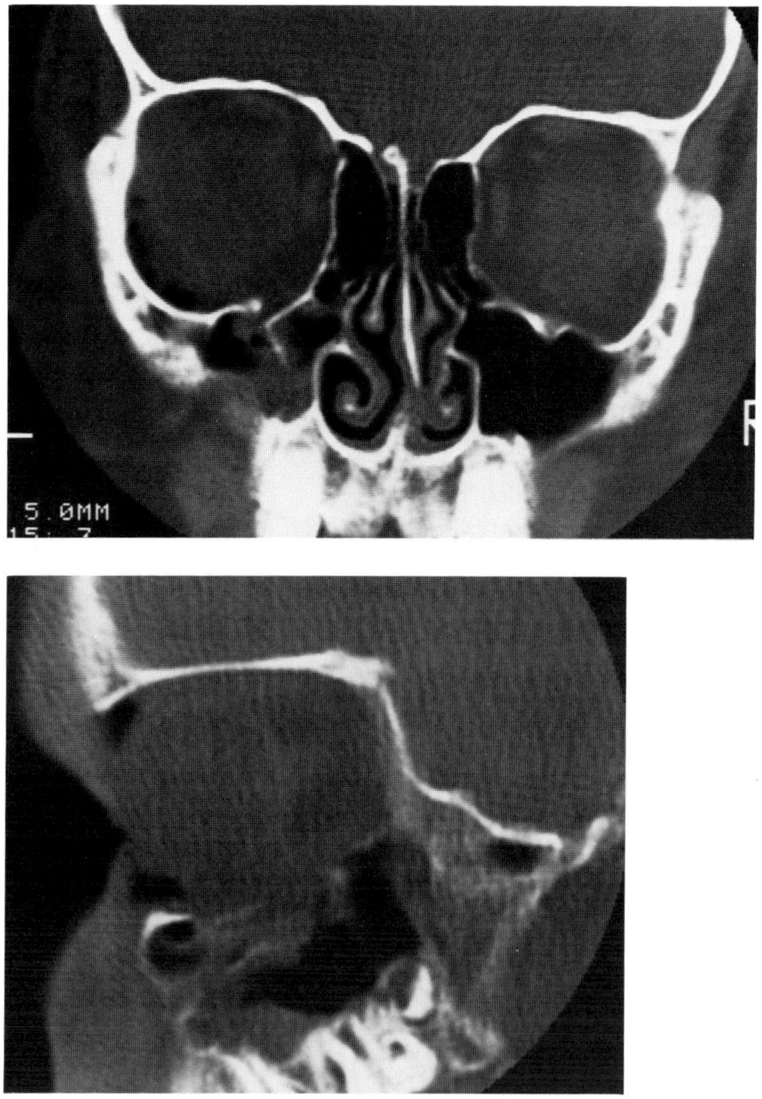

Fig. 2–20 Inferior orbital rim fracture. **(A)** Coronal CT scan demonstrates a left inferior orbital rim fracture with the classic tear drop herniation of the fat into the roof of the left maxillary sinus. Note the air/fluid level in the left maxillary sinus consistent with blood. **(B)** Direct sagittal view demonstrates that the caudal portion of the inferior rectus muscle abuts the fracture fragments.

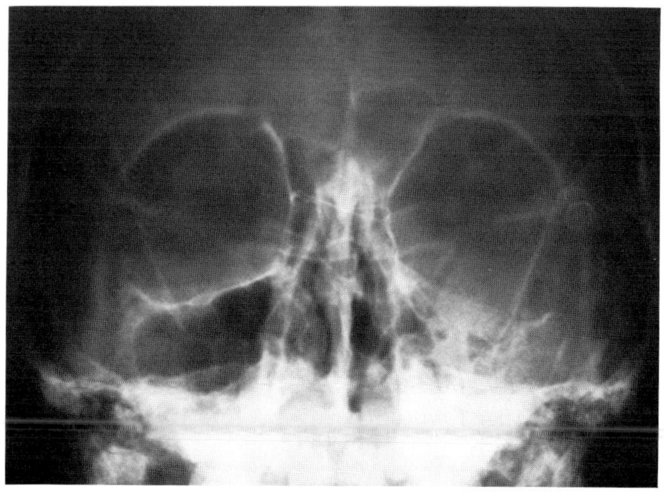

Fig. 2–21 Postfracture deformity. Waters view of a child 1 year after surgical repair of a complex left orbital fracture. Calcified callous at the healed fracture sites and impaired sinus drainage has contributed to the thick, indistinct left maxillary sinus walls.

INCREASED VELOPHARYNGEAL PORTAL

Congenital
- Cleft palate
- Hypoplastic palate
- Enlarged velopharyngeal port
- Bruton's agammaglobulinemia

Iatrogenic
- Postadenoidectomy

INCREASED VELOPHARYNGEAL PORTAL SIZE

Enlargement of the velopharyngeal portal (the posterior portion of the nasopharynx) is usually secondary to surgical removal of an enlarged adenoidal pad (Fig. 2–22). Although adenoid surgery rarely results in speech impediment, if performed in a patient having congenital anomalies that enlarge the velopharyngeal portal, surgery may worsen the hypernasal speech. Congenital abnormalities that may contribute to an enlarged velopharyngeal portal include the hypoplastic maxilla associated with cleft palate, hypoplasia of the velum, or congenital enlargement of the posterior aspect of the nasopharynx. The absence of adenoidal tissue without a history of surgery should bring to mind the possibility of Bruton's agammaglobulinemia. The disease is inherited as an X-linked recessive trait and results in absence of humoral immunity. After the decline in the effect of maternal antibodies in infancy, the child presents with recurrent pneumonia. Chronic sinusitis is a classic feature of the disease. Radiographs reveal absence of the nasopharyngeal and hilar lymphoidal tissue. Affected children have a 6-percent increased risk of either lymphoma or leukemia development.[16]

SOFT TISSUE MASSES OF THE PARAPHARYNGEAL SPACE

Normal
- Neck flexion/expiratory view

Congenital
- Branchial cleft cyst
- Dermoid/teratoma
- Gastrointestinal duplication cyst
- Thyroglossal duct cyst/remnant
- Lingual thyroid
- Thyroid cyst
- Sebaceous cyst
- Cystic hygroma
- Occipital meningocele

Inflammation
- Lymphadenopathy*
- Tonsillitis/uvulitis/adenoiditis
- Salivary gland infection
- Recurrent parotitis/Sjögren's syndrome
- Sinus histiocytosis
- Thyroiditis/thyroid abscess

Neoplasm
- Salivary gland tumor
- Thyroid adenoma
- Parathyroid adenoma
- Hemangioma
- Fibromatosis
- Lymphoma
- Rhabdomyosarcoma
- Fibrosarcoma
- Neuroblastoma

Trauma
- Fracture
- Blunt/penetrating trauma
- Pharyngeal pouch

* Most common.

SOFT TISSUE MASSES OF THE PARAPHARYNGEAL SPACE

The parapharyngeal space is defined as the soft tissues extending from the submucosa of the aerodigestive tract above the thoracic inlet to the skin surface. Prior to the invention of cross-sectional imaging modalities, it was virtually impossible to evaluate this region without surgery. Lateral views of the neck using soft tissue technique during different phases of the respiratory cycle may provide an outline of a soft tissue mass. Ultrasound is useful in delineating solid from cystic masses and defining the organ of origin. Either CT or MRI with contrast enhancement provides the most detailed information about the deep tissues prior to surgery. Specialized invasive proce-

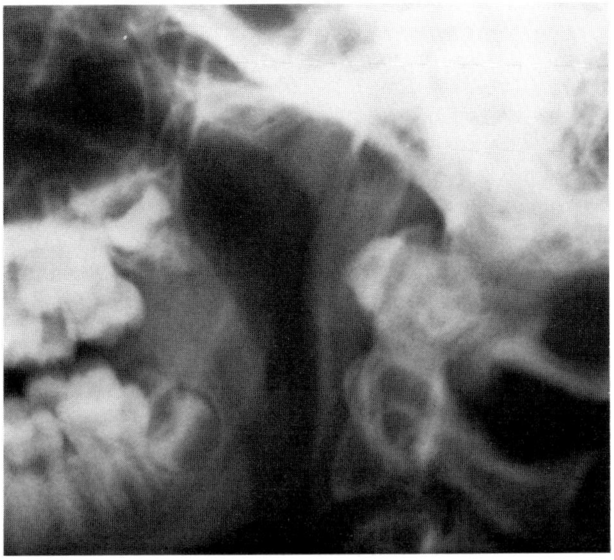

Fig. 2–22 Absent adenoidal pad. Lateral view of this patient's neck demonstrates a large velopharyngeal portal secondary to surgical removal of the adenoidal tissue. The velum is collapsed against the tongue base.

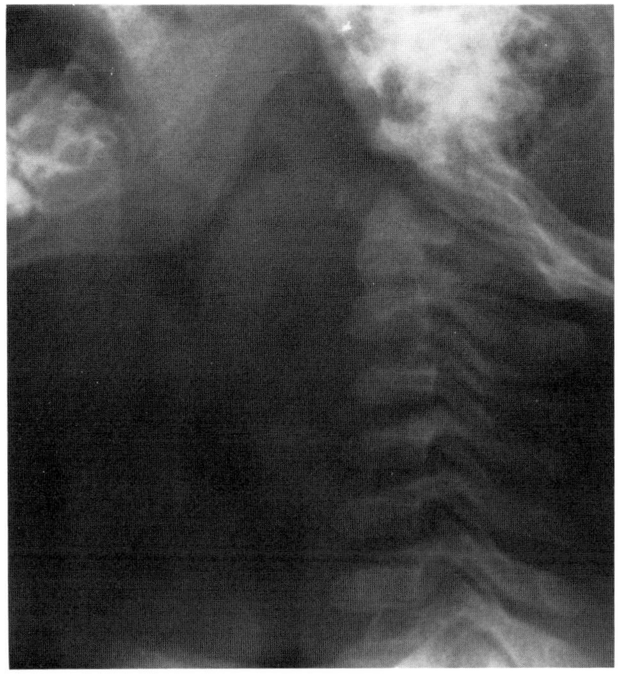

A

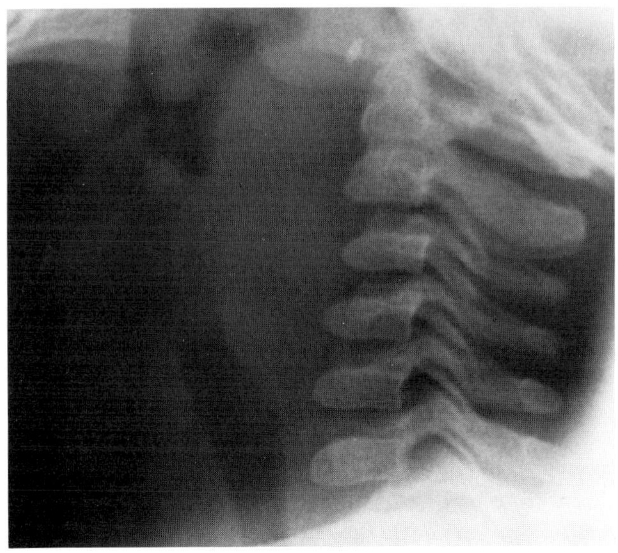

B

Fig. 2–23 Pseudothickening of the retropharyngeal space. **(A)** This child was being examined to rule out a cervical spine fracture. The upper cervical spine is flexed. The prevertebral soft tissues are thickened in the same region. **(B)** A repeat view in a lesser degree of flexion in still suspicious for prevertebral edema. Note that the hypopharynx is collapsed, indicating expiration. (*Figure continues.*)

dures such as sialography and thyroid scintigraphy may be used to evaluate ductal structure or glandular function.

Normal

The most common cause of widening of the retropharyngeal space in children is neck flexion or expiration during the lateral radiograph (Fig. 2–23). It is of vital importance that the lateral view of the soft tissues be obtained with the neck extended during inspiration. Even with the neck in the neutral position, apparent widening of the retropharyngeal soft tissues may result.

Hypertrophy of the adenoidal pad results in a retropharyngeal soft tissue mass. Direct visualization may be required to rule out other more malignant causes of a retropharyngeal mass in symptomatic patients.

Congenital

Most congenital abnormalities of the parapharyngeal space present in infancy as visible asymmetry of the neck, feeding difficulties, or with secondary infection.

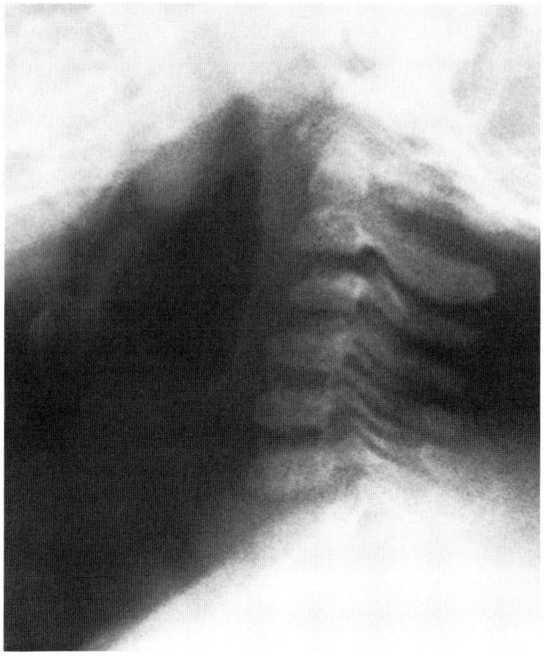

C

Fig. 2–23 (*Continued*). **(C)** Under fluoroscopic control, the neck was straightened and then extended. Note that with inspiration and neck extension, the apparent widening of the prevertebral soft tissues disappears. The child's spine is normal.

The branchial cleft cyst is an embryologic cyst derived from either the first or second cervical arch. It usually presents as an anterior triangle mass with a sinus tract draining to the overlying skin. Although ultrasound easily demonstrates the anechoic fluid characteristic of a simple cyst, communication with the pharynx or piriform sinus may lead to debris accumulation or infection. In these cases, a complex mass is seen with ultrasound. The connecting tract usually passes between the internal and external carotid arteries and may be demonstrated with CT. Because most branchial cleft cysts present after secondary infection, administration of IV contrast material displays a thick, enhancing wall. If CT demonstrates the fistula, the diagnosis may be made with certainty. Branchial cleft cysts occasionally may be intimately related to the salivary glands. Other cystic lesions of the salivary glands include dermoid cyst, simple cyst, and cyst secondary to inflammation.

Dermoid cysts and teratomas usually occur along the midline at the level of the thyroid gland. They may also occur along the tongue and tonsils. While dermoid cysts contain derivatives from the embryologic endoderm and ectoderm, teratomas contain derivatives of all three germ cell layers. Clinically, a dermoid cyst may appear hairy when directly visualized. On CT scans, a unilocular cyst is usually demonstrated containing material that is slightly greater than water density. Teratomas are solid masses that may contain a characteristic toothlike calcification.

The thyroglossal duct runs from the level of the thyroid gland to foramen cecum. Thyroglossal duct cyst is a very common cause of a benign childhood neck mass.[11] Clinically, a child less than 5 years old presents with a palpable midline mass just below the level of the hyoid bone. Ultrasound examination demonstrates a hypoechoic cyst with small internal echos along the midline that moves with swallowing (Fig. 2–24). Surgical resection should include the thyroglossal duct remnants, thyroglossal duct cyst, and the hyoid bone. If not, the recurrence rate is high. The most common site for ectopic thyroid tissue is at the base of the tongue. In the neonate, lingual thyroid may cause respiratory distress. Girls are affected more often than boys. The patient may come to medical attention due to dysphagia or hypothyroidism. Approximately 70 percent of cases have no other detectable thyroid tissue when scintigraphy is performed.[14] Because the ectopic tissue represents the only remnant of thyroid tissue in the majority of cases, it is important to identify functioning thyroid tissue with scintigraphy prior to surgical excision. Ultrasound examination reveals a solid mass of homogeneous hyperechoic tissue when compared to the surrounding muscle. A normal thyroid gland is usually not demonstrated. Simple cysts arising from the thyroid gland are exceedingly rare.

Eighty percent of cystic hygromas arise from the posterior triangle of the neck.[15] Other sites include the mediastinum, the axilla, or the retroperitoneum. Most hygromas are recognized before 1 year of age. Often a cystic mass arising from the posterior neck is identified on prenatal ultrasound examination. Cystic hygroma should be differentiated from an occipital cephalocele, the latter of which is associated with occipital bone defects and an abnormal appearance of the intracranial structures (Fig. 2–25). Congenital

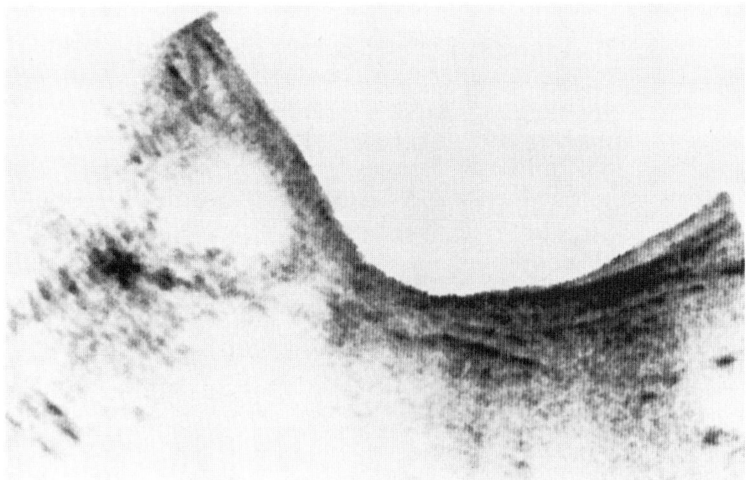

Fig. 2–24 Thyroglossal duct cyst. Longitudinal ultrasound scan demonstrates an anechoic space surrounded by a thick irregular wall. The thickness of the wall is suspicious for superimposed infection.

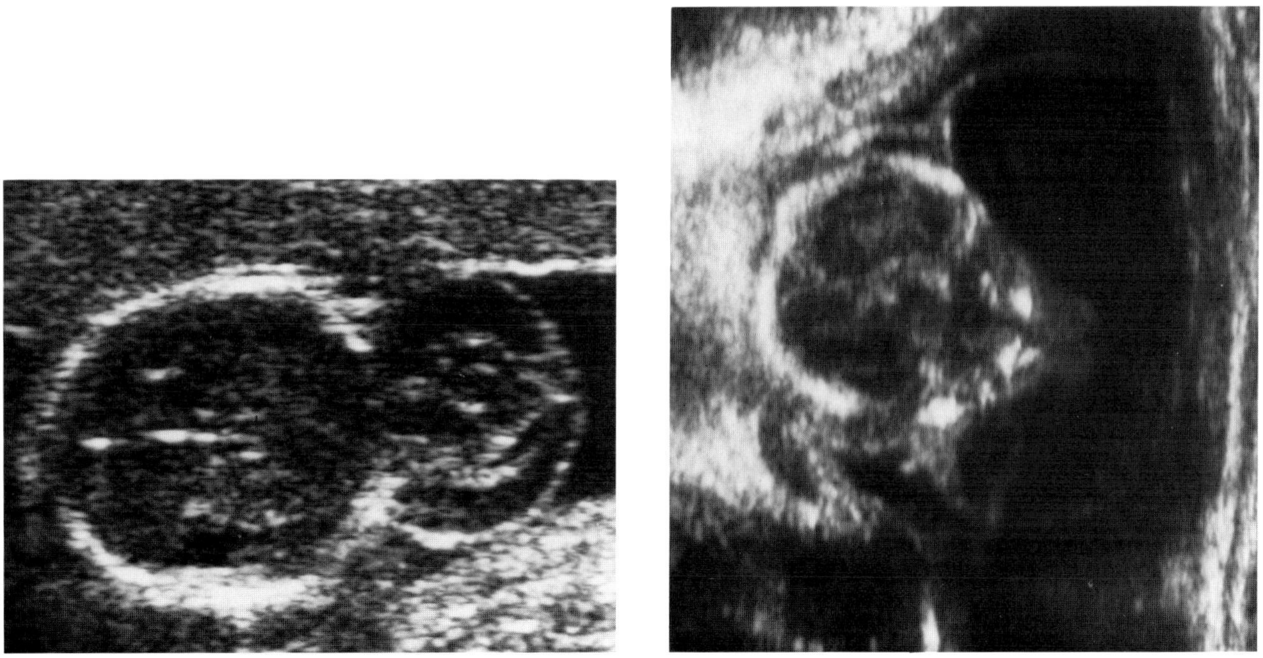

A

B

Fig. 2–25 Occipital cephalocele versus cystic hygroma. (Both patients are oriented in a left lateral debucitus position with the face toward the reader's left.) **(A)** Note the defect in the occipital bone with herniation of the posterior fossa contents into the occipital cephalocele. **(B)** Multiloculated cystic hygroma with intact cervical vertebral bodies and occiput and no herniation of intracranial contents. (Photos courtesy of Dr. Depak Bedi, University of Texas Medical Branch, Galveston, Texas.)

cystic hygroma is associated with fetal Turner's syndrome. Anasarca may be detected on the prenatal ultrasound as well. The histiogenesis of cystic hygroma is disputed. Many authors believe that the mass results from dilatation proximal to congenital stenosis or atresia of the lymphatic channels. Other authors believe that cystic hygroma represents a true neoplasm. The infiltrative nature of the mass, which may surround the trachea and cause airway obstruction, often leads to incomplete surgical resection. Recurrence rates are high with cystic hygroma. While ultrasound is extremely useful in identifying multiloculated, fluid-filled cysts, the full extent of the lesion is better demonstrated with MRI (Fig. 2–26). On T_1-weighted images, uncomplicated cystic hygromas have medium signal intensity. On T_2-weighted images, sharply defined medium intensity cyst walls surround high intensity fluid collections.

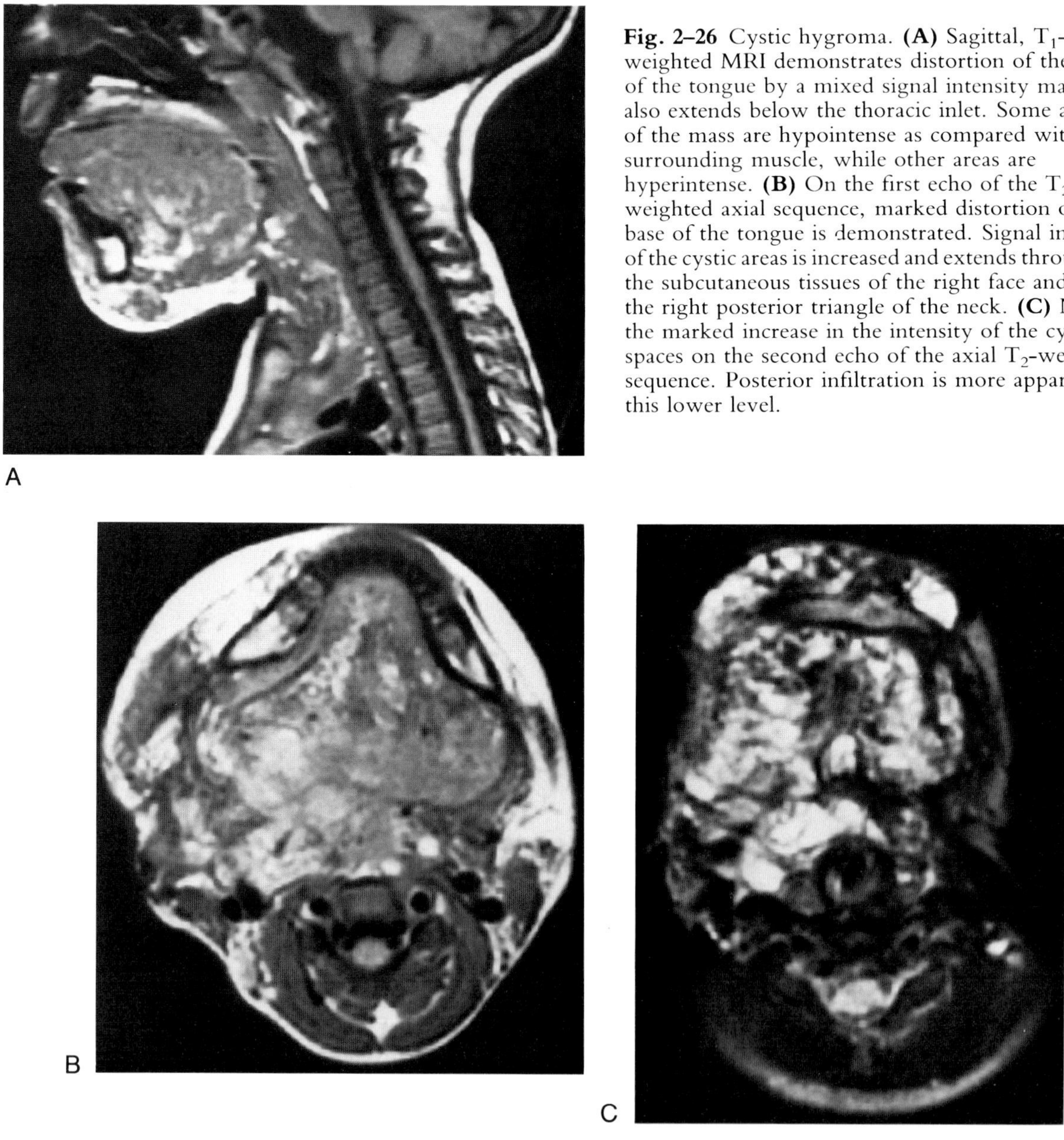

Fig. 2–26 Cystic hygroma. **(A)** Sagittal, T_1-weighted MRI demonstrates distortion of the base of the tongue by a mixed signal intensity mass that also extends below the thoracic inlet. Some areas of the mass are hypointense as compared with surrounding muscle, while other areas are hyperintense. **(B)** On the first echo of the T_2-weighted axial sequence, marked distortion of the base of the tongue is demonstrated. Signal intensity of the cystic areas is increased and extends throughout the subcutaneous tissues of the right face and into the right posterior triangle of the neck. **(C)** Note the marked increase in the intensity of the cystic spaces on the second echo of the axial T_2-weighted sequence. Posterior infiltration is more apparent at this lower level.

Inflammation

The most common cause of a soft tissue mass of the neck in childhood is lymphadenopathy due to either inflammation or neoplasm. By far, inflammatory lymphadenopathy is more common than malignant lymphadenopathy. Patients present with fever, sore throat and, sometimes, torticollis. On lateral radiographic examination of the neck, rounded thickening of the retropharyngeal soft tissues is identified with anterior displacement of the airway (Fig. 2–27). Differentiation from other neck masses is possible with ultrasound examination. Suppurative adenopathy may proceed to abscess formation. Occasionally, calcifications will form after an episode of retropharyngeal abscess. CT is useful in identifying cystic fluid collections that need drainage and gas collections indicative of abscess. Inflammatory adenopathy is classically unilateral. The most common organism associated with inflammatory adenopathy is *Staphylococcus aureus*. Scrofula describes inflammatory lymphadenitis secondary to *Mycobacterium tuberculosis* or atypical mycobacteria. A less common consideration is mucocutaneous lymph node syndrome (Kawasaki disease). An infectious agent is usually not isolated in these patients and the etiology is unknown. Patients present with an acute febrile illness associated with widespread vasculitis, lymphadenopathy, a skin rash, mucous membrane changes, hepatosplenomegaly, jaundice, and gallbladder hydrops. Valvular heart disease and aneurysm formation may result as well. Other inflammatory masses of the neck include enlarged palantine tonsils, adenoids, and uvulitis.

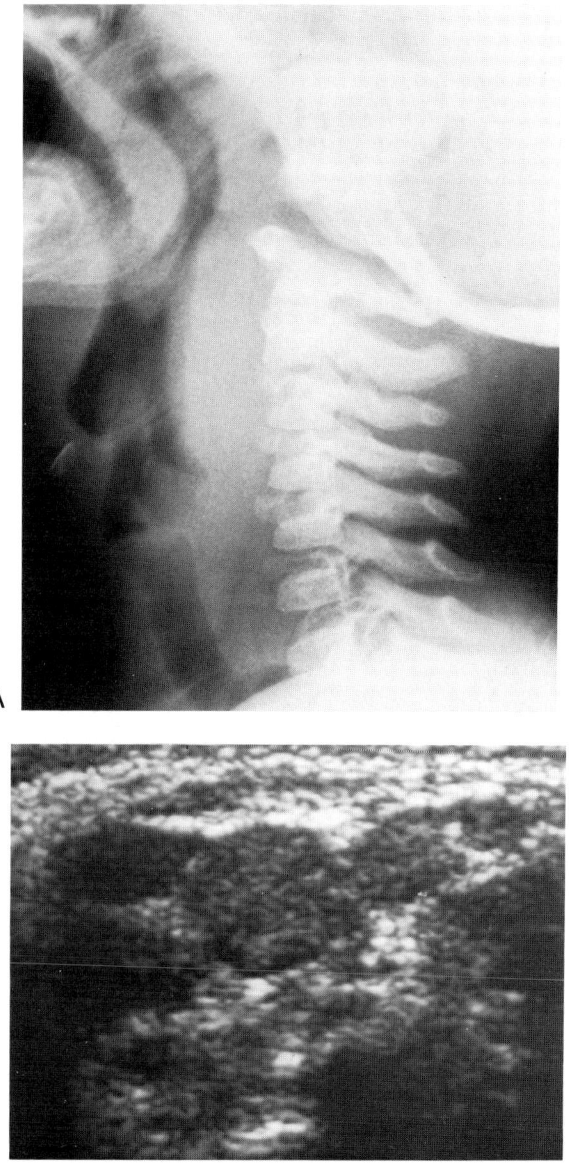

A

B

Fig. 2–27 Retropharyngeal lymphadenopathy. **(A)** Note the profound increase in the thickness of the retropharyngeal soft tissues of this febrile 1-year-old patient. **(B)** Longitudinal ultrasound examination confirmed multiple ovoid hypoechoic masses in a chainlike distribution consistent with lymphadenopathy.

Ascending infections of the salivary glands occur in patients with immunosuppression, dehydration, and ductal narrowing. Mumps virus is the most common infectious etiology. *S. aureus* is a common bacterial cause. Other less common organisms include tuberculosis, fungus, toxoplasmosis, and mixed infections. CT is the method of choice for examination of salivary gland masses. Posting of the scan planes should avoid amalgam fillings and braces, which may degrade the images. Either coronal or axial 5-mm computed tomograms obtained at 5-mm increments provide adequate visualization. CT is able to detect calcifications not seen on plain radiographs. Calcifications of the salivary glands are rare in children and may be associated with previous infection or cystic fibrosis. When infected, the CT appearance is nonspecific and ranges from diffuse enlargement of the gland to focal collections of fluid suggestive of abscess formation (Fig.

2–28). Lymph nodes occur within the salivary glands and become enlarged in the presence of granulomatous disease. Inflammatory conditions of the salivary gland include Sjögren's syndrome (connective tissue disease, xerostomia, and keratoconjunctivitis sicca) and recurrent parotitis. Both conditions demonstrate similar radiologic and pathologic abnormalities. However, recurrent parotitis is usually self-limited and ends with the onset of puberty. CT demonstrates diffuse enlargement of the salivary glands. Soft tissue attenuation stippled with either calcifications or low density fluid collections is similar in appearance to infection. Sialography may demonstrate sialiectasis, calculi, and cysts.

Sinus histiocytosis is a rare lymphadenopathy of unknown etiology producing gross enlargement of the cervical and hilar nodes. The clinical and radiographic findings are undifferentiable from lymphoma. Ultrasound examination reveals multiple, round homogenous hypoechoic masses in a chainlike distribution. Biopsy reveals the benign nature of the lesion.

Enlargement of the thyroid gland in children is usually due to thyroiditis. Infections by either viral or bacterial organisms occur; however, idiopathic and autoimmune thyroiditis are most common. When evidence of either hyperthyroidism or hypothyroidism is present, ^{123}I imaging provides information about iodine uptake and organification. Ultrasound is useful in follow-up of the inflamed thyroid gland for abscess formation or glandular size change (Fig. 2–29). Differentiation between multinodular goiter and thyroiditis of other etiologies is difficult since both imaging modalities provide nonspecific information.

Neoplasm

Cross-sectional imaging has revolutionized differentiation of mass lesions of the parapharyngeal space. However, in children, ultrasound is often the first imaging modality used for differentiation of cystic versus solid masses. This provides easy delineation of the organ of origin. The most common benign tumor arising from the salivary glands is the pleomorphic (mixed) adenoma. There is a high incidence of recurrence of this tumor after surgical excision. Both CT and MRI are extremely useful in evaluating parotid tumors. The most common parotid tumor of

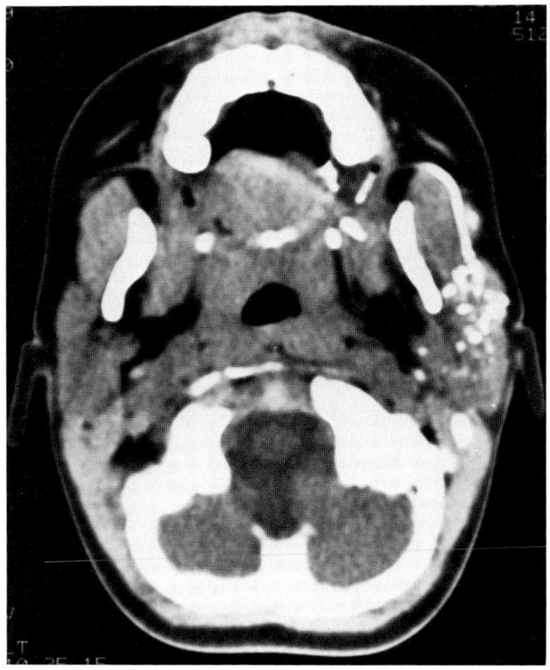

Fig. 2–28 Parotitis. Axial CT scan performed after sialography demonstrates diffuse enlargement of the left parotid gland. While Stenson's duct is normal in size, the smaller branches of the ductal system do not taper normally. Instead, pools of contrast material are seen. These findings are indicative of chronic inflammation.

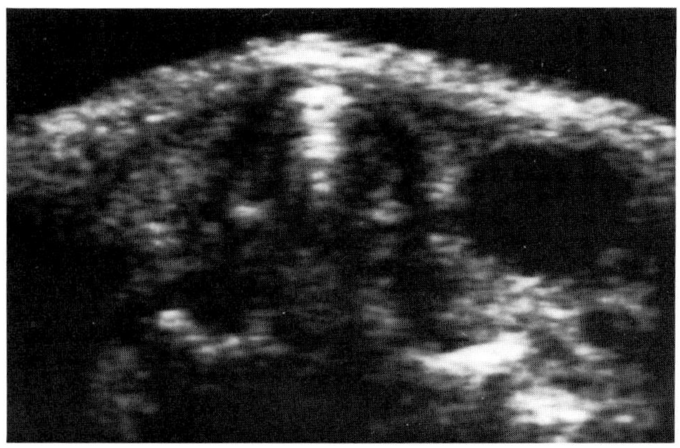

Fig. 2–29 Multinodular goiter. This child had a 2-week history of a painless neck mass. Transverse ultrasound examination demonstrates a large area of cystic degeneration within the left lobe of the thyroid gland. Although the right lobe has maintained its shape, smaller cystic spaces are detectable, especially in the posterior part of the gland.

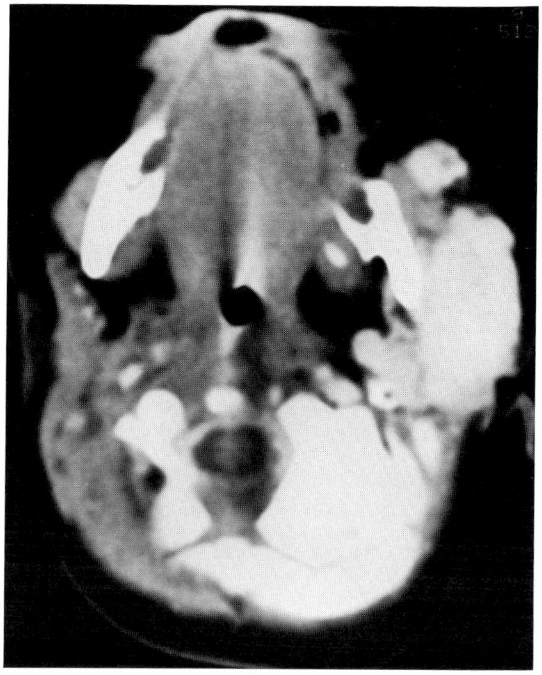

Fig. 2–30 Parotid hemangioendothelioma. Note the densely enhancing mass that enlarges and deforms the superficial lobe of the left parotid gland on axial CT. The size of this hemangioendothelioma prompted surgical resection.

infancy is the hemagioendothelioma (Fig. 2–30). Facial nerve involvement is uncommon in this lesion. The natural history of hemagioendothelioma is spontaneous resolution. The most common primary malignant tumor of the salivary glands is mucoepidermoid carcinoma.

When diffuse or localized enlargement of the thyroid gland is detected clinically, ultrasound, ^{99m}Tc pertechnetate scanning, thallium-201 scanning, and MRI are useful in delineating inflammatory processes from thyroid and parathyroid neoplasms. In both organs, adenomas are more common than carcinomas. Identification of a solid thyroid nodule with any imaging modality is nonspecific with regard to malignancy. Radionuclide scanning provides functional information about the gland. The presence of a "cold" nodule on radionuclide scan is suspicious for malignancy, especially if the patient has a history of external beam radiation therapy to the head or neck. Parathyroid adenomas may also appear as cold nodules on radionuclide scanning. The organ of origin is easily delineated by ultrasound or MRI (Fig. 2–31).

The juvenile angiofibroma is the most common neoplastic parapharyngeal mass. Although this tumor has a tendency to gradually resolve, other hemangio-

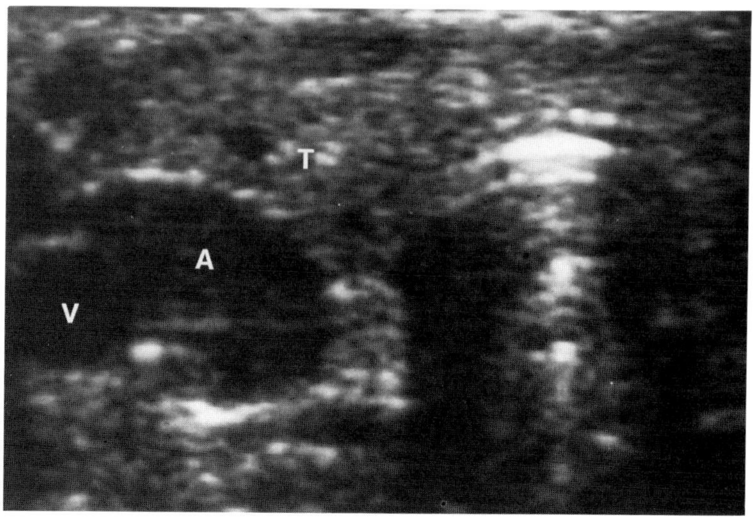

Fig. 2–31 Parathyroid adenoma. The transverse ultrasound image through the neck at the level of the thyroid gland (*T*) demonstrates a hypoechoic mass (*A*) anterior to the jugular vein (*V*) and carotid artery. The demarcation between the mass and the thyroid gland is sharp. At surgery, a parathyroid adenoma was removed.

mas, especially of the tongue, have a predisposition for increasing in size as the patient ages. Ultrasound examination demonstrates a highly echogenic but nonvascular mass. Angiography is useful in delineating the extent of the lesion, source of blood supply, and provides a route for embolization therapy.

Fibromatosis occurring in the neck describes a spectrum of abnormalities ranging from localized soft tissue tumors arising in the sternocleidomastoid muscle of infants, which result in torticollis, to infiltrative lesions with more malignant appearing nuclei (Fig. 2–32). Ultrasound is extremely efficient in identifying fibromatosis coli arising in the sternocleidomastoid muscle. With the more infiltrative variety of fibromatosis, MRI provides excellent soft tissue delineation. If the tumor abuts adjacent bone, CT reliably demonstrates bone destruction.

A

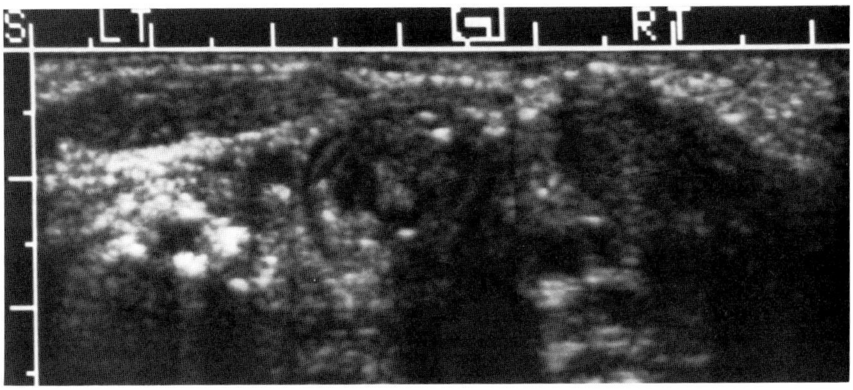

B

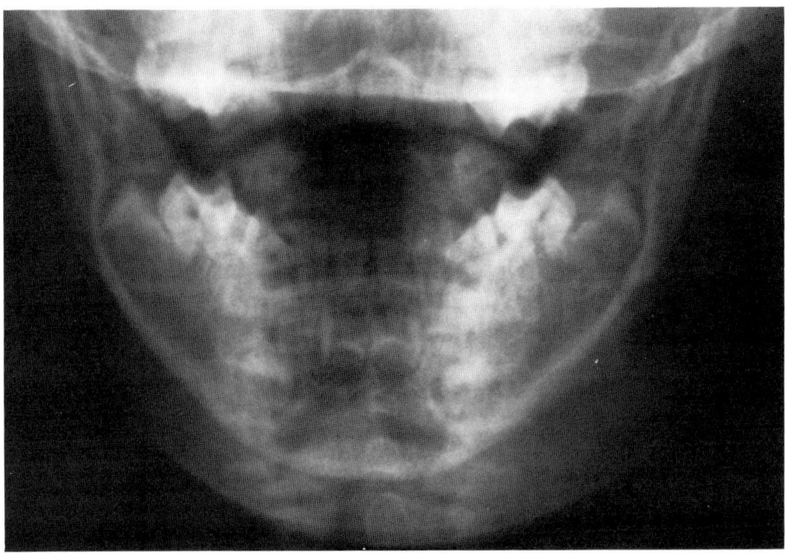

Fig. 2–32 Variations of fibromatosis. **(A)** Fibromatosis coli. Transverse ultrasound examination revealed an increase in the anteroposterior diameter of the right sternocleidomastoid muscle. This child had a 2-month history of torticollis. **(B)** This adolescent presented with painless swelling of the left jaw. The radiograph demonstrates cortical thickening along the inferior lateral aspect of the left mandible. (*Figure continues.*)

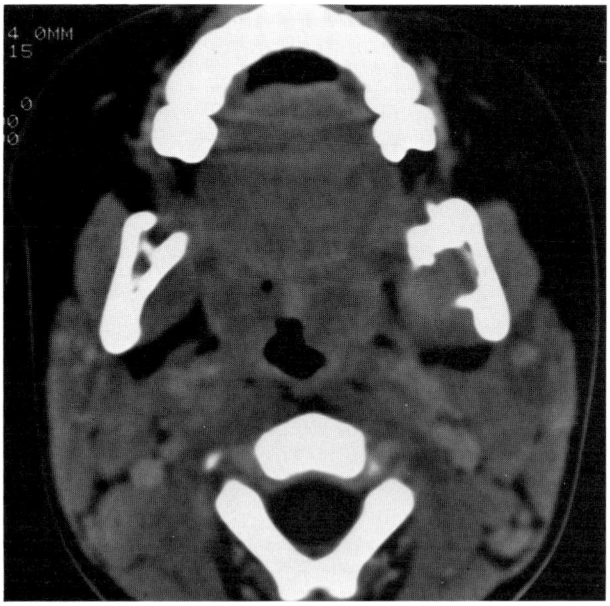

C

Fig. 2–32 (*Continued*). **(C)** CT scan of the same patient demonstrates mandibular destruction by an invansive mass contiguous with the left lateral pterygoid muscle. At surgery, this represented a more aggressive variety of fibromatosis.

The incidence of malignant parapharyngeal tumors in children differs greatly from that in adults. Specifically, malignancy is most likely due to either lymphoma or rhabdomyosarcoma in children. Because of the high incidence of rhabdomyosarcoma of the orbit, this tumor is considered the most common malignant tumor of the head and neck in childhood. Non-Hodgkin's and Hodgkin's lymphoma occur with equal frequency in the head and neck and present as unilateral painless neck masses. Fibrosarcomas are the third most common malignant neoplasm of the head and neck of children. Other less common malignant tumors include neuroblastoma (which usually demonstrates calcifications) and adenocarcinoma of the thyroid, salivary glands, or parathyroid. Ultrasound may be used to identify the solid nature of malignant tumors. However, CT is useful in delineating the extent of malignancy and surrounding bone destruction (Fig. 2–33).

Trauma

Fractures of either the larynx or the cervical spine may result in soft tissue swelling adjacent to the injured site. Blunt trauma to the neck may result in

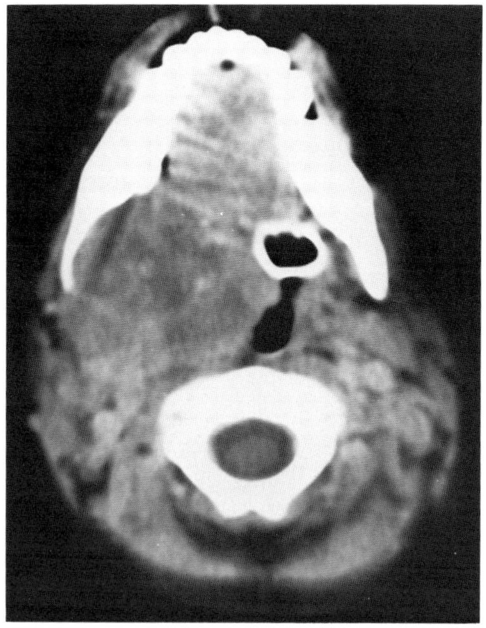

A

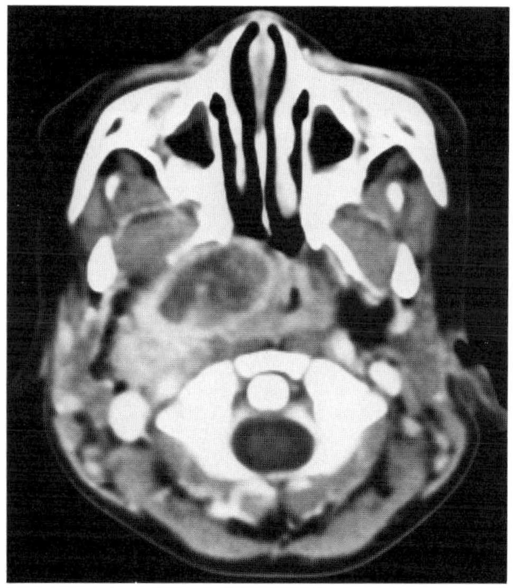

B

Fig. 2–33 Nasopharyngeal rhabdomyosarcoma. **(A)** Contrast-enhanced axial CT scan demonstrates deviation of the patient's endotracheal tube to the left by a low density nasopharyngeal mass that deforms the airway and has eroded the posterior right mandible. **(B)** At a higher level, the mass displaces the right jugular vein and carotid artery posteriorly but does not appear to invade the carotid sheath. (*Figure continues.*)

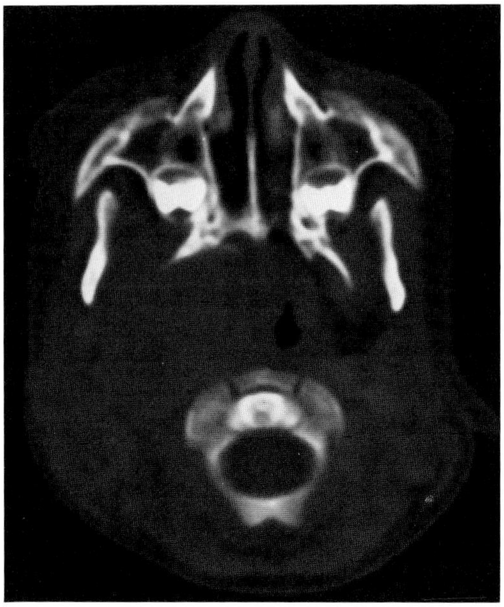

C

Fig. 2–33 (*Continued*). **(C)** Bone window setting taken 5 mm above the last image demonstrates deformity of the right pterygoid plate. The smooth deformity of both the right pterygoid plate and the mandible infer that the mass is slow growing. Nevertheless, this represented a rhabdomyosarcoma.

either subcutaneous emphysema (usually diagnosed clinically by the presence of crepitance) or hematoma formation easily detected with ultrasound examination. Penetrating pharyngeal trauma may be caused by foreign body ingestion, which may result in retropharyngeal abscess formation or hematoma. A barium swallow may be useful in identifying nonradiopaque foreign bodies and associated mucosal injuries.

Pharyngeal pouches are rare in childhood but usually represent acquired dilatations of the pharyngeal wall filled with either air or fluid. Rarely, they may be congenital. These are best demonstrated with a swallow of high density barium. They must be differentiated from the branchial cleft cyst, which arises from a more lateral position along the pharynx.

ABNORMALITIES OF THE HYPOPHARYNX/TRACHEA

Abnormalities of the hypopharynx and trachea may present at birth with symptoms of respiratory difficulty or, later in childhood, with stridor, abnormal cry, or a change in voice quality. The mainstay of radiographic evaluation of the airway is audio-enhanced videofluoroscopy, which allows correlation of the visible dynamic airway with the abnormal sound. For screening purposes, anteroposterior and lateral views of the neck using soft tissue technique are adequate. If both inspiration and expiration are

ABNORMALITIES OF THE HYPOPHARYNX/TRACHEA

- Normal
  - Tracheal buckling
  - "Omega" epiglottis
- Congenital
  - Agenesis
  - Tracheoesophageal fistula
  - Stenosis
  - Web
  - Laryngomalacia
  - Tracheomalacia
  - Vascular rings
  - Bronchopulmonary foregut malformation
  - Ectopic thyroid
  - Tracheobronchomegaly
- Inflammation
  - Epiglottitis
  - Croup
  - Diptheria
  - Subglottic granuloma
  - Mucous retention cyst
- Neoplasm
  - Subglottic hemangioma
  - Laryngeal papilloma
  - Fibroma
  - Schwannoma
  - Lipoma
  - Bronchial carcinoid/adenoid cystic carcinoma
- Trauma
  - Foreign body
  - Vocal cord paralysis
  - Cartilaginous fracture
- Iatrongenic
  - Stenosis
  - Tracheomalacia
  - Laryngospasm

captured, tracheal dynamics may be evaluated. In the past, the usage of a high kilovoltage magnification technique requiring a special filter was advocated by some radiologists. Many pediatric radiologists do not find this technique necessary.

Normal

In infants, buckling of the trachea to the right on expiration is normal and failure to buckle to the right indicates a right aortic arch or other mediastinal pathology.

Portions of the hypopharynx may be redundant in childhood. The classic example of this is redundancy of the aryepiglottic folds resulting in the so-called omega epiglottis (Fig. 2–34). This common variant is often mistaken for epiglottitis, but close scrutiny reveals the aryepiglottic folds to be of normal thickness.

Congenital

Agenesis of the trachea is a lethal condition. Esophageal atresia is commonly associated with tracheoesophageal fistula. Intrinsic congenital abnormalities of the hypopharynx and trachea include agenesis, tracheoesophageal fistula, stenosis, web formation, laryngomalacia, tracheomalacia, and tracheomegaly. Tracheoesophageal fistula is almost always associated with congenital abnormalities of the esophagus including atresia and webs. The H-type fistula is the only type not associated with esophageal atresia and occurs in 5 to 8 percent of cases.[18] Demonstration of the H-type fistula is best performed with the patient first in the lateral position and then prone, with the tip of the nasogastric tube in the hypopharynx. The H-type fistula is usually in the upper third of the esophagus and runs in an upward oblique plane (Fig. 2–35). Vertical defects in the posterior wall of the larynx may allow communication between the hypopharynx and the airway and are termed *laryngeal clefts*.

A B

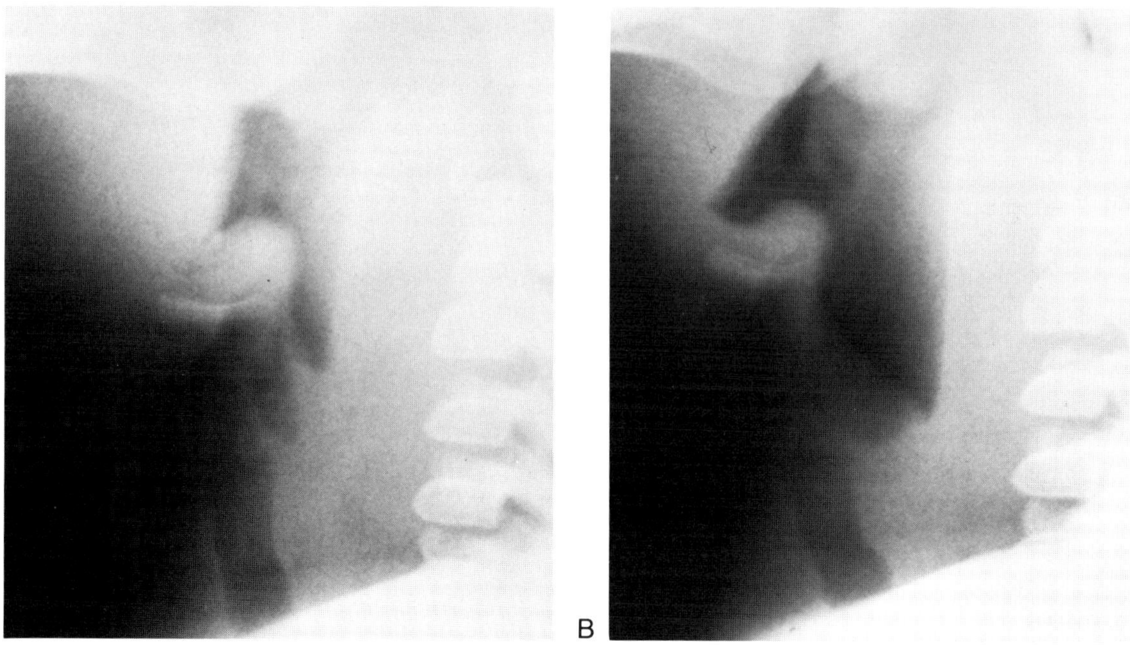

Fig. 2–34 "Omega" epiglottis. **(A)** Note the prominence of the epiglottis but the normal appearing aryepiglottic folds during early expiration. This is consistent with an "omega" epiglottis. **(B)** Inspiration decreases the full appearance of the epiglottis and elongates the aryepiglottic folds. This normal variant should not be confused with epiglottitis.

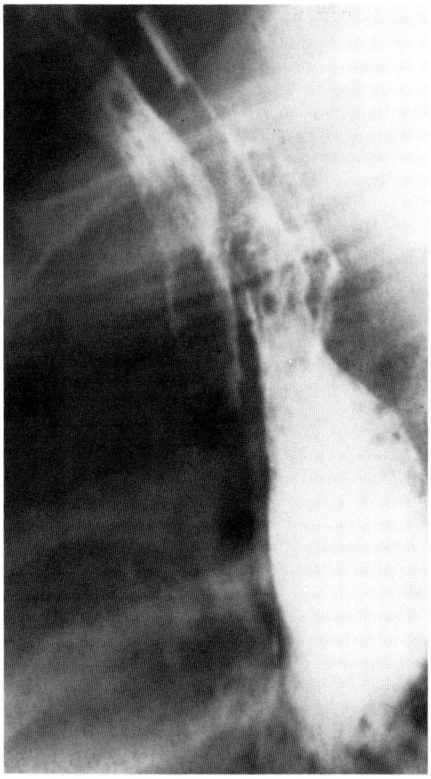

Fig. 2–35 H-type tracheoesophageal fistula. Lateral view after barium has been injected into the proximal esophagus through a catheter. Note the small fistulous tract originating along the anterior wall of the esophagus and extending upward to communicate with the posterior wall of the trachea.

Both laryngeal clefts and congenital webs are best diagnosed using direct laryngoscopy. While web formation may occur at any level along the airway, webs most commonly arise along the anterior glottis.

The most common congenital airway problem in the first year of life requiring a tracheostomy is subglottic stenosis.[12] Videofluoroscopy of the airway reveals fixed circumferential narrowing of the subglottic portion of the trachea during all phases of respiration (Fig. 2–36). This explains the clinical picture of both inspiratory and expiratory stridor that most patients demonstrate. Diffuse hypoplasia of the trachea associated with complete cartilaginous tracheal rings is a less common form of tracheal stenosis. This form is associated with vascular rings and the pulmonary sling. It should be noted that surgical relief of the vascular ring often does not relieve the patient's respiratory difficulty because the underlying portion of the trachea is hypoplastic and flaccid. The diagnosis of tracheal stenosis is best made by MRI in which the superb soft tissue detail demonstrates causes of extrinsic compression while obviating the need for invasive procedures (Fig. 2–37). Both respiratory and cardiac gating may aid in acquiring images with a high signal-to-noise ratio. Tracheal stenosis is rarely an isolated anomaly. Other anomalies of the respiratory, skeletal, cardiovascular and gastrointestinal systems may be present and should be ruled out.

Laryngomalacia and tracheomalacia refer to abnormal collapsibility of the supraglottic or subglottic portions of the airway. Laryngomalacia is considered to be the most common abnormality of the larynx encountered in the young infant.[5] The primary symptom of laryngomalacia is inspiratory stridor presenting in infancy. The patient usually has a normal cry. The stridor is more noticeable when the patient is breathing quietly and decreases with agitation. Videofluoroscopy reveals distention of the hypopharynx during inspiration with downward collapse of the epiglottis and aryepiglottic folds (Fig. 2–38). Laryngomalacia is a self-limiting condition that usually resolves by 1 year of age.

The diagnosis of tracheomalacia is greatly disputed. The normal trachea demonstrates a wide range of responses to abnormal airway pressures. It is difficult, therefore, to determine how narrow is too narrow for the collapsed trachea. Only when there is evidence of cartilaginous abnormality can the diagnosis of tracheomalacia be made with certainty. If fluoroscopic examination reveals tracheal collapse during inspiration then upper airway obstruction should be suspected. Collapse during expiration usually signifies the presence of small airway diseases such as asthma.

The most common pathologic cause of tracheal compression is the presence of a vascular ring.[2] Although most vascular anomalies are asymptomatic, the most common symptomatic vascular ring is the right aortic arch, aberrant left subclavian artery, and presence of a left ligamentum or ductus arteriosus. A double aortic arch is usually symptomatic as well. Less common symptomatic vascular rings include a left aortic

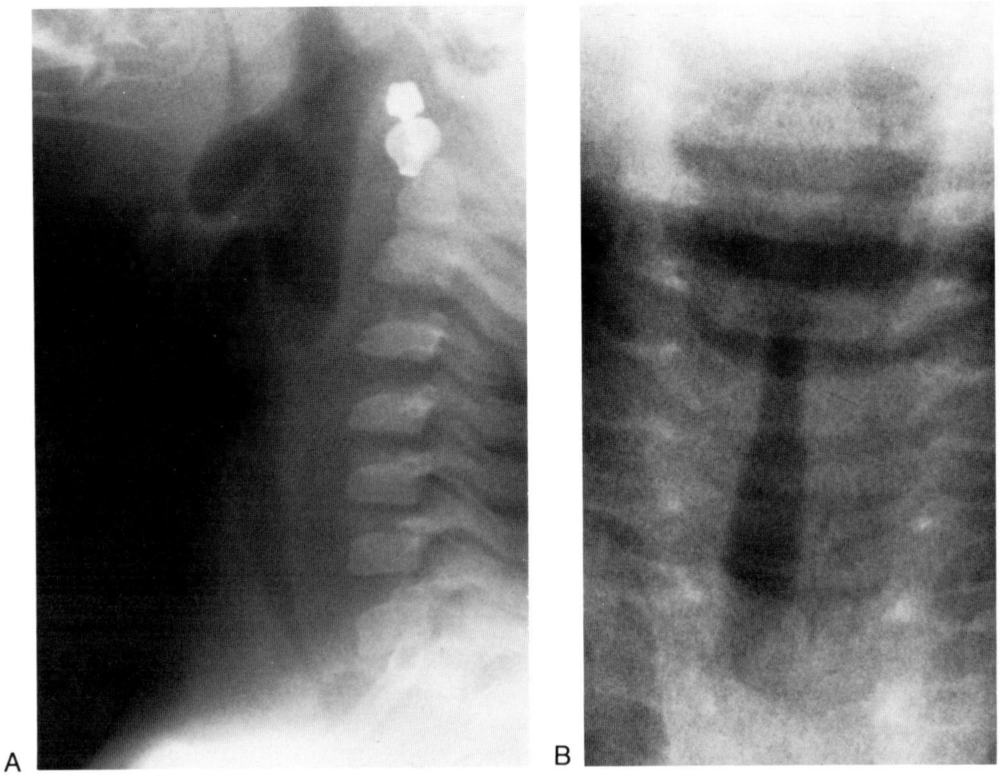

Fig. 2–36 Congenital subglottic stenosis. **(A)** Lateral view of the neck demonstrates concentric narrowing of the subglottic portion of the trachea down to the level of the thoracic inlet. **(B)** Frontal projection demonstrates fixed narrowing of the subglottic portion of the trachea just above the thoracic inlet. The patient had no history of airway trauma.

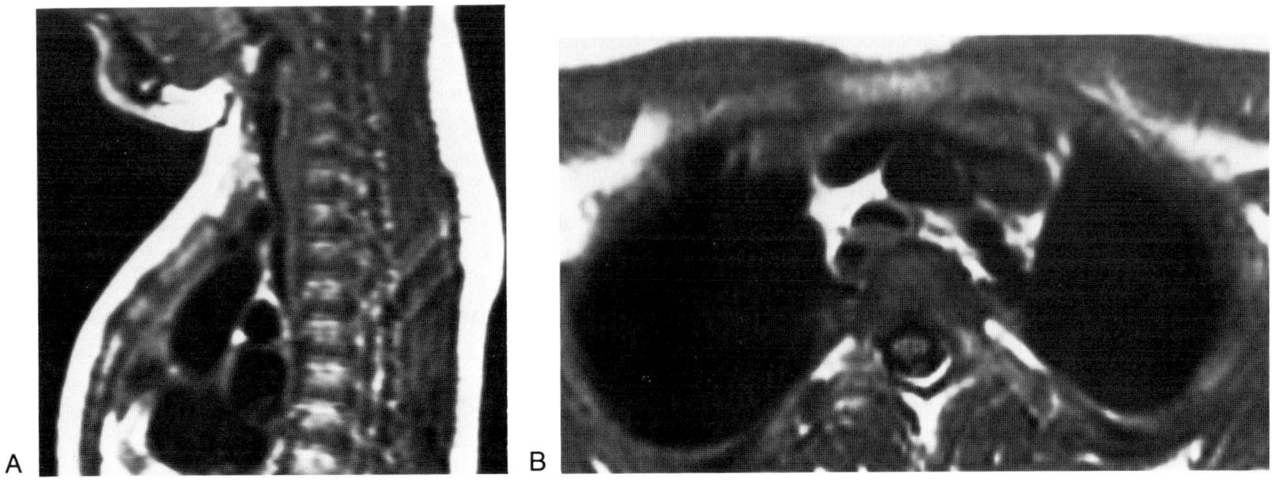

Fig. 2–37 Innominate artery syndrome. **(A)** Sagittal cardiac-gaited T_1-weighted MRI: note the compression of the trachea just below the thoracic inlet by the anomalous innominate artery. **(B)** Axial image demonstrates posterior compression of the trachea by a nondilated esophagus. This is suggestive of tracheomalacia.

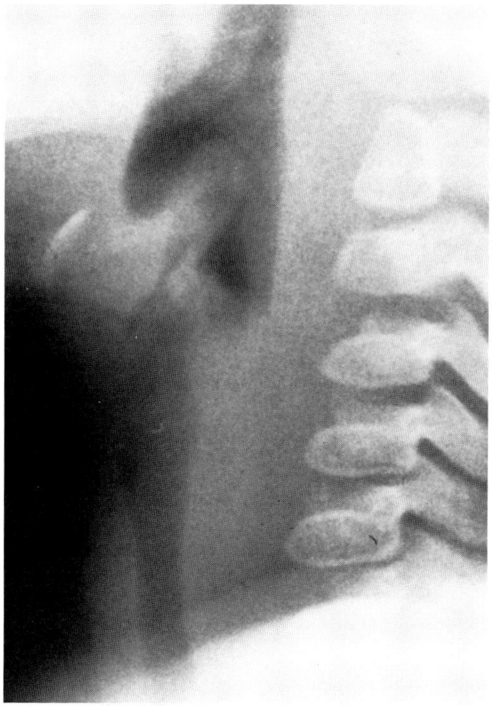

Fig. 2–38 Laryngomalacia. Note the inferoposterior position of the epiglottis with anterior bowing of the epiglottic folds obstructing the airway.

arch, aberrant right subclavian artery with a right ductus or ligamentum arteriosus, and the aberrant left pulmonary artery (pulmonary sling). Barium swallow reveals characteristic esophageal indentations in all cases. The aberrant left subclavian artery produces an oblique posterior esophageal indentation on the esophagus with the presence of a right aortic arch. Obliquity to the opposite side suggests a left aortic arch with an aberrant right subclavian artery. The pulmonary sling causes tracheal posterior and anterior esophageal indentations. Two anomalies of the great vessels commonly present with anterior tracheal narrowing but without symptoms. These are the anomalous innominate artery and an anomalous origin of the left common carotid artery. However, if children are symptomatic, surgery to relieve the tracheal compression usually leads to resolution of the patient's respiratory difficulty. MRI is a noninvasive method of differentiating the vascular rings from rarer causes of extrinsic compression of the trachea, such as bronchopulmonary foregut malformation and mediastinal thyroid tissue.

The most common ectopic location of thyroid tissue is at the base of the tongue. However, extension of the thyroid to the level of the thoracic inlet or the presence of intratracheal thyroid tissue may compromise tracheal function. The presence of intratracheal thyroid tissue is rare and usually comes to clinical attention when the normal thyroid tissue has enlarged due to goiter formation or malignancy.

Congenital tracheobronchomegaly is due to defective elastic and muscle tissue of the airway. The condition may occur as an isolated defect or may be associated with generalized elastic disorders such as Ehlers-Danlos syndrome, acquired cutis laxa, or ataxia telangiectasia. The diagnosis may be suggested on chest x-rays when the diameter of the trachea exceeds 3 cm or the bronchi exceed 2.5 cm. The airway appears corrugated due to excess fibrous tissue between the cartilaginous rings. The abnormal width of the airway may be exacerbated by chronic respiratory tract infections.

Inflammation

While most infections of the hypopharynx and larynx do not require special imaging, if a child presents to the emergency room with symptoms of severe acute upper airway obstruction and fever, lateral radiographs of the airway are sometimes the only method of diagnosing acute epiglottitis without endangering the patient's life. Epiglottitis is due to infection with *Haemophilus influenzae*. The infection usually occurs in patients more than 3 years of age. Dysphagia is an important symptom and most patients present with drooling. Lateral radiography reveals simultaneous thickening of both the epiglottis and aryepiglottic folds (Fig. 2–39). Although the subglottic portion of the airway is usually normal, 10 percent of patients with epiglottitis may demonstrate subglottic edema as well, and present with a radiographic picture similar to croup. Treatment includes antibiotic therapy and intubation until the cherry-red epiglottis returns to a normal size.

In children less than 3 years of age, viral croup is a more common cause of laryngotracheal inflammation. The typical clinical presentation is a young infant with several days history of a runny nose and a barking cough. Inspiratory stridor and chest retractions

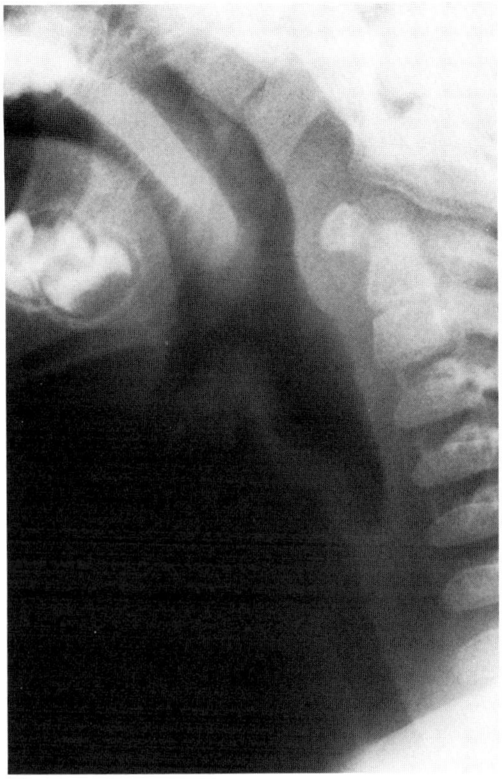

Fig. 2–39 Epiglottitis. This child presented with marked respiratory distress and drooling. The lateral view of the soft tissues of the neck demonstrate uniform swelling of both the epiglottis and the aryepiglottic folds. No evidence of associated croup was seen.

are present. The parainfluenza virus and respiratory syncytial virus are most commonly implicated. The lateral radiograph of the neck demonstrates overdistention of the hypopharynx during inspiration and narrowing of the trachea below the glottis (Fig. 2–40). During expiration, the subglottic trachea widens and the hypopharynx is collapsed. The vocal cords appear thickened and indistinct. On the frontal film, slitlike narrowing of the glottis classically is described as a steeple. If intraluminal membranes are detected on the radiographs, the diagnosis of membranous croup should be suggested (Fig. 2–41). This entity, which occurs in older children, is associated with a more severe clinical course and may be due to bacterial infection. Differential considerations include a non-opaque foreign body in the subglottic region with surrounding edema and intratracheal mucus. Repeat-

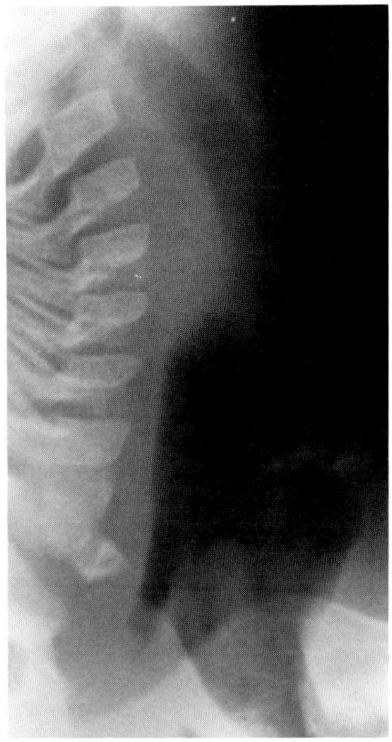

A

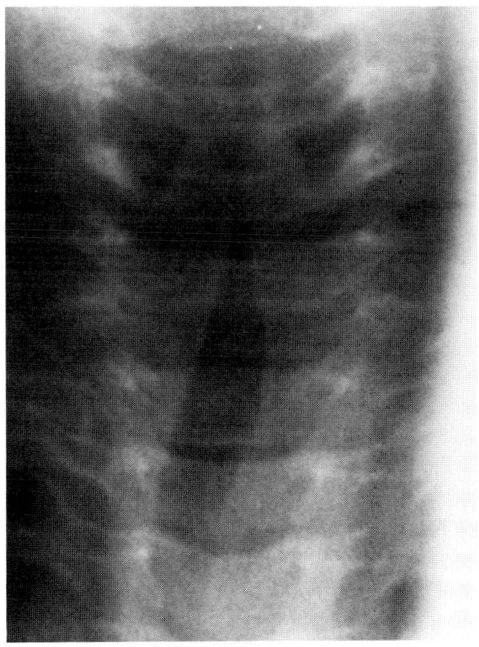

B

Fig. 2–40 Croup. **(A)** Lateral view of the neck demonstrates distention of the hypopharynx and diffuse narrowing of the subglottic portion of the trachea. **(B)** Frontal view demonstrates slitlike narrowing of the glottis.

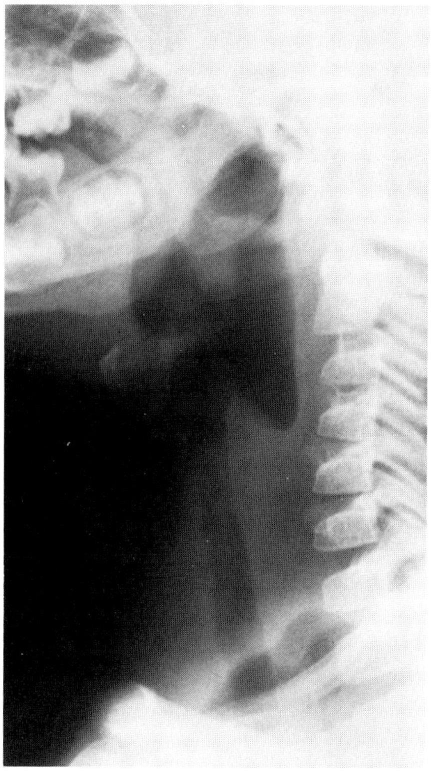

Fig. 2–41 Membranous croup. Note the serpiginous soft tissue density in the subglottic portion of the trachea. This did not clear with coughing and represented a membrane associated with bacterial croup.

ing the lateral view after vigorous coughing will clear mucus simulating an intraluminal membrane.

The presence of membranes within the larynx or hypopharynx may indicate infection by *Corynebacterium diphtheriae*. Since most infants are immunized early in childhood, the disease is more prevalent in adolescents. The bacterial organism produces a necrotizing toxin that is fixed onto the mucosa by the membrane formed. Attempts to remove the membrane hasten the systemic spread of the toxin and may result in neuromuscular effects such as paralysis and myocarditis. Rapid administration of antitoxin may prevent long-term sequelae.

Inflammatory masses are uncommon in the hypopharynx, larynx, and trachea. However, granulomas may form secondary to accidental or iatrogenic airway trauma or are associated with granulomatous diseases such as tuberculosis or Wegener's granulomatosis. Submucosal cysts may develop secondary to mucus retention. In children, these occur most commonly along the aryepiglottic folds. Rarely, a cyst is encountered in the subglottic region. Videofluoroscopy reveals a nonspecific mass of soft tissue density (Fig. 2–42). Direct visualization is necessary for a specific diagnosis. Laser surgery is the treatment of choice for both conditions.

Neoplasm

The most common laryngeal neoplasm in children is the squamous cell papilloma.[20] The juvenile form of laryngeal papillomatosis is thought to be due to hematogenous spread of human papillomavirus infec-

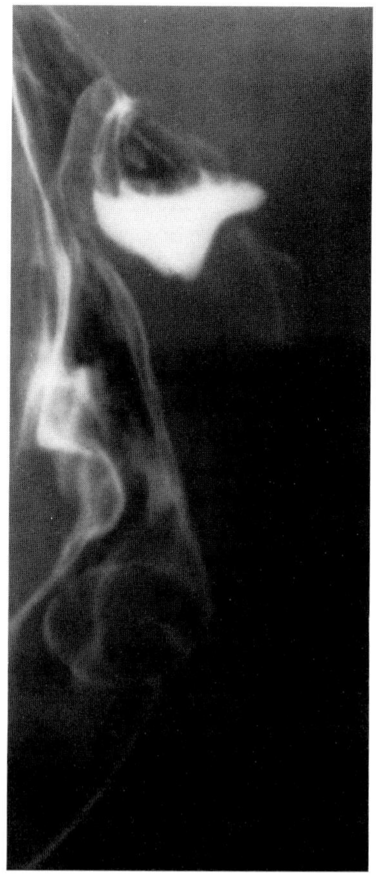

Fig. 2–42 Submucosal cyst. Lateral view from a laryngogram demonstrates a 1-cm rounded mass arising from the anterior trachea at the level of the vocal cords.

tion related to maternal genital condylomas. Clinically, patients present with voice abnormalities of long duration and may or may not have some degree of airway obstruction (Fig. 2–43). If airway obstruction is present, laser obliteration is the treatment of choice to minimize the lower airway seeding that commonly occurs after instrumentation. A careful search of the aerodigestive tract may reveal multiple papillomas. Whether or not these lesions spontaneously regress at puberty remains disputed.

The most common tracheal neoplasm of early infancy is the subglottic hemangioma.[3] The infants present with sporadic episodes of airway obstruction and one-half the patients have associated cutaneous hemangiomas. Radiographic studies reveal asymmetric narrowing of the subglottic portion of the trachea with a soft tissue mass (Fig. 2–44). Growth of the hemangioma usually ceases by 1 year of age and spontaneous involution follows.

Other benign and malignant neoplasms of the larynx and trachea are uncommon and include fibroma, schwannoma, lipoma, bronchial carcinoid, and adenoid cystic carcinoma. On imaging studies, the lipoma is the only lesion that can be reliably differentiated from other neoplasms due to its characteristic density or signal demonstrated on CT or MRI. Malignancies of the tracheobronchial tree are extremely rare in children but bronchial carcinoids and adenoid cystic carcinoma have been reported. Carcinoid syndrome is not associated with the childhood presenta-

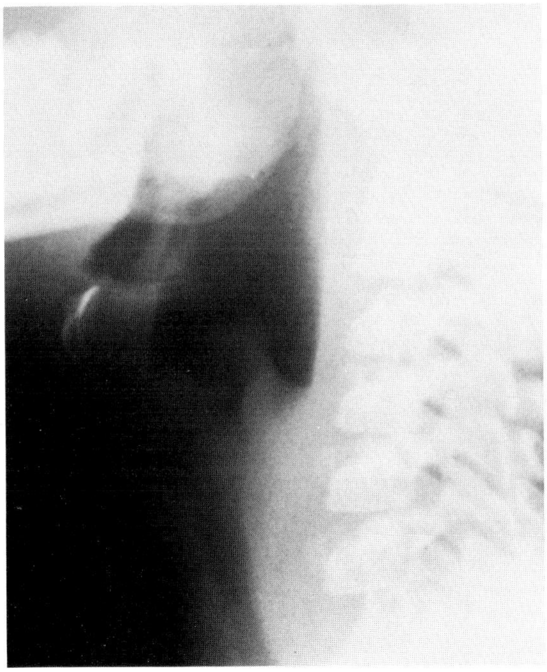

Fig. 2–43 Laryngeal papillomatosis. Note the bilobed soft tissue mass obscuring visualization of the vocal cords on the lateral neck radiograph.

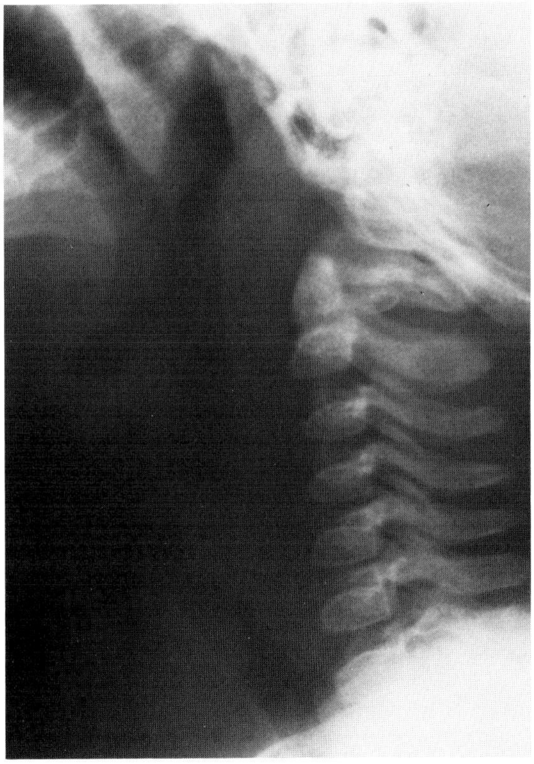

Fig. 2–44 Subglottic hemangioma. Lateral view of an infant's neck with intermittent inspiratory stridor demonstrated a large soft tissue mass arising from the posterior wall of the subglottic trachea. Endoscopy demonstrated a subglottic hemangioma.

tion of these tumors. Treatment includes direct visualization and conservative resection. The adenoid cystic carcinoma is more aggressive than the bronchial carcinoid but is still considered a low grade malignancy. Radiographically it appears as either an intrinsic or extrinsic tracheal mass causing mild upper airway obstruction.

Trauma

When a child presents with acute onset of upper airway obstruction, foreign body aspiration should be considered. A foreign body lodged above the thoracic inlet may incite a profound inflammatory reaction with localized edema and constitutional symptoms mimicking infection. Most aspirated foreign bodies are nonradiopaque and close scrutiny of the plain radiographs is required to recognize them (Fig. 2–45). While a foreign body lodged in the proximal esophagus for less than 24 hours may be removed with the aid of a Foley catheter and fluoroscopic guidance, those lodged within the airway should be removed under general anesthesia by direct visualization.

Unilateral or bilateral vocal cord paralysis is usually secondary to congenital malformation or birth trauma. Central nervous system abnormalities, such as the Chiari malformations and cerebral agenesis, have been associated with vocal cord paralysis. Vascular rings, bronchopulmonary foregut malformations, and other mediastinal masses may compress the recurrent laryngeal nerve and result in unilateral vocal cord paralysis. Birth trauma may result in brain stem injury, intracerebral hemorrhage, or stretching of the recurrent laryngeal nerve. Videofluoroscopy demonstrates decreased motion of the paralyzed cord with failure to approximate the midline during phonation and incomplete relaxation. However, laryngoscopy is the method of choice for demonstrating laryngeal paralysis. The role of the radiologist in the diagnosis of vocal cord paralysis is to determine the etiology by MRI or CT of the head, neck, or mediastinum.

Blunt trauma to the neck may result in fracture or dislocation of the paired cartilages that form the larynx. These injuries are best diagnosed with thin-section axial CT. In noncalcified cartilage, fracture can be inferred by the presence of hemorrhage in the surrounding spaces. Spread of hemorrhage may compromise the airway in the subglottic region. The radiologist often is the first to notice injuries of the larynx since an endotracheal tube may already be positioned in the acutely injured patient and attention is focused on the central nervous system. Prompt treatment reduces the post-traumatic morbidity of the patient.

Iatrogenic

Placement of an endotracheal or tracheostomy tube is almost always accompanied by radiographic evaluation. Complete evaluation includes the location of the tube tip, tube angulation, cuff identification, amount of cuff inflation, and whether fluid has accumulated above the cuff. Endotracheal tubes may migrate up to 2 cm with both lateral and anteroposterior head motion. The tube tip should be located at least 1 cm above the carina but well below the thoracic

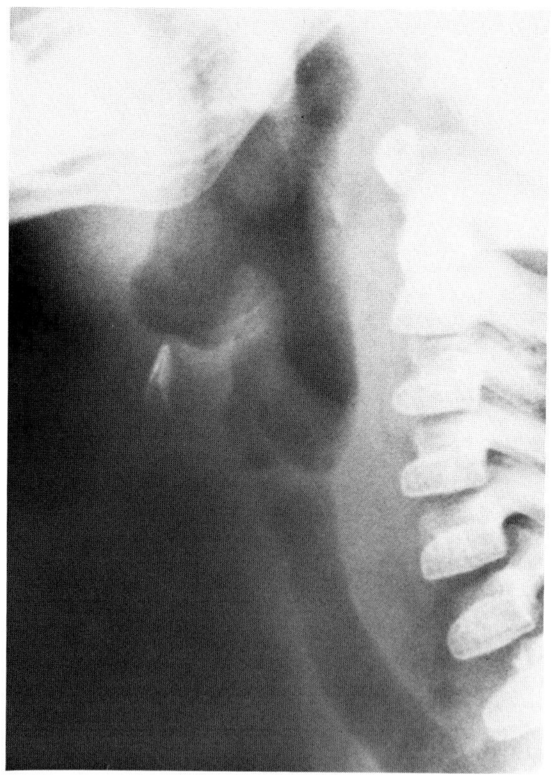

Fig. 2–45 Foreign body. Note the gracile radiopacity extending from the level of the lingual tonsil and velum down the epiglottis. This was a fish bone.

inlet. The cuff is identified as a rectangular air density and should fill but not bulge the trachea. If the cuff is located high at the level of the vocal cords, permanent damage may result. Persistent angulation of a tracheal tube may result in erosion of the tracheal wall and fistula formation with either the esophagus posteriorly or innominate artery anteriorly. If the tracheal air column is replaced by soft tissue density around the endotracheal tube, fluid accumulation should be suspected and suctioning must be performed before the cuff is deflated or aspiration will result.

The most common late complication following intubation is stenosis formation at the level of the cuff or stoma. Segmental stenoses at the level of the cuff may be difficult to differentiate from congenital subglottic stenosis and are usually symmetrical (Fig. 2–46). Tracheomalacia results from over distention of the tube cuff and resultant pressure necrosis of the tracheal wall. With the advent of high volume, low pressure cuffs, the development of this complication is exceedingly rare. Although the diagnosis of acquired tracheal stenosis is usually confirmed with videofluoroscopy, both CT and MRI may be useful in determining the extent of the mucosal abnormality for preoperative planning.

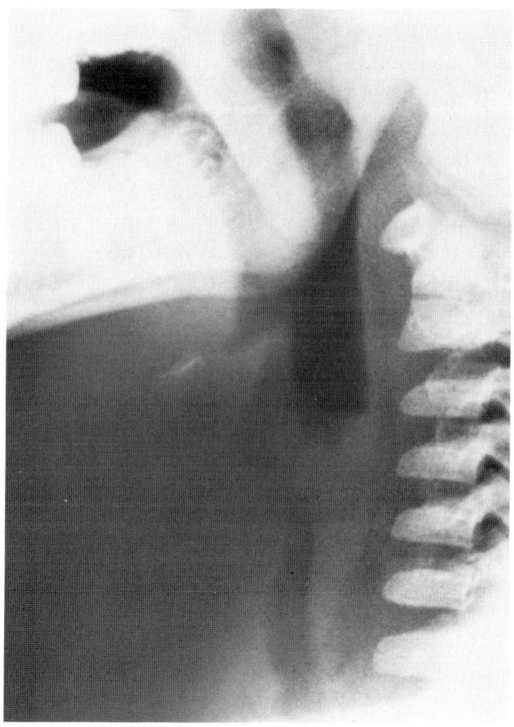

Fig. 2–46 Iatrogenic subglottic stenosis. Note the irregular focal narrowings of the anterior and posterior walls of the subglottic portion of the trachea. Laryngoscopy revealed large inflammatory granulomas secondary to an indwelling in the tracheal tube.

Although laryngospasm does not require radiographic diagnosis, it may be encountered in the radiology department after administration of radiographic contrast material. The advent of nonionic contrast material has decreased the incidence of all complications significantly and most departments are converting to the exclusive use of these low-osmolality agents. Nevertheless, if laryngospasm occurs, prompt administration of oxygen and epinephrine 0.1 to 0.2 ml of a 1:1000 solution subcutaneously every 20 minutes for up to 3 doses as required for relief of airway compromise is the suggested method of treatment.

MANDIBULAR/MAXILLARY ABNORMALITIES

Because both the mandible and the maxilla are tooth-bearing bones, it is not surprising that they share similar pathologic processes. Mandibular views provide adequate demonstration of the respective mandibular condyles but the inherent overlap that is present due to the mandible's shape is inescapable. The panorex view (obtained with special equipment that moves the film about the mandible) displays the mandible, maxilla, and embedded teeth entirely. Dental occlusal radiographs are useful in evaluating the individual teeth. The most sensitive method for evaluating bone destruction of the mandible or maxilla is CT using a bone detail algorithm and axial thin sections. Superior soft tissue detail is provided by MRI. The use of specialized surface coils has made temporomandibular joint arthrography virtually obsolete.

Normal

Twenty deciduous teeth begin erupting at about 6 months of age. The first permanent tooth should

MANDIBULAR/MAXILLARY ABNORMALITIES

Normal
- Supernumerary teeth
- Unerupted/impacted teeth

Congenital
- Dental cysts
- Nondental cystic lesions
- Odontoma
- Syndromes with abnormal dentition

Inflammation
- Dental/periodontal disease
- Radicular cyst
- Osteomyelitis
- Condensing osteitis

Neoplasm
- Odontogenic tumors
- Nonodontogenic tumors

Systemic disease
- Diabetes mellitus
- Hemolytic anemia

Idiopathic
- Infantile cortical hyperostosis

Trauma
- Fracture
- Degenerative joint disease

Iatrogenic
- Surgical ciliated cyst
- Residual cyst

erupt at about 6 years of age. Adults have 32 permanent teeth. Supernumerary teeth are a very common variant. Impaction implies failure of eruption through the gum. The third molars are most likely to be impacted. Tooth impaction weakens the mandible and may predispose patients to fracture. Occasionally, impacted teeth migrate along the mandible. Abnormal occlusal forces may result when the teeth are poorly aligned or in patients with bruxism (jaw clenching and nocturnal grinding). These abnormalities result in accelerated wear on the occlusal surfaces and remodeling of the mandibular condyles.

Congenital

Dental cysts are a variety of well-circumscribed, benign appearing cysts arising from the different cells that form the teeth. The dentigerous cyst is the most likely congenital cyst to present in the first decade of life.[17] This cyst arises from the epithelial sac surrounding an unerupted tooth crown, usually an impacted lower third molar. Radiographically, the unerupted tooth crown is seen within a well-circumscribed unilocular cyst (Fig. 2–47). Multiple dentigerous cysts have been associated with mucopolysaccharidosis type VI. Other findings include calvarial changes, short mandibular rami, paddle-shaped ribs, and wide diaphyses. Rarely, tumors such as the ameloblastoma or carcinoma may arise as a mural nodule in a dentigerous cyst. The primordial cyst (odontogenic keratocyst) makes up 10 to 20 percent of all dental cysts and is most likely to occur in the first two decades of life. The cyst arises from remnants of dental lamina in areas at which tooth formation has been aborted. The posterior aspect of the mandible is the favored location. The cysts may be multiple in about 10 percent of cases. One-half of the cases of multiple primordial cysts are associated with Gorlin's syndrome (basal cell nevus syndrome). The syndrome is an autosomal dominant trait characterized by multiple nevoid basal cell carcinomas, skin lesions, odontogenic keratocysts, ameloblastomas and fibrosarcomas of the mandible, ocular abnormalities, mental retardation, and absence of the internal carotid artery. Radiographic investigation reveals multiple

DENTAL/NONDENTAL CYSTIC LESIONS

Dental
- Dentigerous cyst
- Primordial cyst

Nondental
- Hemorrhagic bone cyst
- Central hemangioma of bone
- Aneurysmal bone cyst
- Epithelial inclusion cysts
- Stafne bone defect

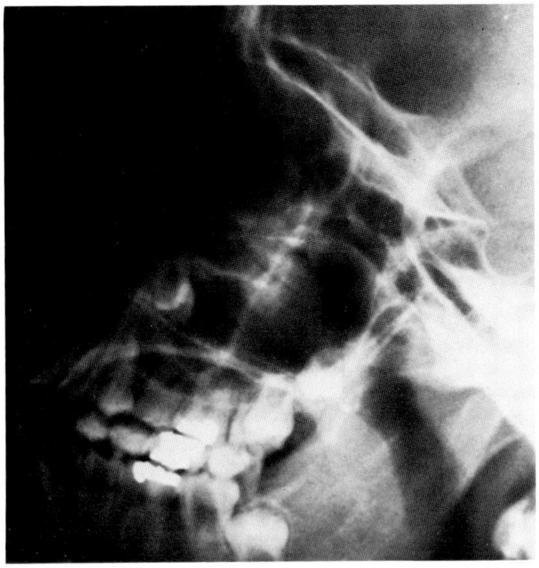

Fig. 2–47 Dentigerous cyst. Lateral view reveals a well-circumscribed cyst occupying one of the maxillary sinuses. In the superoanterior portion of the cyst, a well-formed tooth is identified. Note the sclerotic margin of the cyst inferior to the tooth.

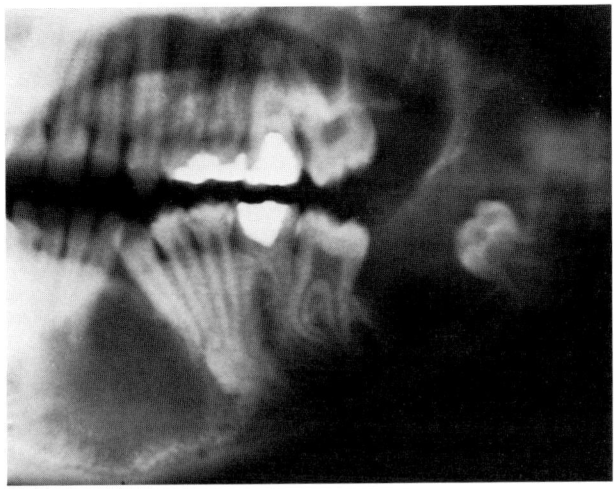

Fig. 2–48 Gorlin's syndrome. Panorex examination of the jaw reveals multiple well-circumscribed cysts that have expanded the body of the mandible and displaced the teeth. Another primordial cyst is identified in the maxilla. This 18-year-old patient had multiple basal cell nevi as well.

odontogenic cysts of the mandible and maxilla, rib and vertebral anomalies, scapular deformities, and lamellar calcification of the falx (Fig. 2–48). The incidence of recurrence of primordial cysts is increased if the cysts are multiple. Other congenital dental cysts are uncommon in children and have both a nonspecific radiographic and pathologic appearance.

Congenital nondental cystic lesions are also common in the mandible and maxilla (see list, p. 44). They present as well-circumscribed radiolucencies that may expand the cortex. The hemorrhagic bone cyst is usually detected in the first two decades of life in an asymptomatic patient. The radiographic appearance is characteristic: a unilocular cyst with well-defined scalloped margins extending between the teeth but not displacing them (Fig. 2–49). Biopsy of the lesion will initiate healing. Recurrence is uncommon.

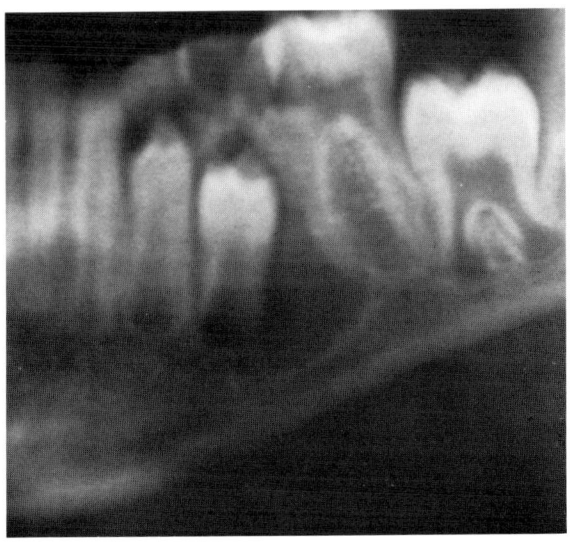

Fig. 2–49 Hemorrhagic bone cyst. A well-defined cyst arises between an unerupted first molar and the second molar.

The mandible and maxilla are also common sites for central hemangioma of bone. This lesion presents as a slow growing mass in the first two decades of life and as a multiloculated lytic lesion with a circumscribed margin on radiographs (Fig. 2–50). Bone destruction may be associated with the lesion. The tumor is highly vascular and biopsy may be fatal.

Rarely, an aneurysmal bone cyst may occur in the mandible or maxilla. This also presents as a multilocular radiolucent defect with a circumscribed margin expanding the mandible or maxilla. Iatrogenic trauma initiates healing.

Epithelial inclusion cysts may form at the fusion sites of the maxillary processes and the frontonasal process. These cysts are named by location and include the nasopalatine duct cyst, medial palatine cyst, and the globulomaxillary cyst, the latter of which is located between the lateral incisor and the canine tooth.

The Stafne bone defect consists of heterotopic salivary gland tissue within a congenital depression of the mandible, which is incidentally noted on radiographs. A well-circumscribed elliptical radiolucency with a sclerotic margin is seen. The appearance of the lesion does not change on follow-up radiographs.

The odontoma is a hamartoma arising from the dental elements and is divided into three major subtypes. Odontomas represent 70 percent of all odontogenic tumors. The compound subtype presents as multiple, poorly formed rudimentary teeth surrounded by a radiolucent dental sheath most commonly located in the anterior maxilla. The complex odontoma appears as a homogeneous bone density surrounded by a thin radiolucent line and occurs with equal frequency in the mandible and maxilla (Fig. 2–51). The third subtype, the ameloblastic odontoma contains odontogenic epithelium and is more aggressive than the other two subtypes.

Syndromes associated with abnormal dentition may be subdivided according to the defective dental component. The primary abnormality in ectodermal dysplasia, epidermolysis bullosa atrophica, and amelogenesis imperfecta in hypoplasia or absence of the enamel of the teeth. The teeth appear discolored and pits are seen in the enamel. Aberrant dentin formation is seen in osteogenesis imperfecta and isolated in dentinogenesis imperfecta. In these entities, the superficial dentin appears normal but the tubular dentin is altered and may result in either absence or enlargement of the pulp chamber. The teeth have an opalescent appearance. Abnormal cementum formation is seen in familial hypophosphatemia (Vitamin D-resistant rickets). In the condition, cementosis, increased secretion of the cementum occurs usually in one quad-

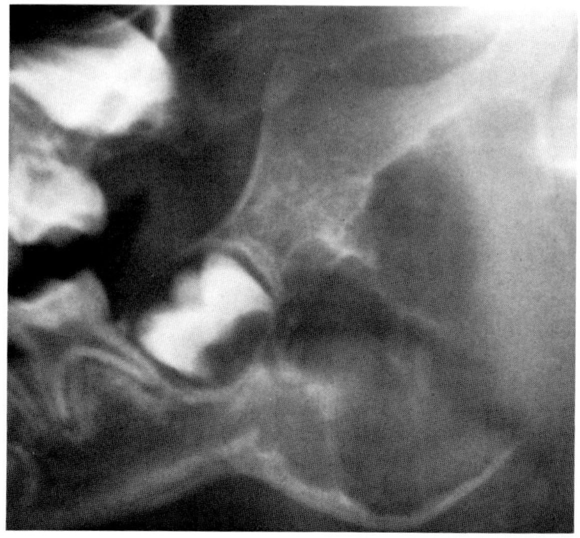

Fig. 2–50 Central hemangioma of bone. Note the multiloculated cystic lesion with a circumscribed margin arising at the angle of the mandible.

SYNDROMES WITH ABNORMAL DENTITION

Ectodermal dysplasia

Epidermolysis bullosa atrophica

Amelogenesis imperfecta

Osteogenesis imperfecta

Dentinogenesis imperfecta

Familial hypophosphatemia

Cementosis

Papillon-Lefevre syndrome

Osteopetrosis

A 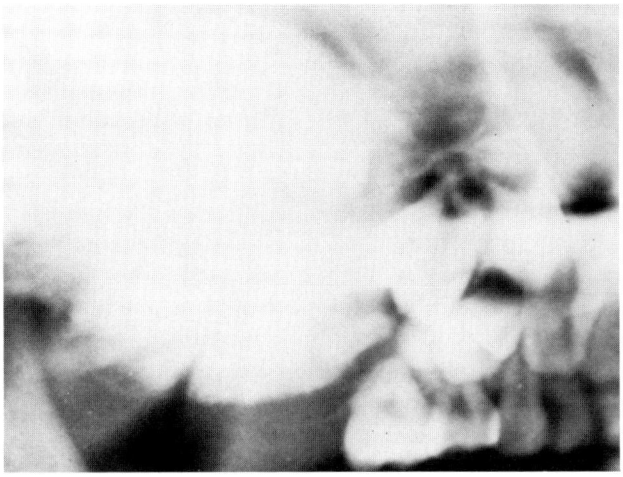 B 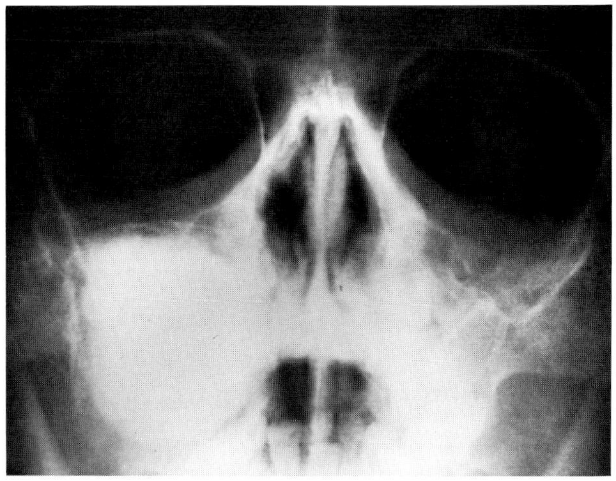

Fig. 2–51 Complex odontoma. **(A)** This 6-year-old child was asymptomatic except for facial asymmetry when she presented to her dentist. The panorex view reveals a homogeneous bone density mass arising in the right maxilla. **(B)** Waters view demonstrates the lucent rim surrounding the odontoma.

rant of the mouth resulting in deposition of amorphous calcified material along the roots of the teeth. The Papillon-Lefevre syndrome is the association of hyperkeratosis of the palms and soles with a preponderance toward periodontal disease. Patients with osteopetrosis (marble bone disease) have a peculiar predilection to osteomyelitis of the jaw.

Inflammation

The most common inflammatory process to involve the mouth is the formation of dental caries. While the advent of antibiotics and emphasis on dental hygiene have decreased the number of severe complications, the problem is still widespread. Dental caries result in demineralization of the dental tissues. Radiographically, they appear as radiolucencies beginning in the crowns of teeth (Fig. 2–52). Extension into the tooth root may lead to loss of the tooth and secondary infection of the surrounding bone. Deposition of breakdown products from pulp decay lead to local inflammation and an increase in the radiolucency of the periapical lamina dura.

Periodontal disease is inflammation of the gingival tissues surrounding the teeth. Chronic inflammation leads to loss of the lamina dura about the tooth crest and widening of the periodontal ligament. The most common cause of periodontal disease is inadequate dental hygiene. This is evidenced on radiographs by calculus deposition below the level of the gingiva. Systemic diseases that increase the likelihood of periodontal disease include Papillon-Lefèvre syndrome, diabetes mellitus, and immunodeficiencies.

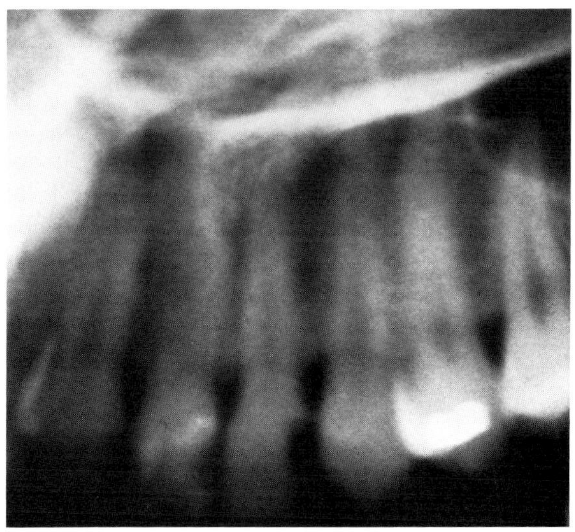

Fig. 2–52 Dental caries. Note the ovoid radiolucencies along the lateral aspects of the incisors. These represent areas of destruction from dental caries.

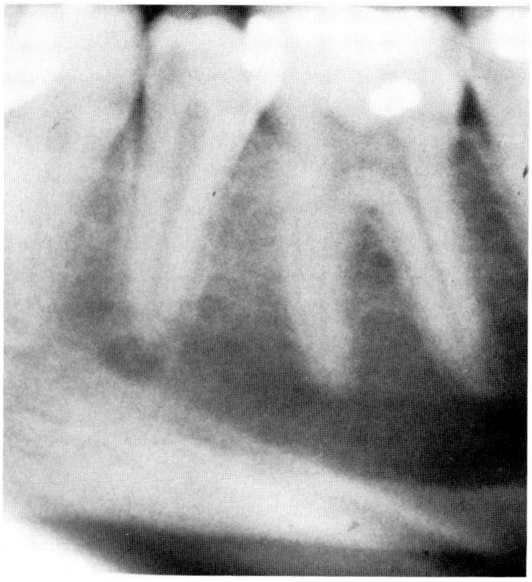

Fig. 2–53 Periapical abscess. The small radiolucency at the base of one of the incisors represents low-grade infection and abscess formation.

When a lucent lesion at the apex of a tooth is identified on dental radiographs, the differential diagnosis includes granuloma formation or periapical abscess (Fig. 2–53). Chronic low-grade infection stimulates the formation of radicular cysts. This is the most frequent cyst of the jaw bones, and accounts for approximately 60 percent of all dental cysts. It is unusual for radicular cysts to form before the shedding of deciduous teeth.

Osteomyelitis is usually secondary to *S. aureus* infection, especially in infants. The spread of infection may be either hematogenous or contiguous. Hematogenous spread is more common in childhood. The mandible is involved more frequently than the maxilla. However, in the neonatal period, osteomyelitis almost exclusively involves the maxilla. Radiographic findings may lag behind the clinical infection. ^{99m}Tc-MDP is useful in identifying infected sites. When low-grade infection or chronic trauma is present, condensing osteitis develops. This is an increase in the radiodensity of the bone adjacent to the tooth roots. The appearance of the amorphous density about the roots of teeth is similar to cementosis (Fig. 2–54). However, in condensing osteitis the periodontal ligament separates the tooth root from the increased bone density. In cementosis, the amorphous material is deposited on the root itself with the periodontal ligament surrounding the abnormal density.

Neoplasm

Odontogenic tumors in children are extremely uncommon with only five tumors having a predilection for patients during the first two decades of life. These are the adenomatoid odontogenic tumor, ameloblastic fibroma, odontogenic fibroma, ameloblastic fibro-odontoma, and odontoma previously described.

The adenomatoid odontogenic tumor or adenoameloblastoma usually arises in the anterior maxilla adjacent to unerupted incisors. Pubescent girls are likely to be affected. Radiographically, a well-circumscribed radiolucent defect intimately related to an unerupted tooth is identified and is difficult to differentiate from a dentigerous cyst (Fig. 2–55). Treatment is surgical excision and recurrence is unlikely.

The ameloblastic fibroma tends to occur in pubescent boys and presents as a slow-growing posterior mandibular mass. Again, the tumor is usually related to an unerupted tooth. The radiolucent defect is multilo-

ODONTOGENIC/NONODONTOGENIC TUMORS

Odontogenic
- Adenomatoid odontogenic tumor
- Ameloblastic fibroma
- Ameloblastic fibro-odontoma
- Odontogenic fibroma

Nonodontogenic
- Osteoma
- Exostosis
- Enostosis
- Giant cell granuloma
- Fibro-osseous tumors
- Brown tumor
- Metastatic malignancies
- Primary bone malignancies
- Nonlipid reticuloendothelioses

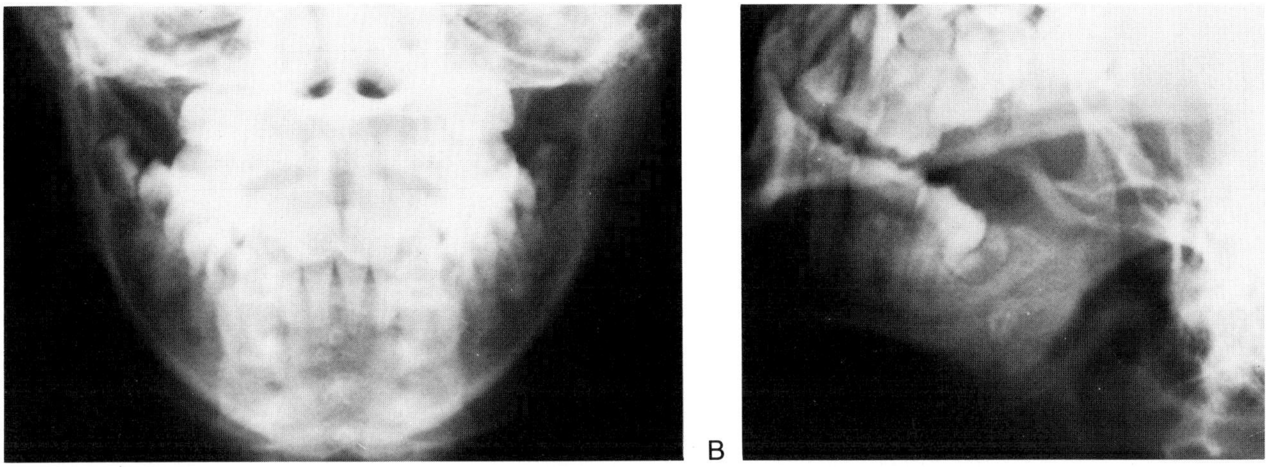

A B

Fig. 2–54 Condensing osteitis. **(A)** Note the soft tissue swelling adjacent to the left mandibular angle. The cortex has been resorbed and an area of increased density has expanded the left mandible. **(B)** An oblique view of the left side of the mandible demonstrates preservation of the periodontal ligament of the second molar and of the third molar, which is just barely erupting. The edge of the bone abnormality is well-defined. These findings are consistent with a low-grade infection.

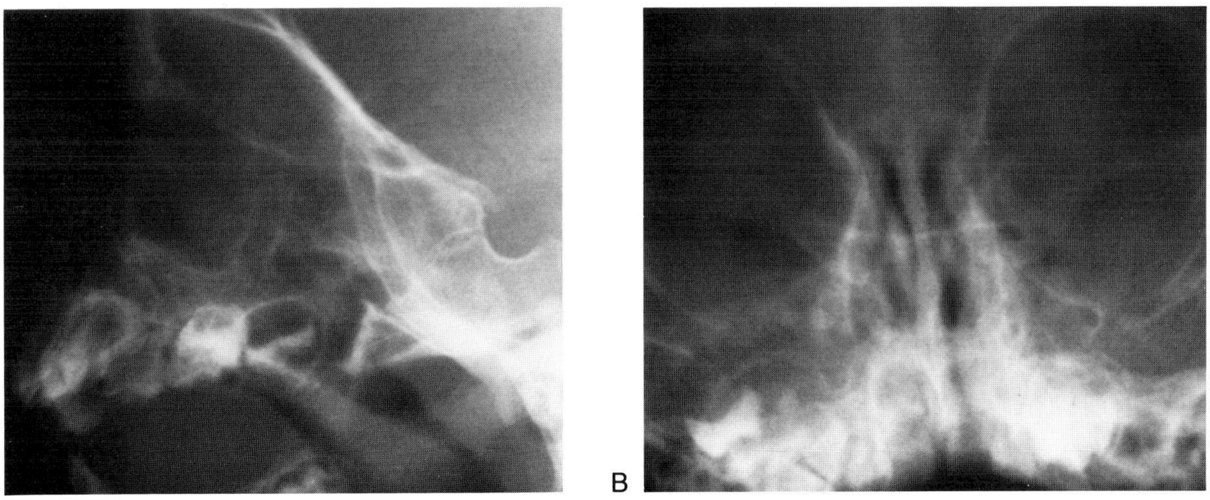

A B

Fig. 2–55 Adenomatoid odontogenic tumor. **(A)** Lateral view demonstrates an area of well-circumscribed radiolucency in the posterior right maxilla with an unerupted tooth arising along the posterior wall of the cyst. **(B)** Waters view demonstrates no displacement of the normal teeth but better demonstrates the unerupted tooth inside the radiolucent neoplasm, which distorts the right maxillary sinus.

culated and similar in appearance to a tumor more common in adults, the ameloblastoma. Both the radiologist and the pathologist are likely to misdiagnose ameloblastic fibroma as ameloblastoma.

If, on pathologic examination, the lesion contains odontomatous elements, the diagnosis of ameloblastic fibro-odontoma is made. This is a tumor of the posterior mandible likely to occur in children of both sexes between the age of 6 and 13. None of the ameloblastic lesions are aggressive and most respond to complete surgical excision without recurrence.

The odontogenic fibroma presents as an expansile multiloculated lesion of the mandible. The mass is slow-growing and primarily fibrous. Pathologically, this lesion is difficult to differentiate from fibromyxoma.

A variety of nonodontogenic neoplasms may arise within the jaw bones (see list, p. 48). If a well-circumscribed radiopacity is seen, the presence of a benign osteoma should be considered (Fig. 2–56). Although these are rare, if multiple, Gardner's syndrome should be suspected. In this syndrome, intestinal polyposis (adenomas with a predilection for malignant transformation) are associated with mandibular cysts, facial osteomas, and desmoid tumors. Gardner's syndrome

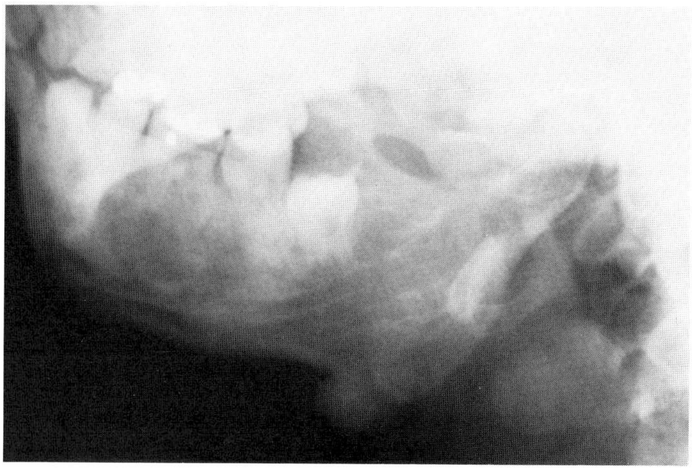

Fig. 2–56 Osteoma. Note the smoothly marginated lesion arising from the angle of the right mandible. The medullary space below the first and second molar is also distorted. These osteomas were associated with colonic polyposis in a patient with Gardner's syndrome.

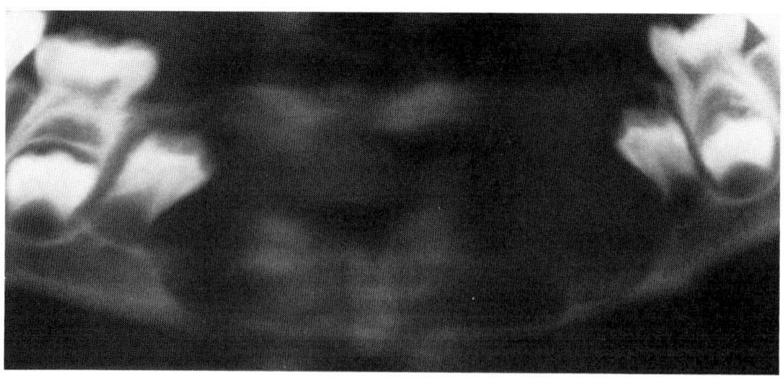

Fig. 2–57 Giant cell granuloma. On the panorex view note the multilocular radiolucency that is expanding but not destroying the cortex of the mandible. Notice how the front teeth are displaced by the expansile lesion, which represents a giant cell granuloma.

is an autosomal dominant trait and screening of other family members is indicated if the syndrome is diagnosed.

Exostosis formation is common along the mandible arising from the mylohiloid ridge (torus mandibularis). From the maxilla, torus palatinus may develop when exostosis formation occurs along the midline. Enostoses are radiopaque densities developing within the medullary space of the mandible.

Intraosseous giant cell granuloma has a radiographic appearance similar to a bone cyst. A multilocular radiolucency is identified at the angle of the mandible. If bilateral, the child presents with cherubic facies in early childhood (Fig. 2–57). The deformity worsens during puberty but regresses during adulthood. The lesion may destroy bone and may be difficult to distinguish from malignancy without biopsy. This lesion does not represent a true giant cell tumor (osteoclastoma) but a giant cell reaction of bone.

A variety of fibromas and fibrous dysplasia are pathologically classified as fibro-osseous tumors. The ossifying fibroma occurs equally in the maxilla and mandible of young adults. The lesion begins as an expansile radiolucency that gradually becomes more radiopaque with age. Radiographically, it may be indistinguishable from monostotic fibrous dysplasia. In ossifying fibroma, the original outline of the involved bone is preserved. The desmoplastic fibroma and mixofibromas are less common and do not have the characteristic radiographic appearance. The most widely recognized of the fibro-osseous tumors is fibrous dysplasia, the most common type of fibro-osseous tumor involving the jaw bone. It may be polyostotic or monostotic. Both forms have been associated with syndromes. McCune-Albright syndrome is the association of café au lait spots on the same side as polyostotic fibrous dysplasia, precocious puberty, and other endocrine disorders. The bone lesions most commonly occur in the femur and pelvis. The radiographic appearance of fibrous dysplasia is variable. A classic "ground glass" appearance to a multilocular radiopaque lesion is most commonly described (Fig. 2–58). Any mixture of radiopacity and lucency may be seen. There is no difference in the appearance of the polyostotic lesions and the monostotic lesions. The monostotic form has a predilection for maxillary involvement in females. The lesions are gradually expansile making complete resection difficult.

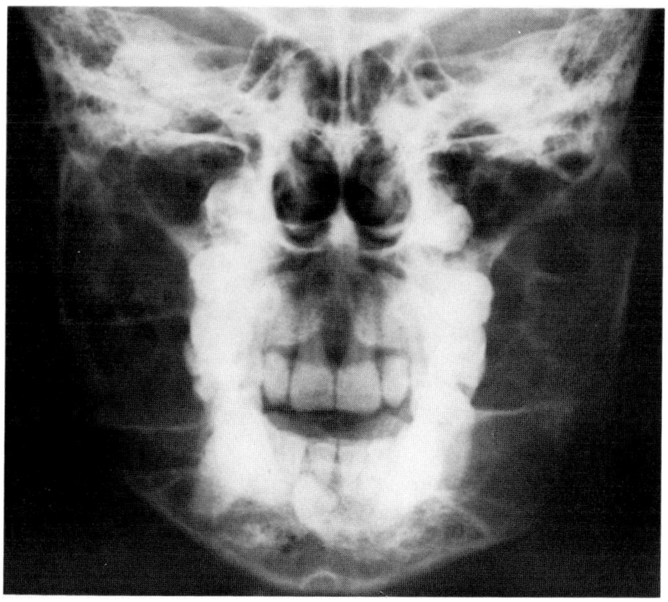

Fig. 2–58 Fibrous dysplasia. Note the multilocular lesion that has deformed the entire mandible. The individual cysts have a "ground glass" appearance. The maxillary sinuses have been replaced by similar multicystic abnormalities consistent with the patient's diagnosis of cherubism.

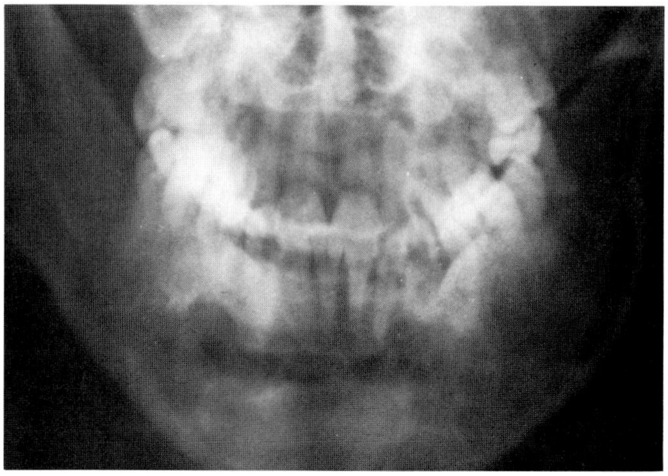

Fig. 2–59 Brown tumor. Note the sharply circumscribed cystic area in the left mandible of a patient with symptoms of hyperparathyroidism.

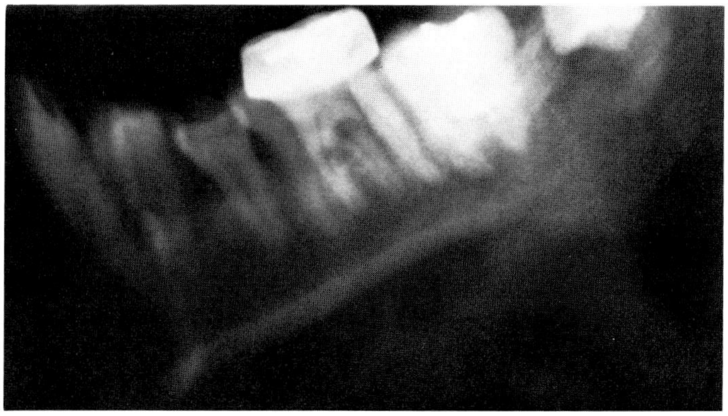

Fig. 2–60 Loss of lamina dura. Note the abscence of thin white lines (lamina dura) surrounding the tooth roots in this child with squamous cell carcinoma of the mandible.

Primary hyperparathyroidism is caused by a hyperfunctioning parathyroid adenoma, carcinoma, or gland. This leads to a wide variety of bone changes including demineralization, bone resorption, erosive arthritis, and brown tumor formation. Brown tumors are radiolucencies that usually are multiloculated and have a well-defined margin (Fig. 2–59). They demonstrate increased uptake on radionuclide scanning and are highly vascular lesions. Occasionally brown tumors occur in the mandible and may be difficult to differentiate from fibrous dysplasia. Secondary hyperparathyroidism, due to chronic renal disease, may rarely cause brown tumor formation. Loss of the lamina dura is another finding that is commonly described in hyperparathyroidism. Other conditions that also demonstrate loss of the lamina dura (or "floating teeth") include Cushing's syndrome, histiocystosis X, hyperparathyroidism, leukemia, metastatic disease, and periodontal disease (Fig. 2–60).

Metastases to the mandible and maxilla are much more common than primary malignancies. Almost any childhood neoplasm has been reported to metastasize to the jaw bones. The mandible is the preferred site and hematogenous spread is the usual route. Although most metastases are osteolytic, medulloblas-

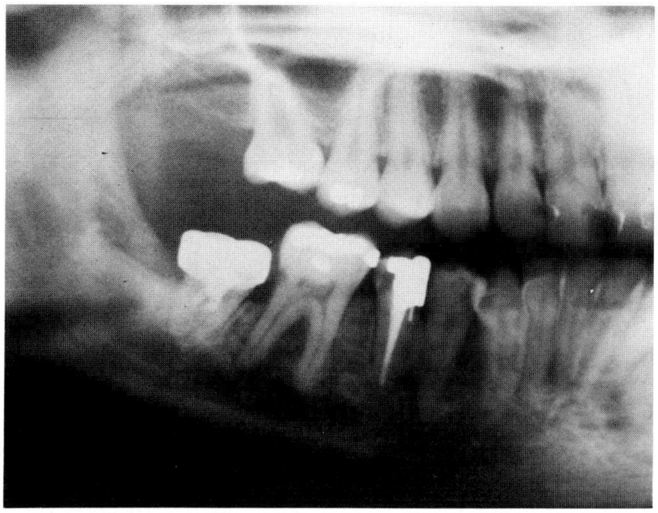

Fig. 2–61 Osteolytic lymphoma. Notice the multiple radiolucent lesions distorting the contour of both the mandible and the maxilla. The lamina dura is no longer apparent around the teeth, representing widespread lymphoma.

toma may cause osteoblastic metastases. Of the lymphomas, the African form of Burkitt's lymphoma has the highest association with mandibular lesions. The majority of African Burkitt's cases are associated with the Epstein-Barr virus. Children with African Burkitt's lymphoma present with massive destructive lesions of the mandible, maxilla, or orbital rims. The bone lesions are radiolucent and multifocal (Fig. 2–61). Early coalescence into large radiolucencies with cortical breakthrough is associated with rapid growth. The appearance is very aggressive and may be confused with osteomyelitis. In fact, secondary infection has been reported. Radionuclide bone scanning identifies other sites of skeletal involvement in metastatic disease.

Primary bone malignancies occurring in the mandible are rare but include osteolytic and osteoblastic osteosarcoma, fibrous sarcoma, malignant fibrous histiocytoma, primary lymphoma of bone (reticulum cell sarcoma), Ewing's sarcoma, primitive neuroectodermal tumor of infancy, and rhabdomyosarcoma. The prognosis with primary osteosarcoma of the mandible is better than that in the long bones. Most patients benefit from a course of preoperative radiation therapy prior to surgery and chemotherapy. Prior radiation therapy may induce the formation of malignant fibrous histiocytoma. Ewing's sarcoma may be osteolytic or osteoblastic and usually is painful. Periosteal reaction is the primary radiographic finding. The tumors are sensitive to treatment with radiotherapy and chemotherapy. Primary lymphoma of bone has a better prognosis than any of the other primary bone malignancies. The lesion is sensitive to radiotherapy. The primitive neuroectodermal tumor of infancy arises from neural crest cells in the first year of life and is pathologically similar to primitive neuroectodermal tumors arising from the posterior fossa. Complete excision is associated with a good prognosis. This lesion presents as a well-circumscribed radiolucency in the mandible.

The nonlipid reticuloendothelioses are systemic derangements of the reticuloendothial system resulting in deposition of histiocytes in tumorlike masses throughout various organ systems. Many believe that Letterer-Siwe disease, Hand-Schuller-Christian disease, and eosinophilic granuloma represent a spectrum of diseases due to the same pathologic process. All three diseases are referred to as histiocytosis X.

Letterer-Siwe disease is the most severe form of the nonlipid reticuloendothelioses and is usually detected before 3 years of age. Patients have lymphade-

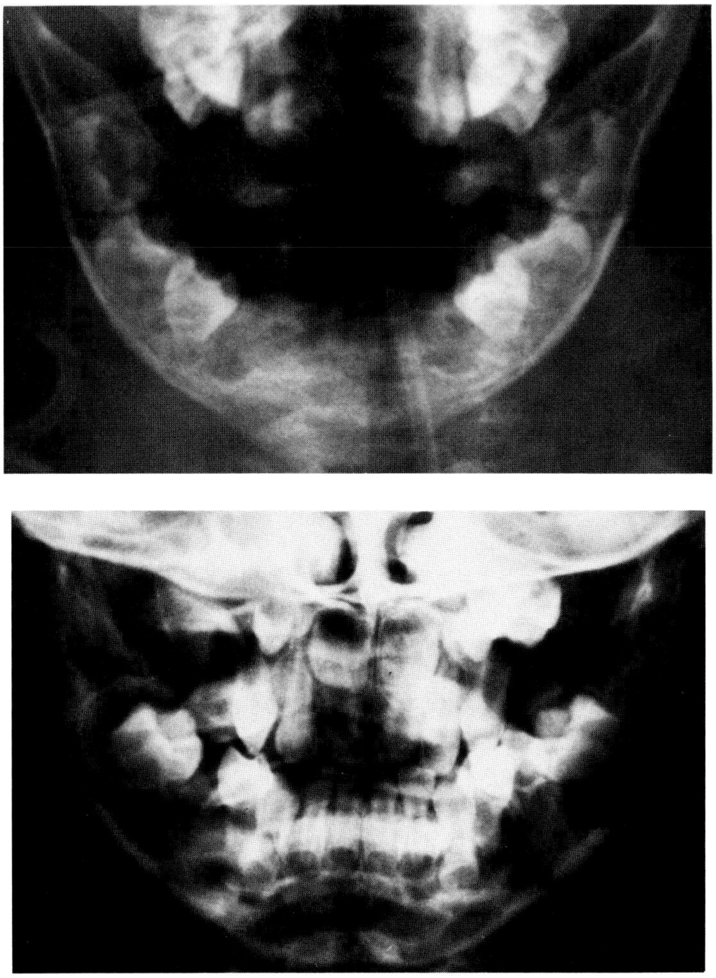

Fig. 2–62 Histiocytosis X. **(A)** Note the absence of the lamina dura surrounding the teeth of the mandible. The diffuse decrease in mineralization was due to infiltration with histiocytosis X. **(B)** Note the multiple lytic lesions that expand the entire mandible in this patient with Letterer-Siwe disease.

nopathy, hepatosplenomegaly, skin rashes, variable amounts of bone involvement, skin involvement, and involvement of the respiratory system. The bone involvement in Letterer-Siwe disease may be minimal. Multiple ill-defined radiolucencies may be identified. Loss of the lamina dura with loosening of the teeth occurs with jaw involvement (Fig. 2–62). Bone involvement is a grave finding.

Hand-Schuller-Christian disease is the triad of diabetes insipidus, exophthalmos, and bone lesions. Usually skin lesions are present as well. Radiologic findings again include loss of the lamina dura, loosening of the teeth, and punched-out lesions without reactive sclerosis throughout the facial bones and calvaria. The onset of Hand-Schuller-Christian disease is usually within the first decade of life.

Eosinophilic granuloma is limited to bone involvement only. Loss of the lamina dura and multiple lytic lesions without sclerotic margins are identified. Eosinophilic granuloma occurs in adolescents. Treatment consists of local curretage or radiation therapy. The prognosis is excellent.

Systemic Disease

Chronic systemic diseases such as diabetes mellitus and anemia may lead to resorption of the alveolar

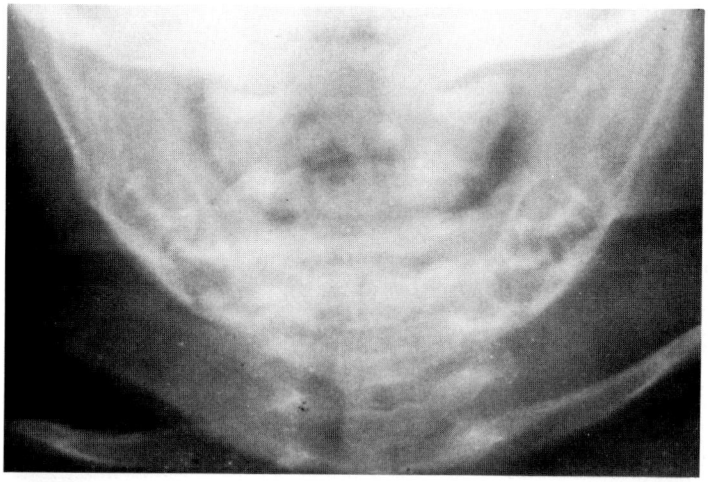

A

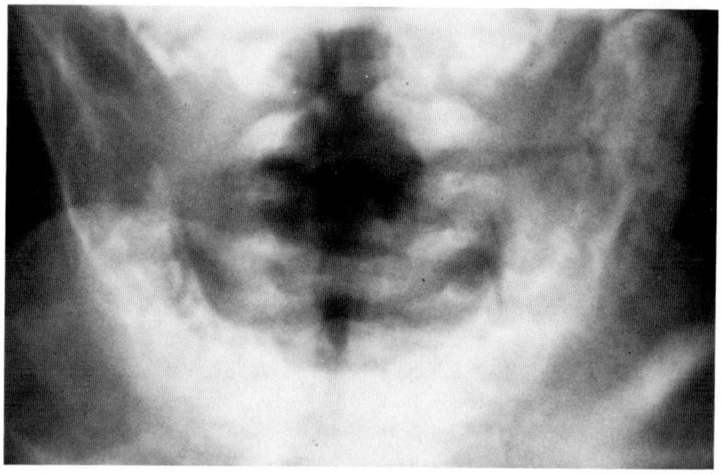

B

Fig. 2–63 Infantile cortical hyperostosis. **(A)** Note the periosteal reaction along the lateral aspect of the left side of the mandible. **(B)** One month later, note the new bone formation that has expanded the left side of the mandible.

process, the cortical bone surrounding the tooth root. In diabetes mellitus, the amount of bone resorption is greater than is normally expected for the patient's age. The hemolytic anemias may cause enlargement of the medullary spaces of the jaw bones and splaying of the trabeculae.

Idiopathic

Infantile cortical hyperostosis (Caffey's disease) is a self-limited condition presenting in the first 6 months of life with fever, iron deficiency anemia, and irritability. A palpable, firm mass is noted over the involved bone. In over 75 percent of patients the mandible is involved. Early in the disease, periosteal reaction is seen. Later, periosteal new bone formation and hyperostosis develop (Fig. 2–63). Other bones commonly involved include the clavicles, ribs, tibia, and ulna. The changes usually occur in the diaphyses of long bones. While the radiographic features may persist for years, the symptoms usually resolve within 1 month after onset.

Trauma

The most common site of mandibular fracture is the neck of the condyle. Because the mandible is a curved structure, ring fractures may occur. Direct blows to the chin may result in simultaneous condylar neck fractures and mandibular angle fractures. Young infants are subject to incomplete bending fractures best

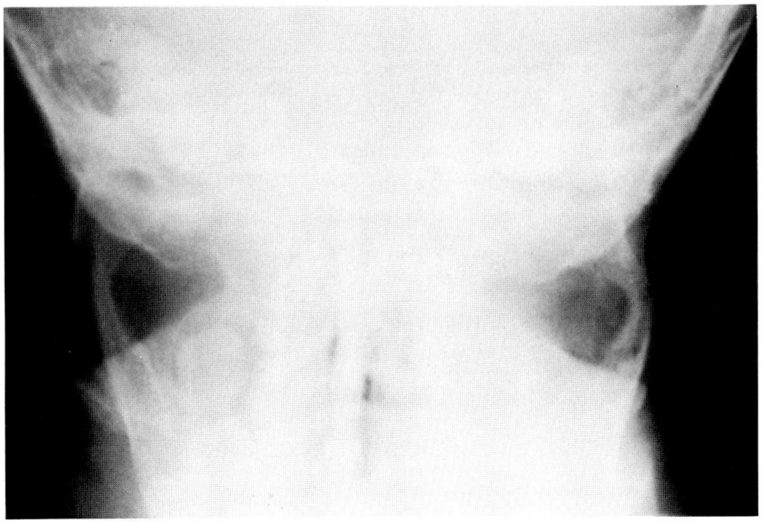

Fig. 2–64 Incomplete mandibular fractures. Towne view demonstrates bilateral bending fractures of the mandibular condyles. The fracture on the left is more apparent than that on the right. (From Ahrendt et al,[26] with permission.)

demonstrated on Towne or Caldwell's views (Fig. 2–64). In comminuted mandibular fractures, CT may be useful for further delineation of the extent of injury.

Joint injuries are the major cause of meniscus derangement of the tempromandibular joint. Symptoms include pain, limitation of motion, and abnormal audible sounds as the condyles move. MRI has virtually replaced temporomandibular joint arthrography for evaluation of internal derangements of the joint. The normal meniscus is positioned between the articular surfaces of the temporal bone and the mandibular condyle (Fig. 2–65). On T_1-weighted images there is a uniform low signal intensity of the meniscus. The posterior aspect of the meniscus is attached to the superior belly of the lateral pterygoid muscle. The inferior belly of the same muscle is responsible for forward condylar motion. The most common internal derangement affecting the temperomandibular joint is anterior displacement of the meniscus. Either coronal or sagittal images may be used to evaluate the accompanying degree of medial or lateral displacement commonly associated with anterior meniscal dislocation. If the meniscus is chronically displaced or structurally abnormal, increased signal is identified and the meniscus may appear thickened (Fig. 2–66). MRI is not as accurate as arthrography in identifying perforation or joint capsule adhesions. A combination of MRI and plain radiographic evaluation allows differentiation of hypointense scar tissue from degenerative calcifications about the joint.

Iatrogenic

Two types of cysts may result from incomplete dental or paranasal sinus surgery. The radicular cyst, which develops at the base of a nonvital tooth, often is completely removed when the tooth is extracted. However, if a cyst persists at the site of tooth extraction, it is termed a *residual cyst*. On radiographs, a sharply demarcated unilocular cyst with a sclerotic border is identified below a gap where the tooth was extracted (Fig. 2–67).

Occasionally, residual epithelium from the maxillary sinus is left after a Caldwell-Luc procedure to drain the sinus. This leads to the formation of a surgical ciliated cyst of the maxilla that is also a radiolucent defect.

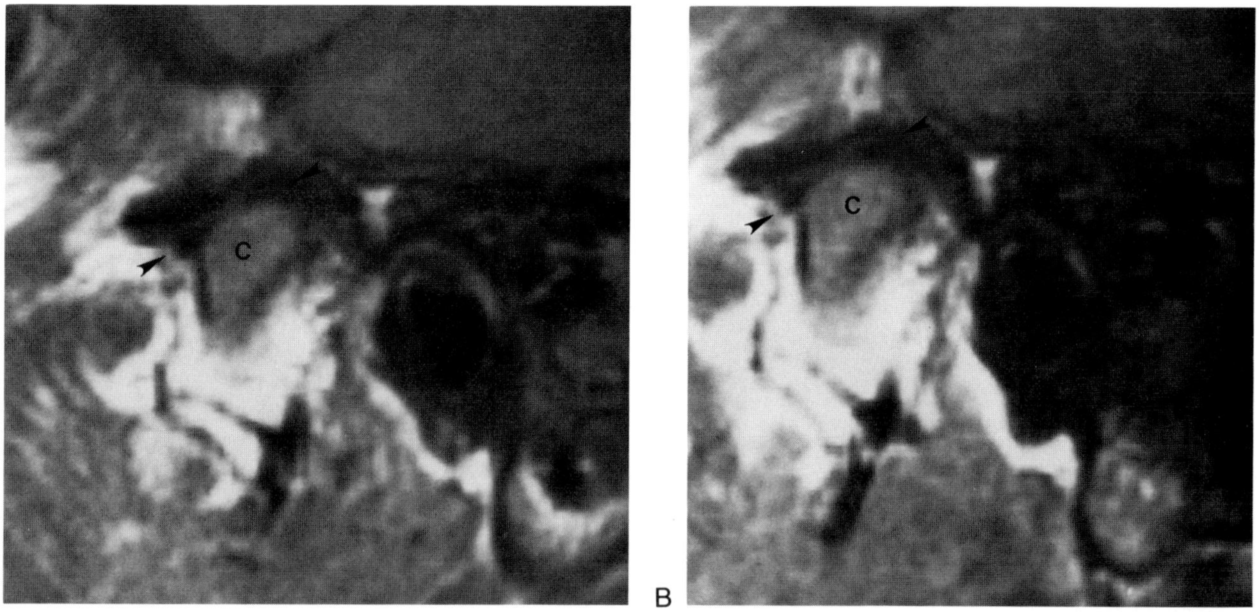

Fig. 2–65 Normal temporomandibular joint. **(A)** Note the isointense meniscus (*arrowheads*) on the T_1-weighted sagittal image covering the articular surface of the left mandibular condyle (*C*) with the mouth closed. **(B)** T_1-weighted sagittal image with the mouth open demonstrates anterior motion of the left mandibular condyle (*C*) but no change in the relationship of the uniformly isointense meniscus (*arrowheads*).

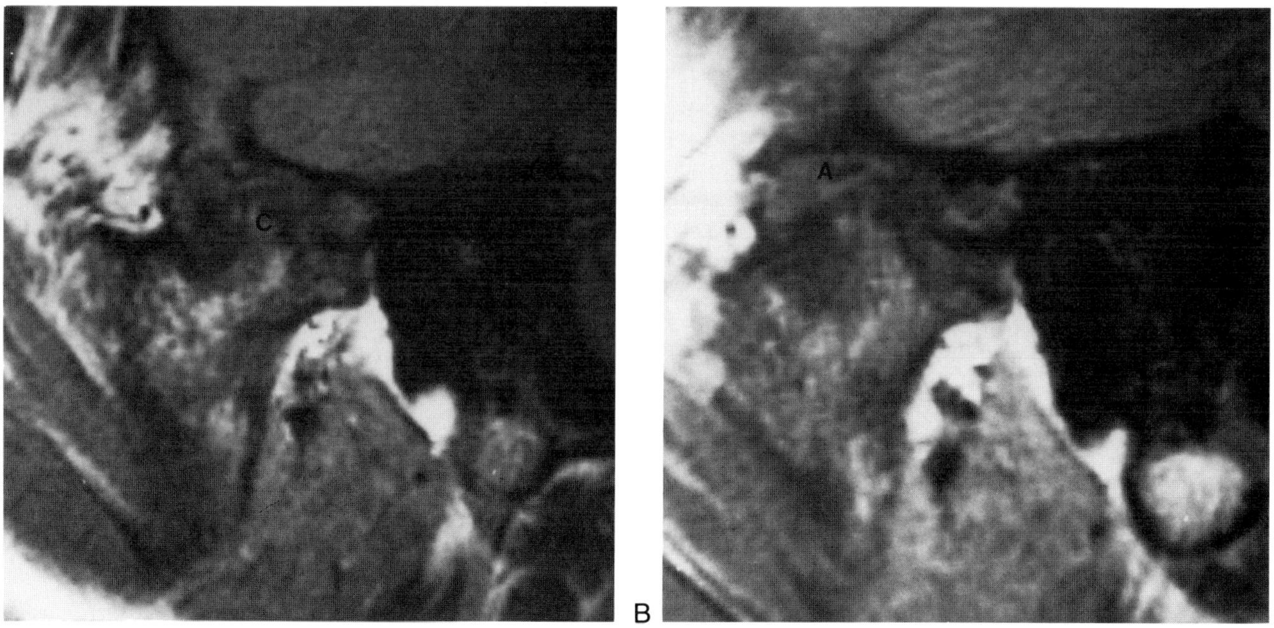

Fig. 2–66 Temporomandibular joint syndrome. **(A)** The closed mouth, T_1-weighted sagittal view reveals a flattened irregular mandibular condyle (*C*) without an identifiable meniscus. **(B)** Opening the mouth causes no change in the relationship of the flattened mandibular condyle and the articular surface of the temporal bone (*A*). The decreased marrow fat due to chronic sclerosis lowers the marrow signal in the involved portion of the mandible. (*Figure continues.*)

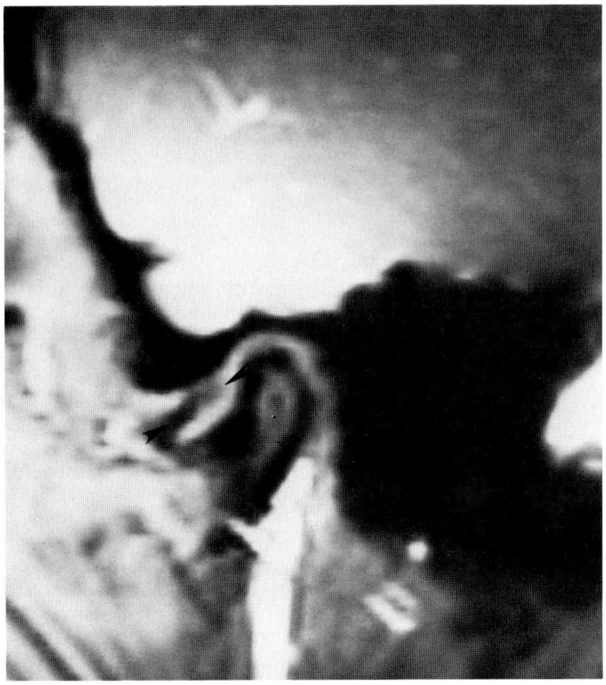

C

Fig. 2–66 (*Continued*). **(C)** T_1-weighted sagittal view of another patient demonstrates anterior displacement of the malformed right meniscus (*arrowheads*), which persisted in both the closed and open mouth positions. This represented meniscal subluxation.

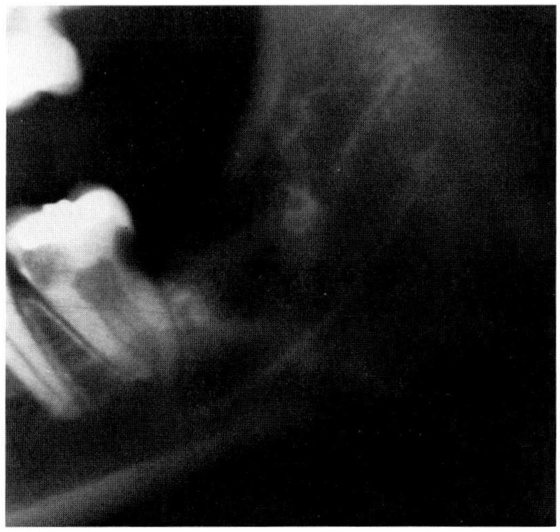

Fig. 2–67 Residual cyst. Note the sharply demarcated area of increased radiolucency at the site where an abscessed third molar was extracted. Note the dental caries in the adjacent molar.

SUGGESTED READINGS

1. Amodio JB, Berdon WE, Abramson S, et al: Cystic fibrosis in childhood: pulmonary, paranasal sinus, and skeletal manifestations. Semin Roentgenol 22:125, 1987
2. Berdon WE, Baker DH: Vascular anomalies and the infant lung: rings, slings and other things. Semin Roentgenol 7:39, 1972
3. Campbell JS, Wiglesworth FW, Latarrocca R, et al: Congenital subglottic hemangiomas of the larynx and trachea in infants. Pediatrics 22:727, 1958
4. Dietrich RB, Lufkin RB, Kangarloo H, et al: Head and neck imaging in the pediatric patient. Radiology 159:769, 1986
5. Dunbar JS: Upper respiratory tract obstruction in infants and children. AJR 109:225, 1970
6. Healy GB: Malignant tumors of the head and neck in children: diagnosis and treatment. Otolaryngol Clin North Am 13:483, 1980
7. Katzberg RW: Temporomandibular joint imaging. Radiology 170:297, 1989
8. Kraus R, Han BK, Babcock DS, et al: Sonography of neck masses in children. AJR 146:609, 1986
9. Lindeberg H, Elbrond O: Laryngeal papillomas: clinical aspects in a series of 231 patients. Clin Otolaryngol 14:333, 1989
10. Lloyd G, Phelps P: Juvenile angiofibroma: imaging by magnetic resonance, CT and conventional techniques. Clin Otolaryngol 11:247, 1986
11. Noyek AM, Friedberg J: Thyroglossal duct and ectopic thyroid disorders. Otolaryngol Clin North Am 14:187, 1981
12. Noyek AM, Shulman HS, Steinhardt ML, et al: The larynx. p. 402. In Bergeron RT, Osborn AG, Som PM (eds): Head and Neck Imaging, Excluding the Brain. CV Mosby, St. Louis, 1984
13. Rapkin RH: The diagnosis of epiglottitis: simplicity and reliability of radiographs of the neck in the differential diagnosis of the croup syndrome. J Pediatr 88:96, 1972
14. Reaume CE, Sofre VL: Lingual thyroid: review of the literature and report of a case. Oral Surg 45:841, 1978
15. Seashore JH, Gardiner LJ, Ariyan S: Management of giant cystic hygroma in infants. Am J Surg 149:459, 1985

16. Shackelford GD, McAlister WH: Primary immunodeficiency diseases and malignancy. AJR 123:144, 1975
17. Shear M: Cysts of the jaws: recent advances. J Oral Pathol 14:43, 1985
18. Singleton EB: X-Ray Diagnosis of the Alimentary Tract in Infants and Children. Year Book Medical Publishers, Chicago, 1959
19. Som PM, Sacher M, Stollman AL, et al: Common tumors of the parapharyngeal space: refined imaging diagnosis. Radiology 169:81, 1988
20. Swischuk LE, Pliny CS, Fagan CJ: Abnormalities of the pharynx and larynx in childhood. Semin Roentgenol 9:283, 1974
21. Unger JM: Head and Neck Imaging. Churchill Livingstone, New York, 1987
22. Weber AL, Mikulis DK: Inflammatory disorders of the paraorbital sinuses and their complications. Radiol Clin North Am 25:615, 1987
23. Wittich GR, Scheible WF, Hajek PC: Ultrasonography of the salivary glands. Radiol Clin North Am 23:29, 1985
24. Zilkha A: Computed tomography in facial trauma. Radiology 144:545, 1982
25. Zinreich SJ, Kennedy DW, Malat J, et al: Fungal sinusitis: diagnosis with CT and MR imaging. Radiology 169:439, 1988
26. Ahrendt D, Swischuk LE, Hayden CK Jr: Incomplete (bending?) fractures of the mandibular condyle in children. Pediatr Radiol 14:140, 1984

3

Respiratory System

Lori L. Barr

Frontal and lateral radiographs of the chest are the mainstay for preliminary surveillance of the cardiovascular and respiratory organs. Special considerations in children include patient positioning, neonatal disease processes, and superimposition of lung and heart disease. In the younger age groups, most frontal chest views are obtained in the anteroposterior position. This is important to consider when evaluating the degree of inspiration and the cardiomediastinal structures. Outside of the neonatal period, the diseases affecting the respiratory system are similar to those in the adult. By evaluating prior chest x-rays, the separation of heart disease from pulmonary abnormalities is somewhat simplified.

Computed tomography (CT) is the cross-sectional imaging modality of choice for evaluation of the lung parenchyma and pleural diseases. Magnetic resonance imaging (MRI) is superior for delineating mediastinal masses because of the natural soft tissue contrast and unlimited reconstruction planes. Chest MRI should be gated to the electrocardiogram. The images are enhanced by using special presaturation techniques to limit the amount of image artifact caused by blood flow and motion.

Various lung patterns seen on pediatric chest x-rays may be sorted out by considering the various mechanisms that cause the finding. Once the mechanism is determined, the underlying causes fall into the familiar categories of congenital, inflammatory, neoplastic, traumatic, systemic, and miscellaneous.

BILATERAL HYPOAERATION

The various mechanisms causing the appearance of bilateral poorly inflated lungs include poor inspiration, extrinsic compression, limited chest wall expansion, pulmomary hypoplasia, impaired air entry, and impaired diaphragmatic excursion (Table 3–1). The most common mechanism encountered is poor inspiration, which is either fortuitous or caused by respiratory depression from a variety of causes (Fig. 3–1). The next most common mechanism is extrinsic compression of the thorax from abdominal distention, which may be secondary to ascites, abdominal masses, or intestinal obstruction. Limited chest wall expansion may be secondary to a variety of neuromuscular diseases including myotonic dystrophy, myesthenia gravis, and dermatomyositis. The bone dysplasias and dwarfism may result in a small chest with short ribs, thus limiting the expansion of the chest wall. Pulmonary hypoplasia may occur as an isolated anomaly or associated with anomalies of the skeletal system, genitourinary tract, or with increased intra-abdominal pressure (Fig. 3–2).

The mechanism of impaired air entry into the thorax should be suspected if one observes paradoxical widening of the superior mediastinum and cardiac silhouette on inspiration. When the airway is not obstructed the heart appears larger during expiration. When the airway is obstructed and obstructive emphysema is present, increased endothoracic pressure results in a decrease in venous blood volume returning to the

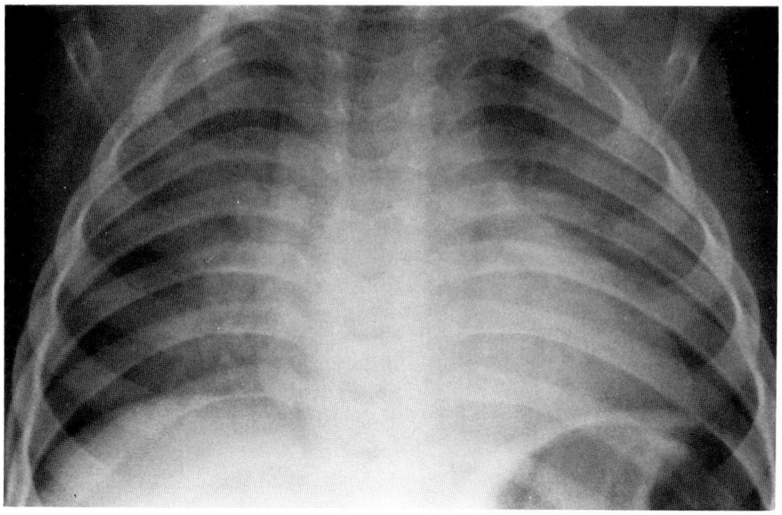

A

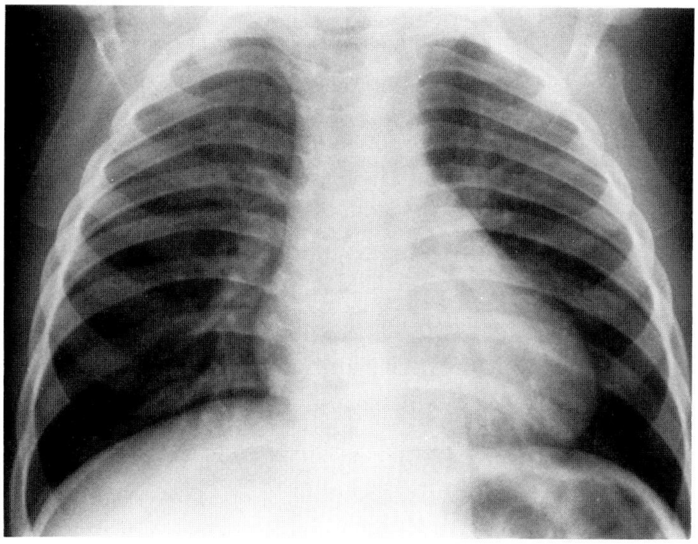

B

Fig. 3–1 Poor inspiration. **(A)** Anteroposterior chest view demonstrates fullness of the hila and cardiac prominence due to expiration. **(B)** With full inspiration, the chest is normal.

heart. Therefore, the heart appears smaller, especially on expiration. However, when obstruction without emphysema is present, inspiratory pressures become more negative and facilitate increased venous blood return to the heart resulting in a larger appearance of the heart during inspiration. Therefore, it is important to evaluate the cardiomediastinal silhouette to determine whether or not the airway is obstructed centrally. Underlying causes of this phenomenon include intrinsic, functional, and extrinsic causes of airway compromise. Congenital tracheal stenosis, epiglottitis, membranous croup, tracheal retention cyst or inflammatory granuloma, subglottic hemangioma, laryngeal papilloma, and iatrogenic scarring all may compromise the lumen of the airway along its inner aspect. The airway may become functionally obstructed during episodes of angioneurotic edema induced by administration of medications, by insect bites, and during sleep apnea. Processes occurring in the neck or mediastinum surrounding the central

Table 3–1 Bilateral Hypoaeration

Mechanism	Cause
Poor inspiration	Fortuitous
	Central nervous system depression
	Intrauterine infection/infarction
	Birth anoxia
	Meningitis
	Ischemia
	Medication
	Accidental poisoning
	Mass effect from tumor/trauma
Extrinsic compression (abdominal distention)	Ascites
	Congenital urinary tract obstruction
	Anasarca
	Trauma
	Hepatic failure
	Peritoneal dialysis
	Abdominal mass
	GI/GU obstructions
	Hepatosplenomegaly
	Ovarian cysts
	Enteric cysts
	Lymphangioma
	Neoplasm (Neuroblastoma, Wilms' tumor)
Limited chest wall expansion	Neuromuscular disease
	Amyotonia congenita
	Myotonic dystrophy
	Myasthenia gravis
	Musculoskeletal disease
	Dermatomyositis
	Dwarfism
	Bone dysplasia
	Trauma
	Flail chest
	Postoperative
Pulmonary hypoplasia	Isolated
	Associated
	Dwarfism
	Bone dysplasia
	Potter's syndrome
	Intrauterine
	Abdominal distention
Impaired air entry	Intrinsic airway compromise
	Congenital tracheal/laryngeal web/stenosis
	Epiglottitis/croup
	Postinflammatory retention cyst/granuloma
	Tumor
	Iatrogenic scarring

Continued

Table 3–1 Bilateral Hypoaeration (*Continued*)

Mechanism	Cause
	Functional airway compromise
	Angioneurotic edema
	Sleep apnea
	Iatrogenic nerve damage
	Extrinsic airway compromise
	Cystic hygroma
	Bronchopulmonary foregut malformation
	Lymphadenopathy (inflammation/tumor)
	Vascular rings
	Trauma
Impaired diaphragmatic excursion	Trauma
	Iatrogenic
	Nerve injury
	Postabdominal surgery
	Mediastinal mass

GI, gastrointestinal; GU, genitourinary.

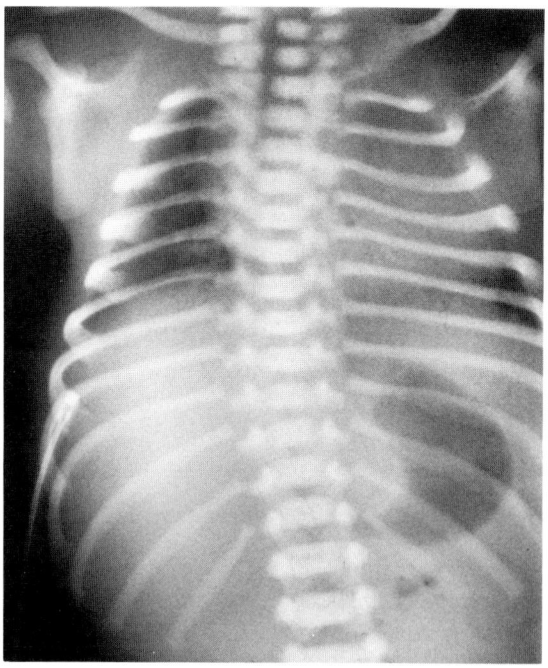

Fig. 3–2 Pulmonary hypoplasia. Frontal view of chest and abdomen demonstrate small lung volumes when compared to the abdominal girth.

Fig. 3–3 Extrinsic compression of the trachea. **(A)** Anteroposterior x-ray of a child presenting with stridor. Note that the trachea is in the midline and a right aortic arch is present. Bilateral hyperaeration is seen. At surgery, the patient had a double aortic arch. **(B)** The anteroposterior chest x-ray of another child with noisy breathing reveals deviation of the trachea to the right and bilateral hyperinflation in all phases of respiration. A cystic mediastinal mass was noted on ultrasound examination that, at surgery, proved to be a bronchogenic cyst.

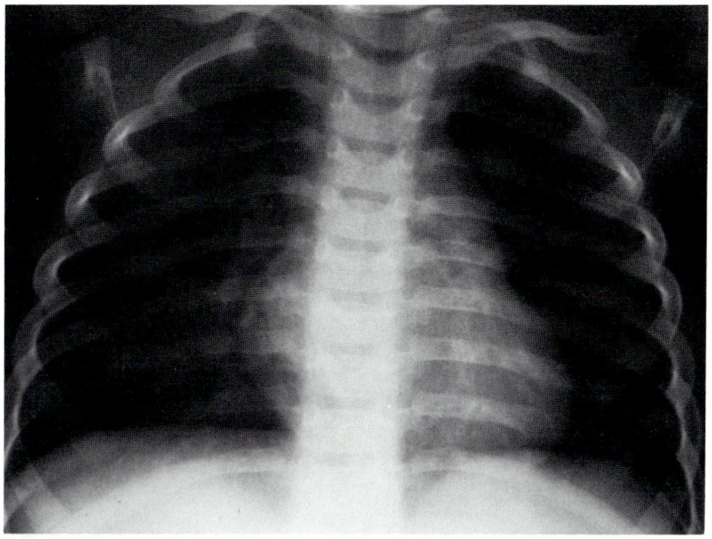

A

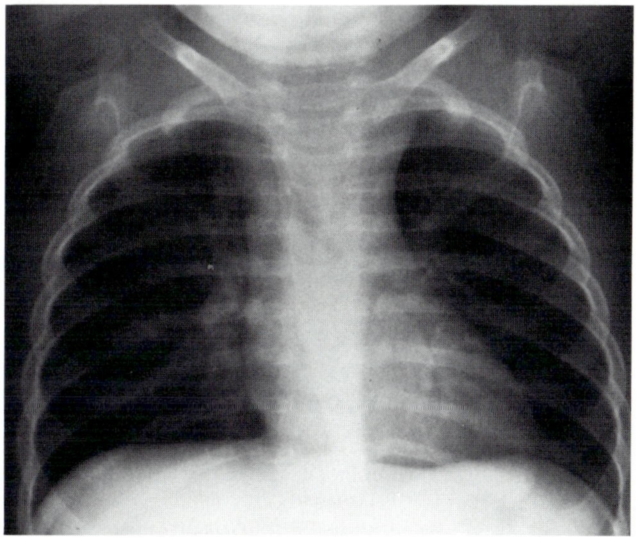

B

airway may extrinsically compress the lumen (Fig. 3–3). These processes include congenital malformations such as cystic hygroma and bronchopulmonary foregut malformation, lymphadenopathy secondary to inflammation or tumor, vascular rings, and blunt or penetrating neck or chest trauma resulting in edema and hematoma formation. Diaphragmatic excursion may be limited if damage to its innervation occurs during chest trauma or surgery or from infiltration by a mediastinal process. Evaluation of the latter two mechanisms, impaired air entry and impaired diaphragmatic excursion, is best accomplished by fluoroscopic evaluation. The diaphragm may be seen to move normally or less than normal in cases of paresis. In paralysis, there is paradoxical diaphragmatic motion during crying, coughing, and sniffing.

BILATERAL HYPERAERATION

The mechanisms leading to bilateral hyperaeration include nonobstructive causes, central airway obstruction, and peripheral airway obstruction (Table 3–2). Often an expiratory radiograph will aid in the differentiation of these causes.

Nonobstructive

The most common cause of nonobstructive hyperaeration is overzealous inspiration. Other causes include overbreathing due to metabolic acidosis, which may be secondary to severe diarrhea or severe dehydration. Dehydration also causes decreased pulmonary vascularity and transient microcardia (Fig. 3–4). Cyanotic heart disease results in hypoxemia and bilateral hyperaeration.

Obstructive

Obstructive emphysema may be secondary to a centrally located process or to peripheral disease of the terminal airways (Fig. 3–5). Common congenital causes of central obstructive emphysema are vascular rings, slings, and bronchogenic cysts. Electrocardiogram-gated MRI is the best noninvasive method of confirming these diagnoses. The most common vascular ring to cause symptoms is a right aortic arch with right descending aorta, aberrant left subclavian artery, and persistent left ductus arteriosus. The second most common vascular ring to cause symptoms is the double aortic arch. Both conditions may lead to compression of the trachea resulting in bilateral hyperaeration. The pulmonary sling (aberrant left pulmonary artery) occasionally causes similar findings but is more likely to cause unequal aeration. Other congenital conditions resulting in peripheral obstructive hyperinflation include alpha$_1$-antitrypsin deficiency and cutis laxa. These conditions are generally not associated with pulmonary infiltrates and are uncommon.

Infections and asthma are much more common causes of peripheral obstructive emphysema. Lower respiratory tract infections caused by viruses or *Mycoplasma pneumoniae* are the usual etiologies. The most common virus associated with this chest pattern is the respiratory syncytial virus, although influenza, parainfluenza, and adenoviruses may cause similar findings.

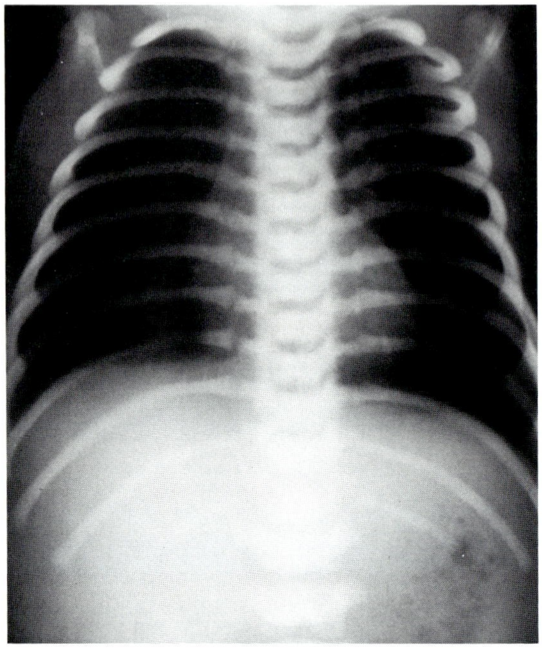

Fig. 3–4 Nonobstructive hyperaeration. Frontal chest view demonstrates decreased pulmonary vascularity and diminished heart size secondary to dehydration and metabolic acidosis.

Infants less than 2 years of age affected with bronchiolitis demonstrate the most profound degree of overaeration. The chest x-ray findings in older children with either viral bronchitis or asthma are virtually identical; parahilar peribronchial infiltrates are present with or without lobar, segmental or subsegmental atelectasis, and hyperaeration. Cystic fibrosis is a systemic disease resulting in a pattern of hyperaeration, parahilar peribronchial infiltrates, and scattered areas of atelectasis. Immunodeficiency is also a rare cause of this pattern.

Central airway compression may be secondary to inflammatory granulomas, infection-induced adenopathy, and endotracheal or paratracheal neoplasms. MRI with cardiac gating is the method of choice for noninvasive evaluation of airway compression because of its superior soft tissue discrimination and ability to easily image in the sagittal and coronal planes. The two most common endotracheal neoplasms to cause this chest pattern are subglottic hemangiomas in infants and laryngeal papillomata in older children. Extrinsic compression may be caused by superior or middle mediastinal masses (see lists,

Table 3–2 Bilateral Hyperaeration

Mechanism	Cause

Nonobstructive	Overzealous inspiration
	Increased respiratory rate
	  Metabolic acidosis
	  Cyanotic heart disease

Central airway obstruction	Vascular rings Pulmonary sling Bronchopulmonary foregut malformation Cystic hygroma Granuloma formation Lymphadenopathy (inflammatory/tumor) Intrisic airway abnormalities

Peripheral airway obstruction	Infection
	  Viruses
	  Mycoplasma pneumoniae
	Cystic fibrosis
	Alpha$_1$-antitrypsin deficiency
	Cutis laxa
	Immunodeficiency
	Assisted ventilation
	Inhalational injury

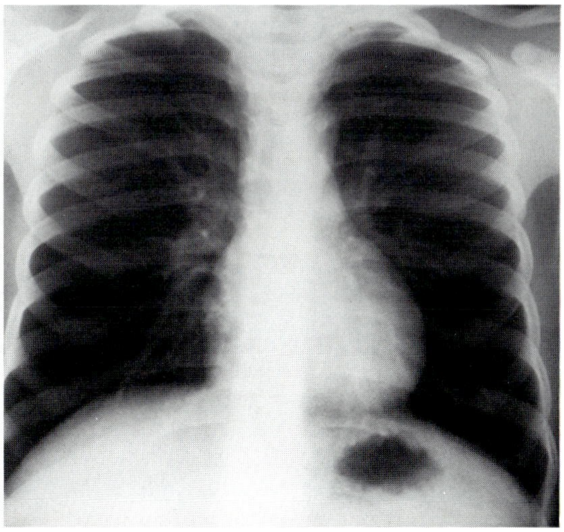

A

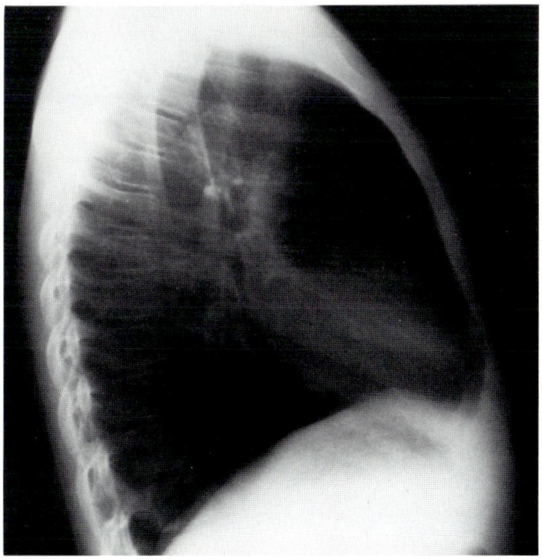

B

Fig. 3–5 Obstructive emphysema. **(A)** Posteroanterior chest x-ray demonstrates symmetrical hyperaeration of both lungs with an increase in the parahilar markings. **(B)** Lateral view demonstrates an increase in the anteroposterior diameter of the chest and flattening of the diaphragm consistent with the diagnosis of cystic fibrosis.

p. 130 and p. 137). A rare traumatic cause of bilateral hyperaeration is inhalational burn injury resulting in thermal bronchiolitis.

UNEQUAL AERATION

One of the most commonly encountered problems on pediatric chest x-rays is that of unequal aeration (Table 3–3). Following observation of an unusually clear or hyperlucent hemithorax, one should attempt to determine whether the hyperlucent hemithorax is small, normal-sized, or enlarged. The mechanisms resulting in the appearance vary with the size of the hemithorax (Table 3–3).

Small Radiolucent Hemithorax

The most common cause of a small hemithorax with increased radiolucency is pulmonary hypoplasia, either congenital or acquired. Congenital pulmonary hypoplasia is associated with ipsilateral hypoplasia or absence of the pulmonary artery. Patients with congenital hypoplasia of the lung are usually asymptomatic and the finding is discovered when a chest x-ray is obtained for other reasons (Fig. 3–6). Decreased pulmonary blood flow due to the hypoplastic or absent pulmonary artery causes the lung to be more radiolucent than usual. More importantly, the affected lung changes size with inspiration and expiration similar to, but not to the same degree as, the normal lung. Congenital hypoplasia of the lung is

Table 3–3 Unequal Aeration

Mechanism	Cause
Small radiolucent hemithorax	
Pulmonary hypoplasia	Congenital Swyer-James syndrome Unilateral pulmonary vein atresia
Pulmonary thromboembolism	Nephrotic syndrome Severe dehydration Indwelling central venous catheter Total parenteral nutrition
Parenchymal damage	Irradiation
Normal-sized radiolucent hemithorax	
Radiographic technique	Overlying artifacts Improper mediastinal filter position
Absent pectoralis muscles	Poland's syndrome Postoperative
Large radiolucent hemithorax	
Obstructive emphysema	Intrinsic bronchial abnormalities Mucus plug Foreign body Tumor Inflammatory mass Extrinsic bronchial compression Mediastinal/hilar lymphadenopathy Tumor Cardiomegaly Aberrant vessels
Compensatory emphysema	Contralateral lung agenesis Total contralateral atelectasis
Space-occupying lesions	Congenital diaphragmatic hernia Congenital lobar emphysema Pneumatocele Pneumothorax

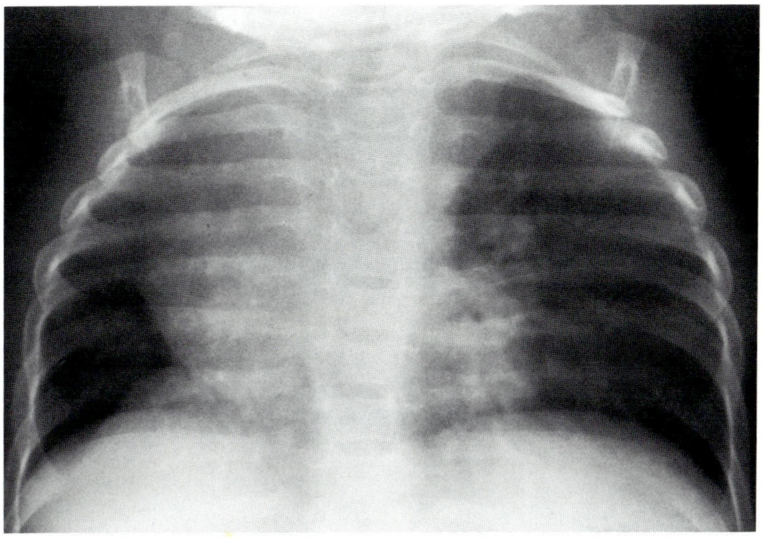

Fig. 3–6 Unilateral pulmonary hypoplasia. Anteroposterior chest x-ray demonstrates a small hyperlucent right hemithorax with deviation of the trachea to the right. The right pulmonary vascularity is decreased. Cardiac catheterization confirmed that the right pulmonary artery was smaller than the left with absence of the artery to the right upper lobe.

more common on the left than on the right, and if associated with congenital heart disease, the underlying defect is usually tetralogy of Fallot or persistent truncus arteriosus. With persistent truncus arteriosus, lung hypoplasia may occur on either side but with tetralogy of Fallot it occurs on the side opposite the aortic arch.

Acquired pulmonary hypoplasia is also called Swyer-James syndrome or MacLeod syndrome. A previous pulmonary insult, usually a viral lower respiratory tract infection results in obliterative bronchiolitis. This causes a small hyperlucent lung that does not change size with respiration, indicating obstructive emphysema (Fig. 3–7). Some authors report a fine reticular pattern of increased interstitial markings in some cases of acquired hypoplasia. Patients with acquired hypoplasia are often plagued by repeated pulmonary infection or cyanosis due to intrapulmonary shunting, while patients with congenital hypoplasia do not have an increased incidence of respiratory distress. Recurring symptoms may warrant further radiographic investigation including cardiac catheterization, pulmonary angiography, and bronchography. Another rather uncommon congenital cause of a small hyperlucent hemithorax is unilateral pulmonary vein atresia or stenosis. Chronic obstruction of pulmonary venous flow results in interstitial pulmonary edema, appearing on radiographs as fine reticularity and, eventually, fibrosis. Cases of pulmonary vein atresia may be difficult to differentiate from Swyer-James lung unless pulmonary arteriography is performed.

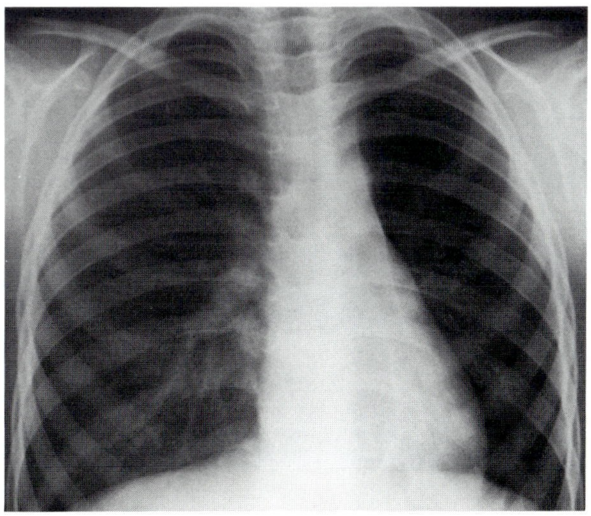

Fig. 3–7 Swyer-James syndrome. Notice the small hyperlucent left hemithorax. Pulmonary arteriography excluded pulmonary vein atresia, thus confirming acquired pulmonary hypoplasia.

Systemic disease, such as nephrotic syndrome, or severe dehydration from any cause can lead to venous thrombosis. If this causes pulmonary embolism, a small hyperlucent hemithorax may result. Pulmonary embolism may be a secondary complication of total parenteral nutrition.

Iatrogenic causes of a small hyperlucent hemithorax include radiation damage to the lung or venous thrombosis and infection caused by indwelling catheters. An irradiated lung may also demonstrate fine reticulations making the differentiation between radiation damage, acquired hypoplasia, and pulmonary vein atresia difficult.

Normal-sized Radiolucent Hemithorax

Poor radiographic technique and Poland's syndrome (unilateral absent pectoralis muscles associated with ipsilateral syndactyly) are miscellaneous causes of a normal-sized hyperlucent hemithorax.

Large Radiolucent Hemithorax

The most common cause of an enlarged hyperlucent hemithorax is obstructive emphysema and the usual etiologies are an endotracheal foreign body or mucus plug (Fig. 3–8). Peanuts are the most commonly aspirated foreign bodies. Obviously, many causes of intrinsic or extrinsic bronchial obstruction could result in this picture but they are considerably less common. On expiration, the size of the obstructed lung does not change. Although the pulmonary vascularity is initially normal, it will eventually decrease. This is due to a combination of increased intrapulmonary pressure and vasoconstriction secondary to hypoxia.

The second most common cause of a large hyperlucent hemithorax is compensatory emphysema. In this condition, the size of the lung changes with respiration just as a normal lung does and the vascularity is normal or increased. Compensatory emphysema involving an entire lung is most often the result of either agenesis or complete atelectasis of the contralateral lung.

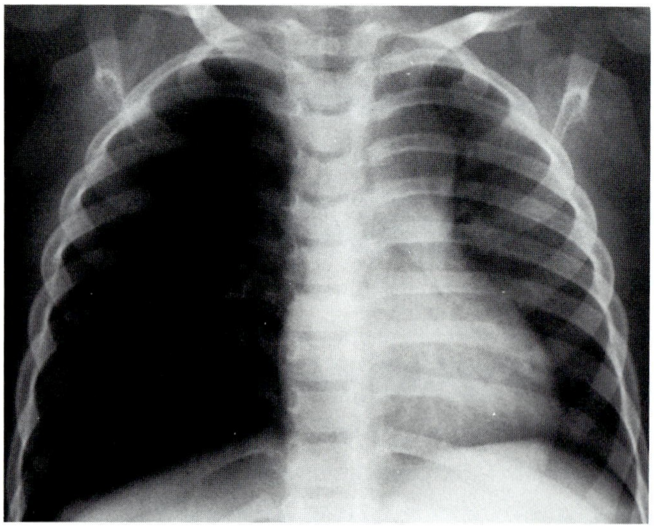

A

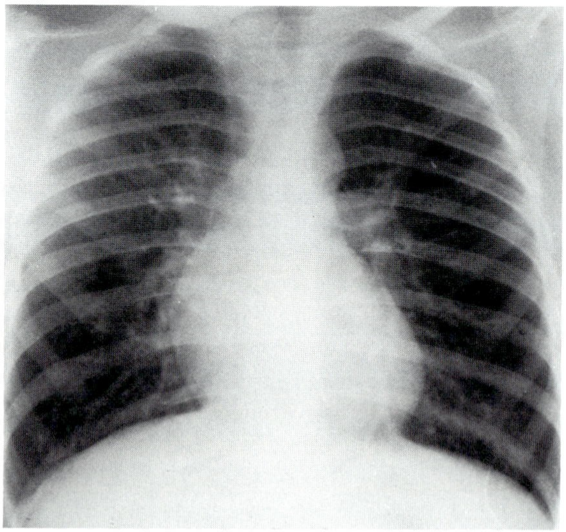

B

Fig. 3–8 Large radiolucent hemithorax. **(A)** Anteroposterior chest x-ray reveals increased radiolucency of the right hemithorax, which is larger than the left. Notice the decreased pulmonary vascularity to the right lung. This child had aspirated a peanut. **(B)** Another patient demonstrates hyperlucency of the enlarged left hemithorax but the pulmonary vascularity is normal. This child had congenital absence of the left pectoralis muscles and ipsilateral syndactyly (Poland's syndrome).

Congenital or acquired diaphragmatic hernia on the left with herniation of an air-filled stomach may result in a similar appearance. Congenital lobar emphysema may affect either of the upper lobes (left is more common), and compensatory emphysema with an ipsilateral, partially hypoplastic lung related to scimitar syndrome or a pulmonary sling should also be considered. A large postinflammatory pneumatocele may appear as a hyperlucent hemithorax, however, a thin wall is usually detectable around the periphery.

Either spontaneous or iatrogenic pneumothorax may result in a large hyperlucent hemithorax. In supine patients, such as neonates, air accumulates anteriorly over the lung (Fig. 3–9). Observation of an extremely sharp ipsilateral mediastinal edge sometimes aids in the diagnosis of an anterior pneumothorax. Erect inspiratory-expiratory, decubitus, and cross-table lateral views are sometimes needed. Spontaneous pneumothorax is uncommon in childhood. Pneumothoraces may be seen with other conditions such as asthma, cystic lung disease, pneumatoceles, cystic fibrosis, endometriosis, histiocytosis X, lymphangiomatosis, Marfan's syndrome, chest trauma, and osteogenic sarcoma metastases to the lungs.

Small Opaque Hemithorax

Another abnormal chest pattern encountered is an opaque hemithorax (Table 3–4). In this case, two important questions must be answered: (1) is the hemithorax totally or partially opaque, and (2) is the hemithorax small or large? If one can determine that the hemithorax is small and totally opaque, the differential diagnosis is limited to total atelectasis or agenesis of the ipsilateral lung (Fig. 3–10).

If the hemithorax is small and partially opaque it is more likely that partial atelectasis or hypoplasia of the lung is present. Partial atelectasis may be primary or may be due to compression by an emphysematous contralateral lung. The combination of right lung hypoplasia, underdevelopment of the right pulmonary artery, and anomalous right pulmonary venous entry into the vena cava is called the scimitar syndrome. The left lung appears large and hyperlucent. Associated anomalies of the right hemidiaphragm that have been reported with the scimitar syndrome include diaphragmatic duplication, congenital diaphragmatic hernia, phrenic cyst, rib anomalies, and absence of the inferior vena cava.

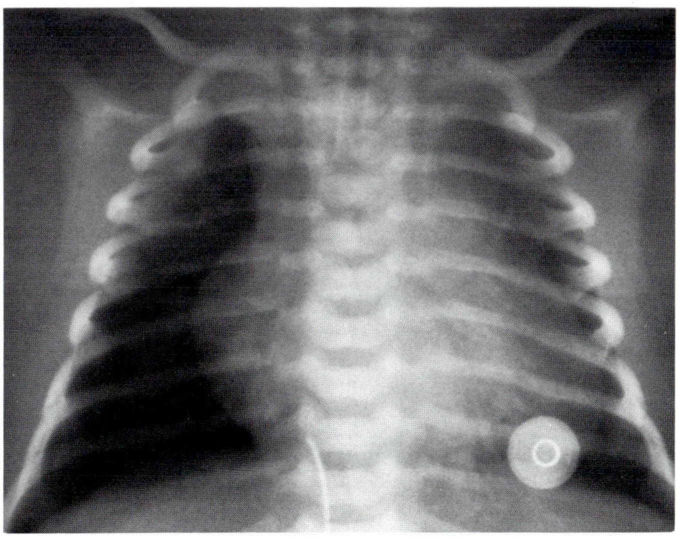

Fig. 3–9 Anterior pneumothorax. Notice the large hyperlucent right hemithorax on this neonatal anteroposterior chest x-ray. The extreme clarity of the right heart border as compared with the left indicates an anterior pneumothorax.

Table 3–4 Opaque Hemithorax

Appearance or Mechanism	Cause
Small opaque hemithorax	
Totally opaque	Agenesis Total atelectasis
Partially opaque	Hypoplasia Partial atelectasis Pulmonary sling Endobronchial obstruction Extrinsic compression
Large opaque hemithorax	
Pleural effusion	Pus Chyle Glomerulonephritis Nephrotic syndrome Sympathetic effusion Pancreatitis Neoplasm Trauma Boerhaave's syndrome Postoperative
Parenchymal fluid	Congenital bronchial obstruction Lobar emphysema Bronchial atresia Bronchogenic cyst Opaque right lung syndrome
Normal-sized opaque hemithorax	
Pleural effusion	Causes listed above under Pleural effusion
Empyema	Bacterial pneumonia

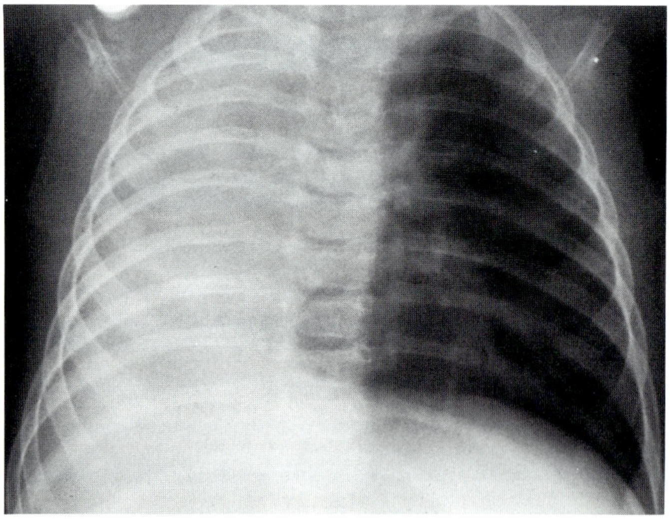

Fig. 3–10 Small opaque hemithorax. Anteroposterior chest x-ray demonstrates a small, totally opaque, right hemithorax suggestive of either total atelectasis or agenesis. The cardiomediastinal silhouette is shifted to the right. The left pulmonary artery is prominent. Cardiac catheterization confirmed abscence of the right pulmonary artery and agenesis of the right lung.

Another common congenital cause of unequal aeration with a small, partially opaque lung is the pulmonary sling (aberrant left pulmonary artery) (Fig. 3–11). The left pulmonary artery arises anomalously from the right pulmonary artery and compresses the right main bronchus as it encircles the carina. This results in partial atelectasis of the right lung. Other causes of partial atelectasis are endobronchial foreign body, neoplasm, and peribronchial lymph node enlargement.

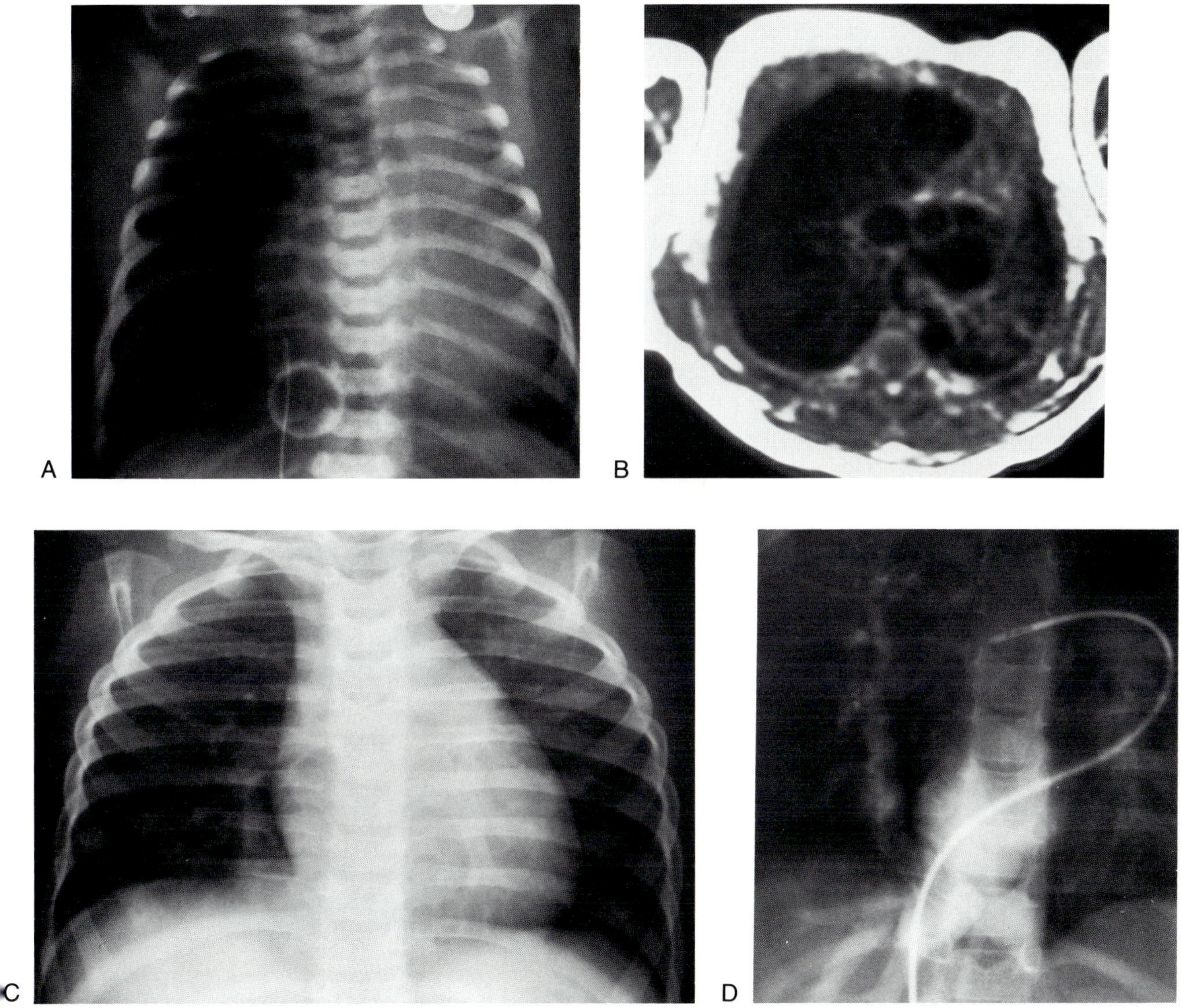

Fig. 3–11 Congenital causes of unequal aeration. **(A)** Anteroposterior chest view of a neonate with mild respiratory distress demonstrates a partially opaque left hemithorax. **(B)** Coronal T_1-weighted MRI demonstrates the anomalous origin of the left pulmonary artery arising from the right pulmonary artery. It courses behind the trachea and passes into the left hemithorax anterior to the aorta. The lateral chest x-ray did not demonstrate characteristic posterior tracheal indentation. **(C)** Anteroposterior chest x-ray in another patient demonstrates a small right hemithorax with increased density in the right lower lobe. **(D)** The diagnosis of scimitar syndrome is confirmed by cardiac catheterization revealing partial anomalous pulmonary venous return to the inferior vena cava. (*Figure continues.*)

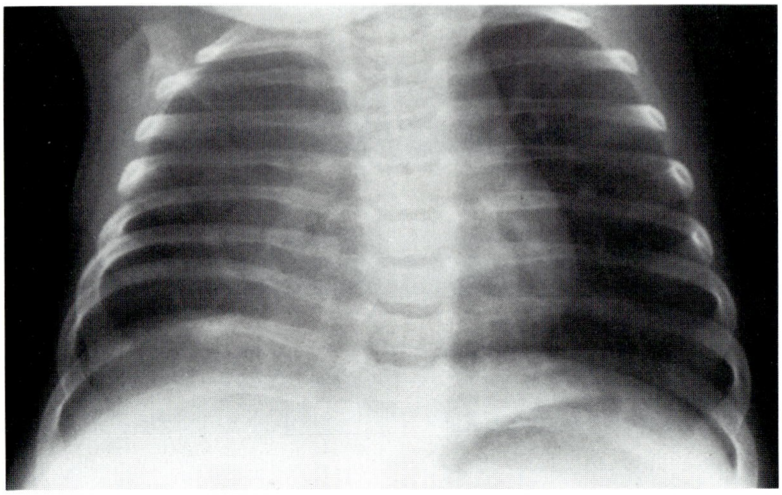

E

Fig. 3–11 (*Continued*). **(E)** Another patient with scimitar syndrome has a small partially opaque right hemithorax. The anomalous vein is less apparent.

Large Opaque Hemithorax

If a large opaque hemithorax is encountered, the most common cause is massive accumulation of pleural fluid. All types of fluid result in the same radiographic appearance, but the most common fluid to accumulate in a child's thorax is pus, most often associated with pneumococcal pneumonia. In the newborn period, however, the fluid is most likely to be lymph or chyle. Chylous effusions may be noted on prenatal ultrasound examination but the etiology remains uncertain. Chylothorax is most likely to occur on the right and is associated with pulmonary lymphangiectasia in Turner's syndrome and Noonan's syndrome (Fig. 3–12).

Other causes of pleural effusion include various infections or inflammatory conditions, most commonly bacterial. Effusion secondary to tuberculosis or fungus is rare. Inflammatory causes include renal disease, such as glomerulonephritis or nephrotic syndrome, subdiaphragmatic abscess, or pancreatitis (usually the effusion is on the left). Pleural effusion may also be secondary to neoplasms, blunt chest trauma, and esophageal rupture. Specifically, neoplasms may arise from the lung parenchyma, chest wall, mediastinum, or represent metastasis (usually from lymphoma or neuroblastoma). Blunt chest trauma results in hemothorax, which may or may not be associated with pulmonary contusions and rib fractures. Esophageal rupture (Boerhaave syndrome) is rare in children except in the newborn period. A hydropneumothorax develops due to the accumulation of esophageal contents. Rupture of the esophagus occurs on the right, except with a right aortic arch, with the right hemithorax being protected by the descending aorta. Fluid may fill a hemithorax immediately following thoracic surgery. This fluid is gradually replaced by fibrosis.

Other causes of a large, opaque hemithorax are less common. Fluid may accumulate in the lung parenchyma due to congenital bronchial obstruction such as is seen in congenital lobar emphysema or bronchial atresia. However, visualization of even the smallest amount of aerated lung, usually in the costophrenic angle, is a subtle clue that a large pleural effusion is not the cause (Fig. 3–13). Pleural effusions obliterate the costophrenic angle. Congenital lobar emphysema is thought to be due to segmental bronchial cartilage underdevelopment. The left upper lobe is the most common location with the right upper lobe and right middle lobes following closely behind. If the patient is symptomatic, emergency lobectomy is the treatment of choice.

Although bronchogenic cysts are commonly thought of as fluid-density middle mediastinal masses, intrapulmonary bronchogenic cysts are two to three times

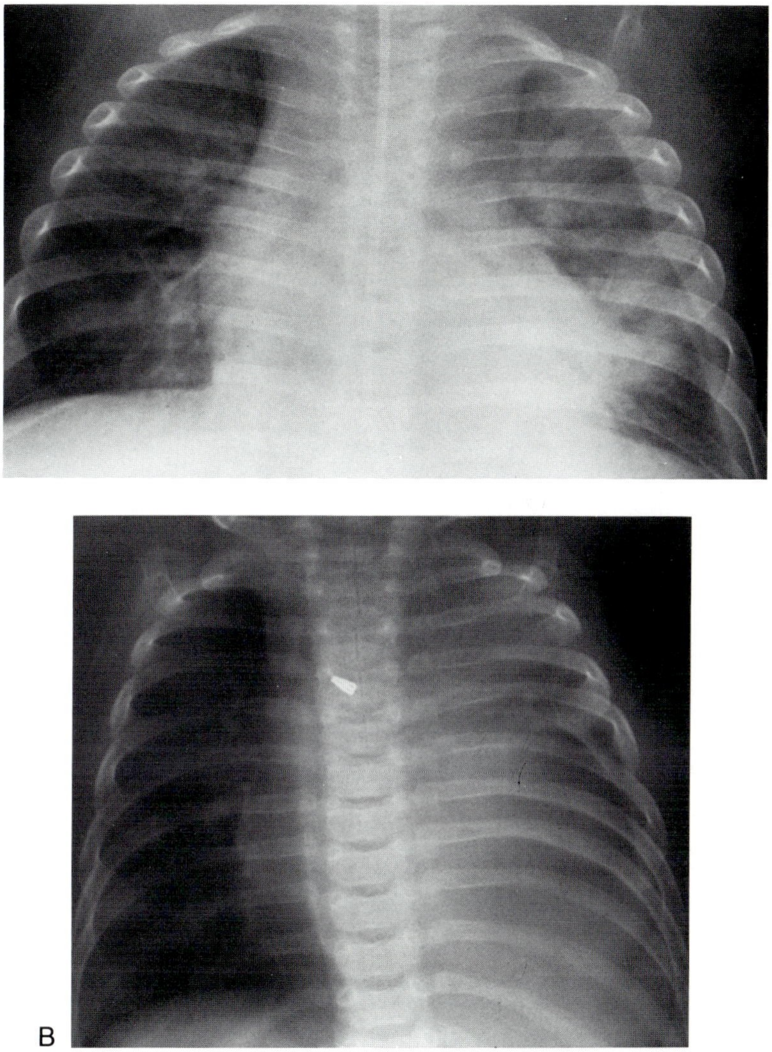

Fig. 3–12 Chylothorax. **(A)** Notice the enlarged left hemithorax and the bilateral increase in the interstitial lung markings in this child with pulmonary lymphangiectasia and chylothorax. **(B)** Another child developed a left chylothorax after cardiac surgery. Note the enlarged, partially opaque left hemithorax.

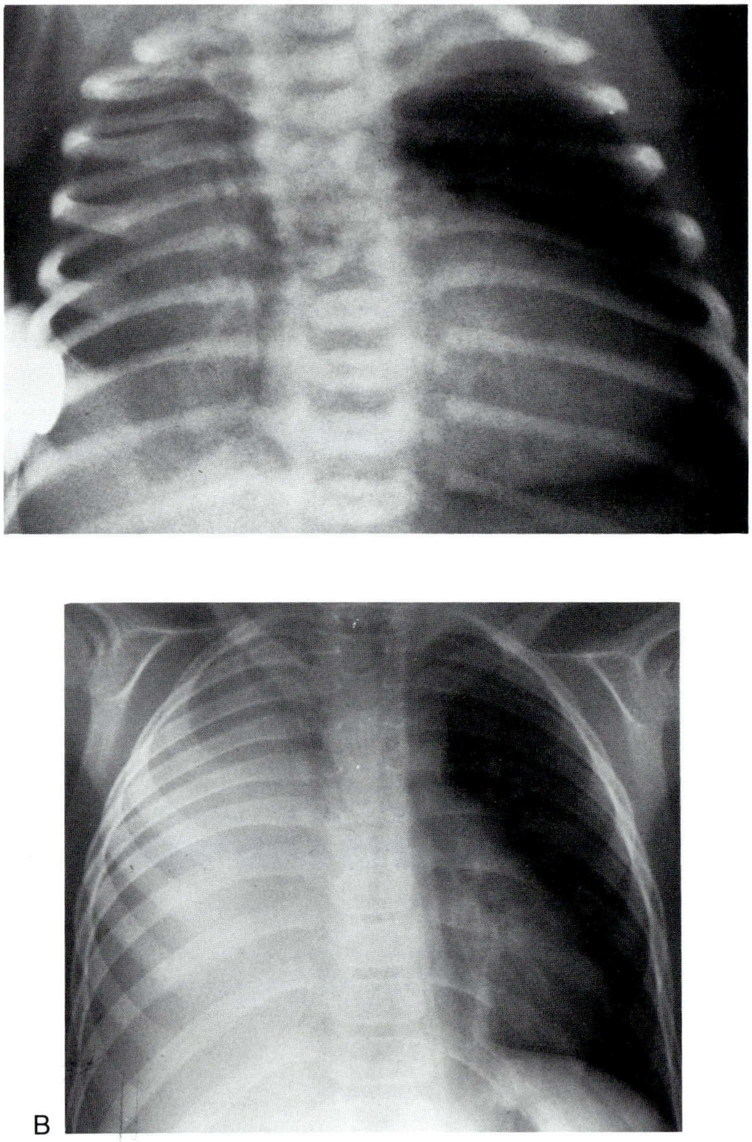

A

B

Fig. 3–13 Large opaque hemithorax. **(A)** Anteroposterior chest x-ray of a newborn in respiratory distress reveals a large opaque right hemithorax. Some aerated lung is present in the right base; suggesting that a pleural effusion is not the cause. The presence of segmentation fusion anomalies of the thoracic spine aid in confirming the diagnosis of a large neurenteric cyst. **(B)** In another patient no residual aerated lung is in the right costophrenic angle, implicating pleural fluid. The opaque hemithorax was secondary to a pneumococcal empyema.

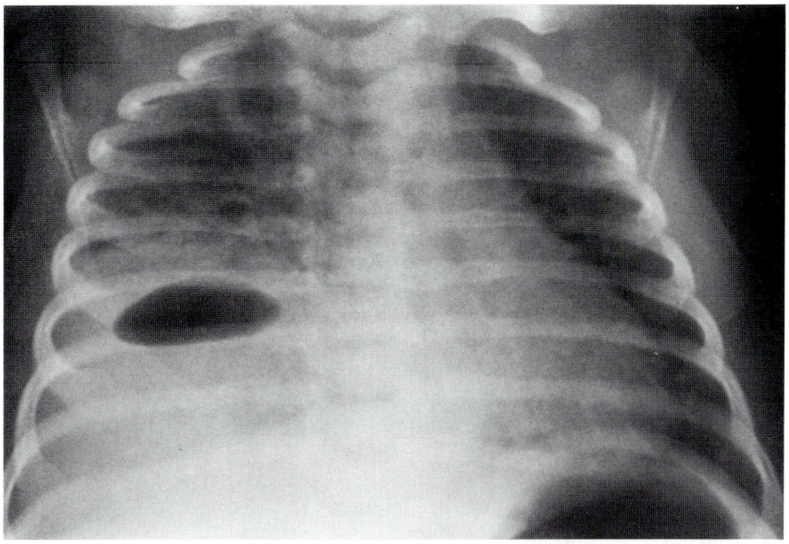

A

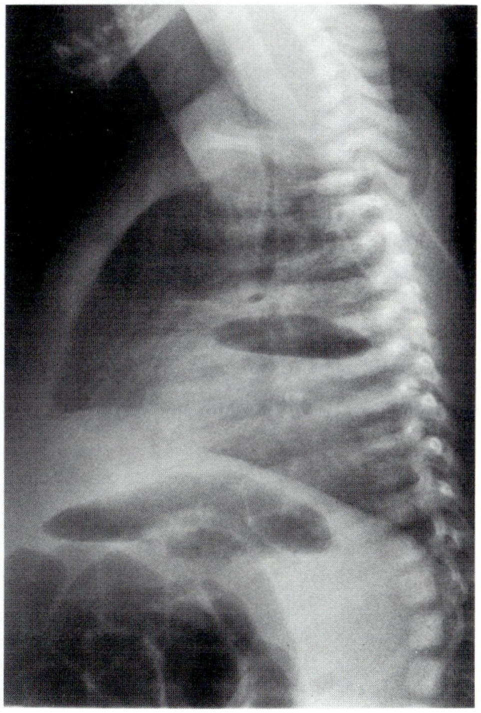

B

Fig. 3–14 Bronchogenic cyst. **(A)** Anteroposterior chest x-ray of an infant presenting with fever. The opaque right lower lobe appears enlarged and an air/fluid level is seen. **(B)** The lateral view confirms the right lower lobe location of an infected bronchopulmonary foregut malformation (bronchogenic cyst).

more common. Bronchogenic cysts may be multiple or may be large enough to approximate the size of an entire lobe (Fig. 3–14). Patients with large cysts commonly present with infantile respiratory distress. While the density of the cyst alone may cause the appearance of a large opaque hemithorax, the bronchogenic cyst may obstruct pulmonary vessels or a main bronchus, thus producing increased density in the affected lung. A neonate presenting with mild respiratory distress and increased density of the right hemithorax may have "the opaque right lung syndrome." This is secondary to transient retention of normal fetal lung fluid that clears within 24 to 48 hours (Fig. 3–15).

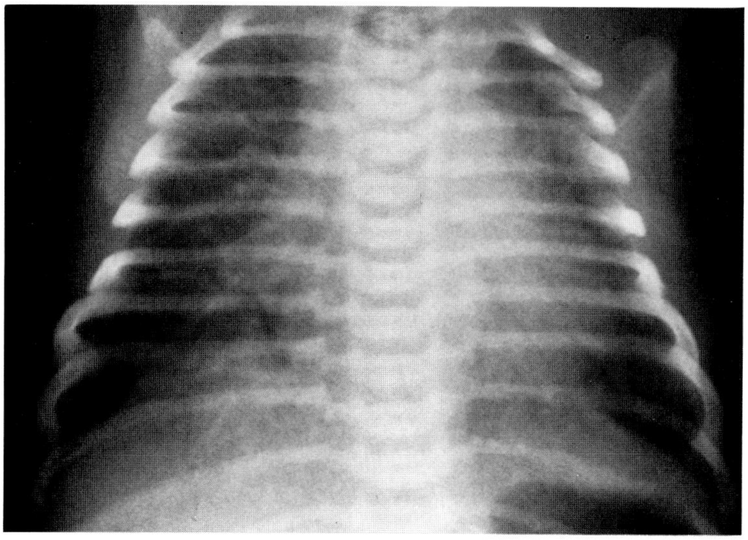

A

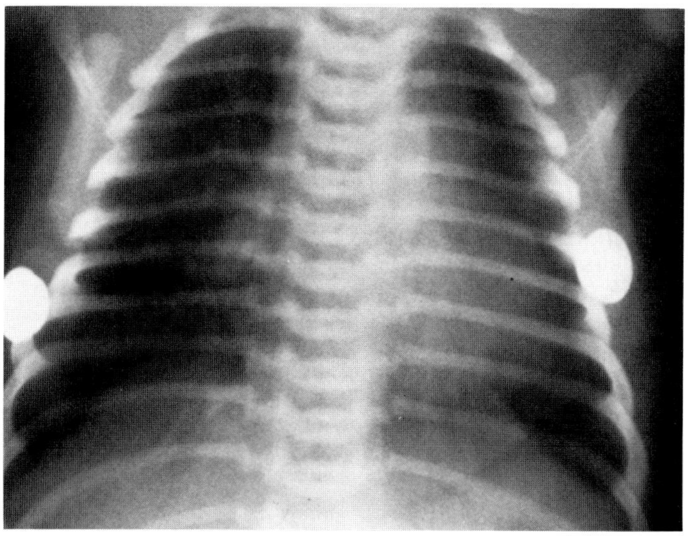

B

Fig. 3–15 Opaque right lung syndrome. **(A)** This newborn with mild respiratory distress demonstrates a reticular pattern of increased density in the right lung as compared with the left. Crowded air bronchograms behind the left heart and nonvisualization of the left hemidiaphragm, indicate left lower lobe collapse. **(B)** A follow-up chest x-ray taken 24 hours later demonstrates resolution of the streaky densities in the right lung. Transient retention of fetal lung fluid is usually bilateral but occasionally it involves only the right side. Incidentally noted is continued left lower lobe collapse.

Normal-sized Opaque Hemithorax

While the most common cause of a normal-sized opaque hemithorax is layering of a small pleural effusion from a variety of causes, it is imperative that the radiologist recognize that the same appearance may signal the development of an empyema. Decubitus chest x-rays may be helpful in demonstrating free pleural fluid. Ultrasound may be helpful in needle localization of a developing empyema. Empyemas are commonly associated with lung abscesses that are easily recognized by air/fluid levels. Both pleural effusions and empyema are commonly associated with bacterial pneumonias. Although bacterial pneumonia may present as a lobar consolidation with corresponding air bronchograms, it is unusual for contiguous lobes to be involved, and only rarely is an entire lung infected.

LUNG PARENCHYMAL DISEASE

In order to differentiate the causes of lung parenchymal disease, one should attempt to characterize the processes based on the type of infiltrate present, the extent of involvement, whether the infiltrates are recurrent, and which part of the parenchyma is involved, the air spaces or the interstitium.

Lobar Alveolar Disease

The radiographic hallmarks of alveolar disease are the same in children as in adults. When the alveoli fill with any type of fluid, air bronchograms are seen. Early alveolar disease appears fluffy and then progresses to a more opaque stage. Complete consolidation usually occurs in a lobar distribution and is most likely secondary to pneumococcal pneumonia when the patient is more than 2 years of age. Statistically, atelectasis occurs more commonly than lobar alveolar disease and often can be differentiated by displacement of the fissures, hilar, or mediastinal structures and a wedge-shaped appearance (Fig. 3–16). Compensatory emphysema may occur in the adjacent lobes. Air bronchograms may also be seen in atelectasis but often appear crowded due to volume loss. It should be noted that in severe interstitial disease air bronchograms also may be seen. However, this is not often confined to one lobe. Other commonly implicated bacterial organisms causing pneumonia in children include *Staphylococcus aureus, M. pneumoniae,* and *Haemophilus influenzae* (most common cause of a lobar pneumonia in infants). Gram-negative organisms, *Klebsiella pneumoniae,* and other bacteria are less common in children. Both *Klebsiella* and gram-negative infections may cause bulging of the fissures of the involved lobe as is seen in adults. One peculiar feature of childhood bacterial lung infections is the early ap-

LOBAR ALVEOLAR DISEASE

- Infection
  - Bacterial
    - *Streptococcus pneumoniae*
    - *Haemophilus influenza*
    - *Staphylococcus aureus*
    - Group B streptococcus
    - Gram-negative bacteria
  - *Mycoplasma pneumoniae*
  - Tuberculosis
  - Fungus
- Aspiration Pneumonia
  - Central nervous system impairment
  - Near-drowning
  - Meconium/amniotic fluid aspiration
  - Familial dysautonomia
  - Accidental ingestion
- Trauma
  - Contusion
- Idiopathic
  - Pulmonary hemosiderosis
- Miscellaneous
  - Thromboemboli/infarction
- Mimics
  - Congenital
    - Lobar emphysema (early)
    - Diaphragmatic hernia (early)
    - Cystic adenomatoid malformation
    - Bronchogenic cyst
    - Arteriovenous malformation
    - Lobar pulmonary vein atresia
  - Normal structures
    - Lower lobe vessels
    - Thymus

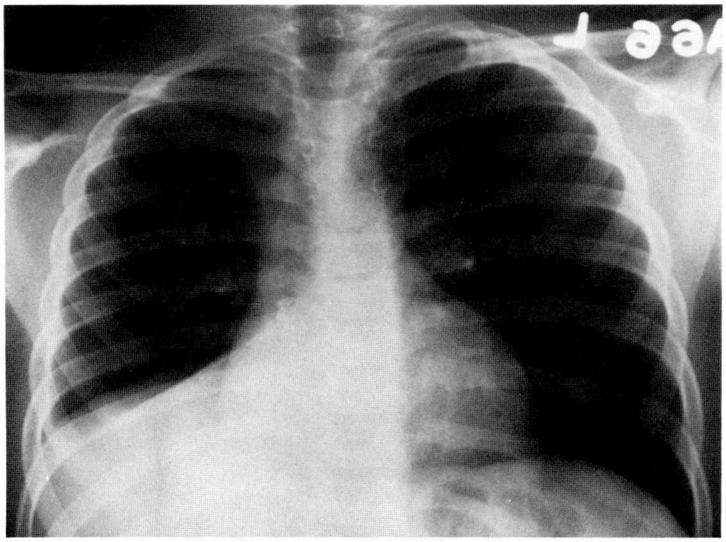

A

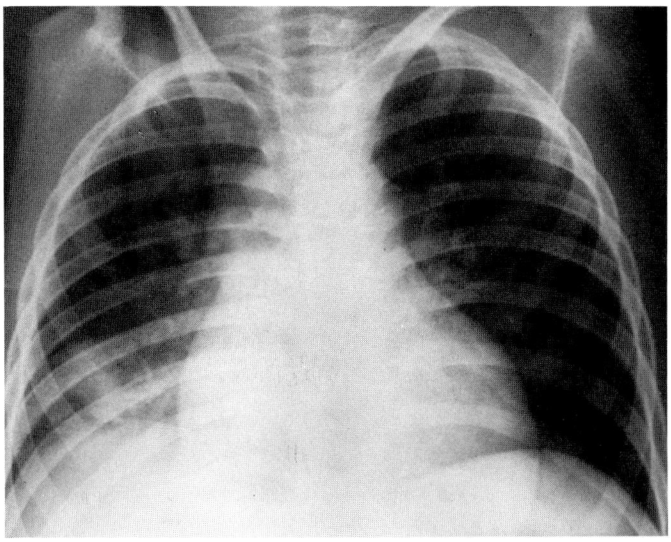

B

Fig. 3–16 Atelectasis. **(A)** This 9-year-old boy presented with shortness of breath. The radiograph demonstrates collapse of the right middle and lower lobes secondary to inhalation of a tooth into the right main stem bronchus. Note the wedge-shaped appearance of atelectasis with compensatory hypertrophy of the right upper lobe and mediastinal shift toward the atelectasis. The right hemidiaphragm is obliterated indicating lower lobe collapse. **(B)** After removal of the tooth, only partial atelectasis persists, causing increased density of the involved lobes but no silhouette sign or mediastinal shift. (*Figure continues.*)

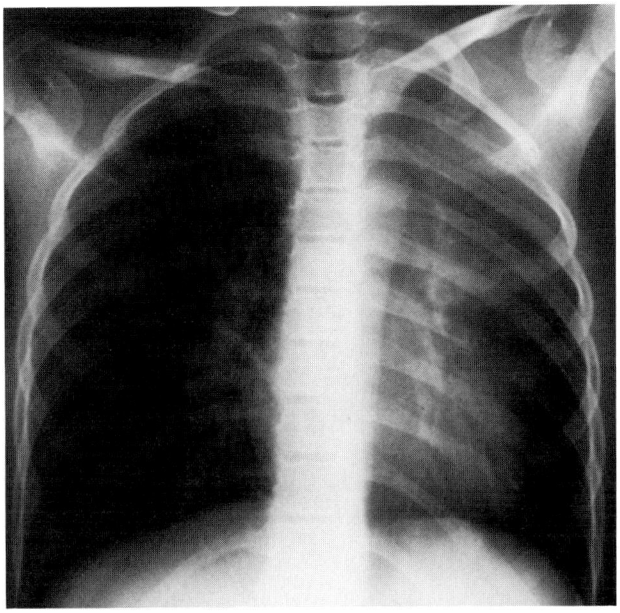

C

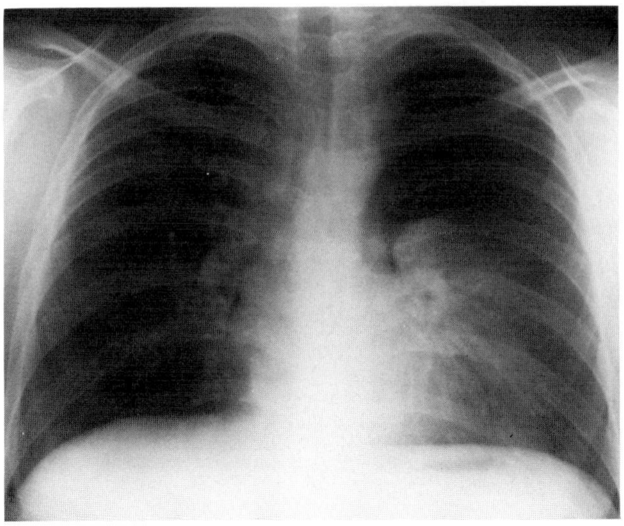

D

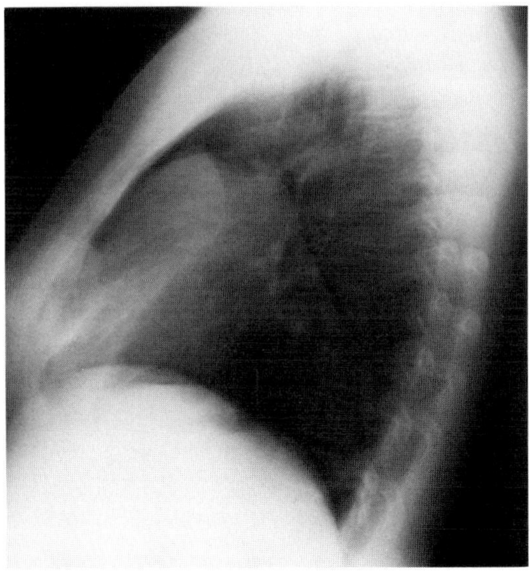

E

Fig. 3–16 (*Continued*). **(C)** Posteroanterior chest x-ray of an asthmatic demonstrates increased density of the left upper lung with upward shift of the left hilum and left deviation of the trachea. These findings indicate left upper lobe atelectasis. **(D)** Posteroanterior chest x-ray in another asthmatic demonstrates total collapse of the left upper lobe, which has rotated downward. Vessels seen in the upper left hemithorax are due to compensatory hypertrophy of the left lower lobe. The sharply marginated curvilinear density at the left hilum represents the left lung apex. The left heart border is obliterated. **(E)** The lateral view confirms increased density in the left upper lobe consistent with complete atelectasis.

pearance of a "solitary pulmonary nodule or mass" that has the classic appearance of lobar consolidation on repeat examinations obtained 24 hours later. This is referred to as a *round pneumonia*. Although *Streptococcus pneumoniae* is the most common cause of lobar consolidation in a child, *S. aureus* has a peculiar ability to present as widespread alveolar infiltrates, usually bilateral. However, the finding of widespread fluffy infiltrates is by no means specific for bacterial pneumonia and is seen in a number of other infectious and noninfectious disease processes.

There are several congenital abnormalities which may mimic alveolar disease confined to a single lobe. These include the early phases of diaphragmatic hernia. congenital lobar emphysema, and cystic adenomatoid malformation. The characteristic location (upper lobes) in lobar emphysema and (lower lobes) in diaphragmatic hernia may aid in the differentiation. Follow-up examinations usually show progression to more characteristic cystic lesions. Intrapulmonary bronchogenic cysts, arteriovenous malformations, and lobar pulmonary vein atresia are other congenital causes. Occasionally, primary tuberculosis and fungal infections may be localized to a single lobe. Hemorrhage into the lung parenchyma from either trauma (pulmonary contusion) or idiopathic pulmonary hemosiderosis should be considered in the differential diagnosis. Pulmonary infarction from any cause may appear as a lobar alveolar consolidation.

Occasionally, normal structures may mimic localized air space disease. The classic example is suspected right upper lobe pneumonia caused by slight rotation of the patient and overlapping of the right border of the thymus and the lung apex. Crowding of the pulmonary vessels in the lung bases may also fool the novice; in fact, some radiologists refer to the lung base of neonates as "the fool's triangle." Occasionally the inferior tip of the scapula may be confused with pneumonia. Lower lobe bacterial pneumonias are often very subtle on chest x-rays and may present with confusing clinical symptoms, such as abdominal pain (Fig. 3–17). For this reason, it is prudent to include the lung bases on one of the multiple anteroposterior views of the abdomen when evaluating a child with abdominal pain. Also, careful scrutiny of the vertebral bodies on the lateral view (the lower levels should be easier to visualize) will confirm the presence of lobar pneumonia in most cases (Fig. 3–18).

Fluffy lower lobe infiltrates may also be seen when aspiration occurs in the upright position. While the

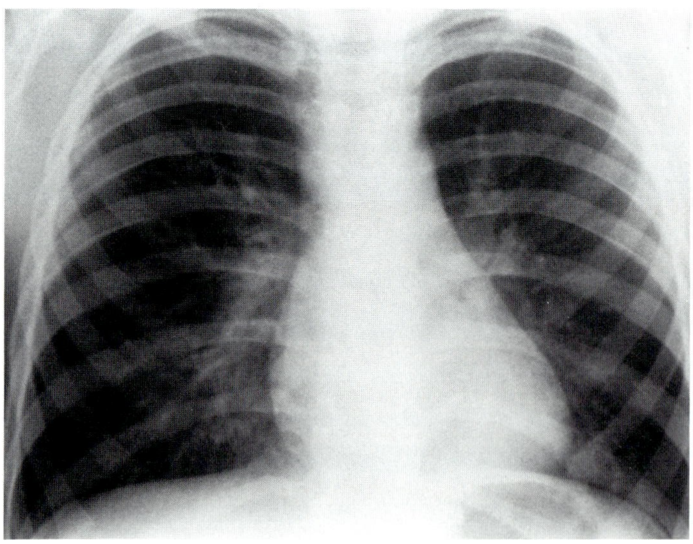

Fig. 3–17 Left lower lobe pneumonia. Posteroanterior chest view shows a subtle wedge-shaped density with air bronchograms behind the heart.

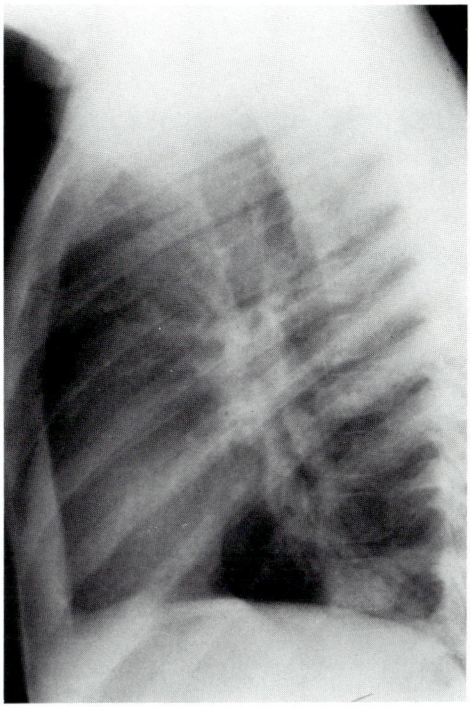

Fig. 3–18 Lateral view of the same patient in Figure 3–17 demonstrates air bronchograms and increased density over the lower thoracic vertebral bodies consistent with left lower lobe pneumonia.

most common aspirated material is gastric contents, hydrocarbon ingestion should be considered also. Classically, the presenting film may show no radiographic abnormality, but bibasilar alveolar infiltrates develop on the subsequent examinations (Fig. 3–19). Local surfactant loss leads to atelectasis, hemorrhage, surrounding pulmonary edema, and pneumatocele formation during healing. In infants, it is not uncommon to see aspiration pneumonia in the right upper lobe indicating that the infant was supine while being fed. Congenital anomalies of the trachea and esophagus, high gastrointestinal tract obstruction, familial dysautonomia, fatigue, and prematurity predispose patients to aspiration pneumonia. Chronic aspiration leads to increased parahilar peribronchial infiltrates due to pulmonary fibrosis. Massive aspiration presents as bilateral fluffy infiltrates in a patient with obvious respiratory distress. If lung destruction occurs due to the acidic gastric contents, the condition is termed *Mendelson syndrome.* Occasionally the abdominal radiograph may be helpful in determining the cause of aspiration or the type of material aspirated. For example, on an erect radiograph, a fluid level may be seen within the stomach after hydrocarbon ingestion. Air-filled distended loops of small and large bowel suggestive of an adynamic ileus have

A

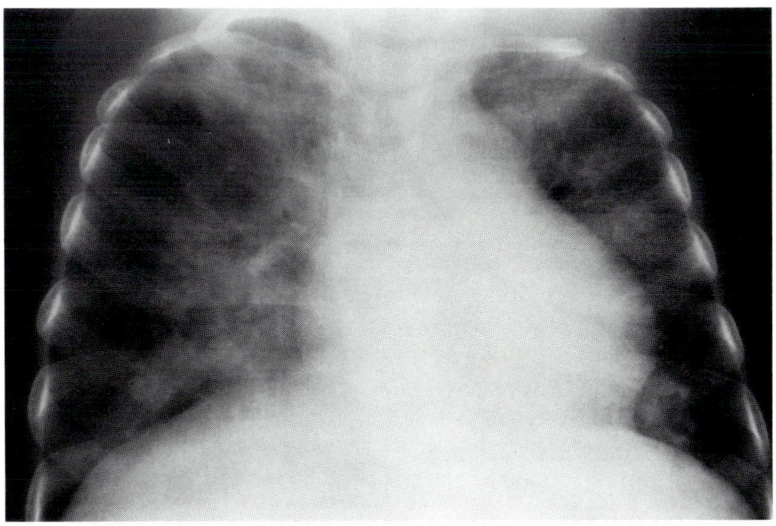

Fig. 3–19 Aspiration changes. **(A)** Anteroposterior view of the chest of a neurologically impaired child demonstrates bilateral fluffy infiltrates predominantly in the bases, consistent with the history of mineral oil aspiration. (*Figure continues.*)

B

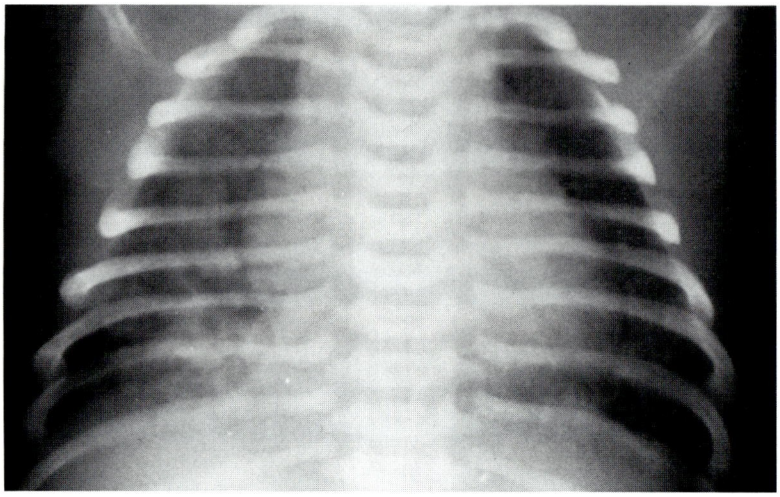

Fig. 3–19 (*Continued*). **(B)** Anteroposterior chest x-ray, taken immediately after birth, of an infant in respiratory distress with meconium seen below the cords. Note the bilateral fluffy infiltrates that cleared slowly, consistent with aspirated meconium.

been associated with Riley-Day syndrome (familial dysautonomia).

Bilateral Patchy Alveolar Disease

When bilateral fluffy infiltrates are present, it may be helpful to determine whether the infiltrates are centrally or peripherally located. The most common cause of widespread patchy alveolar infiltrates is bacterial pneumonia caused by any number of organisms with the *exception* of *S. pneumoniae,* which is more likely to present as a lobar consolidation. Ill-defined but more centrally located infiltrates may be seen in severe subsegmental and segmental atelectasis associated with viral, mycoplasmal, and tuberculous pneumonia. One of the hallmarks of atelectasis is a rapid change in the appearance of a focal abnormality on repeat chest x-rays (Fig. 3–20). Widespread bacterial pneumonia is less likely to change rapidly. One notable infectious cause of widespread patchy alveolar infiltrates that may be centrally located is varicella (chickenpox) pneumonia. Involvement of the lungs is rare in children with normal immunity (Fig. 3–21). Multiple amorphous calcifications may develop following of varicella pneumonia.

Other conditions that may produce bilateral ill-defined alveolar infiltrates include fungal disease, parasitic infestation (visceral larva migrans), sarcoido-

BILATERAL PATCHY ALVEOLAR DISEASE

- Infection
  - Bacteria
  - Virus
    - Varicella pneumonia
  - *Mycoplasma pneumoniae*
  - Tuberculosis
  - Fungus
  - Parasites
    - Visceral larva migrans
- Granulomatous disease
  - Sarcoidosis
- Allergic/eosinophilic pneumonia
  - Löffler's pneumonia
  - Milk allergy
  - Inhaled antigens
  - Drug allergy
- Aspiration
  - Near-drowning
  - Meconium/amniotic fluid
- Systemic disease
  - Uremia (hemorrhage/edema)
- Idiopathic
  - Pulmonary hemosiderosis

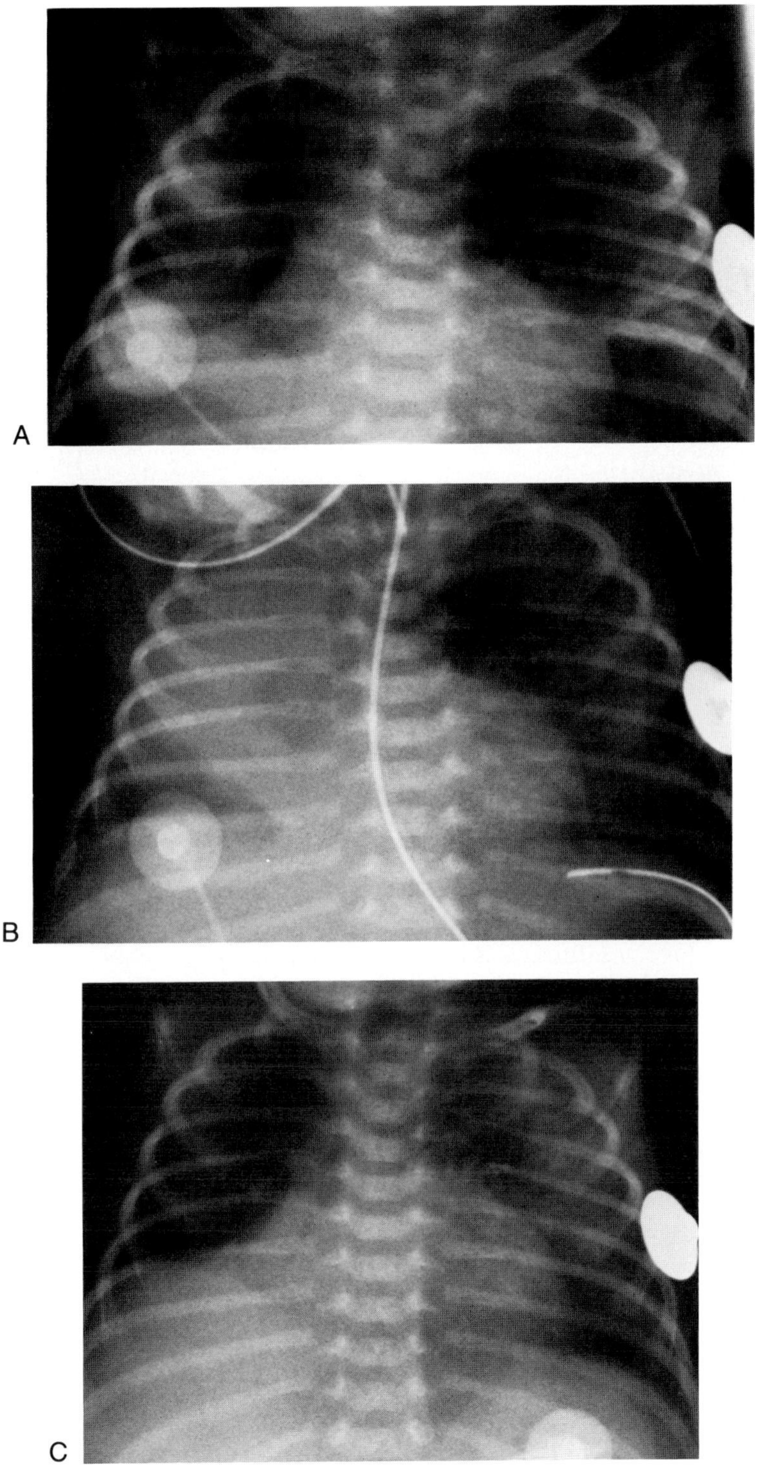

Fig. 3–20 Bilateral patchy infiltrates. **(A)** Radiograph of a neonate in respiratory distress demonstrates bilateral ill-defined patchy opacities. They are wedge-shaped and most likely represent atelectasis. **(B)** Two hours later, the left lung appears clear and the right lung is totally atelectatic. **(C)** The next day a vague area of increased density is seen in the left upper lobe. The right middle and lower lobes are totally atelectatic with compensatory hypertrophy of the right upper lobe. (*Figure continues.*)

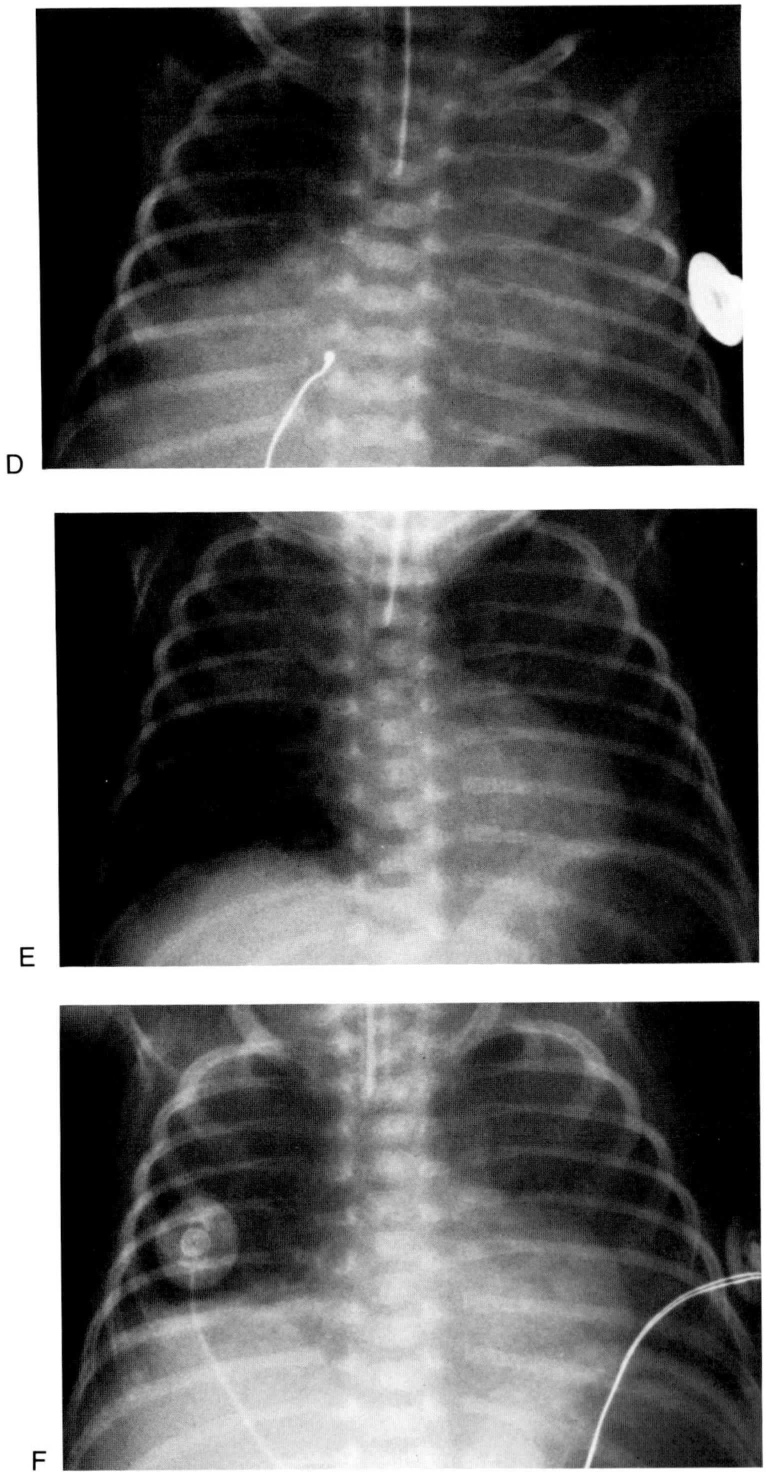

Fig. 3–20 (*Continued.*) **(D)** Twenty-four hours later an endotracheal tube has been placed but abuts the carina. The right lung is unchanged but the left upper lobe has collapsed. **(E)** With retraction of the tube, the atelectasis clears but the right upper lobe collapses. **(F)** Later, both lungs are well-aerated.

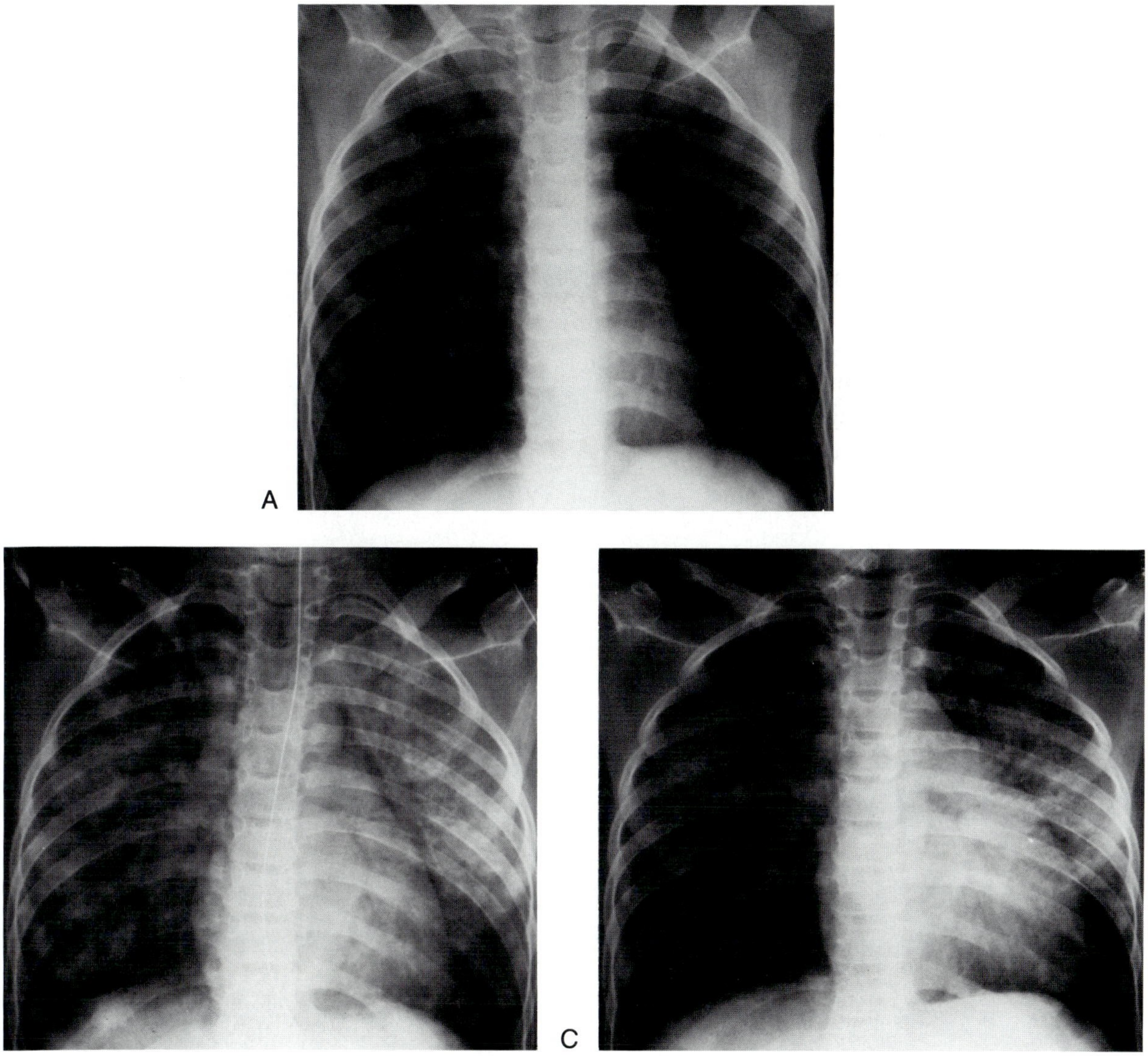

A B C

Fig. 3–21 Bilateral patchy alveolar disease. **(A)** Posteroanterior chest x-ray of a patient undergoing chemotherapy for osteogenic sarcoma. Notice the ill-defined pulmonary nodules present bilaterally. The patient had clinical symptoms of chickenpox. **(B)** Three days later the alveolar nodules have consolidated into widespread alveolar disease. Notice the air bronchograms. Incidentally noted is a pneumomediastinum and subcutaneous emphysema. **(C)** Three more days later, the patient has improved but patchy alveolar disease persists, worst in the left parahilar region.

sis, Löffler's pneumonia, milk allergy, allergic reactions to inhaled substances, early idiopathic pulmonary hemosiderosis, near drowning, and pulmonary hemorrhage or edema secondary to uremia.

Recurrent Bacterial Pneumonia

Recurrent bacterial pneumonia may be the first indication of an underlying immunologic deficiency (Fig. 3–22). The immunodeficiency syndromes that present with recurrent bacterial infections include hypogammaglobulinemia, hyperimmunoglobulinemia E (Buckley syndrome), and the immotile cilia syndromes. Buckley syndrome may present with large recurrent pneumatoceles, skin rashes, and mucocutaneous candidiasis. Bacterial abscesses of other organs, such as the liver and kidneys, have also been reported. The immotile cilia syndrome may occur as an isolated congenital condition presenting with recurrent bacterial infection or may be associated with sinusitis

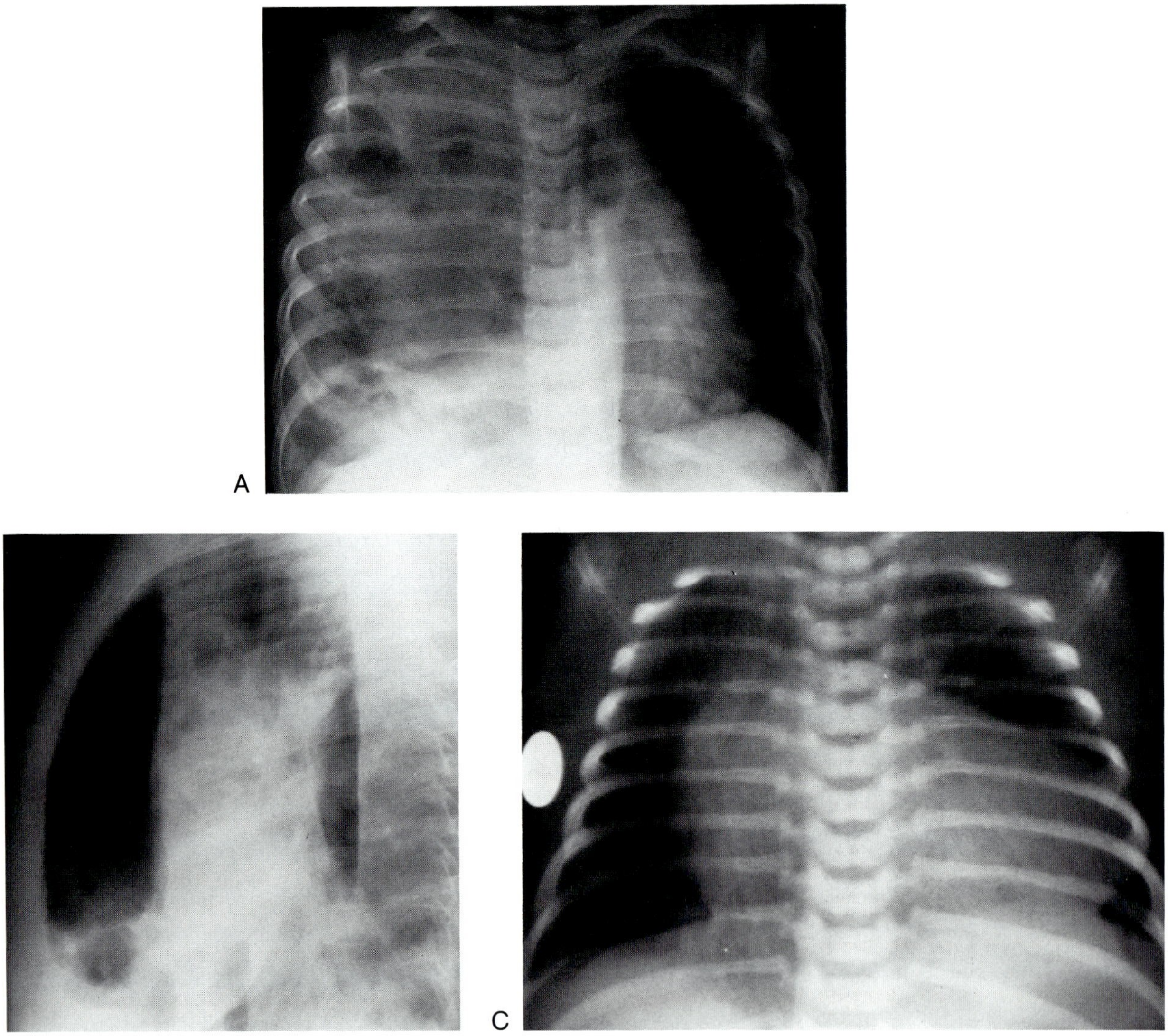

A B C

Fig. 3–22 Recurrent bacterial pneumonia. **(A)** This child had a history of two hospitalizations for pneumonia prior to his current presentation. He had been treated for facial and scalp abscesses several weeks before admission. (*Figure continues.*)

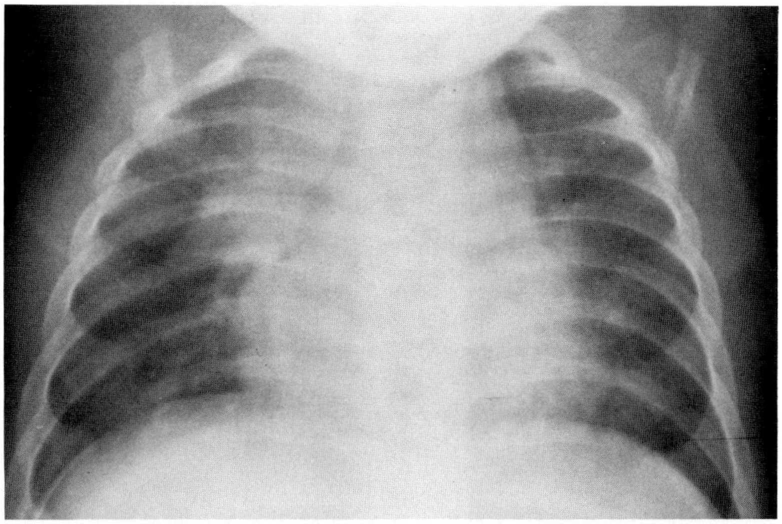

D

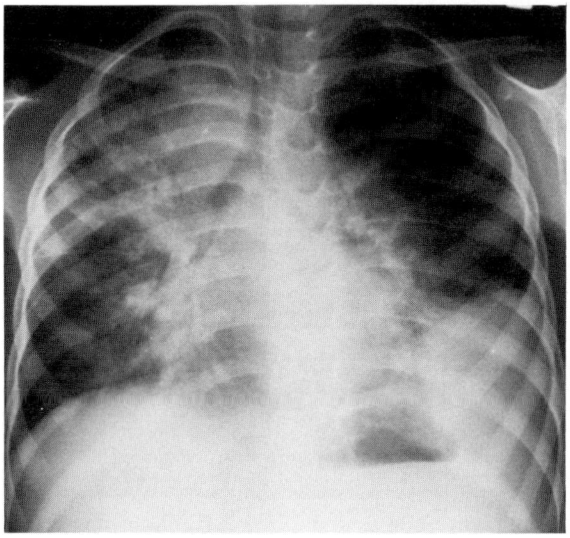

E

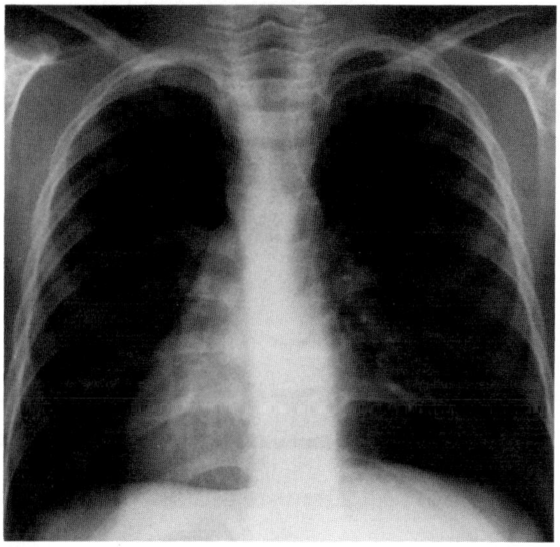

F

Fig. 3–22 (*Continued*). Anteroposterior chest x-ray demonstrates deviation of the trachea away from the hyperexpanded right lung and multiple cystic spaces. Also note the round soft tissue densities in the left lower lobe. **(B)** Supine lateral view demonstrates multiple air/fluid levels in abscess cavities. *Staphylococcus aureus* was cultured from his empyema. The association of recurrent skin and pulmonary infections is consistent with the diagnosis of hyperimmunoglobulinemia E. **(C)** Anteroposterior chest x-ray in a cyanotic neonate with low Apgar scores. Note the conspicuous radiolucency of the superior mediastinum, due to absence of the thymus. The aortic arch is right-sided, the pulmonary vascularity decreased, and the heart enlarged. The combination of arch anomalies and absence of the thymus is suggestive of DiGeorge's syndrome (absent thymus, absent parathyroids, and great vessel anomalies). The lack of T cells results in increased viral and fungal infections. **(D)** By contrast, this neonate has a normal thymus at birth. However, as he grew, he suffered from recurrent bacterial pneumonias. **(E)** At age 11, he presented with fever. Posteroanterior chest x-ray reveals alveolar infiltrates in the right upper lobe, right lower lobe, and left lower lobe. Biopsy revealed *Aspergillus*, an organism often cultured in patients with chronic granulomatous disease of childhood. **(F)** Posteroanterior chest x-ray of a child with a history of recurrent sinusitis shows situs inversus totalis and left lower lobe cysts representing bronchiectasis (Kartagener's syndrome).

and situs inversus (Kartagener's syndrome). One notable sequela to recurrent bacterial infections associated with immunodeficiency states is the development of bronchiectasis with resulting impairment of pulmonary function. If the diagnosis of hypogammaglobulinemia is suspected, lateral views of the soft tissues of the neck and nasopharynx should be obtained to evaluate the presence of adenoidal tissue. Patients with Bruton's disease (X-linked hypogammoglobulinemia) demonstrate a conspicuous absence of lymphoidal tissue in the nasopharynx and will not demonstrate hilar adenopathy (Fig. 3–23). Another genetic syndrome that may present with similar radiographic findings is ataxia-telangiectasia. Aside from absence of enlarged hilar nodes and nasopharyngeal lymphoidal tissue, these patients demonstrate sinusitis and lack a thymic shadow. Associated abnormalities include premature central nervous system atrophy and a predisposition to lymphoreticular malignancies and leukemia. The name of the syndrome is derived from

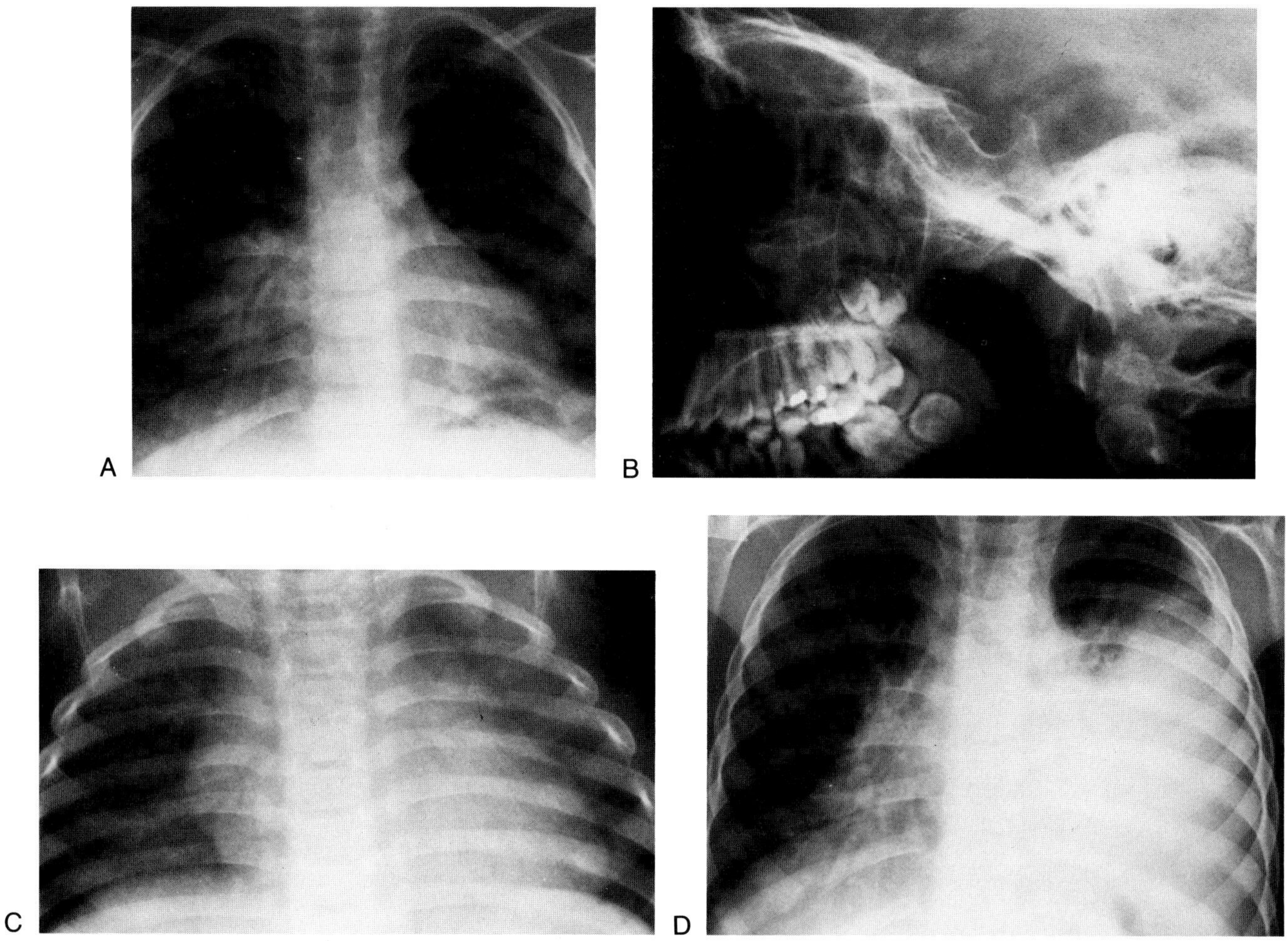

Fig. 3–23 Bruton disease. **(A)** Posteroanterior view of the chest demonstrates right middle lobe pneumonia and bilateral lower lobe bronchiectasis in a patient with known recurrent bacterial infections. **(B)** On the lateral paranasal sinus x-ray, the adenoidal fat pad is conspicuously absent. The patient had no history of surgery. **(C)** A chest x-ray taken at 7 months of age shows a normal thymus. **(D)** At 8 years of age, the patient has left bacterial pneumonia with later development of an empyema. Notice the conspicuous lack of hilar adenopathy on Figures A and D. These findings are consistent with the diagnosis of Bruton disease.

the presence of progressive cerebellar ataxia and oculocutaneous telangiectasia.

Dense Central Alveolar Disease

If the alveolar disease is present in a dense central distribution, pulmonary edema is the most common cause (Table 3–5). Common cardiac causes (left-sided heart failure or valvular disease) and noncardiac causes (renal failure or neurogenic pulmonary edema) should be considered. Other causes of a "butterfly" distribution of alveolar infiltrates in children include pulmonary hemosiderosis, pulmonary alveolar proteinosis, rheumatic pneumonia, hemolytic-uremic syndrome, and lipoid pneumonia (Fig. 3–24).

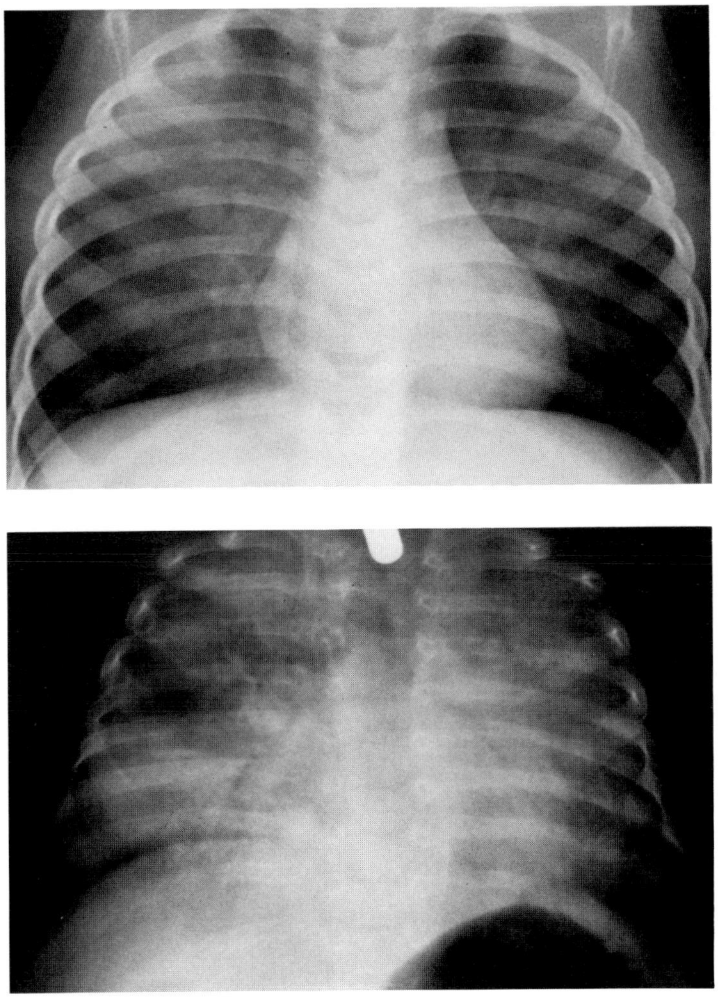

A

B

Fig. 3–24 Dense central alveolar disease. **(A)** Anteroposterior chest x-ray of an infant with frothy sputum. Note the bilateral hazy infiltrates in a central distribution. It is difficult to identify the pulmonary vessels. Alveolar edema was secondary to acute drug overdose. **(B)** Anteroposterior chest x-ray of another patient demonstrates dense alveolar infiltrates. These represented multiple pulmonary infarcts secondary to septic emboli from the patient's ventriculojugular shunt. (*Figure continues.*)

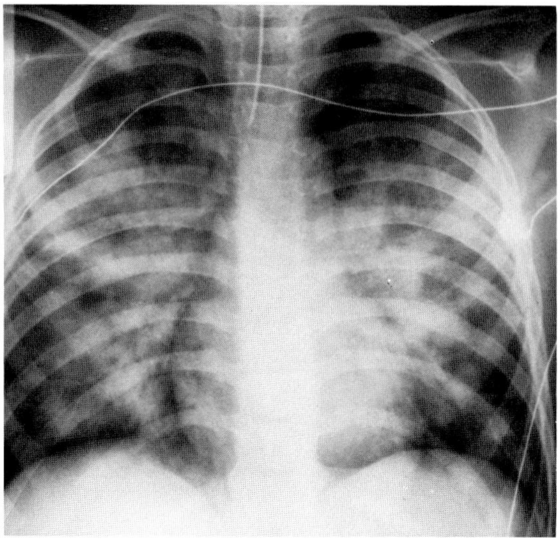

C

Fig. 3–24 (*Continued*). **(C)** Another child 2 hours after nearly drowning has fluffy central alveolar infiltrates. This represents a combination of aspirated water and resultant alveolar edema.

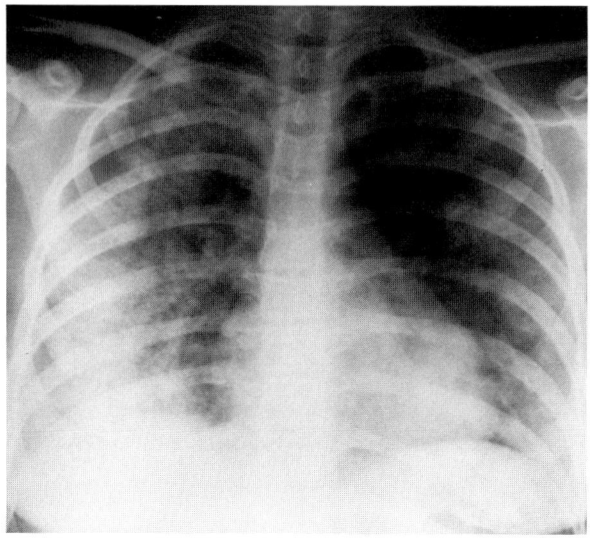

A

Fig. 3–25 Homogeneous parenchymal disease. **(A)** This 13-year-old patient presented with hemoptysis. Note the widespread bilateral ill-defined infiltrates that in some areas appear nodular. Note the air bronchograms present in the lung bases. Pulmonary hemorrhage was secondary to idiopathic hemosiderosis. (*Figure continues.*)

Table 3–5 Dense Central Alveolar Disease

Mechanism	Cause
Edema	Cardiac
	Congenital disease
	Left-sided failure
	Valvular disease
	Noncardiac
	Central nervous system depression
	Trauma
	Ischemia
	Infarction
	Hemorrhage
	Renal failure
	Fluid overload
	Inhalational injury
	Aspiration
	Drug overdose
Idiopathic	Pulmonary hemosiderosis
	Pulmonary alveolar proteinosis
	Rheumatic pneumonia
	Hemolytic-uremic syndrome
	Lipoid pneumonia

Widespread Homogeneous Parenchymal Disease

As previously mentioned, severe interstitial disease may result in a radiographic picture similar to alveolar disease. Often, when interstitial disease is widespread and severe the lungs will have uniform increased density throughout (Fig. 3–25). Whether the disease process is actually confined to the interstitium is uncertain. The most common cause of uniform increased density of both lungs is interstitial pulmonary edema of either cardiogenic or noncardiogenic origin (Table 3–6). Congenital causes of pulmonary edema include pulmonary vein atresia, coarctation of the aorta, large left-to-right shunts, admixture lesions, and arteriovenous fistulas. Infectious and inflammatory causes of pulmonary edema include valvular heart disease, allergies, rheumatic pneumonia, and acute glomerulonephritis. Traumatic causes include neurogenic injury, near-drowning, toxic inhalational injuries, and massive aspiration. Collagen-vascular diseases and idiopathic pulmonary hemosiderosis may also have this appearance.

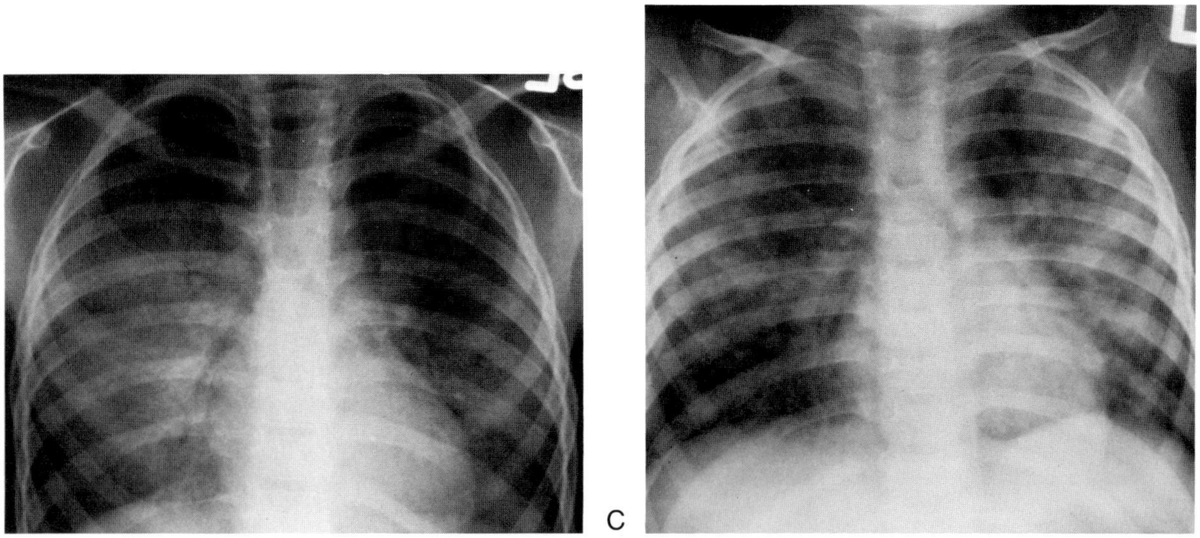

Fig. 3–25 (*Continued*). **(B)** Another patient with idiopathic pulmonary hemosiderosis demonstrates a more diffuse pattern of alveolar infiltrates consistent with bilateral pulmonary hemorrhages. **(C)** Posteroanterior chest x-ray of an immune-compromised child demonstrates widespread parenchymal disease with focal areas of increased density in the upper lobes. In both lower lobes, a nodular pattern is seen, representing interstitial and alveolar involvement in *Pneumocystis carinii* pneumonia.

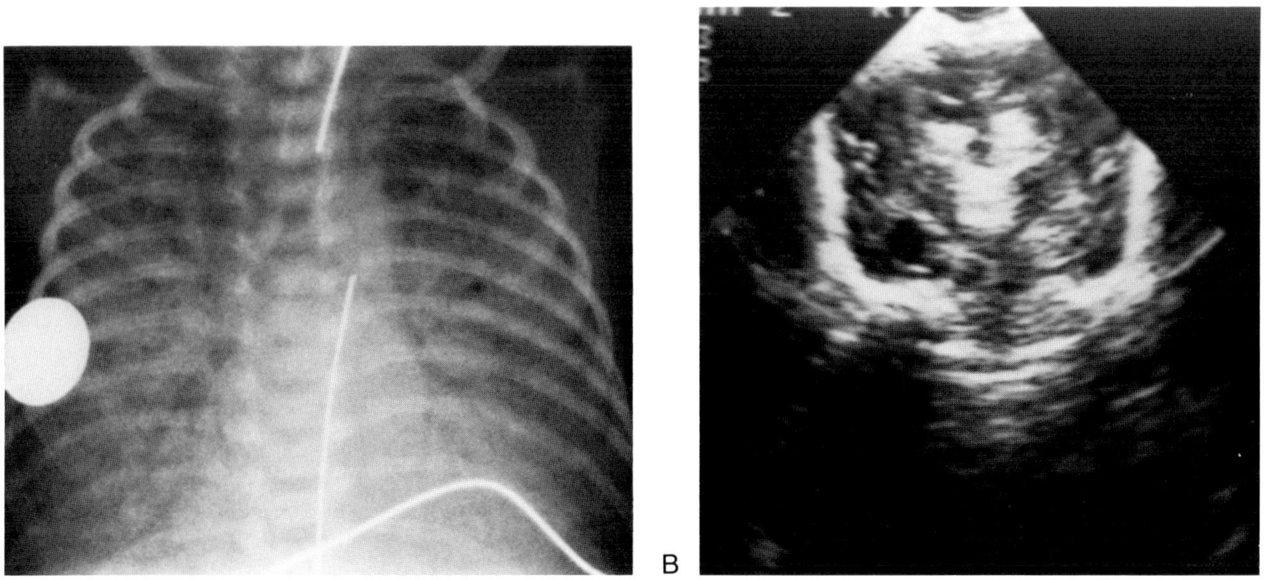

Fig. 3–26 Pulmonary edema. **(A)** Anteroposterior chest x-ray shows diffuse homogeneous parenchymal infiltrates. **(B)** Coronal head ultrasound demonstrates echogenic hemorrhage in both the lateral and third ventricles resulting in neurogenic pulmonary edema.

Table 3–6 Widespread Homogeneous Parenchymal Disease

Mechanism	Cause

Interstitial edema +/− alveolar edema	Cardiac
	  Pulmonary vein atresia
	  Aortic coarctation
	  Left-to-right shunts
	  Admixture lesions
	  Arteriovenous fistulas
	Inflammation
	  Rheumatic heart disease
	  Bacterial endocarditis
	  Rheumatic pneumonia
	  Allergy
	  Acute glomerulonephritis
	Trauma
	  Neurogenic injury
	  Near-drowning
	  Toxic inhalation
	  Accidental ingestion
	Idiopathic
	  Collagen-vascular diseases
	  Pulmonary hemosiderosis

Neonatal infection	Viral pneumonia
Neonatal respiratory distress	Hyaline membrane disease (healing)
Neonatal hemorrhage	Massive pulmonary hemorrhage of the newborn Ischemia

Inflammatory cell infiltration	Opportunistic infection
	  Virus
	  Pneumocystis carinii

Interstitial fibrosis	Any chronic lung disease

Bilateral hazy lungs in the newborn may signify neonatal viral pneumonia, the healing phase of respiratory distress syndrome, pulmonary edema, or pulmonary hemorrhage (Fig. 3–26).

Inflammatory cells may infiltrate the interstitium during infection by viruses or opportunistic infections such as *Pneumocystis carinii*. Cellular infiltration is also seen in idiopathic pulmonary hemosiderosis, Goodpasture syndrome, and the collagen-vascular diseases. Any long-standing interstitial process may result in interstitial fibrosis as the end stage of the disease.

INTERSTITIAL DISEASE

Interstitial disease may present as a variety of patterns including miliary, reticular, reticulonodular, nodular, "honeycomb lung," and parahilar peribronchial infiltrates. The distribution may be localized or widespread. It is interesting to note that in the neonatal period, bacterial pneumonia does *not* present as lobar consolidations. Instead, neonatal bacterial pneumonia (most common organism: group B streptococcus) may demonstrate any of the interstitial patterns described above and is the most common infectious cause mimicking the granular appearance of hyaline membrane disease.

Miliary Interstitial Disease

The most common cause of a diffuse miliary pattern is hematogenous spread of tuberculosis (Fig. 3–27). However, fungal infections such as histoplasmosis, blastomycosis, cryptococcosis, and coccidioidomycosis are not uncommon when one considers the endemic regions for these organisms. Inborn errors of metabolism such as Gaucher's disease (beta-glucosidase deficiency) and Niemann-Pick disease (sphingomyelinase deficiency resulting in storage of sphingomyelin and cholesterol in "foam cells") may result in a miliary pattern of diffuse lung disease. Congenital bacterial pneumonias occasionally appear miliary (Fig. 3–28). Hematogenous spread of metastatic tumors may result in a miliary pattern but this is not as common as a larger nodular pattern. An idiopathic cause of bilateral miliary disease is pulmonary hemosiderosis, which usually occurs in children more than 1 year of age. Clinical signs and symptoms include hypochromic anemia and hemoptysis.

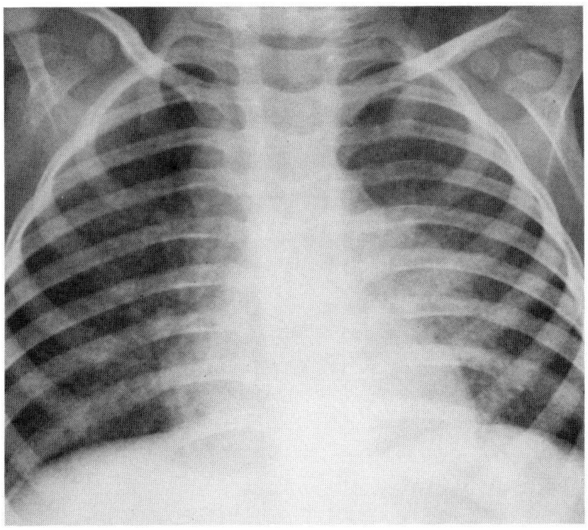

A

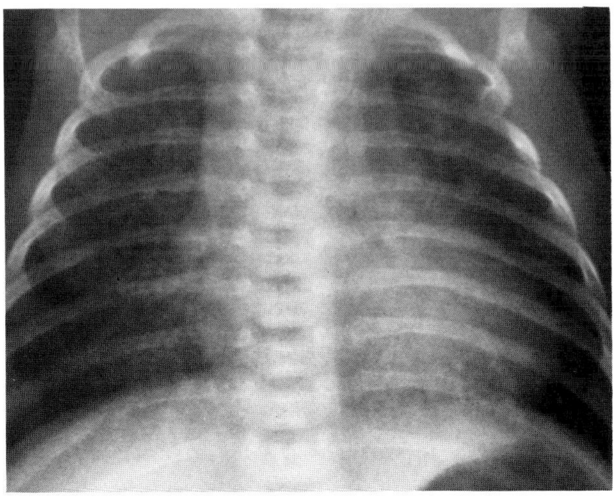

B

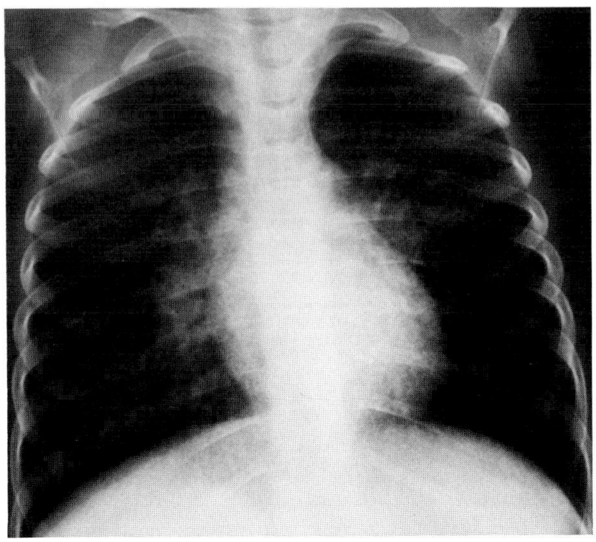

C

Fig. 3–27 Miliary interstitial nodules. **(A)** Anteroposterior chest x-ray of a febrile infant demonstrates bilateral hilar adenopathy associated with stippling of the lungs by tiny soft tissue densities, representing primary tuberculosis with hematogenous spread. **(B)** Anteroposterior chest x-ray in another infant demonstrates diffuse miliary nodules secondary to histiocytosis X. **(C)** This 6-year-old patient had juvenile rheumatoid arthritis with miliary pulmonary involvement evident bilaterally.

MILIARY INTERSTITIAL DISEASE
Tuberculosis
Histoplasmosis
Blastomycosis
Cryptococcosis
Coccidioidomycosis
Gaucher's disease
Neimann-Pick disease
Congenital bacterial pneumonia
Hematogenous metastases
Pulmonary hemosiderosis

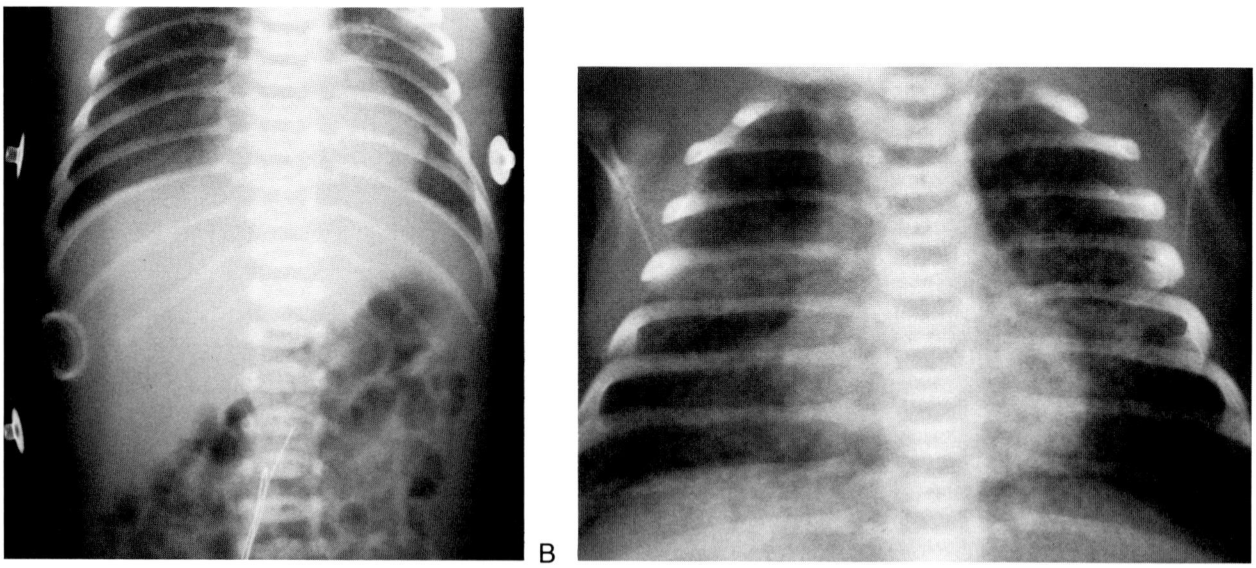

A B

Fig. 3–28 Congenital pneumonia. **(A)** The combined chest/abdomen view demonstrates tiny nodular densities especially apparent in the right lower lobe. The liver is enlarged. These findings are suggestive of bacterial pneumonia. **(B)** Note the diffuse nodules throughout the lungs of this neonate with chlamydia infection.

Nodular Interstitial Disease

The nodular pattern of interstitial lung disease is usually characterized by nodules between 5 mm and 1 cm in size. It is often difficult to differentiate miliary disease from nodular disease and nodular disease from reticulonodular disease.

NODULAR INTERSTITIAL DISEASE

- Neonatal aspiration
- Necrotizing angitis
- Wegener's granulomatosis
- Alveolar microlithiasis
- Thyroid carcinoma metastases

In the neonate, the most common cause of a nodular pattern on the chest x-ray is aspiration of either amniotic fluid or meconium (Fig. 3–29). Rapid resolution is indicative of a large amount of amniotic fluid in the aspirate. Development of widespread subsegmental and segmental atelectasis indicates a high proportion of meconium in the aspirate. Other less common conditions that may rarely present with small nodules include necrotizing angiitis, Wegener's granulomatosis, idiopathic pulmonary alveolar microlithiasis, and metastatic spread of thyroid carcinoma. The last two entities demonstrate calcified nodules. However, the nodules are often so small that the calcifications are difficult to appreciate.

Reticulonodular Interstitial Disease

A more common pattern of interstitial lung disease in children is the reticulonodular pattern. Congenital causes of bilateral diffuse reticulonodular infiltrates include pulmonary lymphangiomyomatosis associated with Turner's syndrome, Gaucher's disease, Niemann-Pick disease, and tuberous sclerosis (Fig. 3–30). Involvement of the lungs in tuberous sclerosis is rarely seen without widespread involvement of other organs (cysts or hamartomas of the kidneys, rhabdomyomas of the heart, intracranial lesions, the characteristic skin lesions of adenoma sebaceum, and subungual fibromas).

A

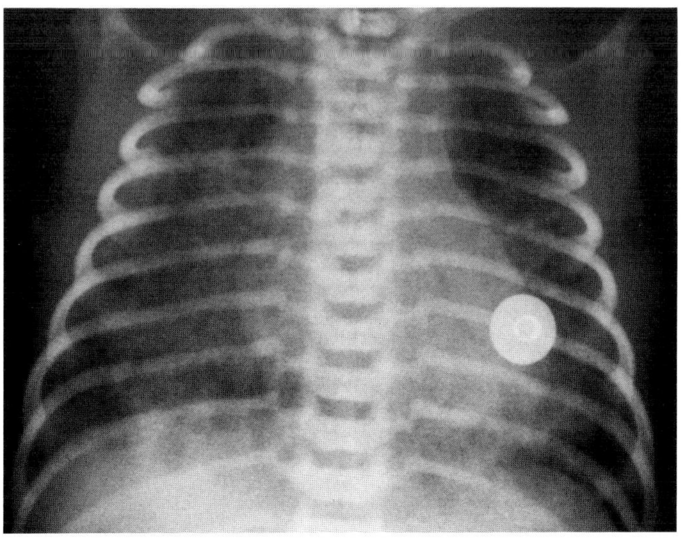

Fig. 3–29 Nodular interstitial disease. **(A)** Anteroposterior chest x-ray of a neonate in respiratory distress demonstrates multiple ill-defined nodular densities scattered throughout the lungs with areas of atelectasis in both bases. This pattern did not resolve promptly and represented meconium aspiration. (*Figure continues.*)

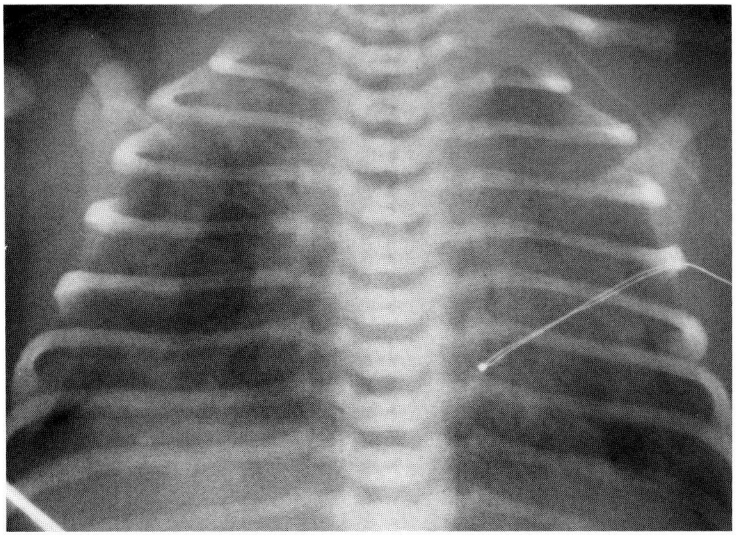

B

Fig. 3–29 (*Continued*). **(B)** Radiograph of another neonate demonstrates large bilateral nodular densities. Volume loss is seen in the left lower lobe. After intubation, the infiltrates cleared rapidly consistent with amniotic fluid aspiration.

RETICULONODULAR INTERSTITIAL DISEASE

Diffuse reticulonodular
- Lymphangiomyomatosis
- Gaucher's disease
- Neimann-Pick disease
- Tuberous sclerosis

Local reticulonodular
- *Mycoplasma pneumoniae*
- Opportunistic viral infection
- Drug reaction
- Leukemia/lymphoma
- Collagen-vascular diseases

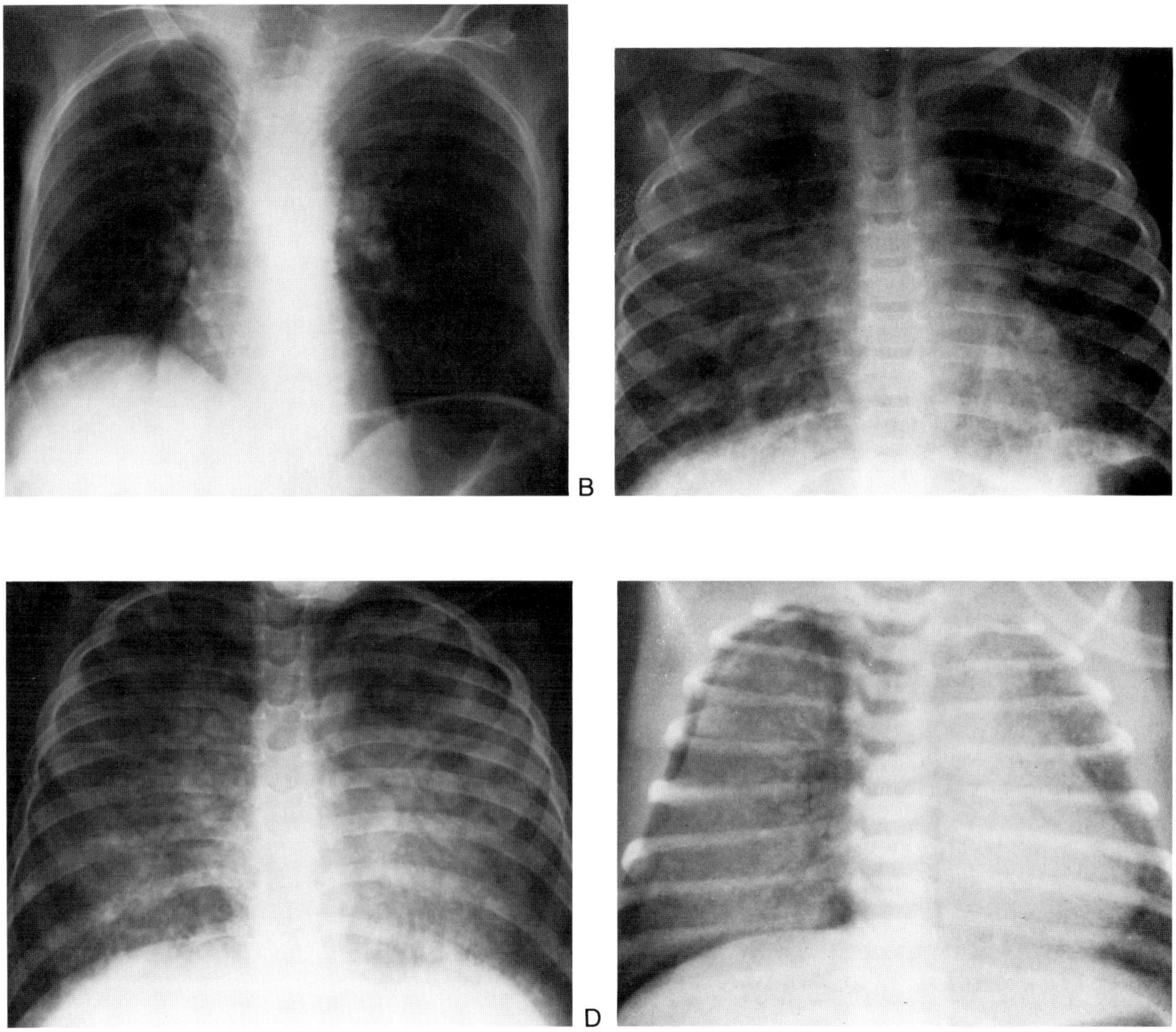

Fig. 3–30 Bilateral diffuse reticulonodular infiltrates. **(A)** Note the fine reticulonodular pattern throughout the lungs in this patient with Gaucher's disease. **(B)** A fine reticulonodular pattern is seen throughout the lungs in this patient with widespread metastasis from neuroblastoma. **(C)** The same patient 6 months later demonstrates an increase in the diffuse reticulonodular lung involvement and development of a right pneumothorax. **(D)** Note the diffuse dense reticulonodular infiltrates opacifying the lungs of this neonate. The autopsy diagnosis was pulmonary lymphangiomyomatosis.

The most common cause of a localized reticulonodular infiltrate is *M. pneumoniae* (Fig. 3–31). Opportunistic viral infections are common in patients with congenital, acquired, and iatrogenic immunodeficiency syndromes. Most patients with combined immunodeficiency of both B and T cell systems have a greater predilection for development of viral pulmonary infections. Although immunization programs have decreased the incidence of severe viral infections in childhood, measles pneumonia is still seen and usually presents as a reticulonodular pattern (Fig. 3–32). Both measles and varicella pneumonia are common in children who have leukemia or lymphoma.

Aside from opportunistic infection, reticulonodular infiltrates may develop in patients with leukemia or lymphoma as reactions to transfusions or chemotherapy, or they may represent pulmonary edema or hemorrhage. The least common cause of pulmonary opacities in patients with leukemia is infiltration of the lung by leukemic cells. This is very rare in children and is most often seen in acute monocytic leukemia. Occasionally leukemic infiltrates develop very rapidly. Surgical biopsy may be required for diagnosis. Collagen-vascular diseases may also cause a reticulonodular pattern.

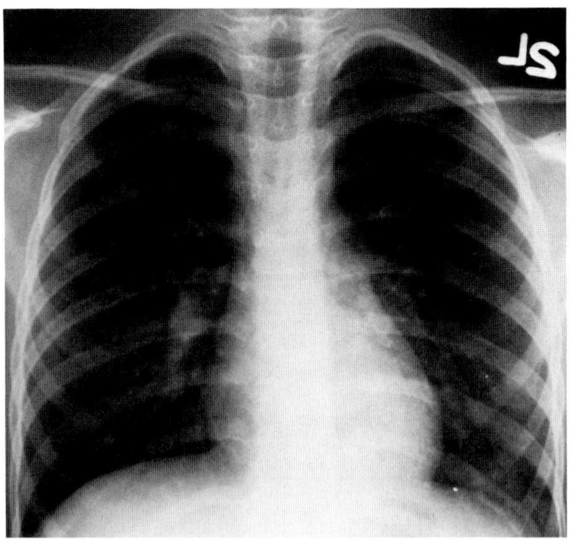

Fig. 3–31 Localized reticulonodular infiltrate. This 9-year-old child presented with a 9-day history of cough and wheezing. Notice the fine reticulonodular pattern in the left lower lobe. The patient responded to erythromycin therapy for *Mycoplasma pneumoniae*.

Fine Interstitial Reticularity

Fine reticularity is recognized in the neonatal period as a granular pattern of diffuse lung involvement (Fig. 3–33). This pattern is most commonly seen with hyaline membrane disease or respiratory distress syndrome. The granular appearance in hyaline membrane disease is caused by the uniform size of over-distended terminal airways (type I bubbles). Occasionally, neonatal pneumonias, tuberous sclerosis, and pulmonary venous obstruction may have the same appearance. Transient tachypnea of the newborn may occasionally appear granular, although bilateral radiating streaks are more common.

In older patients infection is the most likely cause of fine reticularity. Infectious mononucleosis and *P. carinii* pneumonia present with this pattern.

Coarse Interstitial Reticularity

Coarse interstitial reticularity appears as small bubbly lungs in neonates. Congenital causes include lymphangiomyomatosis, tuberous sclerosis, and Wilson-Mikity syndrome. Wilson-Mikity syndrome occurs

RETICULARITY (INTERSTITIAL DISEASE)

Fine reticularity
- Tuberous sclerosis
- Pulmonary venous obstruction
- Neonatal pneumonia
- *Pneumocystis carinii*
- Infectious mononucleosis
- Respiratory distress syndrome (granular)
- Retained fetal lung fluid (transient tachypnea)

Coarse reticularity
- Lymphangiomyomatosis
- Tuberous sclerosis
- Wilson-Mikity syndrome
- Histiocytosis X
- Bronchopulmonary dysplasia

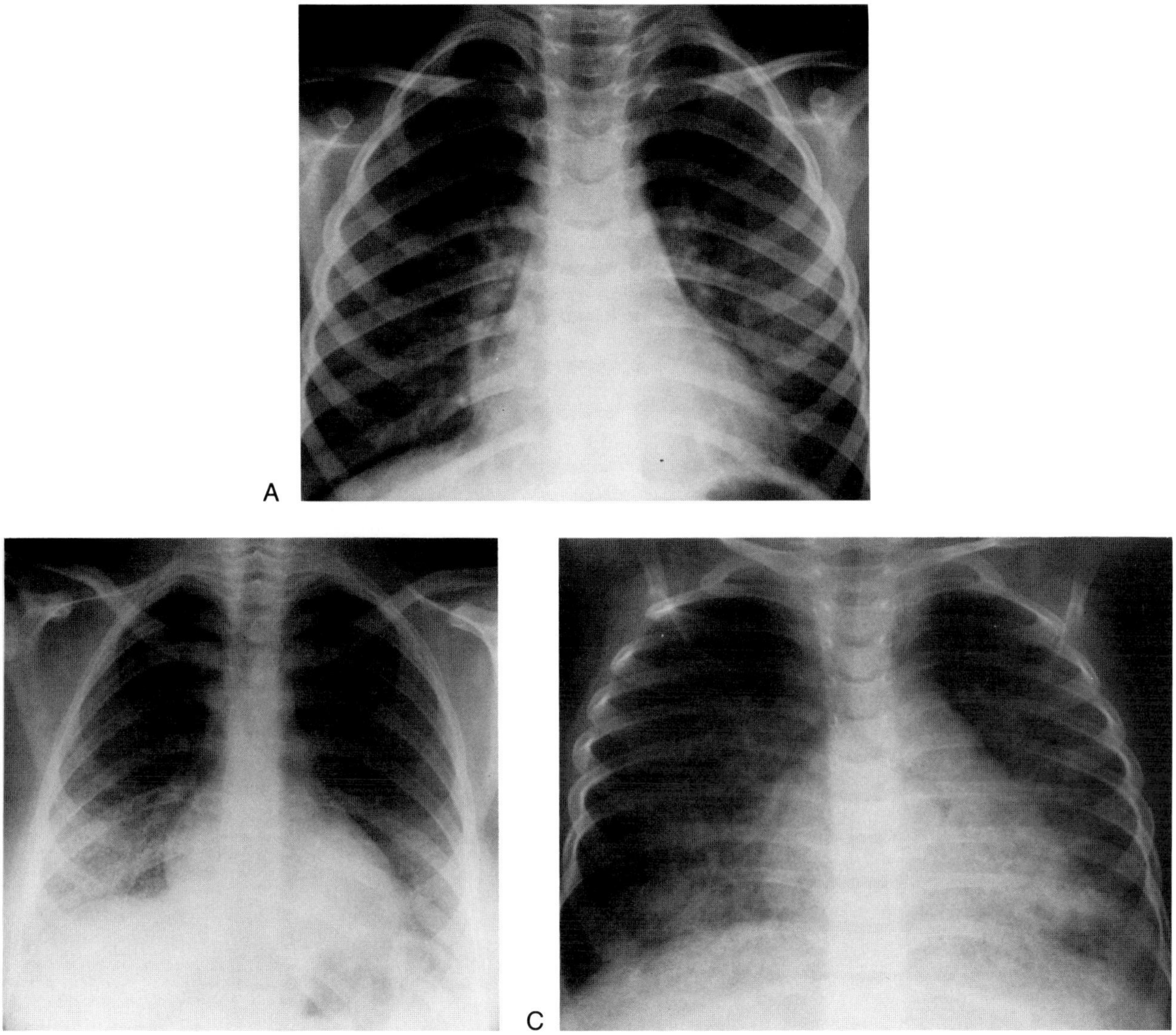

Fig. 3–32 Viral reticulonodular infiltrates. **(A)** Radiograph of a 5-year-old patient demonstrates mild reticulonodular changes bilaterally. Note the indistinctness of the pulmonary vascularity in the upper lobes. He developed a rash typical of measles within hours of the x-ray. **(B)** Note the diffuse reticulonodular pattern throughout the lungs of an immunosuppressed 15-year-old renal transplant patient. The lung changes were due to cytomegalovirus pneumonia. **(C)** Radiographic examination of this 3-year-old AIDS patient demonstrates bilateral diffuse interstitial infiltrates with central nodularity and peripheral reticularity. Lung biopsy revealed lymphoid interstitial pneumonitis, presumed to be a local response to antigenic viral stimuli rather than infection.

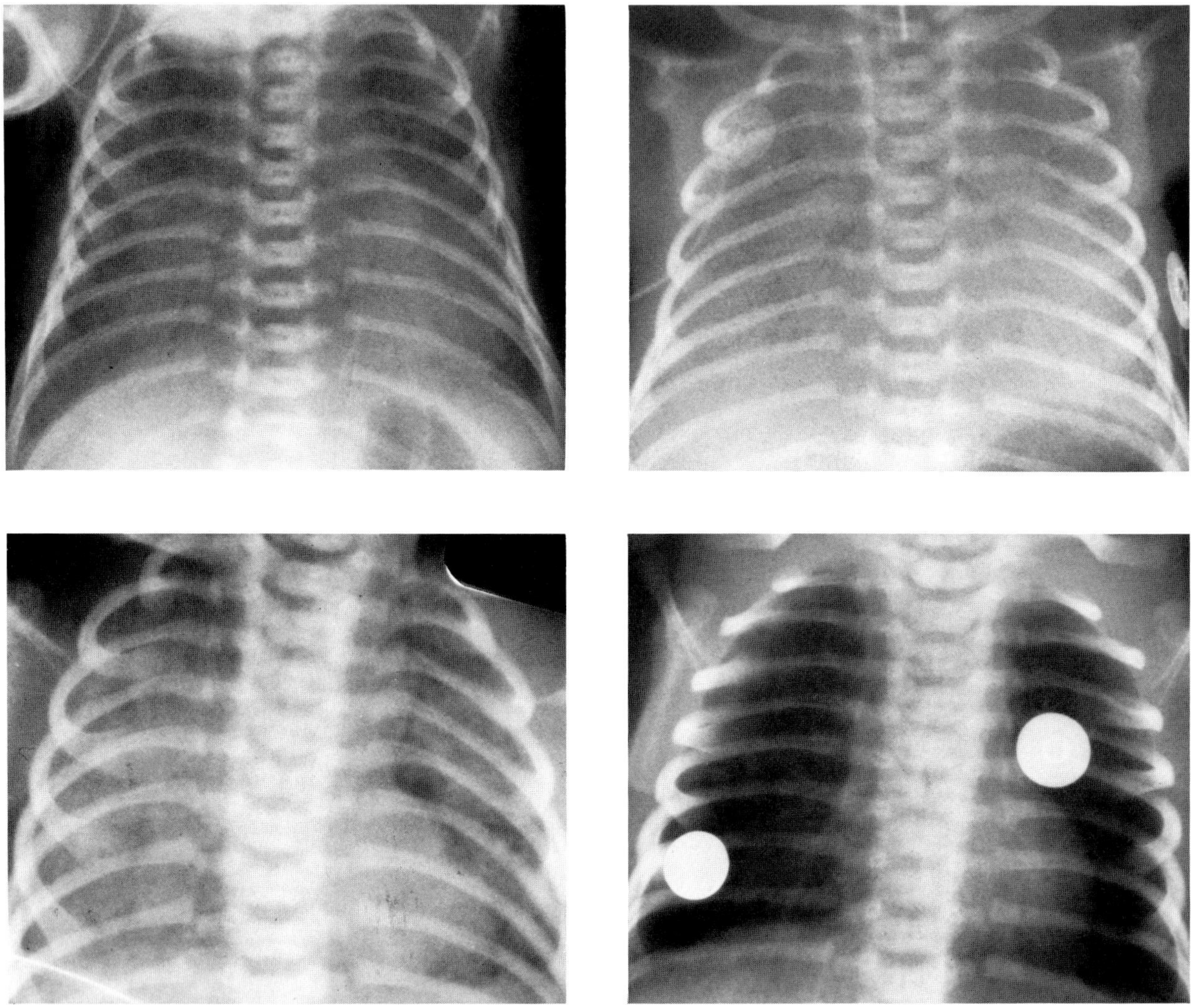

Fig. 3–33 Fine interstitial reticularity. **(A)** Anteroposterior chest x-ray of a neonate with respiratory distress syndrome demonstrates small lungs with a subtle granular pattern and peripheral air bronchograms. **(B)** Anteroposterior chest x-ray of another infant with respiratory distress syndrome demonstrates a granular pattern and typical type I bubbles. **(C)** A third infant also demonstrates respiratory distress and small lungs on the first radiograph obtained after birth. Neither granularity nor air bronchograms are present. The lungs are diffusely hazy. Occasionally, respiratory distress syndrome may present with this pattern. **(D)** Follow-up examination taken 24 hours later demonstrates complete clearing of the lungs consistent with transient tachypnea of the newborn. Hyaline membrane disease will not clear this rapidly.

in premature infants who are normal at birth but develop cyanosis and respiratory distress before 4 weeks of age. Focal nodular infiltrates are seen early on the chest x-rays. The symptoms continue and may increase for several months. In the later stages of the disease coarse reticularity develops, with bubbles of varying sizes on the radiographs. Luckily, complete clinical and radiographic resolution occurs by 2 years of age. The etiology of Wilson-Mikity syndrome remains unknown. It is thought to occur in patients who do not have hyaline membrane disease but who may develop oxygen toxicity under normal atmospheric conditions.

When high concentrations of oxygen are used in the neonatal period, bronchopulmonary dysplasia may result in the formation of type III bubbles, cystic spaces of varying sizes collapsible on expiration (Fig. 3–34). These patients commonly have hyaline membrane disease at birth and rapidly become ventilator-

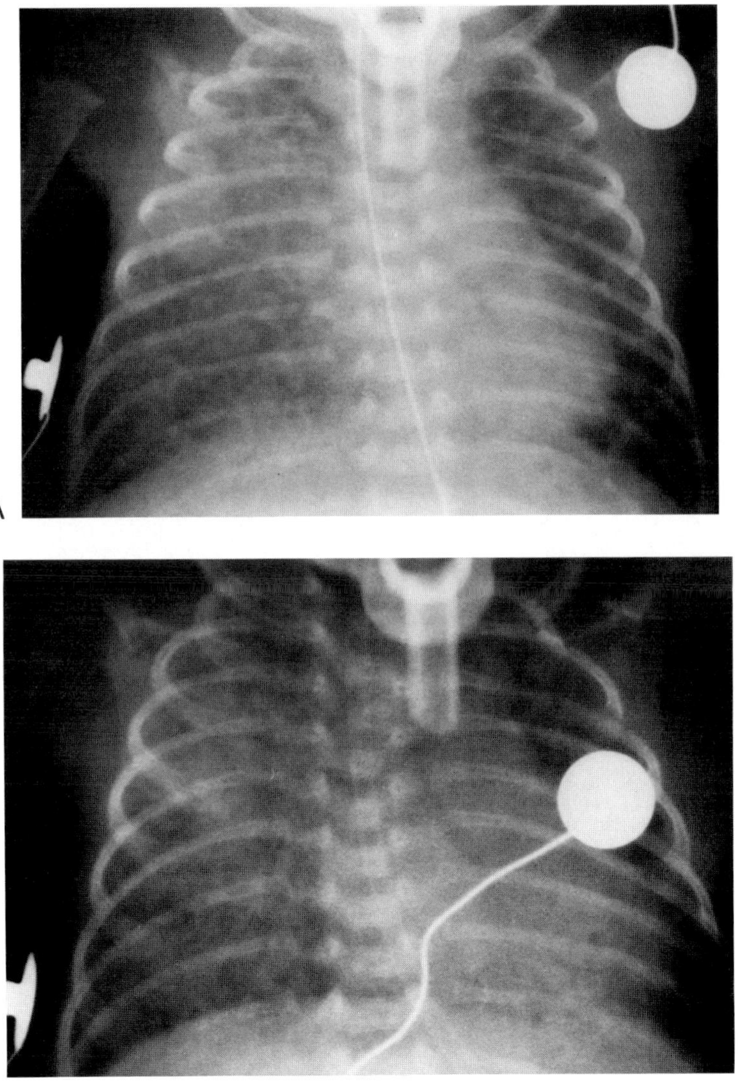

A

B

Fig. 3–34 Coarse reticular infiltrates. **(A)** Inspiratory frontal chest x-ray shows cystic spaces of varying sizes consistent with type III bubbles. **(B)** When the infant exhales, the bubbles collapse. (*Figure continues.*)

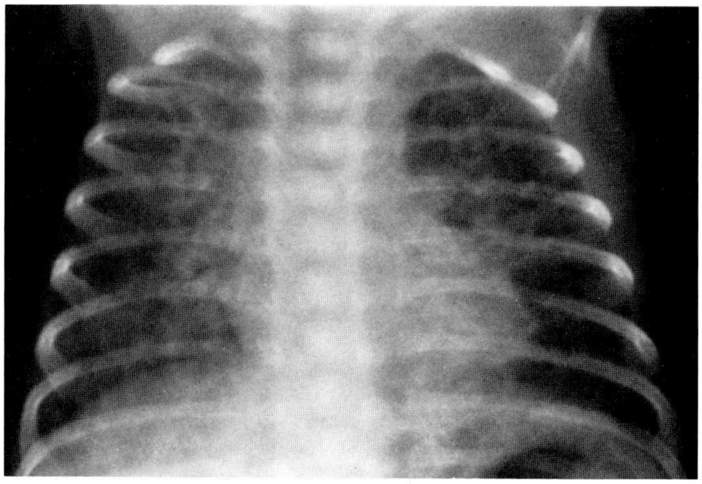

C

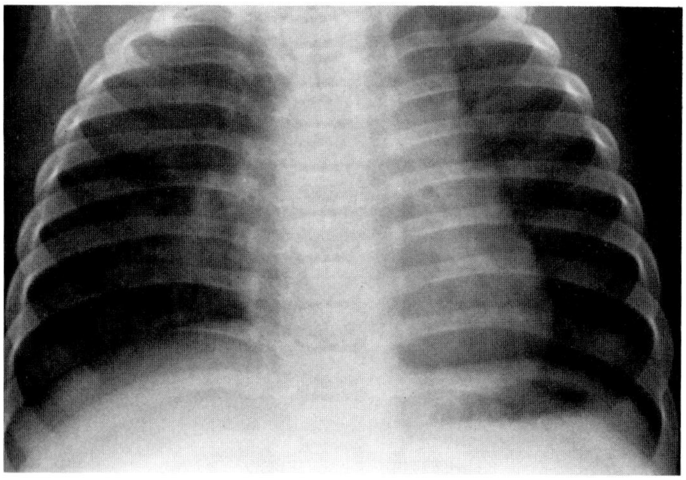

D

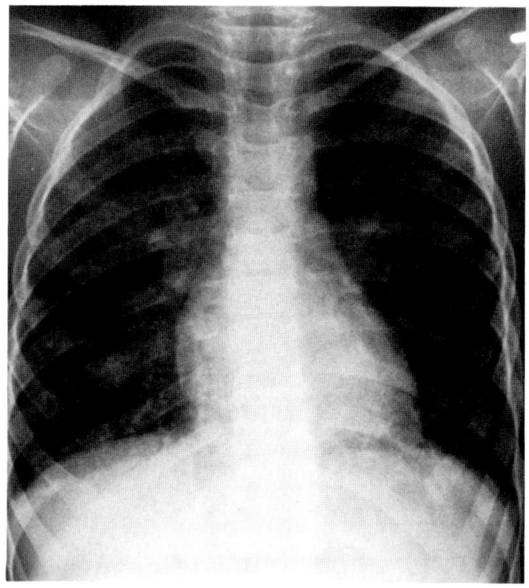

E

Fig. 3–34 (*Continued*). **(C)** Similar findings of diffuse coarse reticularity seen in an infant with Wilson-Mikity syndrome. **(D)** Follow-up posteroanterior chest x-ray 6 years later shows normal lungs. **(E)** Posteroanterior view of a 5-year-old patient demonstrates coarse reticulonodular infiltrates the lung periphery, consistent with histiocytosis X.

dependent. However, bronchopulmonary dysplasia may develop in any neonate requiring high FiO_2 and pressures for adequate oxygenation. As opposed to Wilson-Mikity syndrome, bronchopulmonary dysplasia is associated with long-term pulmonary and cardiovascular complications including recurrent lower respiratory tract infections, pulmonary hypertension, ventricular hypertrophy, and persistent fetal circulation syndrome.

In the older age group, coarse reticular markings appear as honeycomb lungs. This finding may be seen in histiocytosis X. Although eosinophilic granuloma is the most common of the reticuloendothelioses to cause this pattern in the adult, Letterer-Siwe disease and Hand-Schüller-Christian disease are more apt to cause lung involvement in young infants. Honeycomb lungs may develop in any chronic interstitial process that has progressed to fibrosis.

Parahilar Peribronchial Infiltrates

Another common interstitial pattern seen in children is linear opacities radiating from the cardiomediastinal structures; referred to as *parahilar peribronchial infiltrates*. This pattern is most common with viral lower respiratory tract infections and may be associated with hyperinflation and subsegmental and segmental atelectasis (Fig. 3–35). In neonates, streaky infiltrates that clear rapidly (within 6 to 12 hours) may be secondary to retained fetal lung fluid and transient tachypnea. Other considerations in neonates are cytomegalovirus infection and chlamydia pneumonia (Fig. 3–36). Inborn abnormalities that may not be apparent immediately at birth but may result in parahilar peribronchial infiltrates when the patient does become symptomatic include congenital combined immunodeficiency, cystic fibrosis, and familial dysautonomia. Chronic aspiration may result in cicatrization atelectasis and a parahilar peribronchial distribution.

A

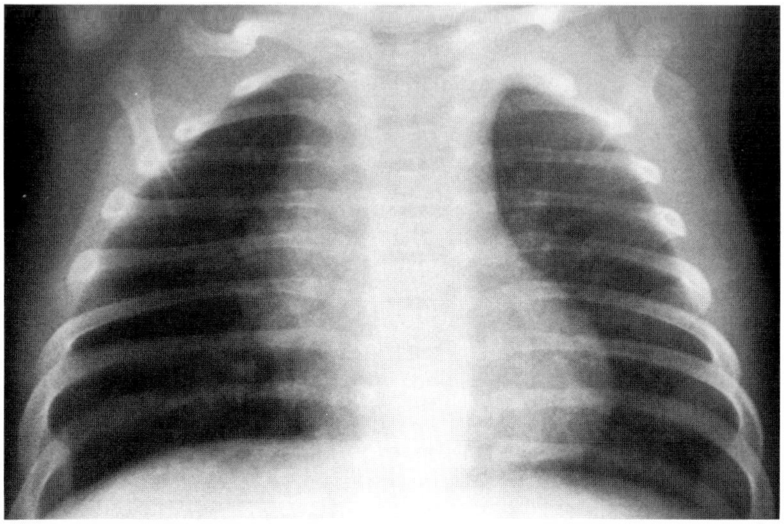

Fig. 3–35 Parahilar peribronchial infiltrates. **(A)** Anteroposterior chest x-ray of an infant with mild respiratory distress symptoms. Note the indistinctness of the pulmonary vessels as they exit the hila. (*Figure continues.*)

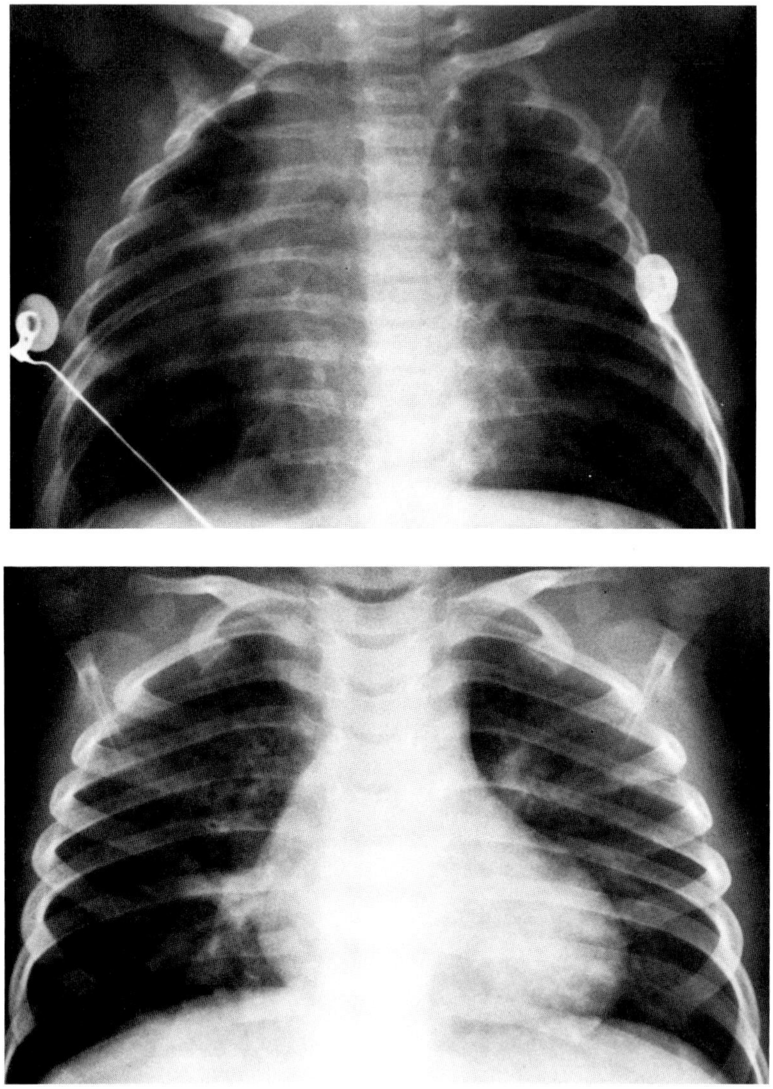

B

C

Fig. 3–35 (*Continued*). **(B)** A repeat chest x-ray obtained several days later demonstrates worsening of the parahilar peribronchial infiltrates and right upper lobe segmental atelectasis. Note subsegmental atelectasis in both bases. The ill-defined opacity overlying the periphery of the right middle lobe is an artifact from the ECG lead. Note a similar artifact in the soft tissues on the left. The lung disease was caused by respiratory synsitial virus. **(C)** Another child with measles pneumonia demonstrates bilateral parahilar peribronchial infiltrates with subsegmental atelectasis in the lung bases. Note the cuffing around the bronchi on end. (*Figure continues.*)

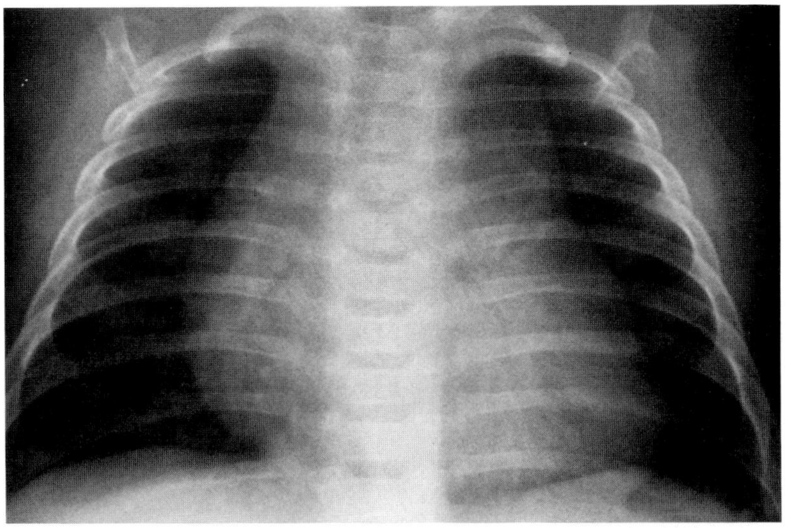

D

Fig. 3–35 (*Continued*). **(D)** Anteroposterior chest x-ray of a child with pertussis demonstrating mild parahilar peribronchial infiltrates.

PARAHILAR PERIBRONCHIAL INFILTRATES (INTERSTITIAL DISEASE)

Viral pneumonia

Neonatal pneumonia (Cytomegalovirus, *Chlamydia*)

Transient tachypnea of the newborn

Cystic fibrosis

Familial dysautonomia

Congenital combined immunodeficiency

Scarring due to chronic aspiration

Mycoplasma pneumoniae

Reticuloendothelioses (early)

Alveolar proteinosis (early)

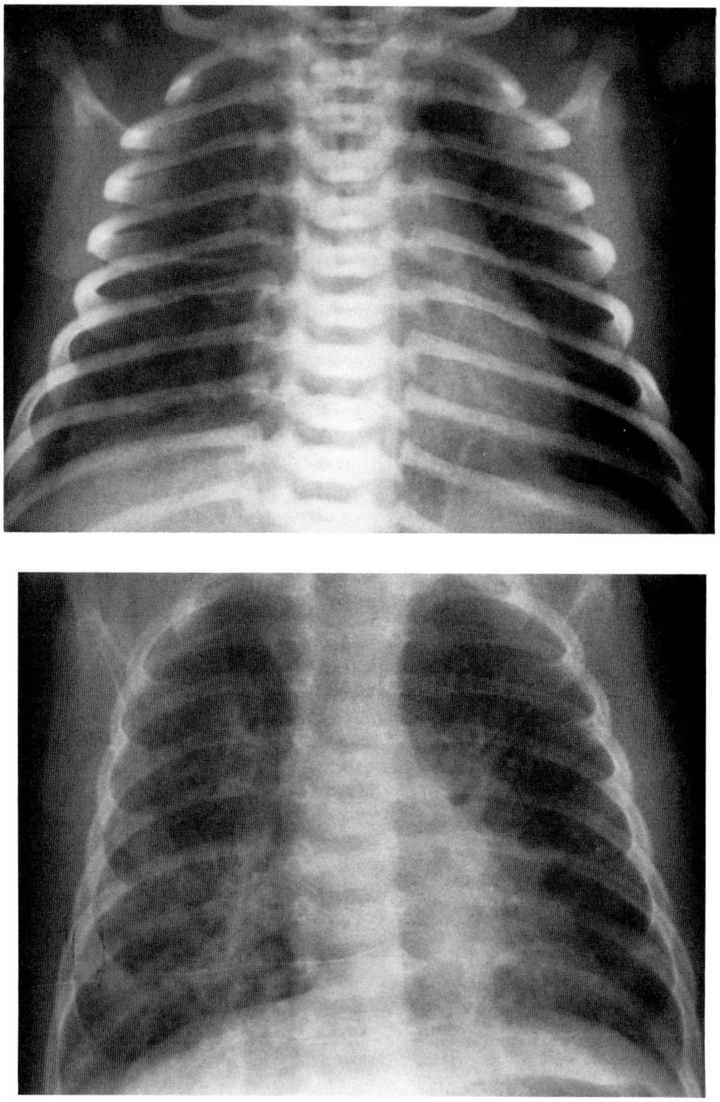

A

B

Fig. 3–36 Neonatal parahilar peribronchial infiltrates. **(A)** This neonate presented with mild respiratory distress. Note the exaggeration of the parahilar peribronchial markings radiating from the mediastinum. This cleared within 24 hours and represented transient tachypnea. **(B)** Another neonate with labored respirations. The severe bilateral parahilar peribronchial infiltrates were due to chlamydia pneumonia.

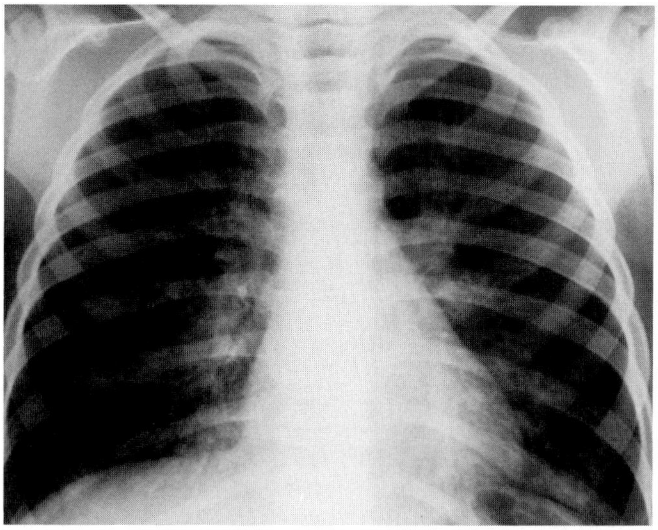

Fig. 3–37 *Mycoplasma pneumoniae.* Note the bilateral parahilar peribronchial infiltrates present. Subsegmental atelectasis is seen behind the heart. A reticulonodular pattern is noted in the right lower lung. This 5-year-old patient had a 2-week history of cough with no fever and responded to erythromycin therapy.

Outside of infancy, *M. pneumoniae* is a common cause of parahilar peribronchial infiltrates (Fig. 3–37). *M. pneumoniae* infection is associated with low grade fever and chronic cough. Treatment is oral erythromycin. In the early stages, both the reticuloendothelioses and alveolar proteinosis have a similar appearance.

SOLITARY CYST

The differential diagnosis for cystic lesions is based on the size, number, and location of the cysts. The most common cause of a solitary cyst is an inflammatory pneumatocele (Table 3–7). Pneumatoceles are usually thin-walled and develop in about 50 percent of children with staphylococcal pneumonia (Fig. 3–38). The occurrence of pneumatoceles associated with other bacterial pneumonias is less common. Pneumatoceles are thought to represent a form of subpleural emphysema. The second most common cause of a solitary cystic lesion in childhood is a lung abscess. Lung abscesses are usually thick-walled with a shaggy inner lining and a hazy periphery due to surrounding edema. After antibiotic therapy is started, the abscess wall may become thin; differentiation between it and a pneumatocele may become more difficult. Abscesses are more likely to contain air/fluid levels than pneumatoceles (Fig. 3–39). Lung abscesses are most frequently caused by staphylococcal sepsis in childhood. *K. pneumoniae* and gram-negative organisms have also been implicated. Occasionally, a neonatal lung abscess may be associated with underlying cystic adenomatoid malformation. Therefore, in the newborn period, surgery is often indicated in addition to antimicrobial therapy. Most lung abscesses are associated with empyemas.

Although relatively rare, congenital causes of solitary cysts include bronchopulmonary foregut malformations, neurenteric cysts, and hiatal hernia.

Aside from bacterial pneumatoceles and abscesses, the inflammatory causes of a solitary cyst include pneumatocele formation secondary to tuberculosis, cavitary tuberculosis, and echinococcus cysts. Hydatid disease is caused by the tapeworm *Echinococcus granulosus,* which is endemic in sheep-raising countries such as Australia, Chile, Argentina, Uruguay, Africa, the USSR, and the Mediterranean coast. In the United States, the tapeworm is encountered in Alaska and in the lower Mississippi River Valley.

Table 3–7 Solitary Cyst

Type	Cause
Pneumatocele	Inflammatory
	Staphylococcal pneumonia
	Other bacteria
	Tuberculosis
	Trauma
	Blunt
	Penetrating
	Accidental ingestion of hydrocarbons
Abscess	Inflammatory
	Staphylococcal sepsis
	Klebsiella pneumoniae
	Gram-negative bacteria
	Congenital
	Cystic adenomatoid malformation
	Aspiration
Congenital	Bronchogenic cyst
	Bronchopulmonary foregut malformation
	Neurenteric cyst
	Hiatal hernia
Cavitary lesion	Inflammatory
	Tuberculosis
	Echnococcus cyst
	Tumor
	Primary
	Metastatic
	Trauma
	Hematoma
	Thromboembolis

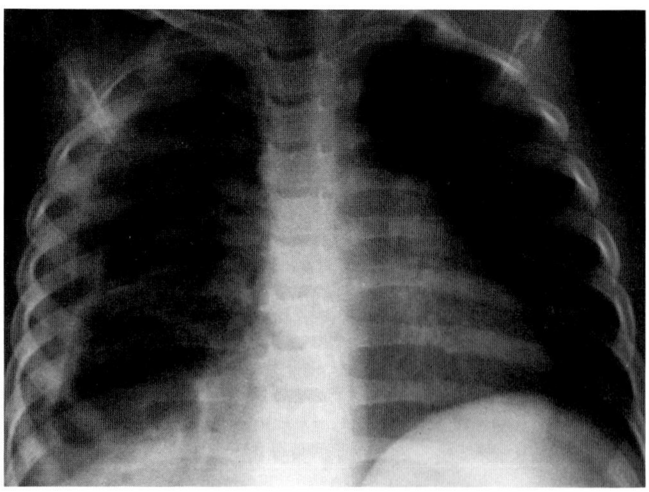

Fig. 3–38 Notice the single thin-walled cavity in the right middle lobe of a patient with resolving staphylococcal pneumonia. The inflammatory pneumatocele and right pleural effusion resolved without residual scarring.

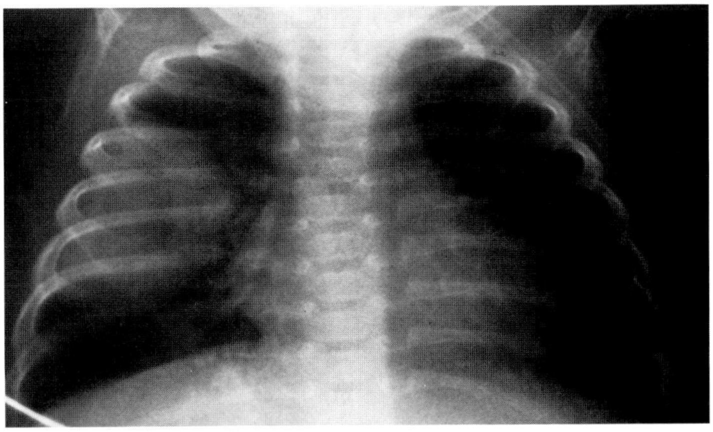

Fig. 3–39 Lung abscess. This infant had a 2-week history of a right-sided well-defined pneumonia that evolved into the right-sided mass seen. Instead of an air/fluid level, a centrally located gas bubble is seen because the patient is supine. Percutaneous drainage of the *Staphylococcus aureus* abscess was curative.

Although the liver is the organ that contains the higher number of worm embryos, it is lung involvement that brings the patient to medical attention. Radiographically, echinococcosis may present as a solitary mass or cyst predominately involving the lower lobes posteriorly, the right more common than the left (Fig. 3–40). Classic radiographic signs occur either when there is rupture between the pericyst and exocyst causing a thin crescent of air around the periphery (air crescent sign) or when the cyst ruptures into the bronchial tree and the membrane floats on the resulting fluid level (camalote sign). Rarely, the cyst wall may calcify.

The least common cause of a solitary cystic lesion in a child's lung is pulmonary tumor. Only rarely has solitary pulmonary metastasis with cavitation been reported in children. Neoplasm would most likely present as a solitary pulmonary nodule.

Traumatic causes of solitary lung cysts are fairly common. Pneumatocele formation may be secondary to blunt or penetrating trauma and are usually multiple.

Occasionally, pulmonary hematomas may cavitate. A miscellaneous cause of pneumatocele formation is hydrocarbon pneumonia. Accidental ingestion of hydrocarbons is a common form of childhood poisoning. Occasionally, neurologically impaired children may aspirate causing abscess formation. Systemic and metabolic causes of a solitary cystic lesion in the lung are very rare. Occasionally a pulmonary infarct may cavitate resulting in this appearance.

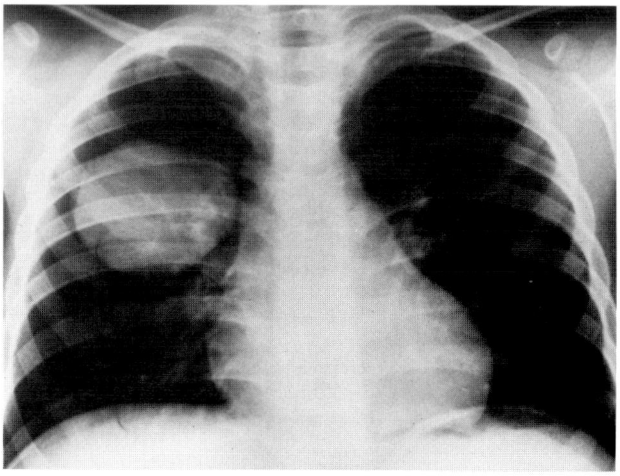

Fig. 3–40 Hydatid disease. Note the round, sharply-demarcated, slightly lobulated soft tissue density in the right upper lobe. The child had a persistent cough. At surgery, an echinococcal cyst was found.

MULTIPLE CYSTS

When one encounters multiple cystic lesions of the lungs, determining whether the cysts are localized or widespread may simplify the differential diagnosis (Table 3–8).

Multiple Cysts Localized to One Part of the Lung

The most common cause of localized lung cysts is multiple inflammatory pneumatoceles usually secondary to staphylococcal pneumonia. A lobar distribution is favored (Fig. 3–41). Pneumatoceles commonly develop within 1 week after the onset of pneumonia and disappear in approximately 6 weeks. Their appearance is characterized by rapid changes, although sometimes pneumatoceles persist for 1 year or longer. Some pneumatoceles are so large they may mimic tension pneumothorax.

Other causes of localized lung cysts are much less common. Congenital abnormalities that merit consideration include cystic adenomatoid malformation, bronchopulmonary foregut malformation, and congenital diaphragmatic hernia.

Table 3–8 Multiple Cysts

Type	Cause
Localized cysts	
Pneumatoceles	Inflammatory
	Staphylococcal pneumonia
	Other bacteria
	Tuberculosis
	Trauma
	Blunt
	Penetrating
	Accidental ingestion of hydrocarbons
Congenital cysts	Cystic adenomatoid malformation
	Bronchopulmonary foregut malformation
	Congenital diaphragmatic hernia
Bronchiectasis	Inflammatory
	Recurrent infection
	Systemic disease
	Cystic fibrosis
Interstitial emphysema	Ventilator assistance
Terminal alveolograms	Hyaline membrane disease
Bilateral cysts	
Chronic disease	Bronchopulmonary displasia
	Wilson-Mikity syndrome
	Cystic fibrosis
Interstitial emphysema	Ventilator assistance
Cavitary lesions	Inflammatory
	Septic emboli
	Neoplasm
	Laryngeal papilloma
	Hematogenous metastases
Pneumatoceles	Immunologic disease
	Wegener's granulomatosis
	Hyperimmunoglobulinema E

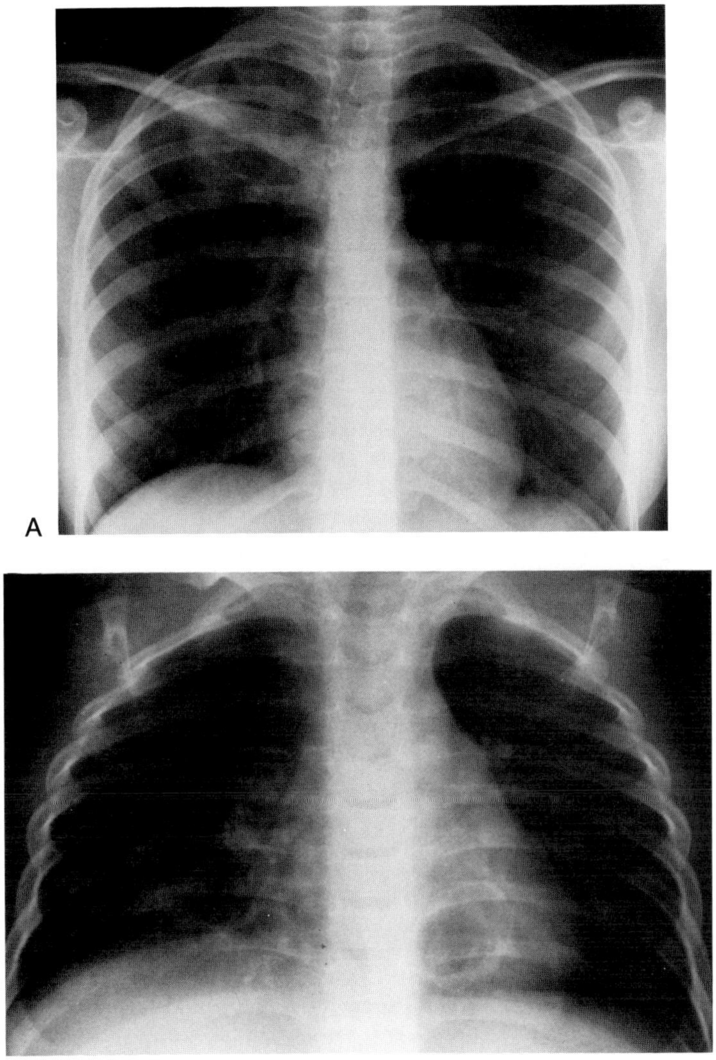

A

B

Fig. 3–41 Multiple localized cysts. **(A)** Note several large thin-walled cavities in the right upper lobe secondary to staphylococcal pneumonia. **(B)** Note the thin-walled cysts present in both lower lobes of another patient. The lower lobe distribution is consistent with the child's history of ingestion of lighter fluid. The inflammatory pneumatoceles developed a week after ingestion.

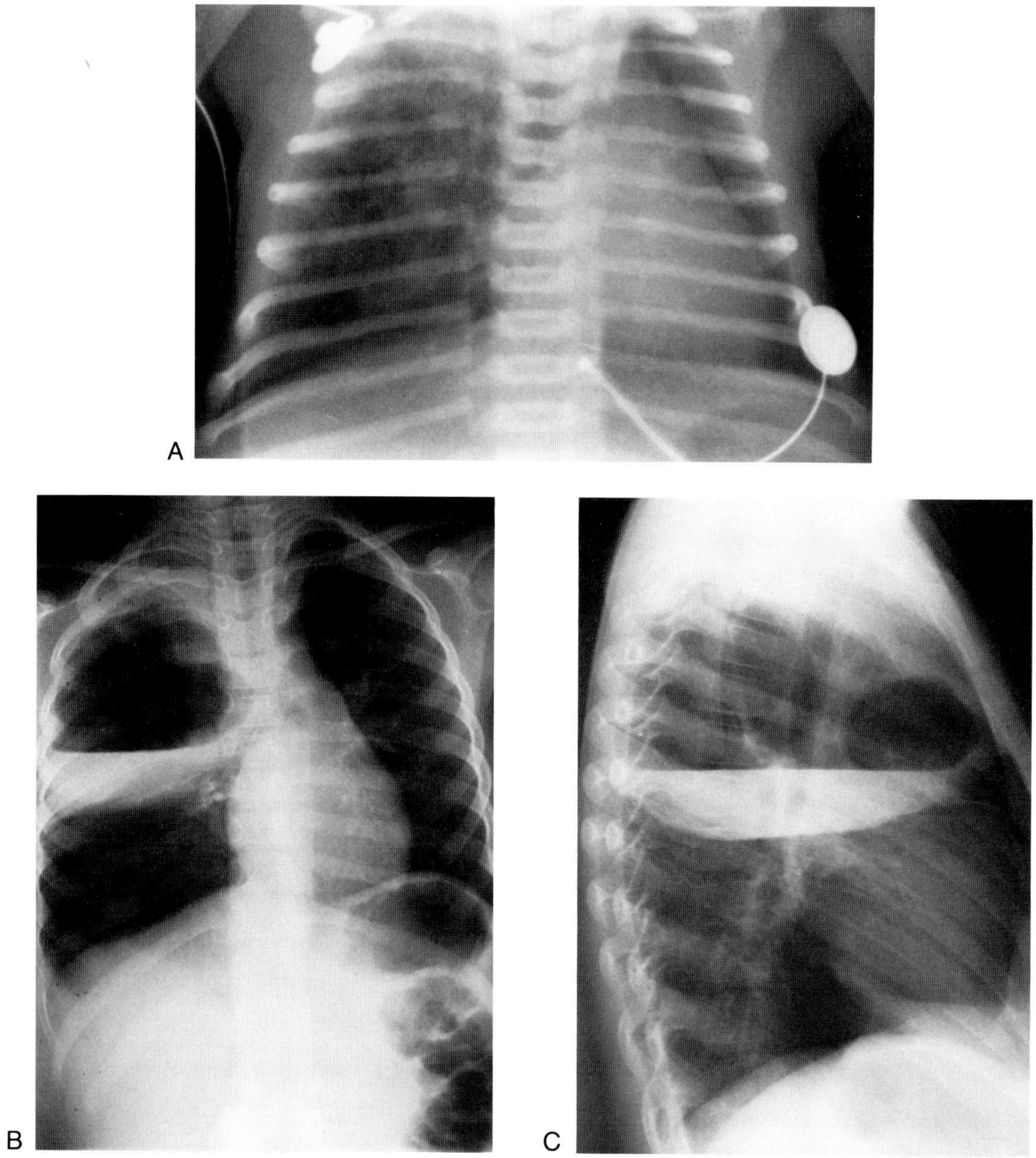

Fig. 3–42 Cystic adenomatoid malformation. **(A)** Frontal chest view of a neonate demonstrates tiny cysts in the right upper lobe. **(B)** Posteroanterior chest x-ray of the same patient at age 6 shows a solitary cystic space with an air/fluid level in the right upper lobe. **(C)** Lateral view confirms the upper lobe location of the cystic adenomatoid malformation.

Cystic adenomatoid malformation is a congenital overgrowth of the terminal respiratory structures manifested by various-sized cysts that communicate with each other. Although a bronchial communication is usually present, the respiratory structures are disorganized. The blood supply is from the pulmonary artery. The clinical hallmark of this anomaly is respiratory distress presenting in the first day of life; this is related to expansion of the adenomatoid cysts. The most common radiographic pattern is multiple cystic lesions of varying sizes (Fig. 3–42). These often demonstrate air/fluid levels. The left lower lobe is most commonly involved, however, any lobe may be affected; multilobar involvement has been reported. Although most cystic adenomatoid malformations are detected in the neonatal period, an increasing number are being discovered on antenatal ultrasound studies for maternal polyhydramnios. A triad of polyhydramnios, fetal hydrops, and either a cystic or solid unilateral lung mass has been described. Rarely, the cysts can enlarge to such a degree that the walls are too thin to be detected and the findings may be confused with congenital lobar emphysema or pneumothorax. These patients are usually asymptomatic. Recently, cases of sarcomatous transformation in cystic mesenchymal hamartomas have been reported. For this reason, surgical resection is recommended.

Bronchopulmonary foregut malformations include a spectrum of abnormalities thought to be caused by a supernumerary lung bud that develops below the normal lung bud. The location, severity, and communication with the gastrointestinal tract appear to be determined by when in embryonic life the supernumerary bud develops. Pulmonary sequestration is defined as nonfunctioning pulmonary tissue without a normal connection to either the bronchial tree or the pulmonary arteries. Extralobar sequestrations are enclosed by visceral pleura that is separate from that of the adjacent lung. In contrast, intralobar sequestration shares the same visceral pleura as the involved lobe. The posterior basal segment of the left lower lobe is the usual site of both types of sequestration although the extralobar variety is more likely to occur below the diaphragm (accessory lung). The arterial blood supply usually arises from the aorta. Venous drainage may flow into the pulmonary veins, azygos system, or portal system. Associated anomalies include congenital diaphragmatic hernia, partial absence of the pericardium, and anomalous pulmonary venous return. Although most bronchopulmonary foregut malformations present as a solid lung mass, those that communicate with the gastrointestinal tract or become infected will present as multiloculated cysts (Fig. 3–43).

While cystic adenomatoid malformation and congenital diaphragmatic hernia present most commonly as surgical emergencies in the neonatal period, pulmonary sequestration usually goes undetected until adolescence or adulthood. MRI is an excellent noninvasive method of identifying the anomalous arterial supply.

Congenital diaphragmatic hernia usually presents as respiratory distress in the newborn period. The most common herniation occurs through the left foramen of Bochdalek (pleuroperitoneal canal). Usually, portions of the gastrointestinal tract, such as the stomach and left colon, herniate through the defect. However, on occasion, solid organs such as the spleen or a kidney may herniate through the defect. Herniations may also occur through the right posterior foramen of Bochdalek, foramen of Morgagni, the diaphragmatic crura, or into the pericardial sac. Rarely, diaphragmatic hernias may be bilateral. If the right hemidiaphragm is defective, solitary herniation of the liver may occur. Occasionally, the omentum or the right kidney may herniate into the right hemithorax as well. Early on, diaphragmatic hernias present as a large opaque hemithorax. With the onset of swallowing, the bowel loops rapidly become air-filled resulting in a multicystic appearance (Fig. 3–44). Examination of the upper abdomen provides the key to the correct diagnosis since the bowel gas pattern is abnormal or, if herniation is on the right, the liver silhouette is absent. Either air or barium may be introduced into the gastrointestinal tract for further evaluation if necessary. Often, a screening ultrasound examination of the involved hemithorax provides the diagnosis.

Although antenatal detection of congenital diaphragmatic hernia is becoming more common, there has been no significant change in the morbidity and mortality associated with this lesion. Pulmonary insufficiency is responsible for the majority of deaths in this condition and is due to associated pulmonary

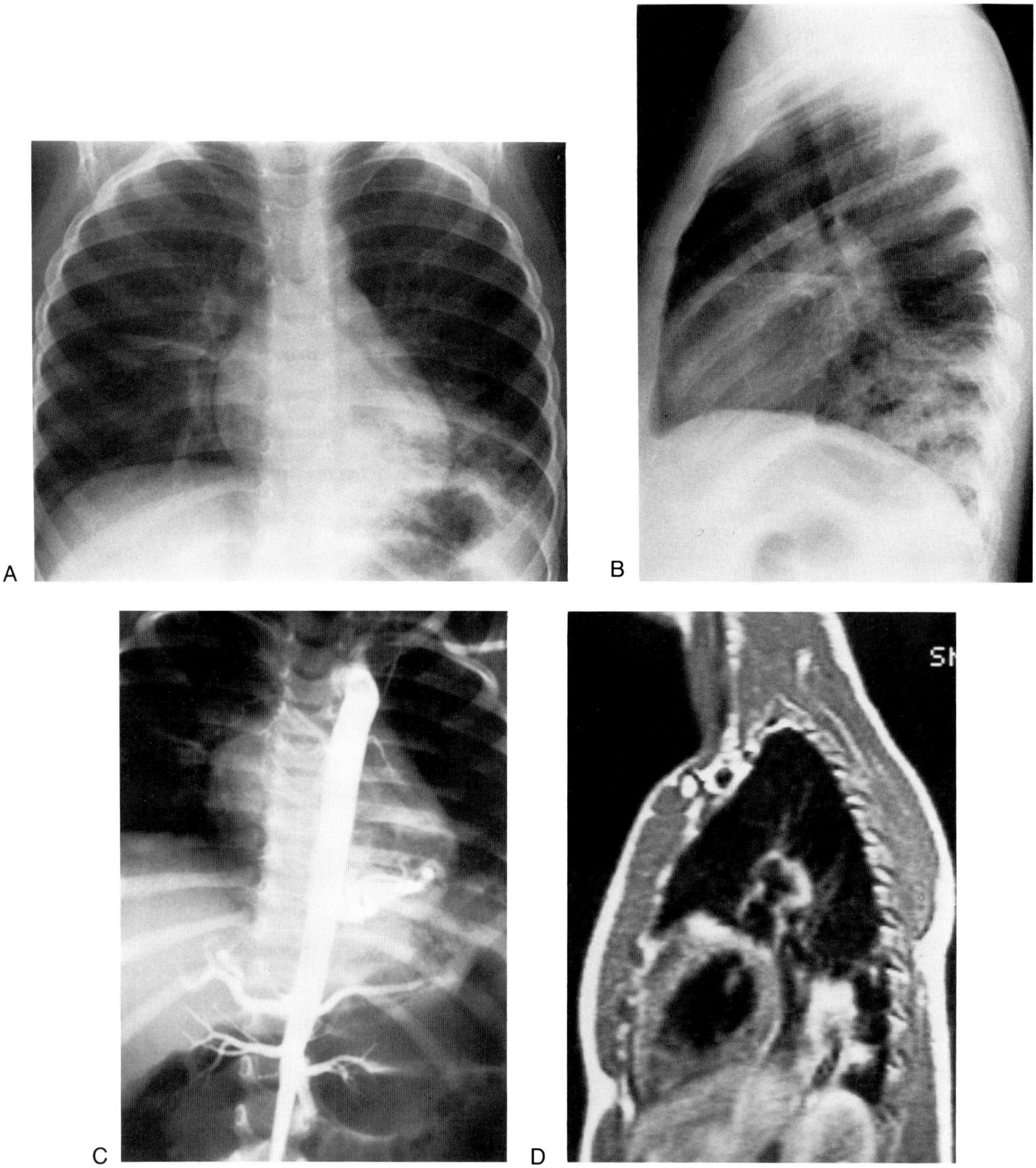

Fig. 3–43 Bronchopulmonary foregut malformations. **(A)** Posteroanterior view of a child's chest demonstrates a mixed density lesion behind the heart with multiple small cysts. **(B)** Lateral view confirms left lower lobe location of pneumonia versus sequestration. **(C)** Aortogram demonstrates the aberrant arterial feeder arising from the distal thoracic aorta. **(D)** Another patient with a left lower lobe sequestration demonstrated on sagittal T_1-weighted MRI. Note the area of increased signal in left lung base with the aberrant vessel denoted by signal void. (*Figure continues.*)

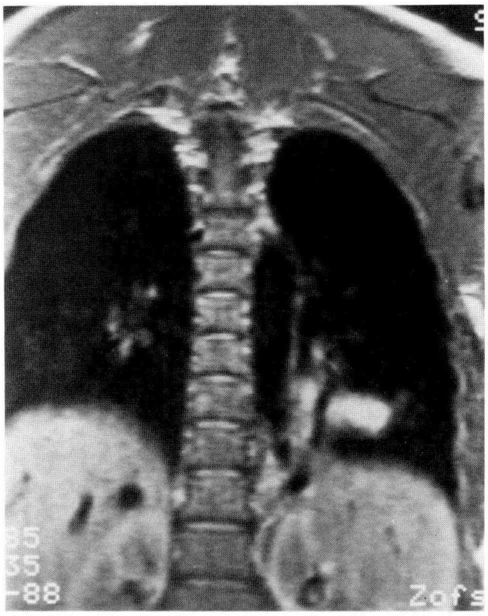

E

Fig. 3–43 (*Continued*). **(E)** Coronal MRI showing the aberrant arterial feeder arising from the proximal abdominal aorta.

hypoplasia and persistent fetal circulation. Utilization of extracorporeal membrane oxygenators (ECMO) for neonatal pulmonary failure may decrease the pulmonary hypertension present before surgical repair of the diaphragmatic hernia. In the future, this may prove efficacious. From an imaging standpoint, infants who are ECMO candidates usually undergo a screening head ultrasound examination to rule out intracranial hemorrhage, a contraindication to ECMO. Because patients are anticoagulated while on ECMO, daily head ultrasound examinations are performed to diagnose any intracranial hemorrhage that may occur during therapy.

An air collection seen in the ipsilateral hemithorax after surgery suggests postsurgical complications such as hernia recurrence and persistence of the hernia sac. However, it is usual for the surgeon to induce a pneumothorax on the ipsilateral side to cushion the hypoplastic lung, which usually expands to meet the size of the hemithorax in the week that follows. Occasionally, anomalies such as ipsilateral upper limb deformity, phocomelia, and congenital heart disease may be associated. Right congenital diaphragmatic hernias have been associated with pleural effusions.

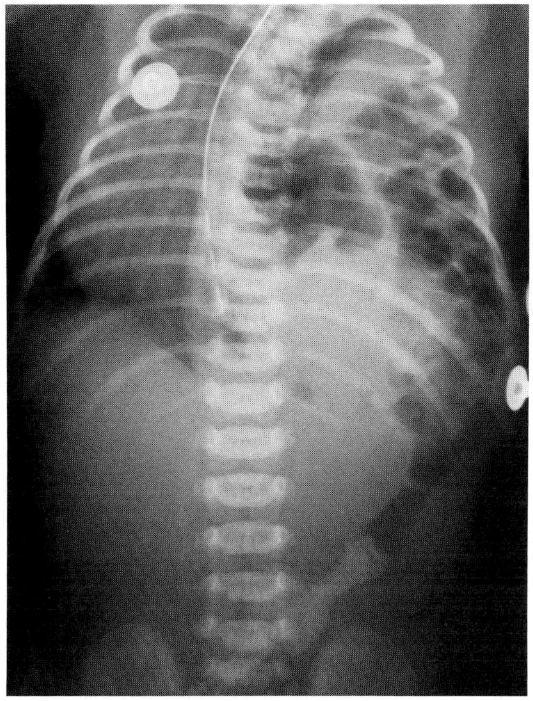

Fig. 3–44 Congenital diaphragmatic hernia. Note that the left lung is not normally aerated and multiple cysts of varying sizes occupy the left hemithorax. The right lung is compressed and the mediastinum is deviated to the right. The abdomen shows a paucity of bowel gas. The nasogastric tube did not advance past T10.

Although sometimes considered a variant of congenital cystic disease of the lungs, bronchiectasis is most commonly associated with recurrent pulmonary infections and is an inflammatory cause of multiple localized cystic lesions (Fig. 3–45). *Bronchiectasis* is bronchial dilatation and can be classified into three groups based on the severity of dilatation and the degree of distal airway obliteration. Cylindrical bronchiectasis is the mildest form. Varicose bronchiectasis is an intermediate phase. Saccular bronchiectasis is the most severe type. In saccular bronchiectasis, the bronchi balloon and cysts extend all the way to the pleural surface. This type is most likely to present as localized cystic lesions, most often involving the lower lobes. Other radiographic findings of bronchiectasis include volume loss, bronchial wall thickening (tram tracking), and increased lung markings. Most patients with bronchiectasis present with symptoms of recurrent lower respiratory tract infections. The presurgical evaluation of patients with suspected

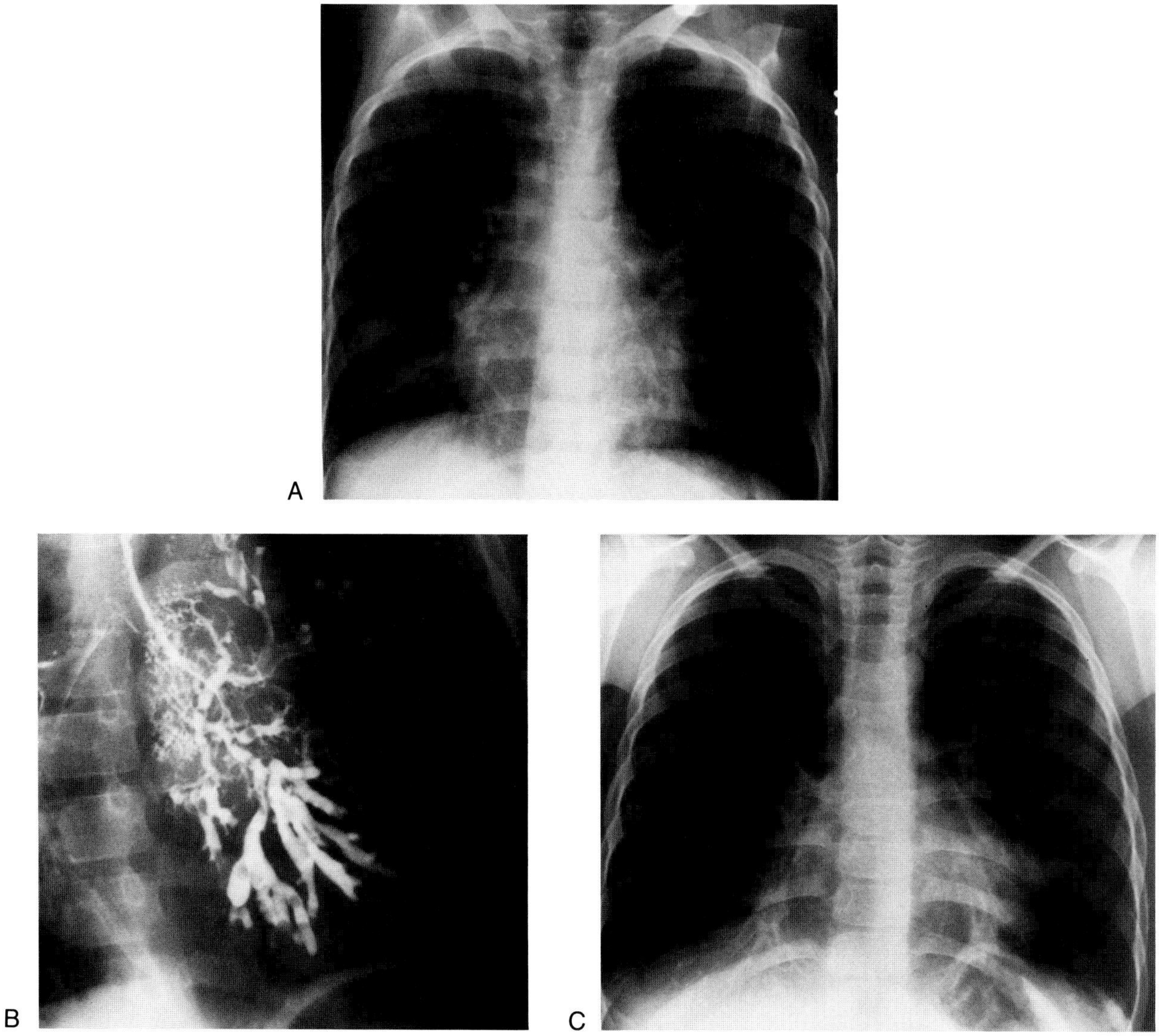

Fig. 3–45 Bronchiectasis. **(A)** Posteroanterior chest x-ray of this 6-year-old patient demonstrates prominent air bronchograms and cystic spaces of varying sizes in the left lower lobe. These findings are consistent with the patient's history of recurrent pneumonias and bronchiectasis. **(B)** Bronchography demonstrated saccular bronchiectasis of the medial basal segment of the left lower lobe. **(C)** In another patient, with Bruton disease, note the volume loss and "tram-tracking" in both lower lobes consistent with cylindrical bronchiectasis.

bronchiectasis varies depending on the geographic location of the medical center and the operating surgeon. Some radiologists advocate the use of high kilovoltage chest x-rays, others, radionuclide ventilation perfusion scans, while still others advocate CT or bronchography. It is sometimes useful for the surgeon to be aware of the functional capacity of the remainder of the lung. With this in mind, radionuclide ventilation perfusion scans will usually provide the necessary information about the diseased segment as well as the normal lung. Most commonly, a lower lobe is involved although the disease may be bilateral.

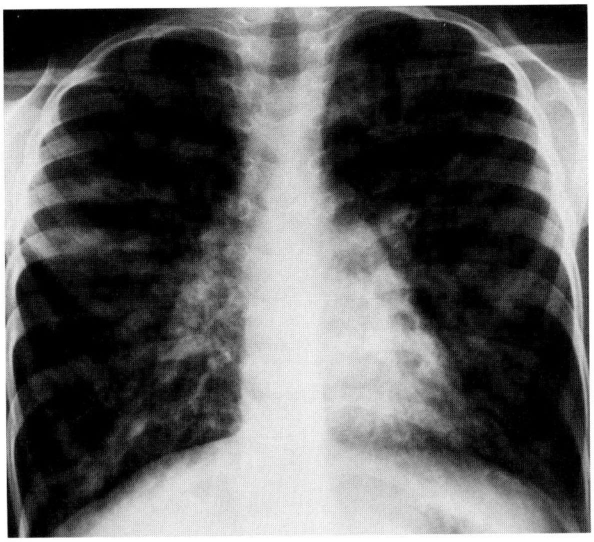

Fig. 3–46 Cystic fibrosis. Note the diffuse increase in the interstitial markings, multiple blebs, and bronchiectasis. Atelectasis is seen in both upper lobes.

Other causes of localized multicystic lung lesions occur less frequently. In the newborn period, pulmonary interstitial emphysema secondary to ventilator assistance may be unilateral. Hyaline membrane disease may occasionally result in a small unilateral multicystic appearance due to type I bubble formation.

Bilateral Cysts

The appearance of multiple bilateral thin walled cysts in a uniform distribution is usually the result of long-standing pulmonary disease. In infancy, this appearance usually results from a process, such as bronchopulmonary dysplasia, Wilson-Mikity syndrome, or pulmonary interstitial emphysema, that began in the neonatal period. Bronchopulmonary dysplasia in the late stages is the most frequent cause of this radiographic appearance. The changes result from respiratory compromise and therapy with high oxygen concentrations. The cysts represent areas of destroyed lung surrounded by fibrous tissue. Wilson-Mikity syndrome results in a radiographic appearance identical to that of bronchopulmonary dysplasia except the cysts in the lower lobes may be slightly larger. Even in the early stages, small cysts may be seen throughout the lungs in all three conditions. After infancy, cystic fibrosis in late or untreated stages can result in a bilateral multicystic appearance. Usually, atelectasis is associated with bilateral blebs and bronchiectasis (Fig. 3–46).

Septic emboli usually occur in children with infected indwelling venous catheters (Fig. 3–47). This is the most recognized form of pulmonary embolic disease in childhood. However, right-sided bacterial endocarditis, staphylococcal osteomyelitis, and intrave-

A

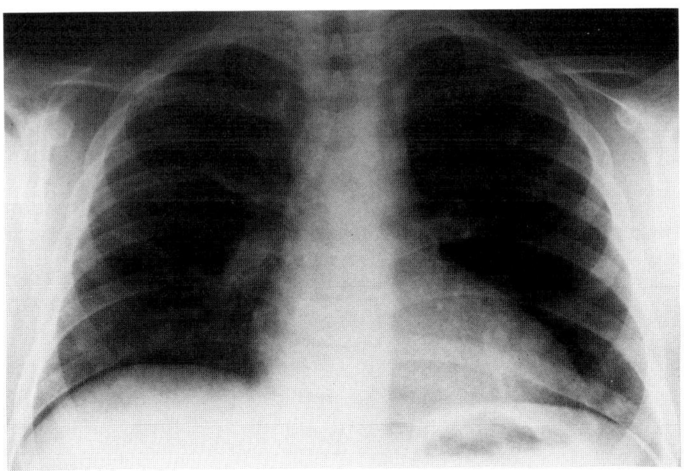

Fig. 3–47 Septic emboli. **(A)** Posteroanterior chest x-ray of a renal transplant patient demonstrates multiple rounded nodules scattered throughout the lungs. No definite cavities are identified on the radiograph. (*Figure continues.*)

B

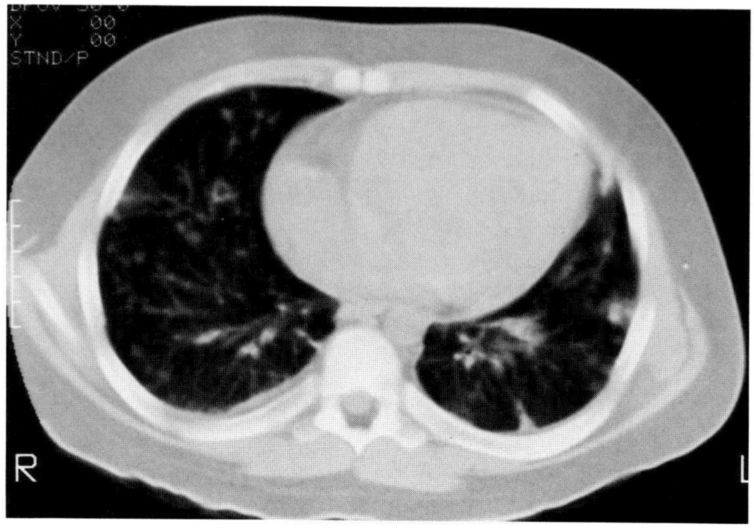

Fig. 3–47 (*Continued*). **(B)** Chest CT scan at lung windows performed the next day demonstrates multiple nodules of varying sizes and small, thick-walled bilateral cysts. These represented septic emboli from an indwelling catheter.

nous (IV) drug abuse are other causes. Occasionally, hilar lymphadenopathy may be associated; it decreases with antibiotic therapy.

Neoplasm, while not a common cause of multiple bilateral pulmonary cavities, is also a consideration. Papillomas are the most common tumor of the larynx in children and may involve the distal airways. They may be single or multiple. Extension down the tracheobronchial tree usually occurs when laryngeal lesions are multiple or after surgical intervention. Spread into the smaller airways occurs in approximately 2.1 percent of patients. Because papillomas usually obstruct airways, scattered atelectasis is commonly seen. The cavitary lesions may resemble cystic bronchiectasis. Multiple solid nodules may be seen (Fig. 3–48). Most patients with reported distal airway involvement have been less than 5 years old. Malignant transformation rarely occurs.

Approximately 4 percent of hematogenous metastases cavitate. The most common hematogenous lung metastases in childhood are from Wilms' tumor (Fig. 3–49). Teratoma and rhabdomyosarcoma also commonly metastasize to the lungs.

Two immunologic diseases may present with multiple bilateral pulmonary cysts. The most common of these is Wegener's granulomatosis, a triad of upper respiratory tract disease, pulmonary involvement, and glomerulonephritis. A form limited to the lung with a slightly better prognosis has also been described. Wegener's granulomatosis most frequently occurs in the fourth and fifth decades of life. However, cases presenting with symptoms of rhinitis and sinusitis have been reported during the second decade. The pathologic hallmark of the disease is the presence of necrotizing granulomas in the paranasal sinuses and nasal passages combined with systemic vasculitis of the small arteries and veins in the lungs and kidneys. Multiple cavitary nodules are frequently identified in both lungs. The chest x-ray appearance may change rapidly (Fig. 3–50), a feature differentiating Wegener's granulomatosis from neoplastic disease.

The triad of skin lesions (boils), abdominal abscesses, and multiple bilateral pneumatoceles (often large) should be recognized as hyperimmunoglobulinemia E or Buckley syndrome. These patients suffer from a defect in neutrophil chemotaxis especially evident when exposed to *S. aureus* or *H. influenzae*. The diagnosis is made when IgE levels exceed 2,000 IU/ml.

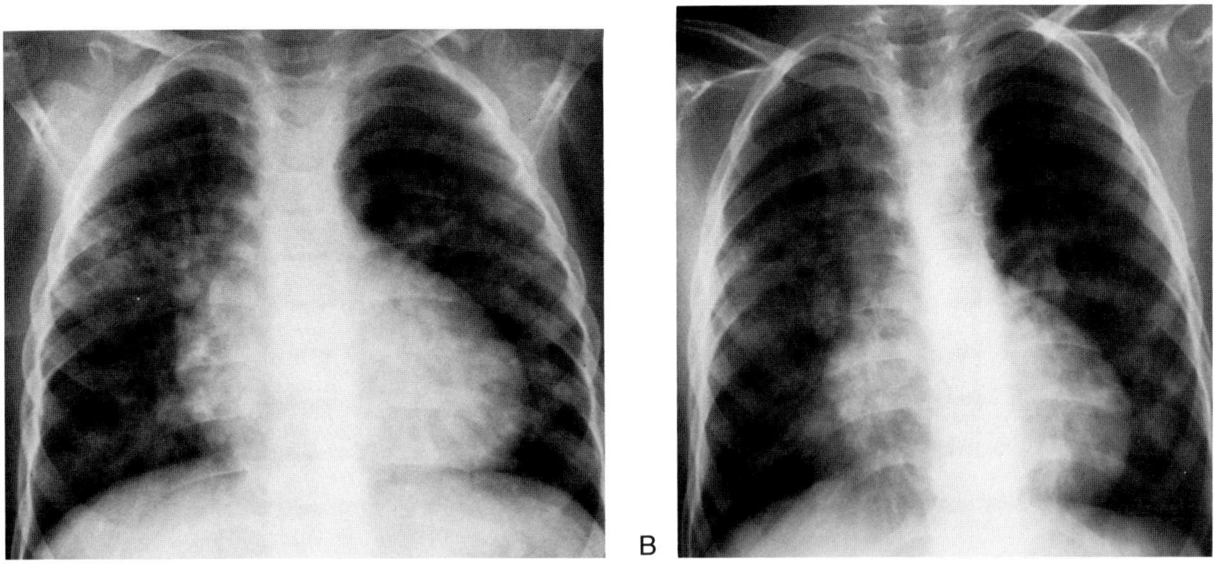

A B

Fig. 3–48 Laryngeal papillomatosis. **(A)** Note the multiple nodules of varying sizes on a posteroanterior chest x-ray of a child diagnosed with laryngeal papillomatosis 2 years earlier. In the periphery of the left lower lobe note that multiple cystic spaces with thick walls suggest cystic bronchiectasis. **(B)** When the child returned 1 year later, the papillomatous lesions are cystic throughout both lungs. Note the right middle lobe atelectasis.

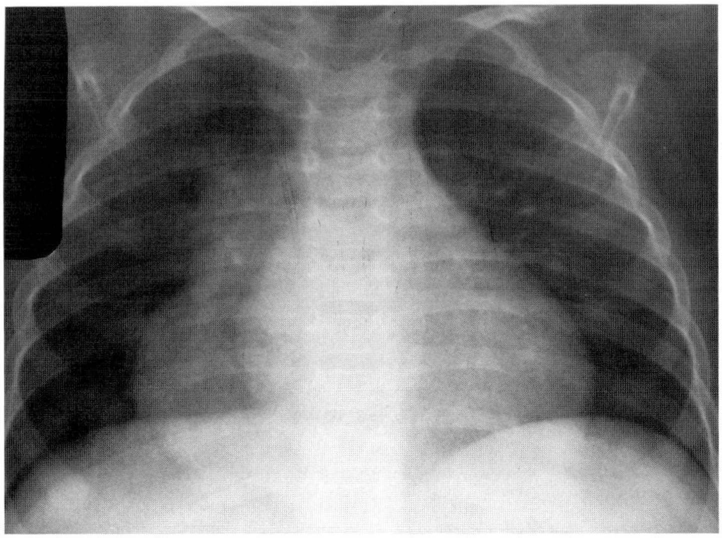

A

Fig. 3–49 Pulmonary metastases. **(A)** Note the multiple soft tissue densities of varying sizes present in both lung bases but more obvious on the right. This 3-year-old patient with Wilms' tumor presented with fever, irritability, and back pain. (*Figure continues.*)

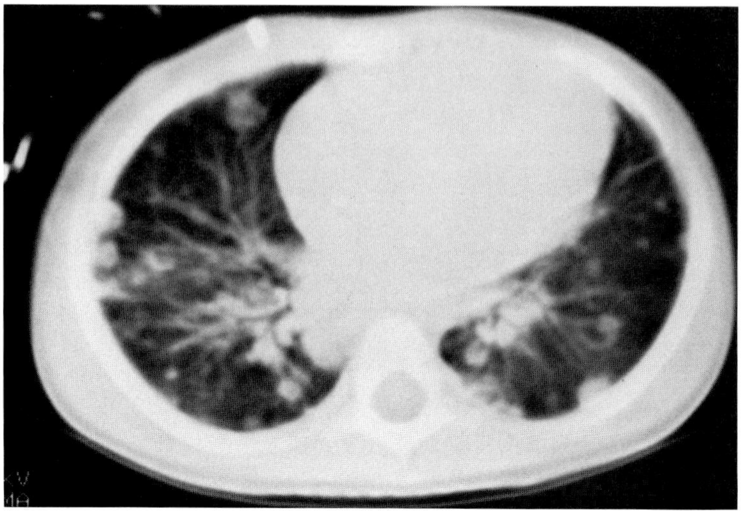

B

Fig. 3–49 (*Continued*). **(B)** Chest CT scan at lung windows of another patient presenting with a large Wilms' tumor demonstrates multiple metastatic pulmonary nodules of varying sizes.

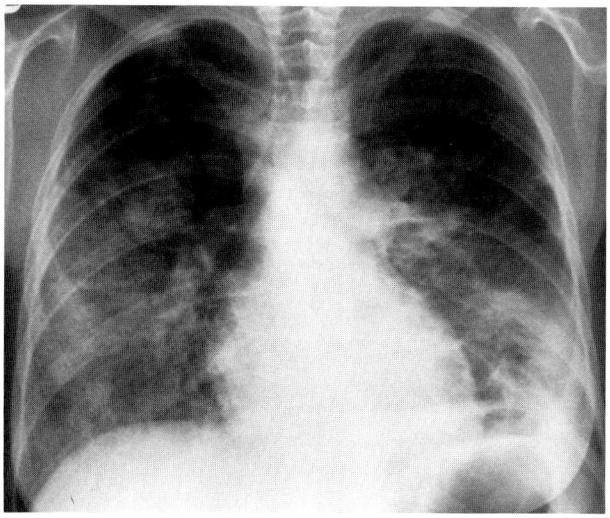

Fig. 3–50 Wegener's granulomatosis. Posteroanterior chest x-ray demonstrates bilateral thick-walled cysts in both lung bases. The necrotizing vasculitis involves the lungs, the sinuses, and the kidneys.

PULMONARY NODULES

The differential diagnosis of pulmonary nodules in childhood is similar to that of cystic lesions. The most useful differentiating feature is the number of nodules present.

Solitary Nodule

When a solitary nodule of soft tissue density is encountered in the lung, the most common cause is granuloma formation secondary to tuberculosis. The other common causes of solitary pulmonary nodules in childhood are also infectious and include round pneumonias and granulomas secondary to other organisms, such as histoplasmosis (Fig. 3–51).

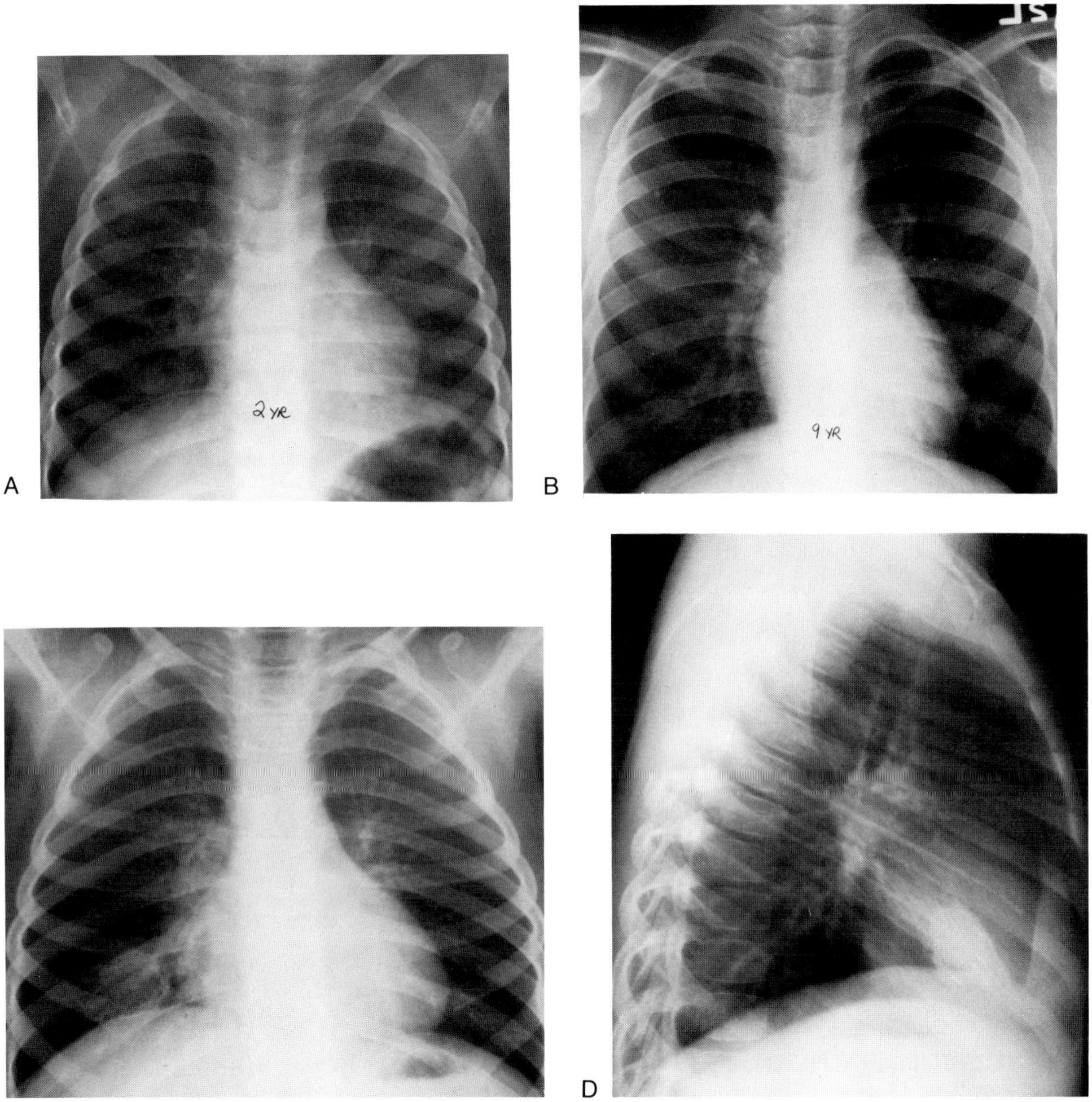

Fig. 3–51 Solitary pulmonary nodule. **(A)** Note the round, sharply-marginated soft tissue density between the second and third anterior right ribs. Right hilar adenopathy is noted. This represented primary tuberculosis. **(B)** Seven years later note the solitary calcified granuloma in the same location. **(C)** This posteroanterior view of an asymptomatic child demonstrates a large well-circumscribed nodule of the right lung base. **(D)** Lateral view confirms a right middle lobe location and calcification within the mass. This represented a granuloma from previous histoplasmosis infection.

SOLITARY PULMONARY NODULES

- Congenital
  - Bronchogenic cyst
  - Pulmonary arteriovenous malformation
  - Bronchial atresia with mucoid impaction
  - Pulmonary varix
  - Bronchopulmonary sequestration
- Inflammatory
  - Granuloma
    - Tuberculosis
    - Fungal infection
  - Round pneumonia
    - Pneumococcal pneumonia
    - Other bacteria
  - Abscess
    - Bacterial pneumonia
- Neoplasm
  - Benign
    - Hamartoma
  - Malignant
    - Bronchial adenoma
    - Sarcoma (primary)
    - Hematogenous metastases
- Artifact
  - Breast bud
  - Neurofibroma
  - Nevus

Round pneumonia represents an early phase of consolidation that rapidly changes into a more typical configuration for bacterial pneumonia. *S. pneumoniae* is the most common organism causing this appearance (Fig. 3–52). Often the pseudotumors occur in a posterior distribution and may simulate mediastinal masses.

The bronchogenic cyst is the most common congenital cause of a solitary pulmonary nodule (Fig. 3–53). Two-thirds of bronchogenic cysts arise in the lung parenchyma with the remainder originating from the tracheobronchial tree. The next most common congenital cause of a solitary pulmonary nodule is arteriovenous malformation. Two-thirds of pulmonary arteriovenous malformations are solitary and one-half the patients diagnosed with arteriovenous malformation have associated hereditary hemorrhagic telangiectasia. The lower lobes are the most common site for both bronchogenic cysts and pulmonary arteriovenous malformations. Identification of the feeding arteries and draining vein of an arteriovenous malformation is possible with either duplex sonography or MRI. Treatment by either surgical resection or

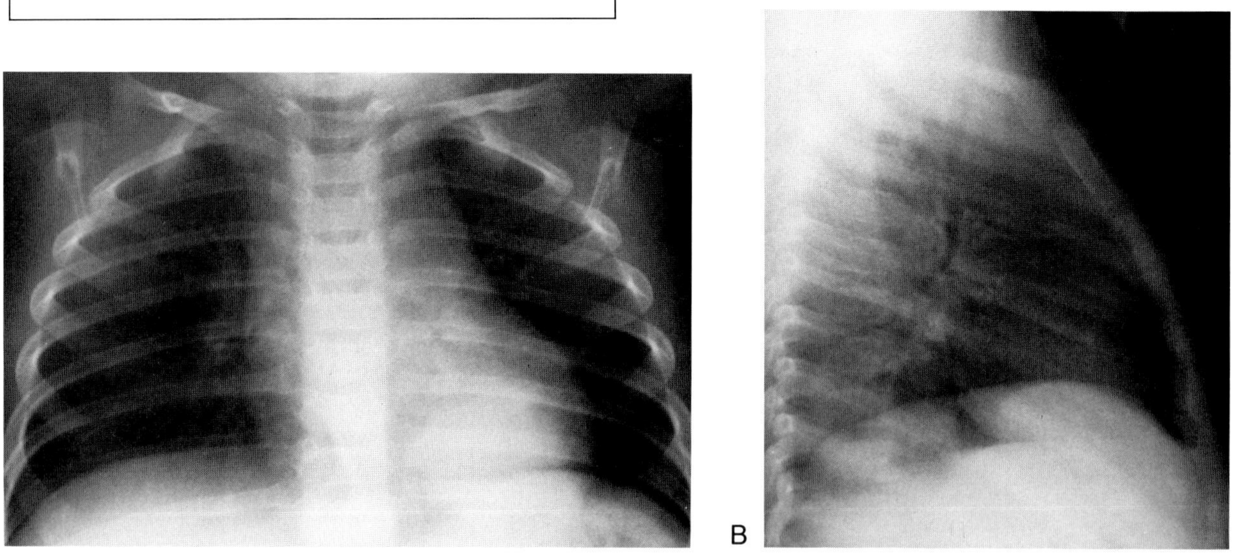

A B

Fig. 3–52 Round pneumonia. **(A)** Posteroanterior chest x-ray of a child with fever demonstrates a round soft tissue density behind the heart. **(B)** Lateral view confirms the round density in a left lower lobe location with air bronchograms. This represented pneumococcal pneumonia.

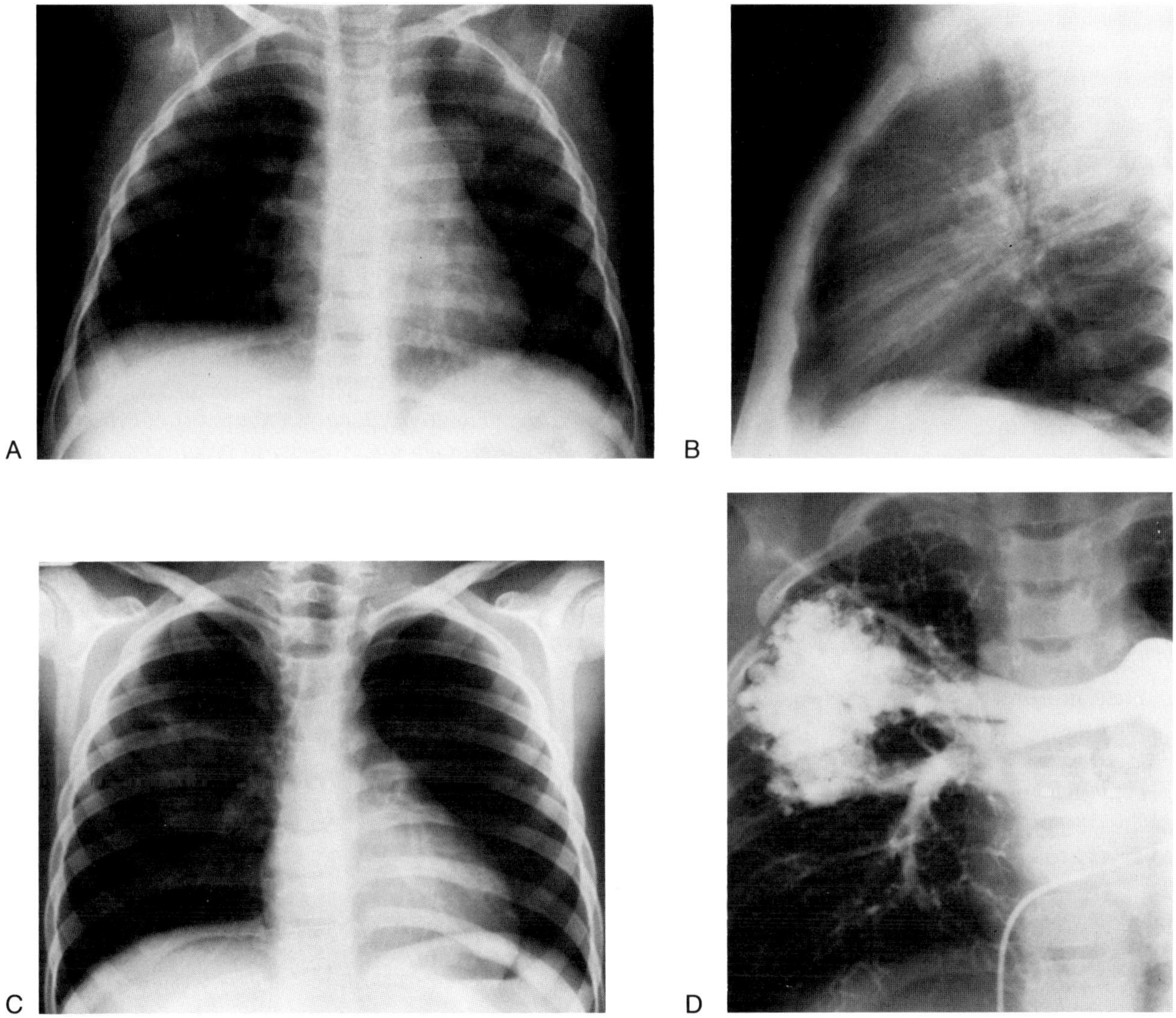

Fig. 3–53 Congenital solitary nodules. **(A)** Posteroanterior chest x-ray of a 2-year-old patient with a known mass since birth. A well-defined area of increased density is seen in the region of the superior segment of the left lower lobe. It obliterates the descending aorta just below the aortic knob. **(B)** Lateral view confirms the position of the mass in the superior segment of the left lower lobe. At surgical resection, a bronchogenic cyst was found. **(C)** The large ill-defined right lung nodule was an unexpected finding in another healthy child. **(D)** A pulmonary arteriogram demonstrates multiple arterial branches supplying a large pulmonary arteriovenous malformation. Note the multiple veins draining toward the left atrium.

embolic occlusion is recommended in all cases of arteriovenous malformation since the available evidence suggests that morbidity and mortality are higher in untreated patients.

Another congenital malformation that causes a soft tissue density nodule in the lungs is bronchial atresia with mucoid impaction. The impacted mucus appears as a pulmonary nodule. The lung parenchyma distal to the obstruction becomes hyperinflated due to collateral air drift and thus appears hyperlucent. Usually bronchial atresia occurs in the apicoposterior bronchus of the left upper lobe. The occurrence of bronchial atresia is exceedingly rare. Likewise, pulmonary varices are also a rare cause of a solitary pulmonary nodule and most often occur in the medial third or in either lung. Although any of the current cross-sectional imaging modalities may be utilized to visualize a pulmonary varix, angiography remains the gold standard. Change in the size of the varix is seen during Valsalva and Muller maneuvers and the entity may be differentiated from pulmonary arteriovenous malformation by filling of the varix on the venous phase of the pulmonary arteriogram. Bronchopulmonary sequestrations may also present as solitary pulmonary nodules but are usually rather large in size.

Infection is by far the most common cause of solitary pulmonary nodules with granulomas and round pneumonias occurring most frequently. Occasionally, lung abscesses from any infectious agent may occur as solitary pulmonary nodules and are most often large in size.

One benign tumor, the hamartoma, and several malignant primary tumors should be considered in the differential diagnosis of a solitary pulmonary nodule. The spectrum of lung hamartomas includes the cystic adenomatoid malformation and chondromatous hamartomas. Cystic adenomatoid malformation has been previously described. Chrondromatous hamartomas appear as round or lobulated soft tissue masses. The characteristic "popcorn" calcification associated with hamartomas is much more likely to occur in adults than in children. The reported incidence of calcification varies widely but is definitely less than 50 percent.

The outdated term *bronchial adenoma* describes a group of low-grade malignancies known for local invasiveness and distant metastases. The bronchial carcinoid arising from Kulchitsky cells is the most common of the group. The other tumors in order of decreasing frequency are cylindromas, mucoepidermoid tumors, and pleomorphic tumors. Eighty percent of adenomas are centrally located, arising from major bronchi. The radiographic findings vary depending on whether the tumor is endobronchial or a peripheral pulmonary nodule (Fig. 3–54). A lesion that obstructs the bronchus may be associated with atelectasis or recurrent pneumonia. The most common presenting symptom is hemoptysis. Both the carcinoid syndrome and Cushing syndrome associated with adult bronchial carcinoids are absent in childhood.

Primary lung sarcomas occur 10 times more frequently than do primary bronchogenic carcinomas in children. This relationship is reversed in adults. Sarcomatous transformation has been associated with cystic adenomatoid malformation. Less than 1 percent of all bronchogenic carcinomas occur during the first two decades of life.

Hematogenous metastases to the lungs present as a solitary lung nodule in less than 25 percent of cases. The most likely primary malignancies with lung metastases include Wilms' tumor, teratoma, and rhabdomyosarcoma. If a child is diagnosed with primary malignancy, high resolution CT scans are obtained with overlapping thin cuts to diminish respiratory motion.

Artifacts, which may appear as solitary or multiple pulmonary nodules, include the breast buds in prepubescent females and skin lesions such as neurofibromas. These lesions classically disappear on the lateral view.

Multiple Nodules

The most common cause of multiple pulmonary nodules in children is granuloma formation secondary to fungus infection (histoplasmosis). Tuberculosis is also a common cause of multiple granulomatous nod-

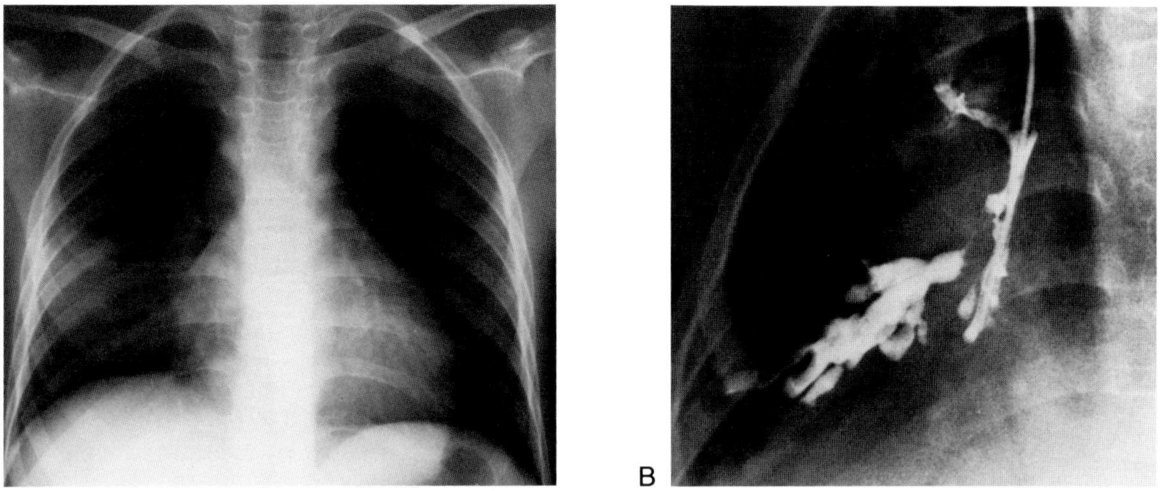

Fig. 3–54 Mucoepidermoid tumor. **(A)** Posteroanterior chest x-ray demonstrates irregularity of the right heart border consistent with right middle lobe disease. Small cystic spaces are seen within the right middle lobe. This may indicate bronchiectasis. The bronchus intermedius appears smaller than corresponding bronchi on the left. **(B)** Oblique view from a thoracic bronchogram demonstrates considerable narrowing of the right middle lobe bronchus and poststenotic dilatation consistent with cylindrical bronchiectasis. At resection, an endobronchial mucoepidermoid carcinoma was found.

MULTIPLE PULMONARY NODULES

- Congenital
  - Pulmonary arteriovenous malformation
- Inflammatory
  - Infectious granulomas
    - Histoplasmosis
    - Tuberculosis
  - Noninfectious granulomas
    - Sarcoidisis
    - Wegener's granulomatosis
  - Septic emboli
- Neoplasm
  - Benign
    - Laryngeal papillomatosis
  - Hematogenous metastases
    - Osteosarcoma
    - Thyroid carcinoma
    - Yolk sac tumors
- Idiopathic
  - Collagen-vascular diseases

ules (Fig. 3–55). Pulmonary densities associated with histoplasmosis are uniformly small in size and may calcify. Similar calcifications are seen in the liver and spleen.

Congenital causes of multiple pulmonary nodules are multiple pulmonary arteriovenous malformations. These tend to occur in the lower lobes and may be round or oval in size (Fig. 3–56).

Aside from tuberculosis and histoplasmosis, other fungi, multiple septic emboli, and multiple lung abscesses may appear as pulmonary nodules early in their course. When lung abscesses are present, early CT scans will reveal cavitation (Fig. 3–57). Sarcoidosis represents an idiopathic form of granulomatous disease that is not common in children but has the same radiographic appearance seen in adults. The most common neoplastic cause of childhood multiple pulmonary nodules is hematogenous metastasis from Wilms' tumor. Osteosarcoma, thyroid carcinoma, and yolk sac tumors may also result in hematogenous metastasis to the lungs. Metastatic nodules rarely calcify, with the exception of osteosarcoma. Laryngeal papillomatosis is usually considered a benign neoplasm. Nevertheless, endobronchial spread after surgical manipulation may result in multiple pulmonary nodules with or without cavitation. A similar appearance is seen with either Wegener's granulomatosis or the collagen-vascular diseases.

Wegener's granulomatosis and collagen-vascular diseases may present as multiple soft tissue density nodules within the lung parenchyma.

MEDIASTINUM

The mediastinum may be divided into four compartments: superior, anterior, middle, and posterior.

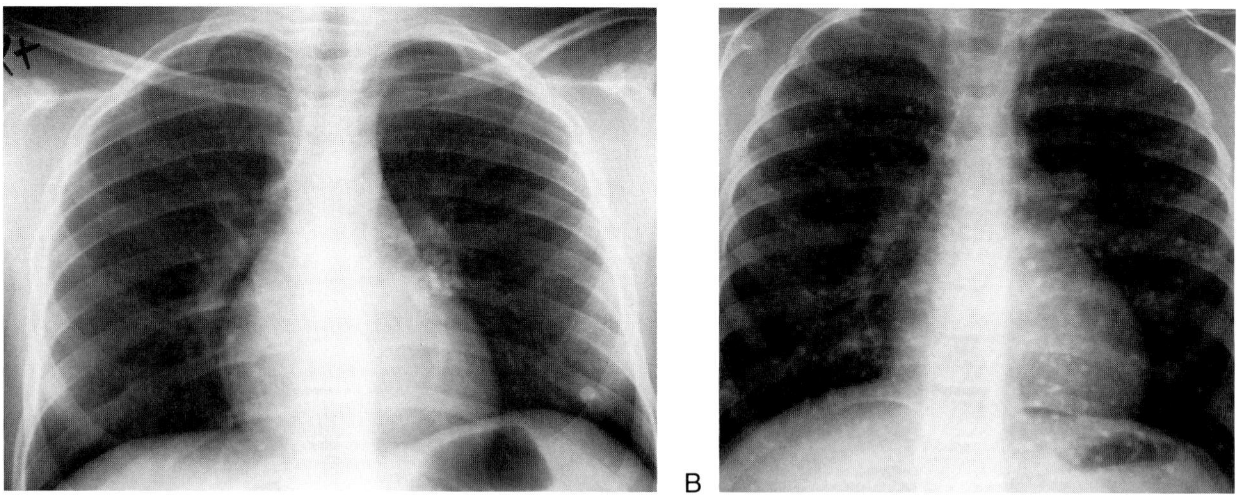

A B

Fig. 3–55 Multiple pulmonary nodules. **(A)** Note the lobulated, dense mass in the left hilar region and the well-circumscribed nodule in the left lung base. This represents a calcified granuloma from previous tuberculosis. Calcification is also present in the left hilar lymph nodes. **(B)** Multiple calcified nodules are scattered throughout both lungs in a child previously infected with histoplasmosis. Note calcification of the left hilar lymph nodes as well.

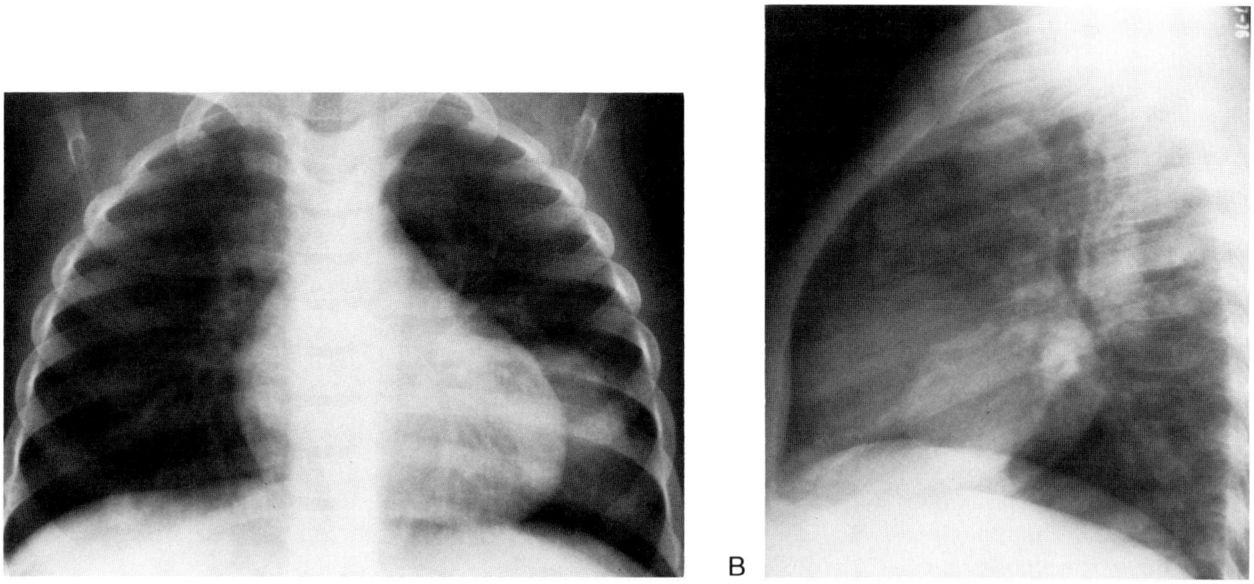

Fig. 3–56 Multiple arteriovenous malformations. **(A)** Posteroanterior chest x-ray demonstrates multiple rounded nodules in both upper and lower lobes. Note that the nodules lie in close proximity to large pulmonary vessels. **(B)** Lateral view confirms the feeding and/or draining vessels to the upper lobe nodules. Cardiac catheterization shortly after birth diagnosed multiple pulmonary arteriovenous malformations in this patient with Osler-Weber-Rendu syndrome.

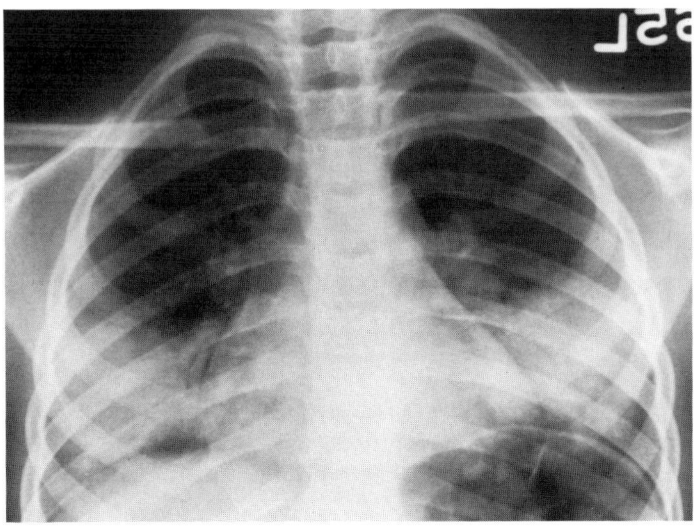

Fig. 3–57 Multiple infectious pulmonary nodules. Note the soft tissue densities present in both lower lobes. The lateral margins of both lesions are ill-defined. Air bronchograms are seen medially. This child was diagnosed with bilateral round pneumonias and responded to prompt antibiotic therapy.

Superior Mediastinum

Abnormalities of the superior mediastinum are most often noted incidentally during plain radiographic analysis of the chest. Signs include widening of the paramediastinum or deviation of the trachea from its normal position. The most common cause of superior mediastinal widening, whether unilateral or bilateral, is the normal thymus gland. This is less of a consideration after 3 years of age. Congenital causes of superior mediastinal widening include cystic hygroma, hemangioma, aortic dilatation due to aortic stenosis or persistent truncus arteriosis, dilated great vessels due to intracranial arteriovenous malformations, persistent left superior vena cava, type I total anomalous pulmonary venous return, bronchopulmonary foregut malformation, and teratomas (Fig. 3–58). Cystic hygromas often extend into the superior mediastinum from the neck and are easily diagnosed either with ultrasound or MRI. All the vascular anomalies can be well outlined using MRI. Intracranial arteriovenous malformations cause enlargement of both the carotid arteries and the jugular veins, seen as bilateral superior mediastinal widening. Teratomas usually occur shortly after the onset of birth and contain calcifications. Inflammatory conditions include lymphadenopathy, mediastinitis, and idiopathic or mycotic aneurysms of the aorta due to predisposing conditions such as periarteritis nodosa, neurofibromatosis, Kawasaki disease, homocystinuria, Marfan's syndrome, and Takayasu's arteritis. The most common cause of arterial aneurysm in the pediatric age group is umbilical artery catheterization in young infants. Neoplasms may cause enlargement of the superior mediastinum by infiltration of lymphoma or leukemia into thymus, thyroid neoplasms, fibroma, neurofibroma, and neuroblastoma. However, involvement of the superior mediastinum is less common than involvement of the lower portions of the mediastinum. Blunt chest trauma may be responsible for mediastinal hemorrhage. Birth trauma has been associated with thymic hemorrhage. Traumatic interruption of the great vessels should be suspected if the clinical history of blunt chest trauma to the sternum is associated with acute mediastinal widening. Iatrogenic hematomas may be caused by placement of central venous lines. Catheter placement outside of one of the great vessels may result in mediastinal fluid collections or frank mediastinitis. Miscellaneous causes of superior mediastinal widening include aortic dilatation due to systemic hypertension, retrosternal thyroid tissue, and an overabundance of mediastinal fat. The latter may be diagnosed on plain radiographs by radiolucency in the superior mediastinum. Dilatation of the upper esophagus from any cause may present as widening of the superior mediastinum. Common causes include foreign body obstruction of the esophagus, achalasia, and esophageal stenosis following corrosive ingestion.

SUPERIOR MEDIASTINAL MASS

- Normal variant
  - Thymus
  - Thyroid
- Congenital
  - Cystic hygroma
  - Hemangioma
  - Aortic stenosis
  - Persistent truncus arteriosus
  - Intracranial arteriovenous malformation
  - Total anomalous pulmonary venous return (type I)
  - Bronchopulmonary foregut malformation
  - Teratoma
- Inflammatory
  - Lymphadenopathy
  - Aortic aneurysm
  - Mediastinitis
- Neoplasm
  - Lymphoma/leukemia
  - Thyroid tumor
  - Fibroma
  - Neurofibroma
  - Neuroblastoma
- Trauma
  - Great vessel dissection
  - Hemorrhage
    - Mediastinal
    - Thymic
  - Esophageal stenosis
- Iatrogenic
  - Hematoma
  - Parenteral fluid leak
- Idiopathic
  - Hypertension
  - Achalasia

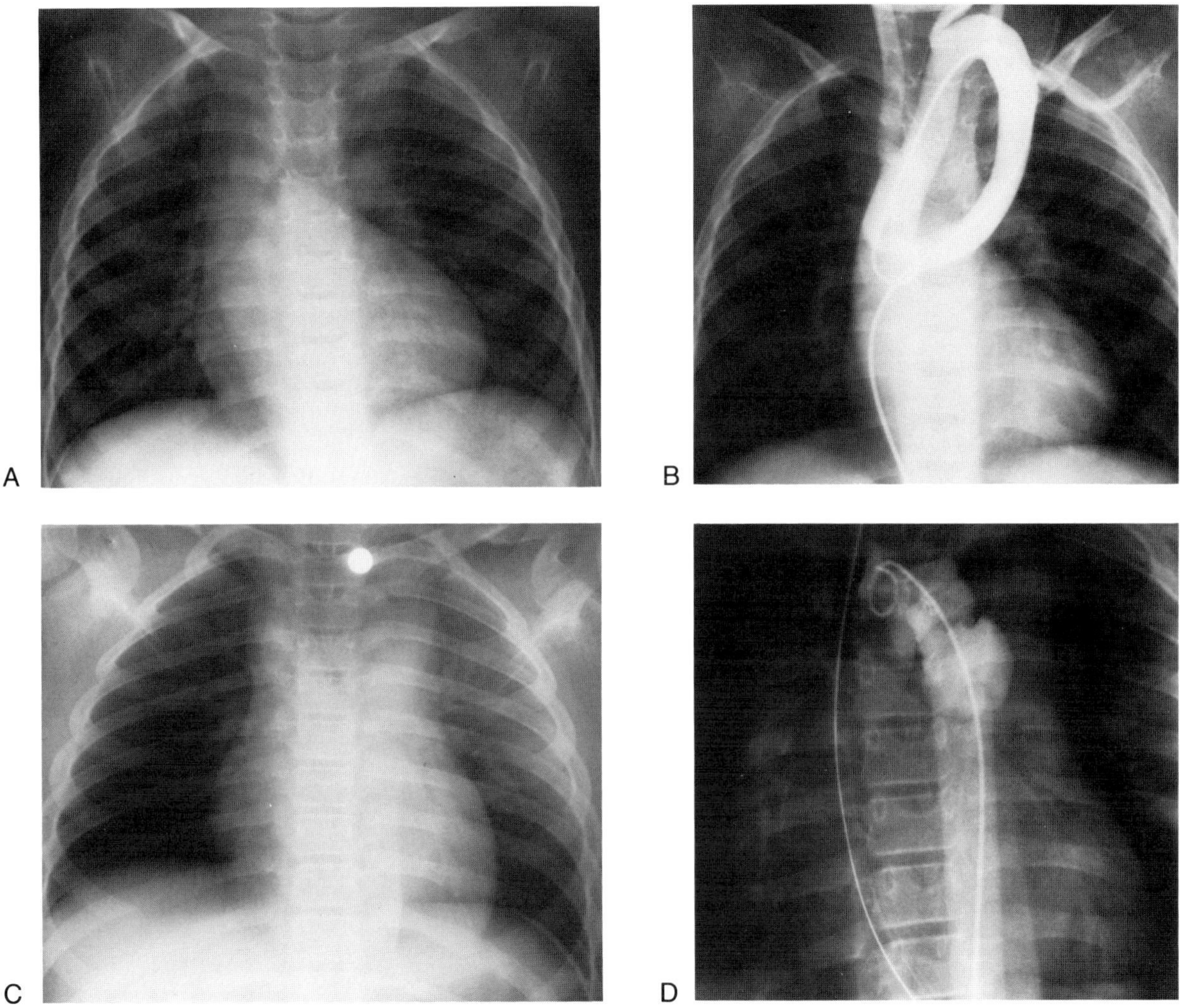

Fig. 3–58 Superior mediastinal widening. **(A)** Posteroanterior chest x-ray of an asymptomatic 4-year-old child demonstrates prominence of the superior mediastinum. The aortic knob is not clearly visible and a right aortic arch is suggested. **(B)** The aortogram reveals a cervical aortic arch with an aberrant right subclavian artery. There was also a right patent ductus arteriosus forming a vascular ring. **(C)** Another child demonstrates widening of the upper mediastinum, left apical pleural capping, and widening of the left paraspinous stripe after a motor vehicle accident. This is suspicious of great vessel injury. **(D)** The aortogram demonstrates an aortic tear at the level of the ligamentum arteriosum. Note the extravasation of contrast material outside of the expected lumen. *(Figure continues.)*

E 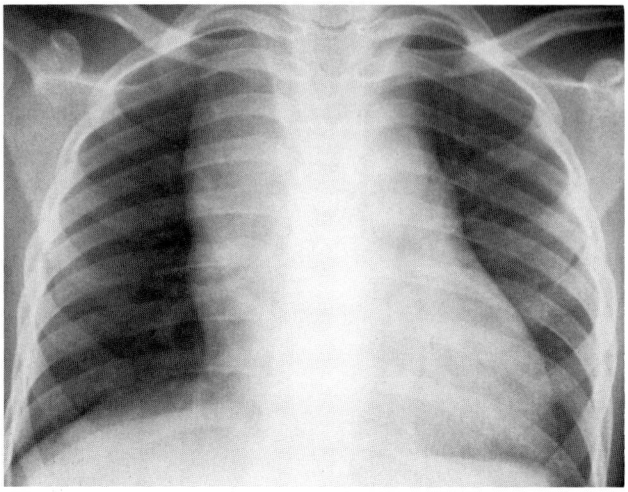

F 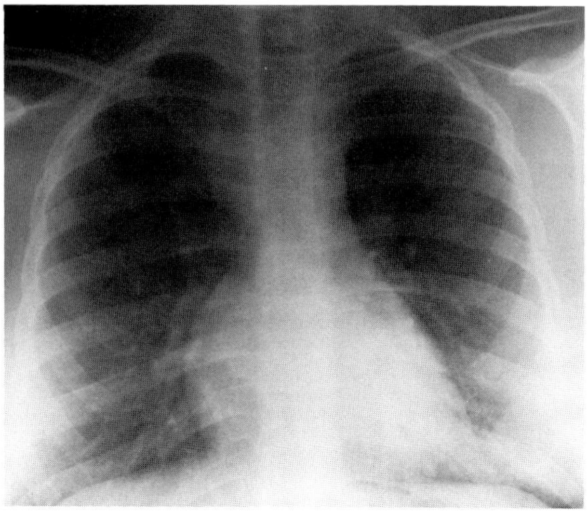

Fig. 3–58 (*Continued*). **(E)** Posteroanterior chest x-ray of an 11-year-old patient demonstrates superior mediastinal widening and lateral displacement of the posterior pleural lines. The lines extend above the clavicles indicating that the mass is posterior. Acute lymphoblastic leukemia had infiltrated her superior mediastinal lymph nodes. **(F)** Posteroanterior chest x-ray of another child demonstrates widening of the superior mediastinum, which is not quite as dense as the adjacent soft tissues. This 14-year-old patient had been on steroid therapy for idiopathic thrombocytopenic purpura. The superior mediastinum was infiltrated with fat secondary to steroid therapy as diagnosed by CT attentuation coefficients of −45 to −50. Lipomatous tumors may have similar attenuation coefficients.

Anterior Mediastinum

In the consideration of anterior mediastinal masses, one must again think of the thymus. The variability of the normal thymus is limitless (Fig. 3–59). Moreover, the thymus atrophies under stress and rebound hypertrophy occurs after resolution of the stress. This physiologic thymic enlargement is by far the most common abnormality involving the thymus. Thymic cysts and tumors are exceedingly rare in children. Several reports of hemorrhage into thymic cysts in children with aplastic anemia are found in the literature. The other normal structure that may cause an anterior mediastinal mass is ectopic thyroid tissue. This occurs more commonly in the superior mediastinum than in the anterior mediastinum.

Rare congenital causes of anterior mediastinal masses include right congenital diaphragmatic hernia through the foramen of Morgagni, pericardial cysts, and type I total anomalous pulmonary venous return with the vertical vein forming the anterior mediastinal mass. A much rarer congenital cause of an anterior mediastinal mass is an aneurysm of the sinus of Valsalva due to deficiency of the supporting structures of the aortic valve cusps. The rare rupture of an aneurysm of the sinus of Valsalva is clinically heralded by acute onset of chest pain and shortness of breath. Since an acute left-to-right shunt develops, increased pulmonary vascularity is seen and, usually, biventricular enlargement. On the lateral view, an anterior mediastinal mass may be seen. The right aortic sinus usually ruptures with leakage of arterial blood into the right ventricular outflow tract.

Inflammatory conditions resulting in anterior mediastinal masses include chronic mediastinitis secondary to granulomatous diseases such as tuberculosis and histoplasmosis, parasternal cellulitis, and sternal osteomyelitis. Thyroiditis may also cause anterior mediastinal enlargement when a retrosternal thyroid is present.

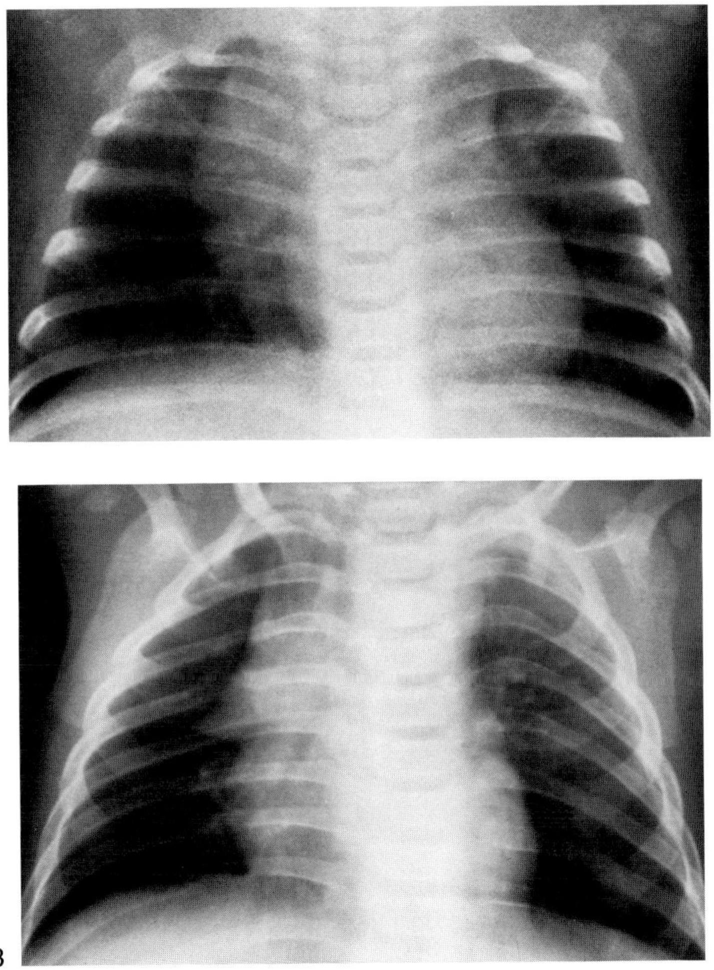

Fig. 3–59 Normal thymus. **(A)** Radiograph of a 3-month-old infant demonstrates prominence of the upper mediastinum, especially on the right, which represents the normal thymus gland. **(B)** Another infant, with the classic "thymic sail" sign demonstrated on the right.

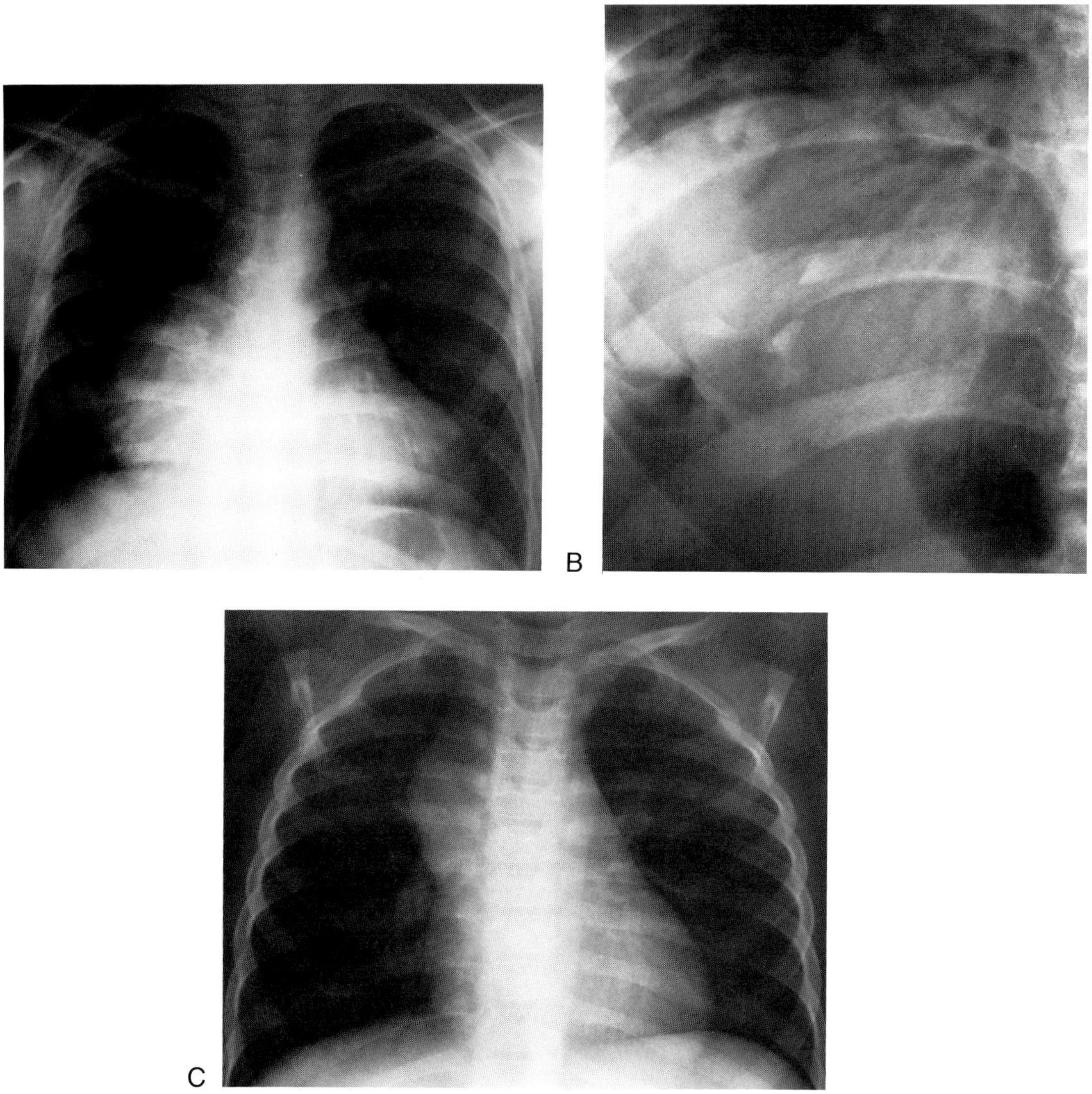

A B C

Fig. 3–60 Anterior mediastinal masses. **(A)** This young man was virtually asymptomatic when his chest x-ray was obtained. Note the widened inferior mediastinum. The right pulmonary artery and its branches can be seen through the mass (hilum overlay sign). This indicates the mass is more likely to be in the anterior mediastinum. **(B)** Changing the radiographic technique allowed better visualization of the lobulated mass and multiple tooth-shaped calcifications highly suggestive of a teratoma. Crowded air bronchograms are caused by extrinsic compression of the right lower lobe bronchus by the teratoma. **(C)** Posteroanterior chest x-ray of another child demonstrates a smoothly marginated right mediastinal mass and visualization of the right pulmonary artery and its branches. Note that the superior margin of the mass fades out at the level of the clavicles, indicating its location in the anterior mediastinum. (*Figure continues.*)

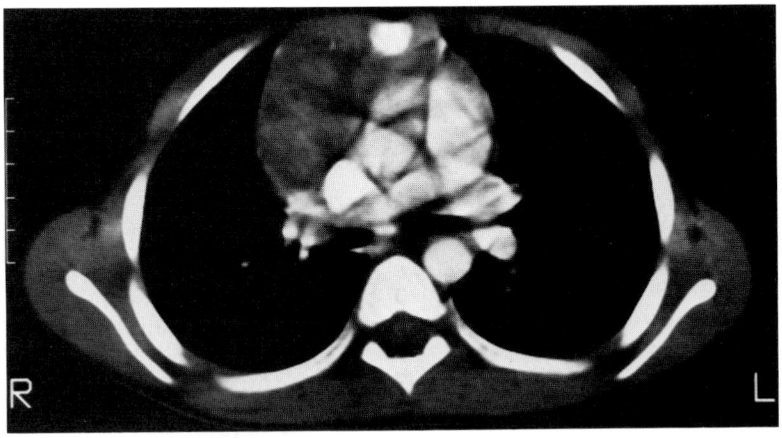

D

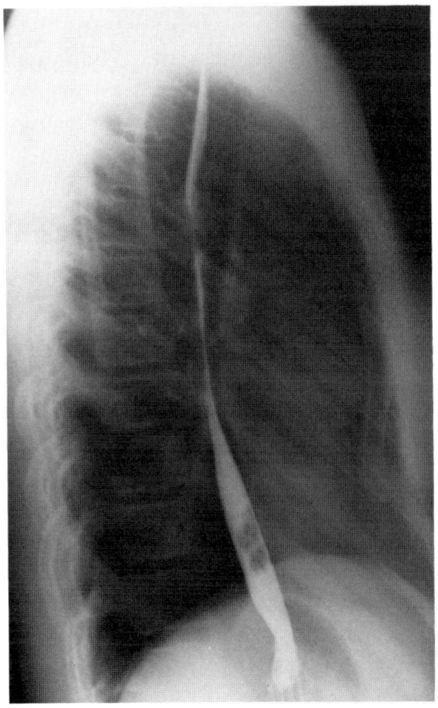

E

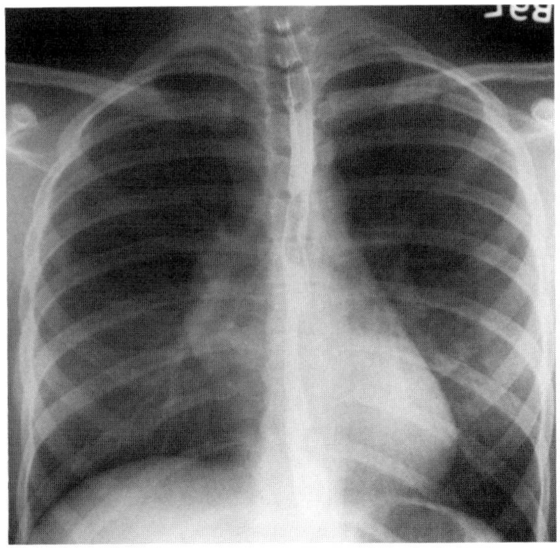

F

Fig. 3–60 (*Continued*). **(D)** Chest CT scan at soft tissue windows reveals a mixed attenuation anterior mediastinal mass with no apparent calcifications and moderate enhancement with contrast material injection. These findings are nonspecific but represented a lymphangioma. **(E)** Lateral view of another patient demonstrates a pectus excavatum deformity, which may compress the mediastinal structures. A subtle increase in the density of the retrosternal space is present. **(F)** While a pectus deformity may alter the appearance of the right heart border, one would not expect to clearly see the right pulmonary artery and its branches unless a mass of the anterior mediastinum is present. Note the sharply marginated right mediastinal mass that fades imperceptibly into the right heart border. This patient's CT scan looked almost identical to the previous case; however, this mass was a thymolipoma.

ANTERIOR MEDIASTINAL MASS

Normal variants
- Thymus
- Rebound thymic hypertrophy
- Ectopic thyroid

Congenital
- Cystic hygroma
- Congenital diaphragmatic hernia
- Pericardial cysts
- Total anomalous pulmonary venous return (type I)
- Sinus of Valsalva aneurysm

Inflammatory
- Mediastinitis
- Parasternal cellulitis
- Sternal osteomyelitis
- Thyroiditis (ectopic thyroid)
- Infectious mononucleosis

Neoplasm
- Teratoma
- Mesenchymal tumor
- Germ cell tumors
- Metastatic seminoma
- Lymphoma

Idiopathic
- Histiocytosis X
- Sarcoidosis

Trauma
- Hemorrhage
  - Mediastinal
  - Thymic
- Ruptured sinus of Valsalva aneurysm

The most common tumors involving the anterior mediastinum of children include dermoids and teratomas (Fig. 3–60). Dermoids, containing elements of two dermal layers, are much less common than teratomas, which contain elements of all three dermal layers. Dermoids are classically cystic, while teratomas may be cystic, solid, or mixed. Benign teratomas are much more common than malignant teratomas. The characteristic finding of mature calcifications may be difficult to see without cross-sectional imaging. Mesenchymal tumors, the most common of which is the cystic hygroma, may involve the anterior mediastinum. As previously mentioned, cystic hygromas are more common in the neck. Other mesenchymal tumors involving the anterior mediastinum include lipomas, lipomatosis, fibromas (most common), hemangiomas, and sarcomatous mesenchymal tumors. Germ cell tumors other than teratomas are much less common, but primary seminomas of the anterior mediastinum have been reported in childhood. The possibility that anterior mediastinal involvement by seminoma is the result of metastatic spread from a gonadal lesion must be excluded. Yolk sac tumors also have been reported, most commonly presenting as large anterior mediastinal masses in boys. These patients demonstrate an elevated level of serum alpha-fetoprotein. Hodgkins's lymphoma tends to extend into the anterior mediastinum from the middle mediastinum. Lymphomatous involvement of the anterior mediastinum may also be secondary to lymph node enlargement or infiltration of the thymus. Other causes of anterior mediastinal lymphadenopathy include histiocytosis X, sarcoidosis, chest wall inflammation, and infectious mononucleosis.

Accidental or iatrogenic trauma to the thymus or vascular structures may result in thymic or mediastinal hemorrhage.

Middle Mediastinum

The most common middle mediastinal mass in childhood is lymphadenopathy secondary to lymphoma or leukemia. Congenital causes of middle mediastinal masses include bronchopulmonary foregut malformations (bronchogenic cysts, enteric duplications), hiatal or intrapericardial hernias, pleuropericardial cysts, and cervical aortic arch. Lymphadenopathy may be secondary to infections of any type (viral or respiratory tract infections most common). Pertussis, bacteria, mycoplasma, and the granulomatous diseases may also cause lymphadenopathy. Hilar adenopathy may be difficult to assess on plain radiographs and CT. However, the natural contrast between the

MIDDLE MEDIASTINAL MASS

- Congenital
  - Bronchopulmonary foregut malformation
  - Hiatal hernia
  - Intrapericardial hernia
  - Pleuropericardial cyst
  - Cervical aortic arch
- Inflammatory
  - Lymphadenopathy
    - Infectious
    - Viral lower respiratory tract infection
    - Bacterial pneumonia
    - Tuberculosis
    - Pertussis
    - *Mycoplasma pneumoniae*
    - Noninfectious
    - Sarcoidosis
- Neoplasm
  - Lymphadenopathy
    - Lymphoma
    - Leukemia
- Idiopathic
  - Histiocytosis X
- Trauma
  - Diaphragmatic hernia
  - Failed hiatal hernia repair
  - Aortic aneurysm
  - Pancreatic pseudocyst
- Miscellaneous
  - Azygous vein dilatation
  - Superior vena cava dilatation

vessels and lymph nodes provided by electrocardiogram-gated MRI provides superior visualization of the middle mediastinal lymph nodes (Fig. 3–61). Mycotic aneurysms of the aorta may be responsible for large middle mediastinal masses. Endothoracic extension of pancreatic pseudocysts may rarely present as a middle mediastinal mass.

Lymphomatous involvement of lymph nodes is the most common cause of hilar and mediastinal lymph node enlargement. Classically, Hodgkin's lymphoma demonstrates asymmetric bilateral involvement. Involvement of the adjacent anterior mediastinal and retrosternal nodes is frequently associated. Ninety percent of patients with Hodgkin's lymphoma will demonstrate endothoracic involvement at some time during the course of their disease. Non-Hodgkin's lymphoma is less common in children than Hodgkin's lymphoma but has a poorer prognosis. Endothoracic involvement is not as common in non-Hodgkin's lymphoma. There is a predilection for development of non-Hodgkin's lymphoma in patients with both congenital and acquired immunodeficiencies. Lymphoma is the third most common malignancy of childhood. Calcifications may be seen in infiltrated lymph nodes after therapy.

Leukemia is the most common cause of cancer deaths in children less than 15 years of age. The peak incidence of acute lymphocytic leukemia is 4 years; peak incidence of acute myelocytic leukemia is the end of the second decade. The classic symptoms of fatigue, fevers, and petechiae or bleeding are caused by the associated anemia. Lymphadenopathy may

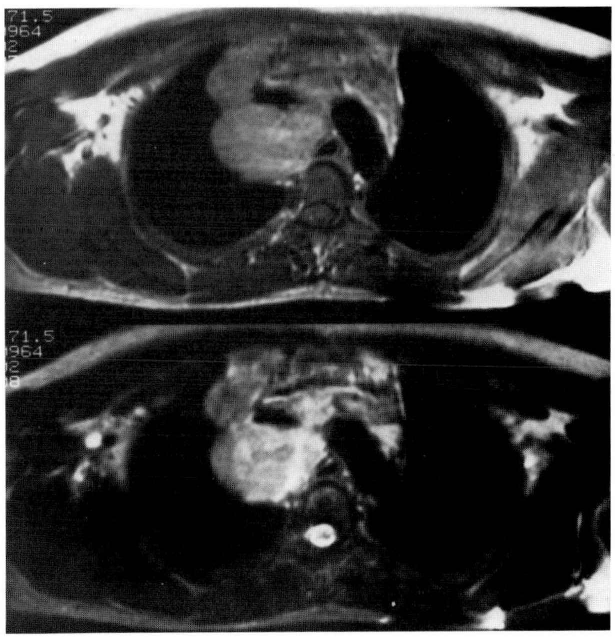

A

Fig. 3–61 Middle mediastinal lymphadenopathy. **(A)** Axial T_1-weighted cardiac-gated MRI demonstrates compression of the right pulmonary artery and trachea by multiple rounded homogeneous masses. The lymphadenopathy was secondary to Hodgkin's disease. (*Figure continues.*)

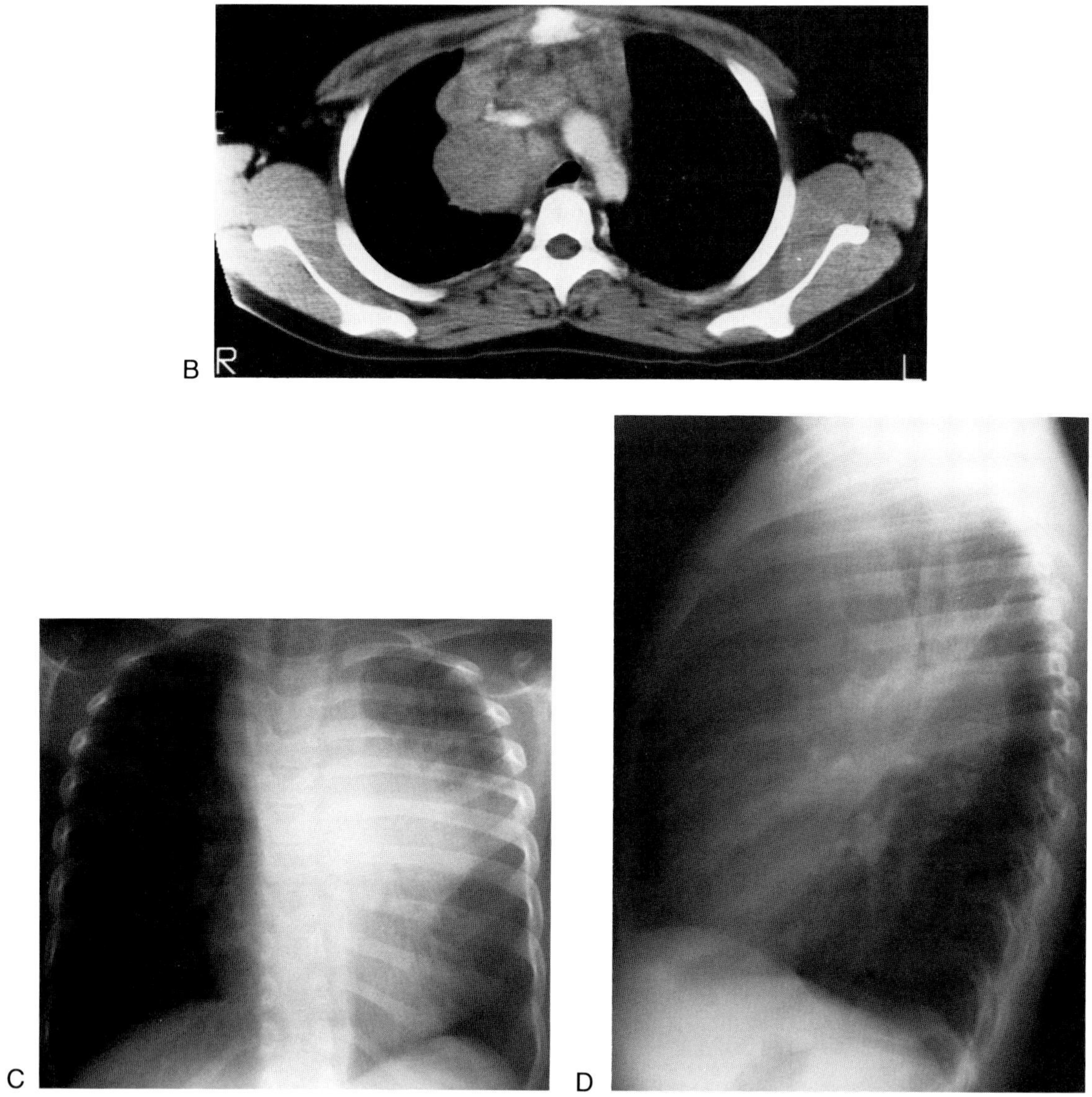

Fig. 3–61 (*Continued*). **(B)** Contrast material must be administered in order to gain the same information by CT. The patient's lymphadenopathy extended into the anterior mediastinum and neck. **(C)** Posteroanterior chest x-ray of another child demonstrates involvement of both the anterior and middle mediastinal compartments. Note the deviation of the trachea to the right and symmetrical widening of the upper half of the mediastinum. A large asymmetrical soft tissue density obscures visualization of the left pulmonary artery and its branches indicating middle mediastinal involvement. **(D)** Lateral view demonstrates soft tissue density filling the retrosternal air space and posterior displacement of the trachea. Biopsy revealed non-Hodgkin's lymphoma.

be noted on physical examination. The most common chest x-ray finding associated with leukemia is mediastinal and hilar lymph node enlargement. This is seen at the onset of the disease in more than one-third of cases. Acute myelocytic leukemia has a predilection for lung infiltration. Malignant lymphadenopathy may be secondary to metastasis from primary sites outside of the thorax. Benign lymphadenopathy may be secondary to the reticuloendothelioses. Traumatic diaphragmatic hernia, aneurysms of the aorta, and pancreatitis (pseudocyst formation) are other causes of middle mediastinal masses. Miscellaneous causes include dilatation of azygos vein secondary to infrahepatic inferior vena cava anomalies, thrombosis, and congestive heart failure. Dilatation of the superior vena cava for any reason may appear as a superior or middle mediastinal mass.

Posterior Mediastinum

Up to 40 percent of posterior mediastinal masses in children are of neurogenic origin. Neuroblastoma/ganglioneuroblastoma/ganglioneuroma represent a complex of neurogenic tumors varying in maturity of the cells. Forty percent of neuroblastomas are discovered before the age of 2 years; the other two cell types are more common in older children. When thoracic neuroblastoma is discovered, it is more likely to be primary than mestastatic. Primary neuroblastoma is associated with rib erosions, intraspinal extension, posterior scalloping of the vertebral body, and widening of the neural foramen in the majority of cases (Fig. 3–62). While the incidence of calcification within primary abdominal neuroblastoma approaches 50 percent, the incidence is 40 percent in primary thoracic neuroblastoma. Neuroblastoma metastatic to the thorax does not demonstrate calcifications or rib erosions. Displacement of the trachea and esophagus by a lobulated mass is common. Surgical excision is the treatment of choice.

Congenital causes of posterior mediastinal masses include neurenteric cysts resulting from incomplete separation of the notochord and endoderm during embryonic life. Sometimes only a meningeal stalk remains. In other cases, direct communication between the esophagus and thoracic spinal canal are possible. Frequently the soft tissue mass is associated with segmentation fusion anomalies of the adjacent spine (Fig. 3–63). Bronchopulmonary foregut malformations (enteric cyst, pulmonary sequestration) also occur in the posterior mediastinum. Lateral meningoceles associated with neurofibromatosis are rare con-

POSTERIOR MEDIASTINAL MASS

- Congenital
  - Neurenteric cyst
  - Enteric duplication
  - Bronchopulmonary foregut malformation
  - Lateral meningocele
  - Diaphragmatic hernia
  - Azygous continuation of the inferior vena cava
  - Ectopic thymus
  - Hemolytic anemia
  - Ectopic kidney
- Inflammatory
  - Pancreatic pseudocyst
  - Spine osteomyelitis (Pott's disease)
- Neoplasm
  - Neural tumors
    - Neuroblastoma
    - Ganglioneuroblastoma
    - Ganglioneuroma
    - Neurofibroma
  - Mesenchymal tumors
    - Lipoma
    - Fibroma
  - Sarcoma
  - Pheochromocytoma
  - Bone tumors
    - Osteoblastoma
    - Osteogenic sarcoma
    - Ewing's sarcoma
    - Lymphoma/leukemia
    - Osteoblastic metastases
    - Aneurysmal bone cyst
    - Hemangioma
- Trauma
  - Fracture
  - Diaphragmatic hernia
- Postoperative
  - Spinal surgery

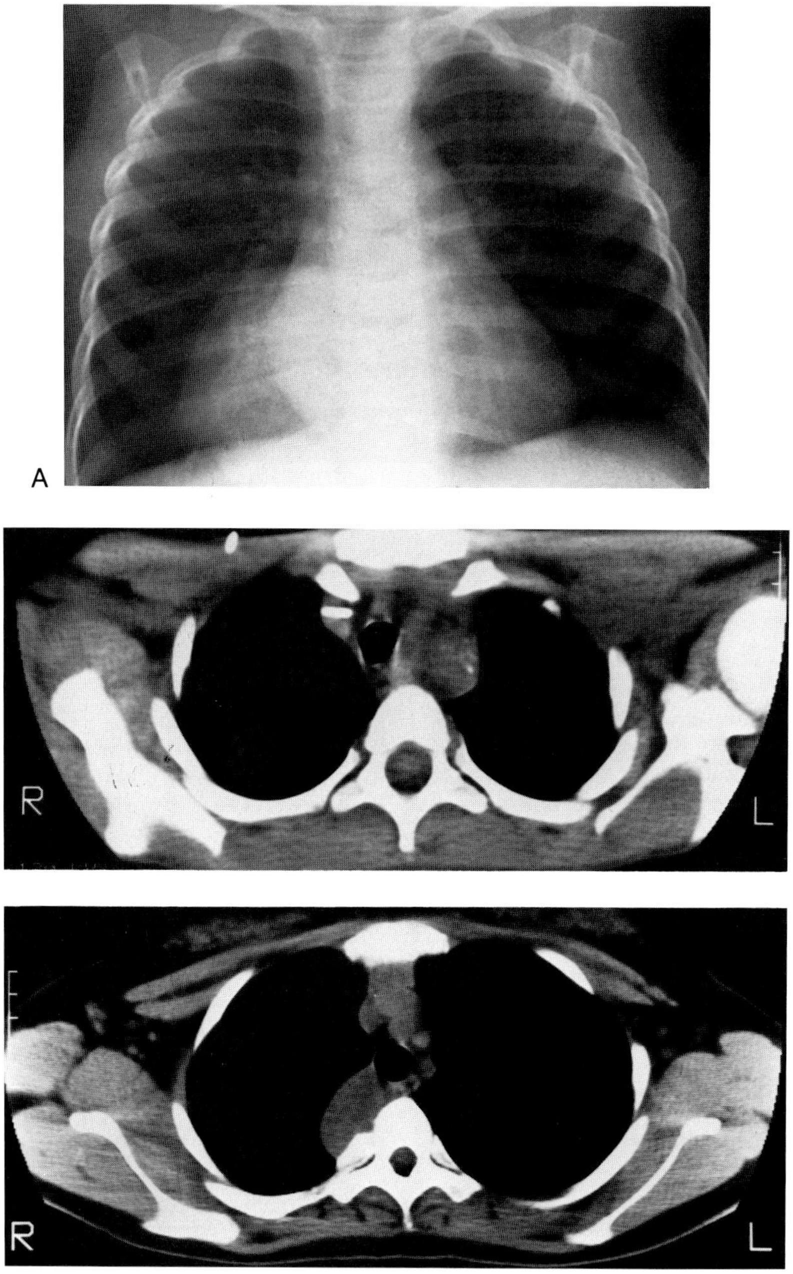

A

B

C

Fig. 3–62 Neurogenic posterior mediastinal masses. **(A)** This 1-year-old patient presented with fever. Her anteroposterior chest x-ray demonstrates a smoothly marginated right paraspinous mass extended from T7 through T12. Note the slight widening of the rib interspaces on the right, calcifications within the mass, and indistinctness of the right pedicle of T7. These findings are highly suspicious for thoracic neuroblastoma. **(B)** Another patient with intrathoracic neuroblastoma demonstrates a smoothly marginated left paraspinous mass by CT that displaces the trachea to the right. CT allows detection of smaller calcifications within the mass. Either CT or MRI may be used to evaluate involvement of the spinal canal. **(C)** Another patient incidentally noted to have a right posterior mediastinal mass when a chest x-ray was taken for a rib injury. CT scan demonstrates a well-defined homogeneous mass with no evidence of bone destruction, consistent with the diagnosis of ganglioneuroma.

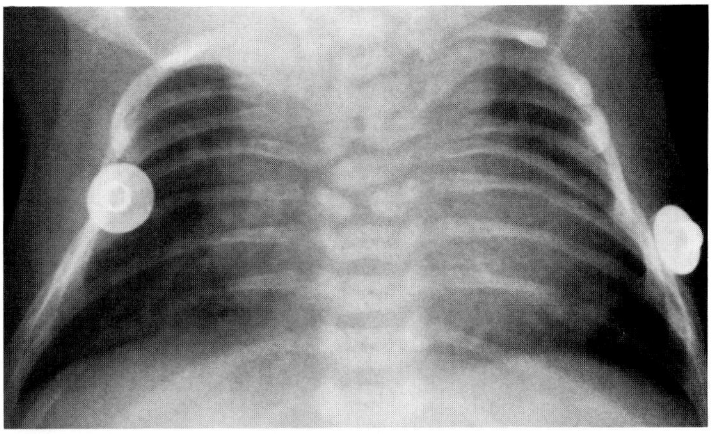

A

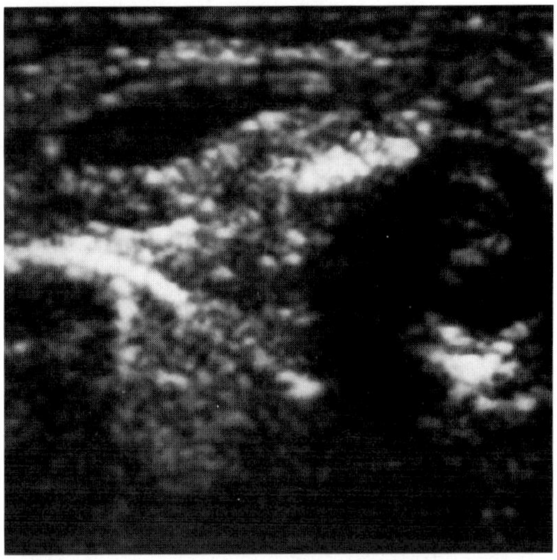

B

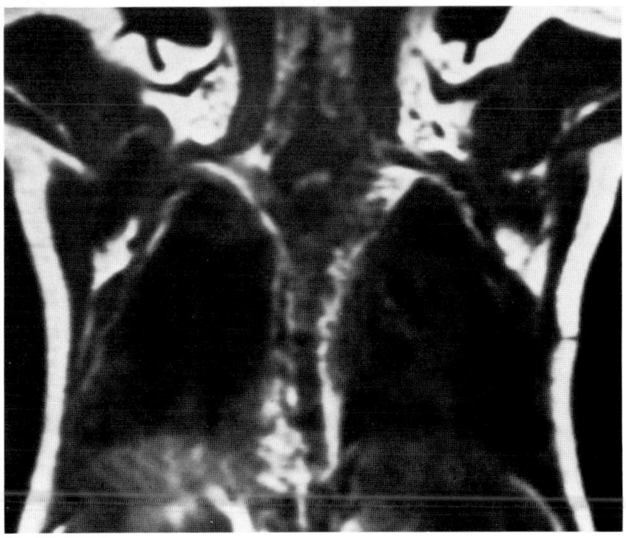

C

Fig. 3–63 Neurenteric cyst. **(A)** Anteroposterior chest x-ray demonstrates multiple segmentation-fusion anomalies in the midthoracic spine that were associated with kyphosis. **(B)** Transverse ultrasound image of the thoracic spine shows displacement of the spinal cord to the right by a cystic intraspinal mass. **(C)** Coronal T_1-weighted MRI demonstrates bilateral widening of the spinal canal and a multicystic mass. (*Figure continues.*)

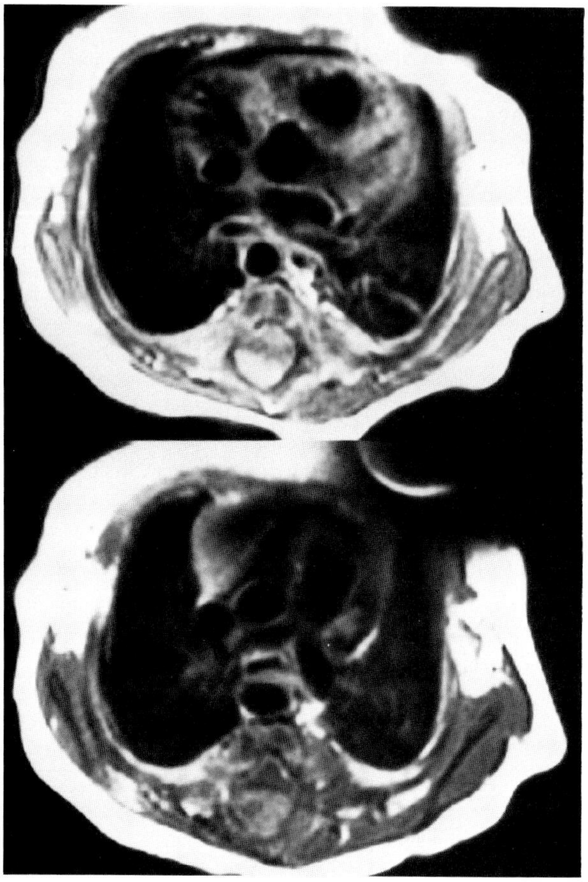

D

Fig. 3–63 (*Continued*). **(D)** Transverse T_1-weighted cardiac-gated MRI demonstrates the heterogeneous nature of the intraspinal mass. The fluid collections behaved like cerebrospinal fluid on various pulse sequences. At surgery, an intraspinal neurenteric cyst was found.

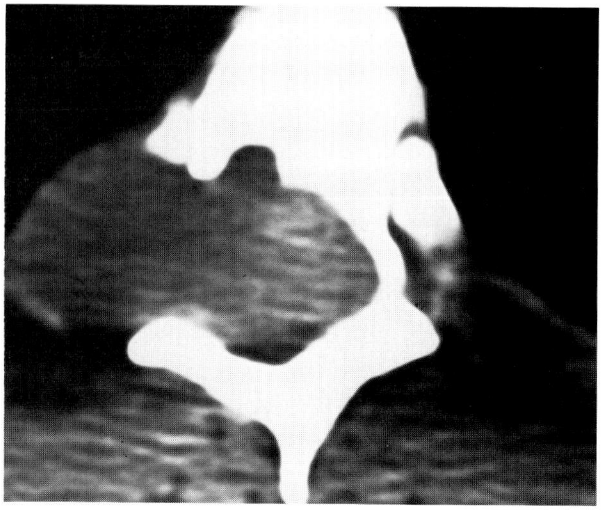

A

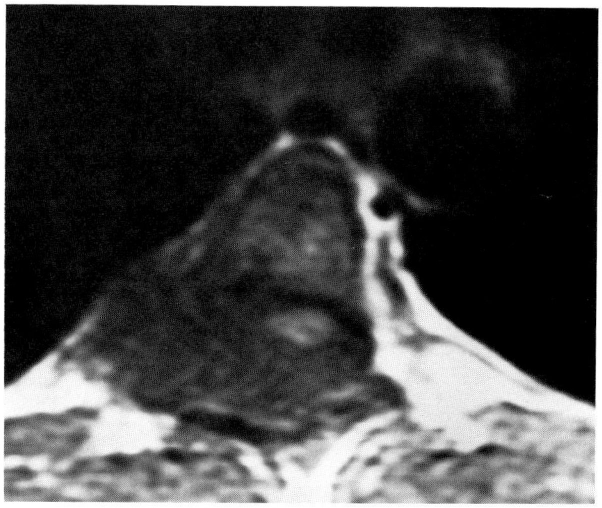

B

Fig. 3–64 Lateral thoracic meningocele. **(A)** Axial nonenhanced CT scan demonstrates widening of the right T5 neural foramen. A low density mass spans the gap. **(B)** The mass is filled with fluid with the same signal intensity as the cerebrospinal fluid surrounding the hyperintense spinal cord on this T_1-weighted axial MRI.

genital causes of posterior mediastinal masses (Fig. 3–64), and are usually associated with kyphoscoliosis. Myelography coordinated with CT is the diagnostic modality of choice in these cases. Congenital diaphragmatic hernias through the foramen of Bochdalek and hiatal hernias may present as posterior mediastinal masses. Azygous continuation of the inferior vena cava presents as irregular dilatation of the azygos vein on the frontal view and the absence of the inferior vena cava shadow on the lateral view (Fig. 3–65). Ectopic thymus occurs most commonly in the posterior mediastinum and may lie posterior to the superior vena cava. Congenital hemolytic anemias or thalassemia may lead to extramedullary hematopoiesis presenting as lobulated masses, usually bilateral, in the lower half of the thorax.

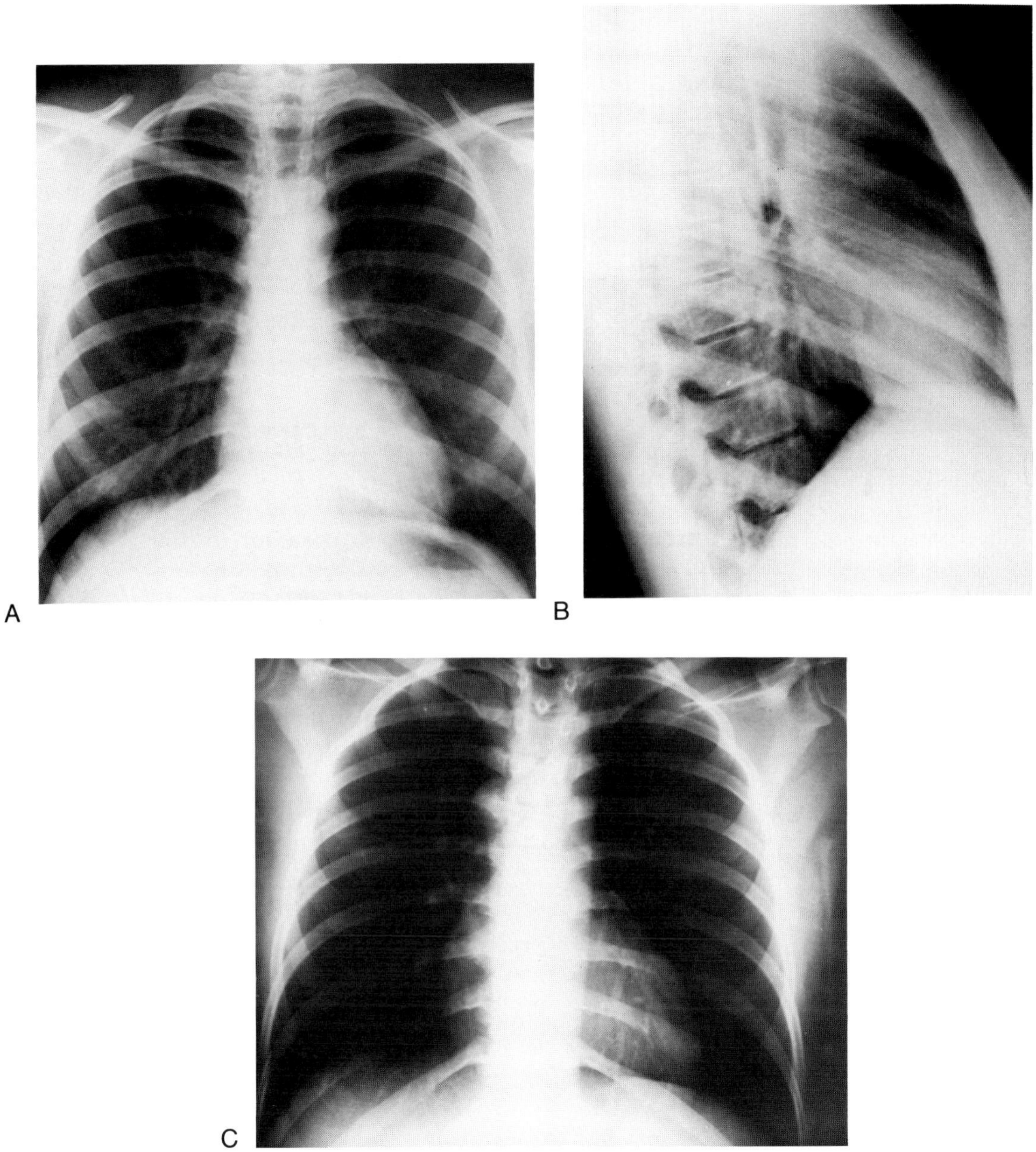

Fig. 3–65 Azygous continuation of the inferior vena cava. **(A)** Posteroanterior chest x-ray of an asymptomatic teenager appears normal. **(B)** Lateral view demonstrates absence of the inferior vena cava. **(C)** An over-penetrated chest x-ray demonstrates a prominent, irregular azygos vein. The combination of findings is suggestive of the diagnosis of azygos continuation of the inferior vena cava. *(Figure continues.)*

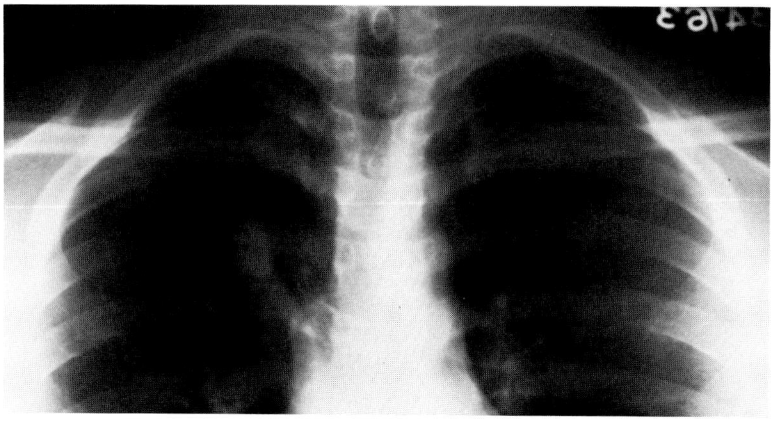

D

Fig. 3–65 (*Continued*). **(D)** Notice the prominence of the azygos vein and the azygos lobe in the close-up view of the upper thorax of another patient with azygos continuation of the inferior vena cava.

Inflammatory conditions affecting the posterior mediastinum include endothoracic extension of pancreatic pseudocysts and spinal osteomyelitis usually caused by granulomatous infections. Although Pott's disease is associated with tuberculosis, other fungal infections involving the spine tend to spare the disk spaces (Fig. 3–66).

Neoplastic conditions aside from neuroblastoma/ganglioneuroma include neurofibromas, lipomas, other mesenchymal tumors and their sarcomatous counterparts, pheochromocytoma, and neoplasms of the bony spine (giant osteoblastomas, osteogenic sarcoma, Ewing's sarcoma, lymphoma, leukemia and osteoblastic metastases, and aneurysmal bone cysts).

Spinal trauma or posterior rib fractures may result in a posterior mediastinal hematoma. Traumatic diaphragmatic hernia may be difficult to differentiate from the congenital variety unless previous radiographs are available for comparison. Other miscellaneous causes include malposition of solid organs, such as herniation of a kidney through the foramen of Bochdalek, and small posteriorly situated pneumonias.

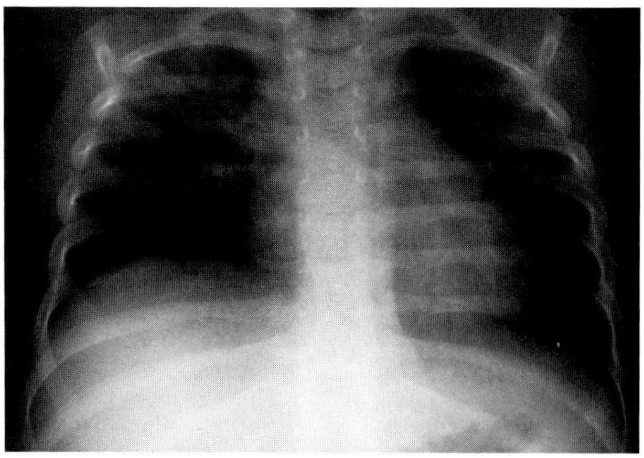

A

Fig. 3–66 Spinal osteomyelitis. **(A)** Anteroposterior chest x-ray demonstrates right upper lobe disease and a left paraspinous mass. There appears to be loss of height of the lower thoracic vertebral bodies. The combination of lung disease and a paraspinal mass is suspicious for tuberculosis with subsequent development of Pott's disease. (*Figure continues.*)

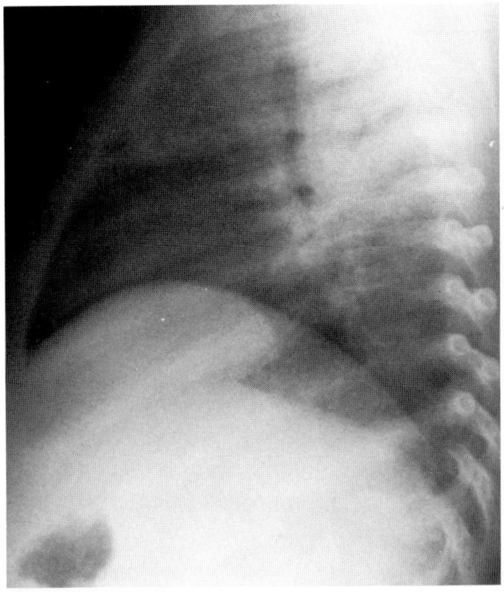

B

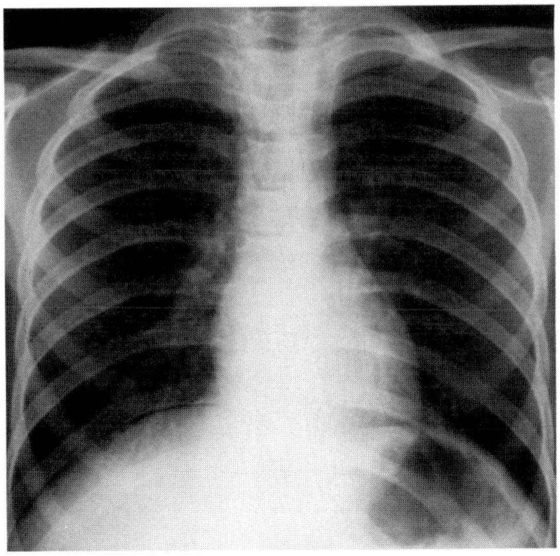

C

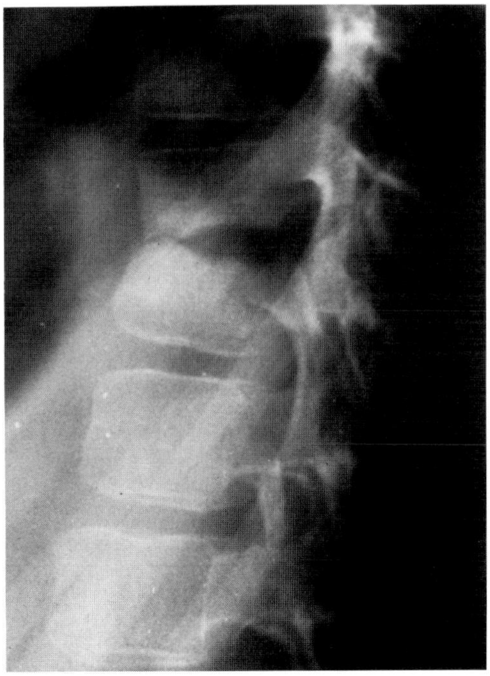

D

Fig. 3–66 (*Continued*). **(B)** Lateral view confirms profound destruction of the vertebral bodies of T9 to T11. **(C)** Another child who presented with back pain. Note the subtle bilateral paraspinous masses at the level of the diaphragm. The lungs are clear. **(D)** Lateral view of the lower thoracic spine demonstrates destruction of the disk space and adjacent vertebral bodies at T10-T11. Disk space destruction is suggestive of osteomyelitis caused by tuberculosis or bacteria. Other fungi spare the disk space.

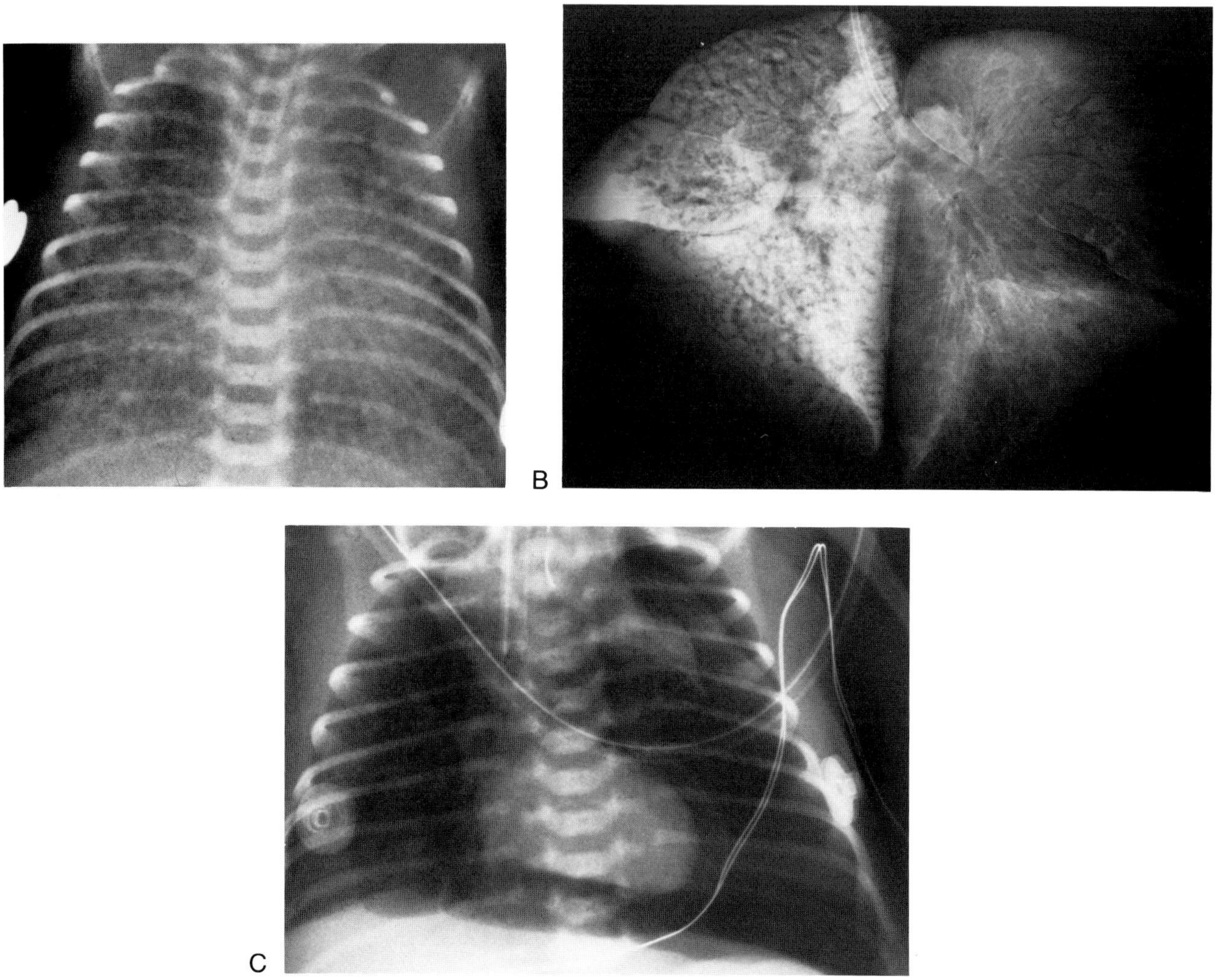

Fig. 3–67 Pulmonary interstitial emphysema. **(A)** Anteroposterior chest x-ray reveals serpiginous air collections throughout both lungs, characteristic of pulmonary interstitial emphysema. Respiratory distress syndrome made mechanical ventilation necessary and resulted in this complication. **(B)** Postmortem specimen of another infant demonstrates pulmonary interstitial emphysema that is worse on the right than the left. Notice the serpiginous lines coursing throughout the lung parenchyma, which do not correspond to normal bronchioles. **(C)** Another patient required high ventilatory settings for aeration of his immature lungs. This resulted in a left pneumothorax, pneumopericardium, and a pneumomediastinum ("continous diaphragm" sign). The thymus is bilaterally uplifted by the mediastinal air ("angel wing" sign).

Mediastinal Air

Air may occupy the mediastinal space and may extend either into the neck or into the abdominal cavity. In the newborn, pneumomediastinum results in elevation of both thymic lobes (the angel wings sign), and is a frequent complication of pulmonary interstitial emphysema (Fig. 3–67). Pulmonary interstitial emphysema often results after high pressure ventilation is used on patients with hyaline membrane disease. Tiny serpiginous air collections are seen in the distal lung parenchyma. These collections are trapped on expiration and eventually lead to pneumothorax,

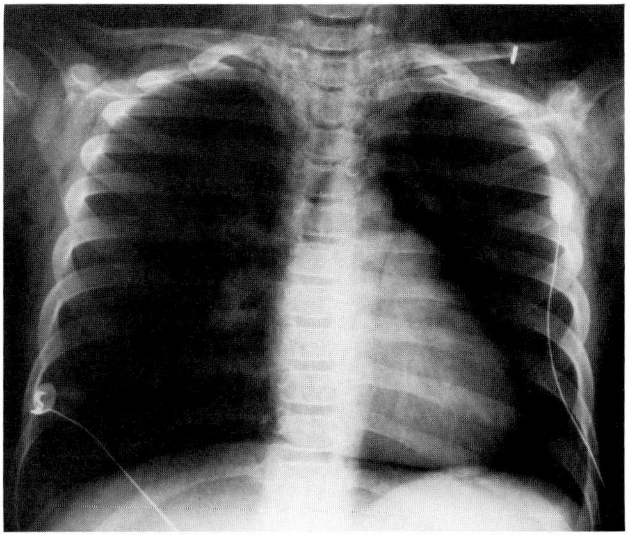

Fig. 3–68 Pneumomediastinum. Posteroanterior chest x-ray reveals the lower margin of the heart to be outlined by air. Also note the pleuropericardial air, air silhouetting the aortic knob and descending aorta, and subcutaneous emphysema. The spontaneous free air accumulations were secondary to a severe cough.

pneumomediastinum, or pneumopericardium. The most common cause of pneumomediastinum in children is asthmatic airway obstruction. Paroxysmal coughing may occasionally lead to spontaneous pneumomediastinum formation. Either accidental or iatrogenic trauma to the chest wall, esophagus, tracheobronchial tree, and lung parenchyma may result in mediastinal air collections. The continuous diaphragm sign is characteristic of pneumomediastinum (Fig. 3–68).

SUGGESTED READINGS

1. Ablow RC, Gross I, Effman EL, et al: The radiographic features of early onset group B streptococcal neonatal sepsis. Radiology 124:771, 1977
2. Amodio J, Abramson S, Berdon W: Primary pulmonary tuberculosis in infancy: a resurgent disease in the urban United States. Pediatr Radiol 16:185, 1986
3. Buck JR, Connors RH, Coon WW, et al: Pulmonary embolism in children. J Pediatr Surg 16:385, 1981
4. Buntain W, Woolley M, Mahour GH, et al: Pulmonary sequestration in children: a 25-year experience. Surgery 81:413, 1977
5. Chudley AE, Barmada MA: Diaphragmatic elevation in neonatal myotonic dystrophy. Am J Dis Child 133:1182, 1979
6. Couchard M, Polge J, Bomsel F: Hyaline membrane disease: diagnosis, radiologic observation, treatment and complications. A radiological study of 589 cases. Am Radiol 17:669, 1974
7. Day DL, Gedgaudas E: The thymus. Radiol Clin North Am 22:519, 1984
8. Fagan CJ, Swischuk LE: The opaque lung in lobar emphysema. AJR 114:300, 1972
9. Faure C, Verderi D, Schmit P, Sirinelli D: Chest x-ray findings in children with congenital ciliary abnormalities. Pediatr Radiol 15:269, 1985
10. Felman AH, Rhatigan RM, Pierson KK: Pulmonary lymphangiectasia: observations in 17 patients and proposed classification. AJR 116:548, 1972
11. Felson B: Pulmonary agenesis and related anomalies. Semin Roentgenol 7:17, 1972
12. Fisher JE, Nelson SJ, Allen JE, Holzman RS: Congenital cystic adenomatoid malformation of the lung. Am J Dis Child 136:1071, 1982
13. Franken EA Jr, Smith JA, Smith WL: Tumors of the chest wall in infants and children. Pediatr Radiol 6:13, 1977
14. Gregory GA, Gooding CA, Phibbs RH, Tooley WH: Meconium aspiration in infants—a prospective study. J Pediatr 85:848, 1974
15. Hall JA Jr, Hartenburg MA, Kodroff MB: Chest radiographic findings in neonates on extracorporeal membrane oxygenation. Radiology 157:75, 1985
16. Hartman GE, Schochat SJ: Primary pulmonary neo-

plasms of childhood: a review. Ann Thorac Surg 36:108, 1983
17. Hungerford GD, Williams HBL, Gandevia B: Bronchial walls in radiologic diagnosis of asthma. Br J Radiol 50:783, 1977
18. Kassner EG, Kauffman SL, Yoon JJ, et al: Pulmonary candidiasis in infants: clinical radiologic and pathologic features. AJR 137:707, 1981
19. King RM, Telander RL, Smithson WA, et al: Primary mediastinal tumors in children. J Pediatr Surg 17:512, 1982
20. Kirkpatrick JA, Fleisher DS: Roentgen appearance of chest in acute glomerulonephritis in children. J Pediatr 64:492, 1964
21. Kuhn JP, Fletcher BD, DeLemos RA: Roentgen findings in transient tachypnea of the newborn. Radiology 92:751, 1969
22. MacPherson RI, Cumming GR, Chernick V: Unilateral hyperlucent lung: a complication of viral pneumonia. J Can Assoc Radiol 20:225, 1969
23. McCook TA, Kirks DR, Merten DF, et al: Pulmonary alveolar proteinosis in children. AJR 137:1023, 1981
24. Merten DF, Bowie JD, Kirks DR, Grossman H: Anteromedial diaphragmatic defects in infancy: current approaches to diagnostic imaging. Radiology 142:361, 1982
25. Mikity VG, Taber P: Complications in the treatment of the respiratory distress syndrome: bronchopulmonary dysplasia, oxygen toxicity and the Wilson-Mikity syndrome. Pediatr Clin North Am 20:419, 1973
26. Moskowitz PS, Griscom NT: The medial pneumothorax. Radiology 120:143, 1976
27. Neumann G, Benz-Bohn G, Rister M: Wegener's granulomatosis in childhood. Pediatr Radiol 14:267, 1984
28. Othersen HB Jr, Lorenzo RL: Diaphragmatic paralysis and eventration: newer approaches to diagnosis and operative correction. J Pediatr Surg 12:309, 1977
29. Reed JC, Sobonya RE: Congenital lung cyst. Radiology 117:315, 1975
30. Riggs W Jr, Benton C, Wood B: Cervical neurogenic tumors presenting as thoracic apical masses in infants and children. Pediatr Radiol 5:201, 1977
31. Sumner TE, Volberg FM, Kiser PE, Shaffner L: Mediastinal cystic hygroma in children. Pediatr Radiol 11:160, 1981
32. Swischuk LE: Bubbles in hyaline membrane disease: differentiation of three types. Radiology 122:417, 1977
33. Swischuk LE, Hayden CK Jr: Lower respiratory tract infection in children (is roentgenographic differentiation possible?) Pediatr Radiol 16:4278, 1986
34. Swischuk LE, Hayden CK Jr, Richardson CJ: Neonatal opaque right lung: delayed fluid resorption. Radiology 141:671, 1981
35. Westcott JL, Cole SR: Interstitial pulmonary emphysema in children and adults: roentgenographic features. Radiology 111:367, 1974
36. Wood BP: Infantile chlamydia trachomatis pneumonia: radiographic features. Ann Radiol 22:213, 1979

4

Heart and Great Vessels

Janet L. Strife

APPROACH

By far, the most common cause of cardiovascular abnormalities in children is congenital heart disease. The chest x-ray remains the major screening tool for suspecting cardiac anomalies. In an era of color flow Doppler echocardiography, axial angiography, magnetic resonance imaging (MRI), and in vivo myocardial metabolism, blood flow and perfusion studies, it is simplistic to think that a specific definitive diagnosis can be made on the basis of the plain radiograph. However, since the plain radiograph is the major screening tool, familiarity with the normal and abnormal structures improves one's diagnostic acumen in delineating those patients suspected of having congenital heart disease; knowing where normal structures are and the relation of the vessels to the lung greatly facilitates the interpretation of chest x-rays.

As in all areas of radiology, a systematic approach is essential in evaluating a chest x-ray to discern all the clues necessary for proper interpretation. One must evaluate heart size, configuration, pulmonary blood flow, chamber enlargement, situs abnormalities, and bony and soft tissue changes. This chapter presents an ordered approach to the plain radiograph diagnosis of congenital heart disease and anomalies of the great vessels. In addition, appropriate clinical information, radiographic appearance, and various imaging modalities are discussed as they relate to specific common congenital lesions. Eight lesions, which account for 80 percent of all congenital heart disease, are listed in Table 4–1.

Table 4–1 Incidence of Congenital Heart Defects

Defect	Percentage
Ventricular septal defect	29
Atrial septal defect	11
Pulmonic stenosis	9
Patent ductus arteriosus	8
Tetralogy of Fallot	6
Aortic stenosis	5
Coarctation	5
D-transposition of the great vessels	4
Other	23
Total	100

Percentage averaged from multiple studies.
(Modified from Condon,[4] with permission.)

Pulmonary Vascularity

Congenital heart lesions are categorized by pulmonary vascular patterns and the presence or absence of cyanosis. Pulmonary arterial flow is described as increased, diminished, symmetric, asymmetric, or demonstrating systemic collateral flow. The radiographic assessment of pulmonary flow is difficult, occasionally even for the experienced observer. One method is to evaluate the diameter of the right descending pulmonary artery and correlate it to the diameter of the trachea at the level of the aortic knob. The tracheal diameter of normal children increases directly with age and the absolute tracheal diameter closely corresponds to the absolute diameter of the right descending pulmonary artery (Fig. 4–1). However, in patients with left-to-right shunts with an increase in volume and size of the pulmonary arteries, the right descending pulmonary artery will not be smaller than the tracheal diameter and frequently is larger. The normal pulmonary artery in the periphery has a constant relationship to the diameter of the adjacent bronchial lumen. The arterial bronchial index is independent of age or sex. Therefore, on standard chest x-rays one can compare the diameter of the vessel seen on end with that of the adjacent bronchus (Fig. 4–2).

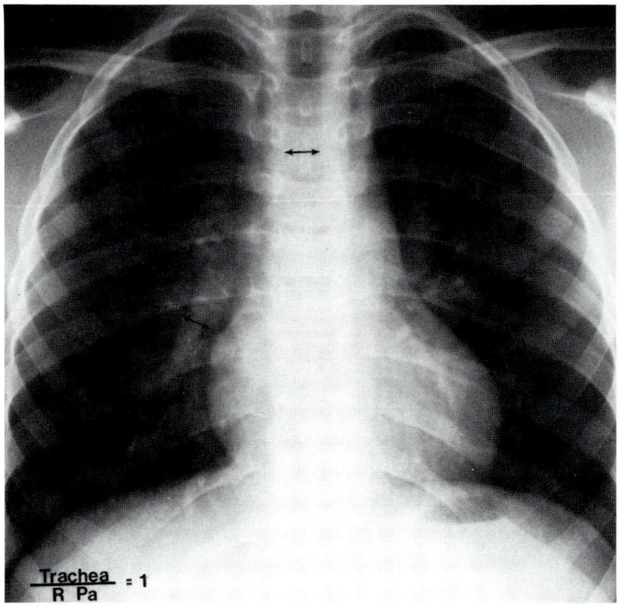

Fig. 4–1 A normal chest radiograph. The transverse diameter of the trachea at the level of the aortic arch (top arrow) is the same as the diameter of the right descending pulmonary artery (bottom arrow).

CATEGORIZING CONGENITAL HEART DISEASE BASED ON ASSESSMENT OF PULMONARY FLOW

Acyanotic: increased flow
- Ventricular septal defect
- Patent ductus arteriosus
- Atrial septal defect
- Atrioventricular canal defect
- Aortic pulmonary window
- Partial anomalous pulmonary venous return

Cyanotic: decreased pulmonary flow
- Tetralogy of Fallot
- Tricuspid atresia
- D-transposition of the great vessels with pulmonic stenosis

Cyanotic: increased pulmonary flow
- D-transposition of the great vessels
- Truncus arteriosus
- Total anomalous pulmonary venous return
- Single ventricle

Heart disease with normal pulmonary flow
- Pulmonic stenosis
- Aortic stenosis
- Coarctation of the aorta
- Mitral stenosis

Decreased pulmonary arterial flow occurs when blood is diverted away from the pulmonary circuit. In these circumstances, the main pulmonary artery segment is decreased in size and the peripheral portions of the right and left pulmonary arteries are small and thinned. It may give a hyperlucent appearance to the lung. Systemic collateral or aortic pulmonary anastomosis flow can be seen when the normal arborization of vessels from the right and left hilum does not occur. The systemic collateral vessels have abnormal direction and appear more tortuous. Occasionally, the origin of the systemic collateral vessels from the descending aorta is apparent (Fig. 4–3).

Normally, the right and left pulmonary arteries are of similar size and close inspection should determine whether they are symmetric. Familiarity with causes of asymmetric enlargement will aid in making a specific diagnosis. For example, in pulmonary valvar stenosis, enlargement of the left pulmonary artery due to a jet phenomenon occurs, with poststenotic dilatation involving the left pulmonary artery more than the right. Unequal blood flow also occurs in

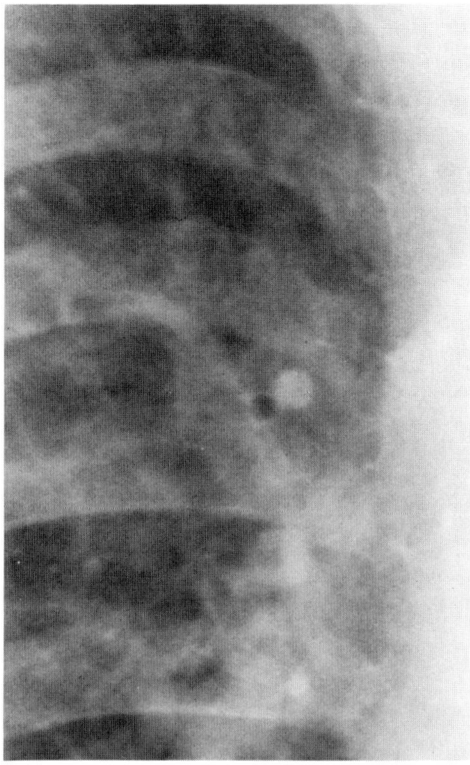

Fig. 4–2 This patient has a left-to-right shunt. Note the diameter of the artery is larger than the diameter of the adjacent bronchial lumen.

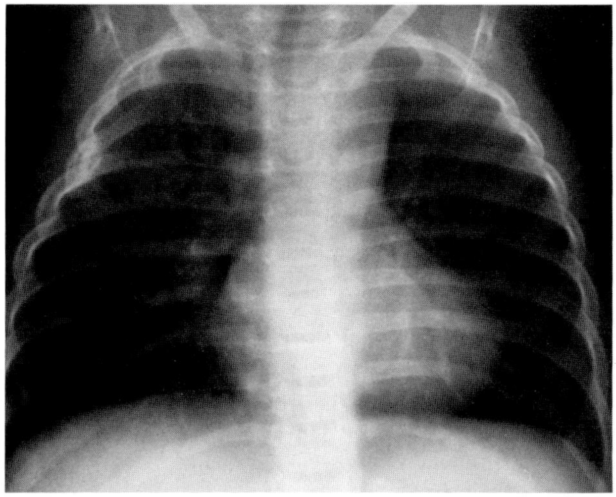

Fig. 4–4 Asymmetric pulmonary flow with the right pulmonary artery larger than the left. This patient has tetralogy of Fallot and has postoperative rib changes involving the 4th and 5th ribs, along the right lateral chest wall, secondary to a palliative Blalock-Taussig shunt.

patients that have had systemic-to-pulmonary palliative anastomosis. If surgical rib changes on the side of increased pulmonary flow are seen, systemic-to-pulmonary palliative anastomosis is a likely diagnosis (Fig. 4–4).

A 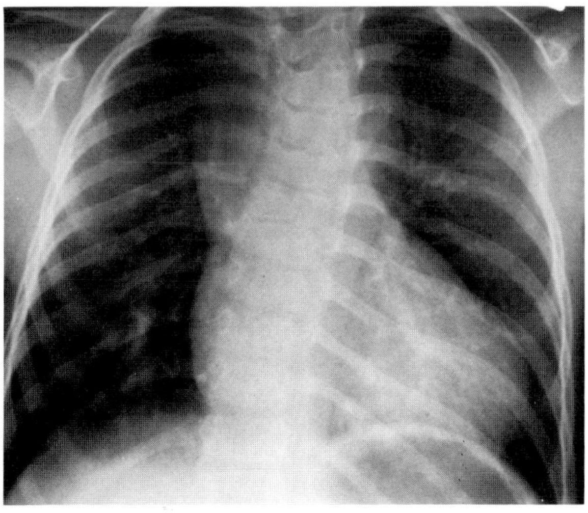

B 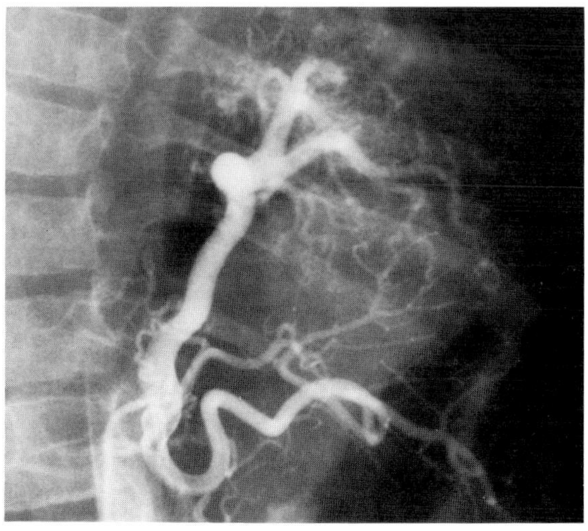

Fig. 4–3 This patient has pulmonary atresia, ventricular septal defect, and systemic collateral vessels arising from the descending aorta to the lungs. **(A)** There is abnormal arborization of vessels. The pulmonary arterial vessels do not appear to have a hilar origin. **(B)** Selective injection of a systemic vessel off the descending aorta. The tortuous vessels extend into the lung and have abnormal vascular distributions.

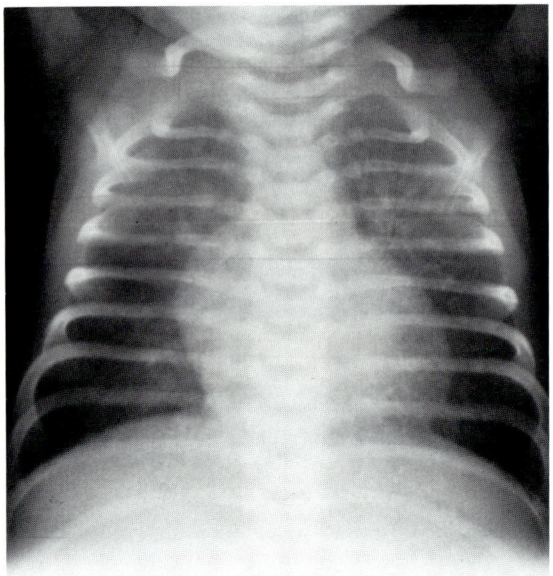

Fig. 4–5 An example of pulmonary edema in an 8-day-old child who has total anomalous pulmonary venous return. Note the blurred, indistinct appearance of the vessels.

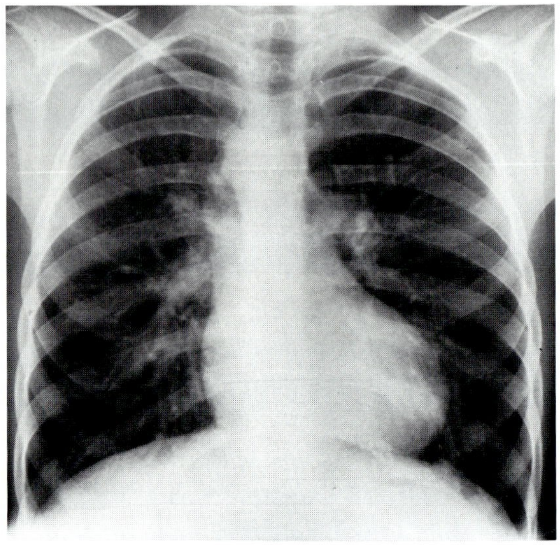

Fig. 4–6 In patients with right aortic arch, the trachea is displaced to the left and indented on its right lateral border. The aortic knob and descending aorta can also be visualized.

Pulmonary venous prominence is suggested by a lacy reticulated appearance. Pulmonary edema in young infants is recognized with an indistinctness of vessels and a reticulated-like pattern of the lungs (Fig. 4–5).

The size and position of the aortic knob is important in a systematic approach to congenital heart lesions. In infancy, the site of the aortic arch is frequently difficult due to the presence of the thymus. Close inspection of the chest x-ray should be made for indentation of the aortic knob on the trachea, site of the aortic knob, and the position of the descending aorta. As the child becomes older, the position of the aortic knob is easier to recognize. The trachea in a child with a right aortic arch is frequently displaced to the midline or towards the left (Fig. 4–6). The finding of a right aortic arch suggests cyanotic heart disease. The most common lesions having a right aortic arch include truncus arteriosus (30 to 35 percent), tetralogy of Fallot (30 percent), pulmonary atresia with ventricular septal defect (30 percent), double outlet right ventricle (20 percent), and tricuspid atresia (3 to 5 percent). The size of the aortic knob is also important; when significant right-to-left shunt is present, the aorta is usually enlarged.

Heart Size and Specific Chamber Enlargement

Assessment of heart size is difficult in young infants due to the presence of the thymus and the lateral view is useful in assessing cardiomegaly. When there is left atrial enlargement, posterior displacement of the left main stem bronchus may be noted on lateral views. In normal children, the posterior border of the heart is partially formed by the posterior wall of the inferior vena cava as it enters the right atrium; it is unusual to have any chamber posterior to the inferior vena cava. However, with left ventricular dilatation and occasionally with left ventricular hypertrophy, there will be prominence of a chamber posterior to the inferior vena cava (Fig. 4–7). Occasionally, patients with severe right ventricular hypertrophy will displace the left ventricle posteriorly and give a similar appearance. Right ventricular enlargement is

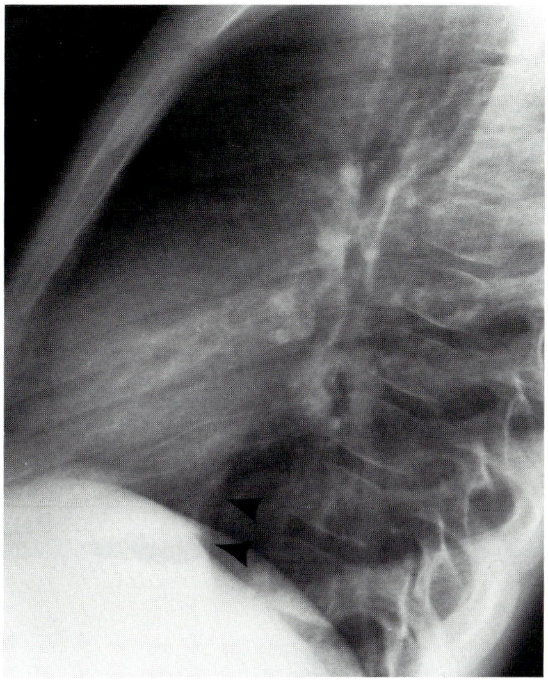

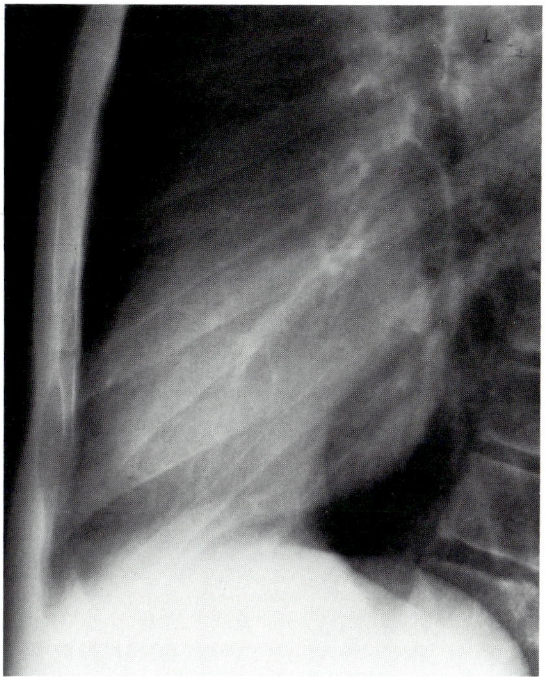

Fig. 4–7 (A) Lateral view of the chest demonstrating the posterior wall of the inferior vena cava in a normal patient (arrows). **(B)** The patient has left ventricular enlargement with aortic insufficiency.

recognized by uplifting of the apex of the heart. On the lateral view in older patients a filling in of the retrosternal clear space occurs.

Extracardiac Structures

The most common cause of rib notching in children is coarctation of the aorta. The rib notching is due to collateral blood flow from the subclavian arteries to the internal mammary arteries to the intercostal arteries to the aorta below the level of obstruction.

Close inspection for evidence of prior heart surgery should be made by examining the ribs for sclerosis or bony or soft tissue changes indicating a prior thoracotomy (see Fig. 4–4). Surgical procedures involving a left thoracotomy include palliative shunts, of which the Blalock-Taussig is the most common. A left thoracotomy approach is also used in repair of coarctation, ductus arteriosus ligation, and occasionally pulmonary artery banding. Postoperative radiographs demonstrating midline sternotomy sutures usually involve total repairs such as total repair of tetralogy of Fallot, repair of transposition of the great vessels, repair of intracardiac shunts, and surgical repair of the aortic valve or pulmonary valve. A right thoracotomy approach is seen less frequently. It may be associated with a systemic-to-pulmonary anastomosis. Occasionally, atrial septotomies are performed via a right thoracotomy.

Situs Considerations

The term *situs* defines the position of the normally asymmetric organs such as the lungs, atria, liver, spleen, and stomach in relation to the midline or sagittal plane. In situs solitus, the normal situation, the trilobed lung, venous atrium, and liver are in the right side and the bilobed lung, arterial atrium, stomach, and spleen are on the left. Situs inversus is the mirror image of normal. The incidence of congenital heart disease in situs inversus is 3 to 5 percent. Situs ambiguous is an unusual condition in which the previously noted asymmetric structures may be symmetric. Therefore, one can have bilateral left-sidedness, seen in polysplenia syndromes, or bilateral right-sidedness, seen in asplenia syndromes. In a condition of situs solitus with right-sided cardiac apex or situs inversus with left-sided cardiac apex, there is discordance between the cardiac apex and the abdominal situs. When discordance occurs, 95 to 98 percent of patients have congenital heart disease that is frequently complex heart disease. The best indication of situs is tracheobronchial anatomy. The right mainstem bronchus has a more acute angle at the bifurcation than the left bronchus. Close inspection for venous anomalies of either systemic or pulmonary venous return should be made. Patients that have bilateral right-sidedness have more severe congenital anomalies than ones that have bilateral left-sidedness.

CONGENITAL HEART DISEASE WITH INCREASED PULMONARY ARTERIAL FLOW

Ventricular Septal Defect

Ventricular septal defect is the most common congenital heart lesion associated with an increase in pulmonary arterial flow. In overall incidence, it is second only to bicuspid aortic valve and accounts for 29 percent of all congenital cardiac anomalies. Ventricular septal defects may occur alone or in association with a number of other lesions. Of the four types of ventricular septal defects, the most common is a defect in the *membranous* portion of the ventricular septum, which is high in the interventricular septum beneath the aortic valve (Fig. 4–8). *Muscular defects* occur lower in the ventricular septum and can be multiple. Up to 20 percent of muscular defects may close spontaneously as the child grows. A defect that is above the crista supraventricularis, immediately inferior to the anterior leaflet of the aortic valve, is called a *supracristal ventricular septal defect.* This type of defect is associated with aortic insufficiency. Even though the left-to-right shunting in this lesion is not severe, the lesion may cause turbulence and injury to the aortic valve and necessitate surgery. The ventricular septum also has a defect, which is posterior and part of the *atrioventricular canal defect.*

Radiographically, small left-to-right shunts appear normal. Patients with moderate shunts demonstrate moderate cardiomegaly and increase in pulmonary arterial flow. In those patients with large left-to-right shunts, there may be marked cardiomegaly, enlargement of the main pulmonary artery, peripheral pulmonary arteries, and mild changes of heart failure. In infants and young children, when the main pulmonary artery enlarges it encroaches on the superior mediastinum and is high in position. In fact, the main pulmonary artery may be at the same level of the transverse portion of the aortic knob (Fig. 4–9). There also may be hyperinflation of the lungs as the increase in pulmonary arterial flow decreases pulmonary elasticity and recoil. Patients with large left-to-right shunts have an increased incidence of recurrent pneumonia and pulmonary infections. Left atrial enlargement may be evident by posterior displacement of the left main stem bronchus on lateral view (Fig. 4–10).

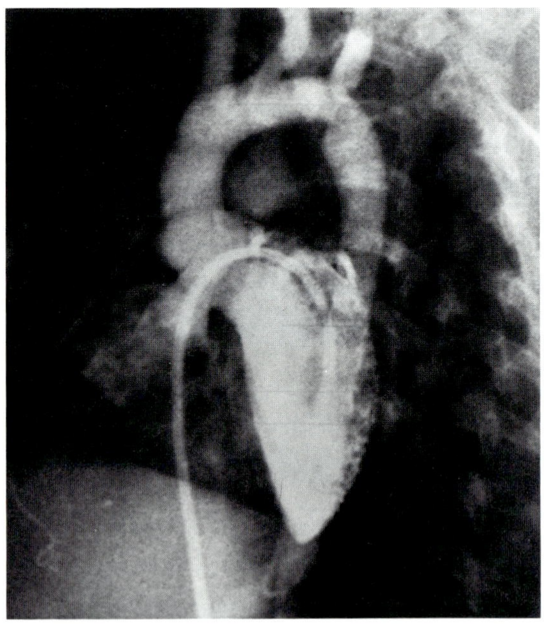

Fig. 4–8 Membranous ventricular septal defect. Left ventriculography with 70 degree left anterior oblique and 30 degree cranial angulation demonstrating a high membranous ventricular septal defect.

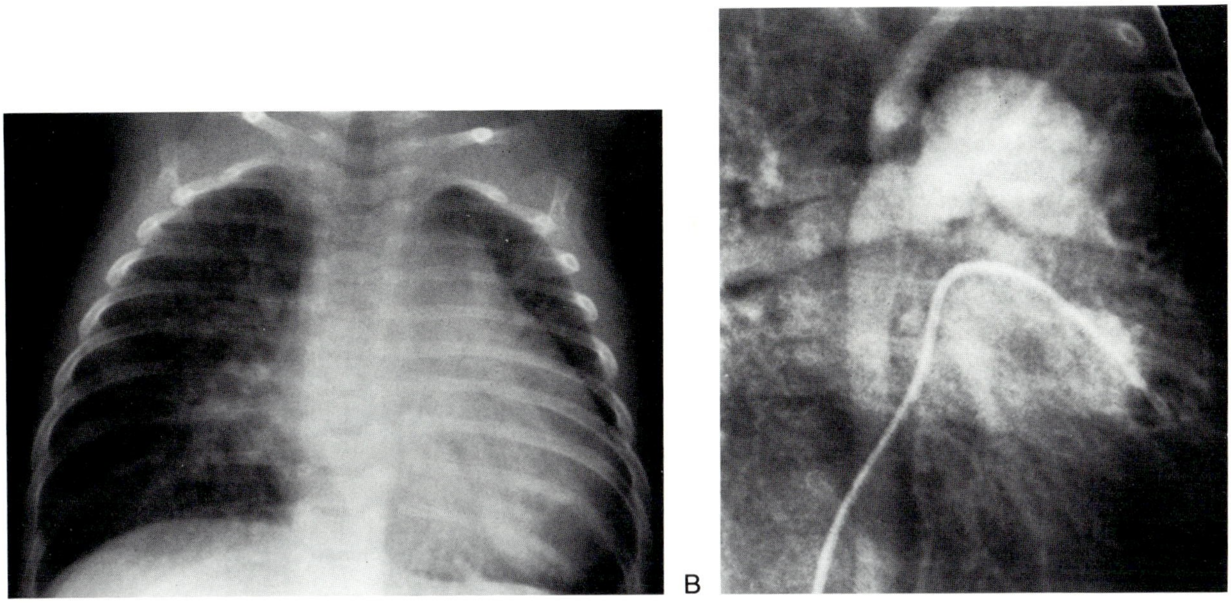

A B

Fig. 4–9 Moderate ventricular septal defect. **(A)** The cardiac pericardial silhouette is enlarged and there is prominence of the main pulmonary artery and increased flow. **(B)** Left ventriculography in 30 degree right anterior oblique view demonstrates filling of both the pulmonary artery (via ventricular septal defect) and the aorta. Notice that the main pulmonary artery encroaches on the superior mediastinum as it enlarges.

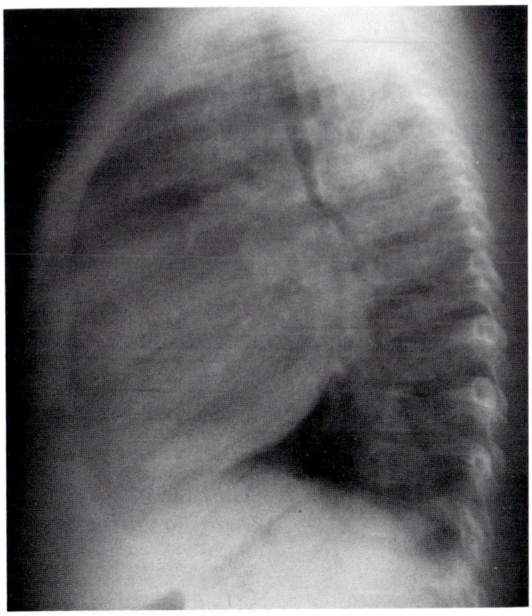

Fig. 4–10 The left mainstem bronchus is displaced posteriorly due to left atrial enlargement.

In approximately one-third of patients with ventricular septal defects, the defect closes spontaneously. Treatment depends on the size of the defect. In large shunts, a surgical approach with placement of a Dacron patch or pericardial patch on the ventricular septal defect is usually performed.

Patent Ductus Arteriosus

A patent ductus arteriosus is a communication between the aorta and pulmonary artery. The ductus arteriosus in premature infants is dynamic and there may be right-to-left shunting, left-to-right shunting, bidirectional shunting, or transient closure. The exact mechanisms responsible for the initial closure of the ductus arteriosus are not fully understood.

In certain individuals, the normal mechanism for closure of the ductus arteriosus does not occur in infancy resulting in persistent communication between the aorta and pulmonary artery. As the aortic pressure is higher in both systole and diastole, continuous left-to-right shunting through the ductus arteriosus occurs.

The typical chest x-ray shows mild cardiomegaly with increased size of the main pulmonary artery and increase in pulmonary arterial flow. In patients with small-to-medium left-to-right shunting, the left atrium and left ventricle may be of normal size, however, in large shunts, there is a large pulmonary artery, large left atrium, left ventricle, and prominence of the ascending aorta.

In newborns or premature infants, a patent ductus arteriosus is a common cause of congestive heart failure. During the first week of life, physiologic pulmonary arterial hypertension in association with respiratory distress syndrome may be present and shunting at the ductal level may be bidirectional. As the hyaline membrane disease improves and pulmonary artery pressure begins to fall, left-to-right shunting may occur. This delayed closure of ductus arteriosus in preterm infants is well recognized radiographically. Evaluation of serial chest x-rays is important as there may be a mild increase in heart size and an indistinctness of the pulmonary vascularity suggesting pulmonary edema.

The treatment of premature neonates with respiratory distress syndrome and a patent ductus arteriosus has been both surgical and pharmacologic using prostaglandin inhibitors. In older patients, surgical ligation requires a left thoracotomy (unless there is a right aortic arch) with division of the ductus. Approaches to percutaneous closure of the ductus using expandable umbrellas has met with some success.

A patent ductus arteriosus may be associated with left-sided congenital lesions such as aortic valve stenosis, coarctation of the aorta, interruption of the aorta or hypoplastic left heart syndrome. Bidirectional shunting may be present. On the other hand, left-to-right shunting occurs in patients who have marked decrease in pulmonary artery flow, such as pulmonary atresia, severe tetralogy of Fallot, or tricuspid atresia.

Atrial Septal Defect

The atrial septal defect is the third most common cause of increase in pulmonary arterial flow. Usually, atrial septal defects occur in girls and present later in childhood. The left atrial pressure is only slightly higher than the right atrial pressure and, even in the presence of a large defect, the patients are rarely symptomatic. Isolated atrial septal defects may be subdivided according to their position within the atrial septum. A patent foramen ovale is commonly present, particularly in the neonate. This is simply a defect in apposition of the septum secundum to the septum primum. This defect becomes functional only if sufficient elevation of pressure occurs in the right atrium, allowing a right-to-left shunt. The ostium secundum defect is the most common of all atrial septal defects and accounts for 60 percent of cases. It is a single opening of 1 to 3 cm in diameter and is located near the fossa ovalis. The sinus venosus atrial septal defect is located high in the atrial septum at the junction of the superior vena cava and right atrium. It is almost always associated with anomalous drainage of the upper lobe pulmonary vein into the superior vena cava.

The chest x-ray will demonstrate a slightly older child, who has increase in pulmonary arterial flow. There may be slight straightening of the left cardiac contour because of dilatation of the pulmonary outflow tract and main pulmonary artery. Filling in of the retrosternal clear space may indicate right ventricular enlargement.

The treatment for atrial septal defects involves elective surgical repair for moderate-to-large shunts. Transcatheter closure using expandable umbrellas that are placed fluoroscopically and guided echographically have increasingly been utilized in some centers.

Atrioventricular Canal Defects

The atrioventricular canal is sometimes referred to as an endocardial cushion defect and is among the most common symptomatic congenital left-to-right heart lesions. Patients with trisomy 21 (Down's syndrome) account for 40 percent of all patients with atrioventricular canals.

The atrioventricular septum contributes to the formation of the ventricular septum, the lower part of the atrial septum, and the septal leaflets of the mitral and tricuspid valves. Abnormalities of growth and fusion of the endocardial cushion or atrioventricular portion of the septum leads to partial or complete defects. There may be various combinations of low atrial septal defect (ostium primum), high ventricular septal defect (posterior defect of the cushion type), and common atrioventricular valve. These patients are prone to develop congestive heart failure early in infancy due to significant left-to-right shunting. The radiographs may demonstrate cardiomegaly, which may be due to insufficiency of the valves in addition to the significant left-to-right shunting (Fig. 4–11). The left-to-right shunting can occur at the atrial level, ventricular level, and left ventricular-right atrial level. Angiographically, there is an abnormality of the mitral valve, which may be cleft, and a "gooseneck" deformity of the left ventricular outflow tract, which is due to an abnormal insertion of the mitral valve leaflets. (Fig. 4–12)

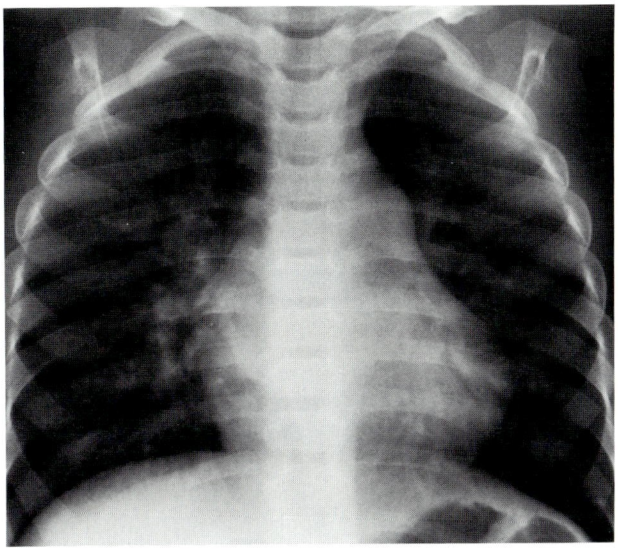

Fig. 4–11 Ostium primum atrial septal defect: mild cardiomegaly, prominence of the main pulmonary artery, and increased pulmonary arterial flow bilaterally.

Other Left-to-Right Shunts

Other causes of congenital heart disease with increased pulmonary vascularity include isolated left ventricular-to-right atrial shunts, aortic pulmonary window, ruptured aortic sinus aneurysm, coronary artery fistula, and partial anomalous pulmonary venous return.

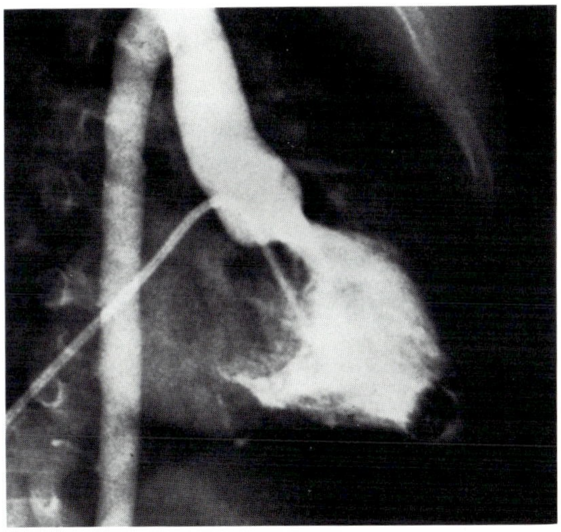

Fig. 4–12 Left ventriculography in a patient with atrioventricular defect performed in the 30 degree RAO view. There is a gooseneck deformity of the left ventricular outflow, and abnormal attachment of the mitral valve with a small left ventricular-right atrial shunt.

CYANOSIS WITH DECREASED PULMONARY FLOW

Tetralogy of Fallot and tricuspid atresia are the most common causes of cyanosis with decreased flow. However, many congenital heart lesions that have associated severe pulmonic stenosis will demonstrate decrease in pulmonary artery flow. Thus, D-transposition of the great vessels with pulmonic stenosis will have diminished flow. In addition, single ventricle or double outlet right ventricle with pulmonic stenosis will have diminished flow. In general, with decreased pulmonary vascularity, the heart size is frequently normal.

Tetralogy of Fallot

The hallmarks of tetralogy of Fallot are (1) right ventricular outflow tract obstruction, (2) subaortic large ventricular septal defect, (3) overriding aorta, and (4) right ventricular hypertrophy. Tetralogy of Fallot is the most common cyanotic congenital heart lesion in childhood and is the fifth most common congenital heart anomaly accounting for 6 percent of congenital heart lesions. The right ventricular outflow tract obstruction can occur at multiple levels and involve

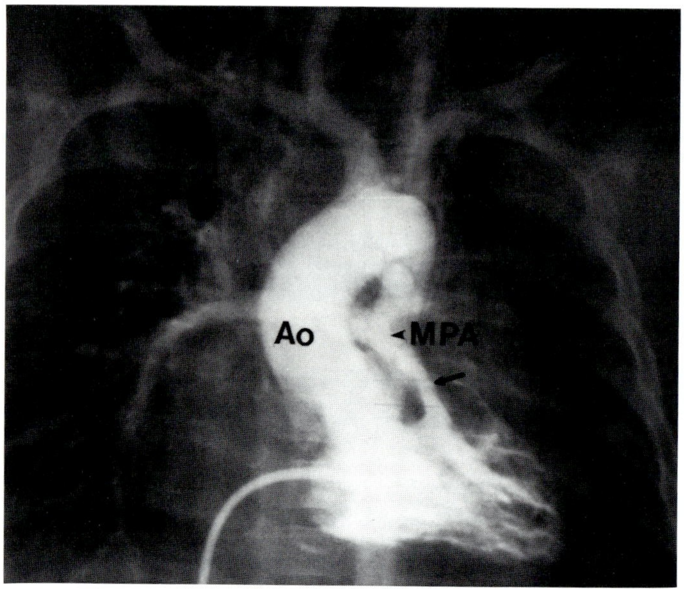

Fig. 4–13 Right ventricular injection demonstrating infundibular narrowing (arrow) and small main pulmonary artery (MPA) (arrowhead). There is significant right-to-left shunting with an enlarged aorta (Ao).

the infundibulum of the right ventricle, the pulmonary annulus, pulmonary valve, main pulmonary artery, and the peripheral pulmonary vessels (Fig. 4–13). Infundibular stenosis is invariably present and relates to anterior displacement of the body of the crista supraventricularis or infundibular septum. The degree of right ventricular outflow tract obstruction determines the severity of the patient's symptoms. Those patients with mild outflow tract obstruction may have left-to-right shunting across the ventricular septal defect. These patients are referred to as "pink tets." However, infundibular stenosis progresses and, eventually, right-to-left shunting across the ventricular septal defect occurs. Right ventricular hypertrophy occurs because of obstruction to outflow of the right ventricle or hypertrophy secondary to ejection of blood via the ventricular septal defect into the aorta.

The chest x-ray is frequently characteristic and demonstrates a normal sized heart with abnormal configuration (Fig. 4–14). Right ventricular hypertrophy rotates the heart in a clockwise rotation and elevates the cardiac apex upward and laterally. This creates the coeur en sabot appearance of the heart. Because of decrease in pulmonary arterial flow, the main pulmonary artery segment may be concave. The aorta is always prominent, secondary to the right-to-left shunt, which occurs at the ventricular level (Fig. 4–13). A right aortic arch is found in 20 to 30 percent of cases.

The cardiovascular history of the entity of tetralogy of Fallot reflects significant advances over the last 50 years in the diagnosis, treatment, and surgical approaches in cardiovascular disease. Dr. Helen Taussig was the pediatric cardiologist who suggested to the surgeon Dr. Howard Blalock that he create a ductus arteriosus in a young cyanotic child with tetralogy of Fallot. The first "blue baby" operation occurred in 1942. A Blalock-Taussig shunt was originally performed using the left or right subclavian artery anastomosed to the right or left pulmonary artery (Fig. 4–15). Currently, a Gortex graft is usually used. As the systemic pressure is always higher than the pulmonary artery pressure, a small shunt creates significant pulmonary artery flow. Definitive repair of tetralogy of Fallot involves closure of the ventricular septal defect and reconstruction of the right ventricular outflow tract to bypass or replace deficient or stenotic pulmonary valves. Due to long-standing right ventricular enlargement, these patients may have dysrhythmias or right bundle branch block following

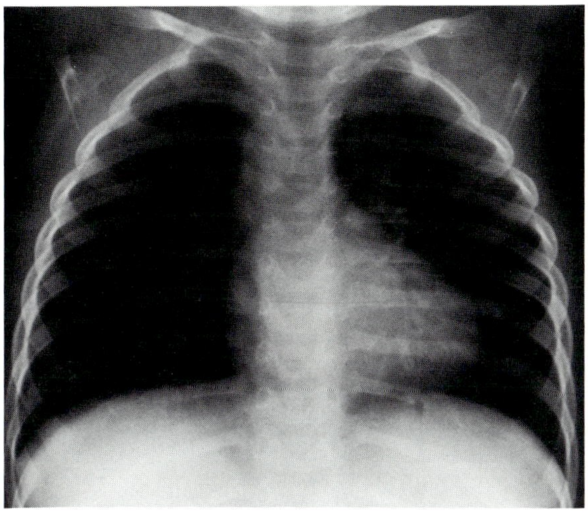

Fig. 4–14 Tetralogy of Fallot. The patient has a boot-shaped heart secondary to right ventricular enlargement, decrease in pulmonary arterial flow bilaterally, and a right aortic arch.

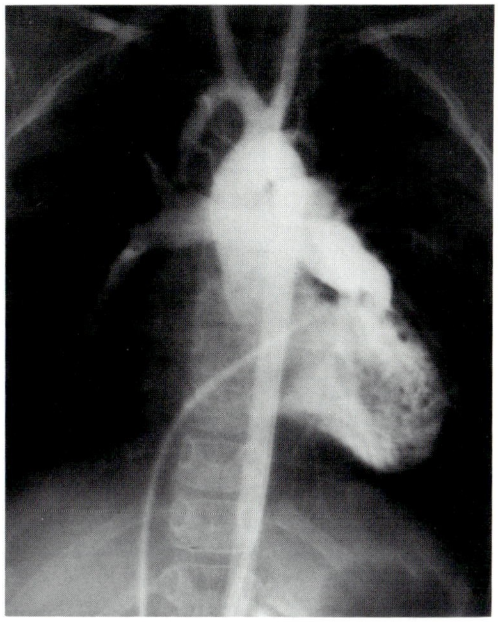

Fig. 4–15 The subclavian artery bilaterally has been used to create a systemic-to-pulmonary artery shunt. The arrow indicates the small left Blalock-Taussig shunt.

surgical repair. Their long-term prognosis has improved significantly since the early 1940s when palliative surgery was first attempted.

There is much confusion concerning the use of the term "severe" tetralogy of Fallot. This term is reserved for use when there is no forward flow through the pulmonic valve into the main pulmonary artery. Another term to describe this lesion is *pulmonary atresia with a ventricular septal defect.* The pulmonary arterial supply to the lungs is via a ductus arteriosus or systemic collaterals or aortic pulmonary collaterals from the descending aorta. To add further confusion, this was originally described as persistent truncus arteriosus type IV of Collett and Edwards. It has now been shown that persistent truncus arteriosus type IV is not a "true truncus" as it does not involve an embryologic abnormality of the conal septum division. As it is not a true truncus, it has been described as a "pseudotruncus." Therefore, the terms *pseudotruncus arteriosus, truncus arteriosus type IV, severe tetralogy of Fallot,* and *pulmonary atresia with ventricular septal defect* all describe conditions in which there is no forward flow into the pulmonary arteries and a ventricular septal defect is present with an overriding aorta.

In neonates, a large patent ductus arteriosus may supply pulmonary arterial flow to both lungs and retrograde flow back to the pulmonary valve. When the ductus begins to close, profound cyanosis ensues. Treatment with prostaglandin will dilate the ductus arteriosus. Subsequently, an emergency modified Blalock-Taussig shunt is performed. In older patients, MRI has increasingly been used in diagnosing the extent of systemic collateral vessels off the descending aorta (Fig. 4–16). In order to do a total repair of these patients, the pulmonary artery anatomy must be of sufficient size to allow systemic venous return. There may be atresia of the main pulmonary artery and the left and right pulmonary arteries may not be connected. The term *nonconfluent pulmonary arteries* refers to pulmonary arteries that are not connected. MRI has been useful in evaluating sequential growth of pulmonary arteries, the position of the systemic pulmonary collaterals, and the presence or absence of confluence.

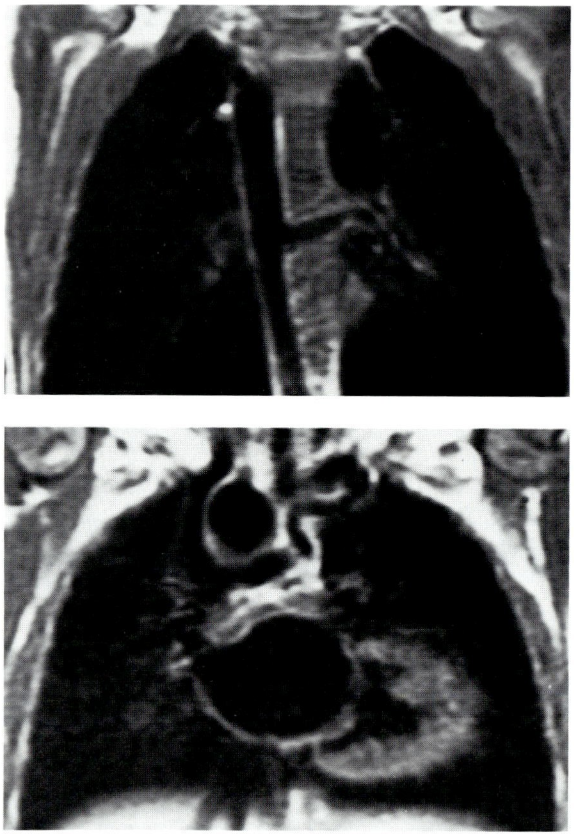

A

B

Fig. 4–16 (A) Coronal MRI demonstrating large bronchial collateral off descending aorta. **(B)** The patient has a patent left palliative shunt from innominate to pulmonary artery. (From Bisset,[2] with permission.)

Tricuspid Atresia

In tricuspid atresia there is complete agenesis of the tricuspid valve with no direct communication between the right atrium and the right ventricle. All the right atrial flow crosses a large atrial septal defect into the left atrium. Associated lesions include a ventricular septal defect with blood flowing from the left ventricle to the right ventricle and subsequent filling of the main pulmonary artery. An increased incidence of D-transposition of the great vessels also occurs in one-third of patients with tricuspid atresia. In patients that do not have a ventricular septal defect, tricuspid atresia is part of a hypoplastic right heart syndrome. There may be associated pulmonary atresia, and small right ventricle and tricuspid atresia. Palliative surgery (placement of a modified Blalock-Taussig shunt) is performed to increase pulmonary blood flow. The definitive surgical repair for tricuspid atresia is called a *Fontan procedure* and is performed in older patients. In this procedure the right atrium is connected to the main pulmonary artery with or without a valve.

Ebstein's Anomaly

Ebstein's anomaly is downward displacement of the septal leaflet of the tricuspid valve that results in a decrease in size and function of the right ventricle. The right atrium is the chamber proximal to the tricuspid valve. Therefore, when the tricuspid valve is displaced within the right atrium (somewhat like a diverticulum), a "three chambered" right side is present (e.g., the true right ventricular chamber, the right atrial portion of the right ventricle, and the right atrium). The abnormally positioned valve leads to functional obstruction of right atrial emptying and the right heart grossly enlarges.

In the neonate, there may be massive cardiomegaly with the right heart markedly enlarged. In older children, there is a "squared" appearance to the heart, which on the left side is due to elevation and horizontal positioning of the right ventricular outflow tract and on the right side, is due to massive right atrial enlargement (Fig. 4–17). The appearance on echocardiography is characteristic, showing the displaced insertion of the abnormal septal leaflet.

Occasionally, ECMO (extracorporeal membrane oxygenation) has been used transiently to sustain appropriate oxygenation in newborns with severe pulmonary hypertension in Ebstein's anomaly. Older infants may be relatively asymptomatic, depending on the degree of obstruction. When surgery is indicated, plication of the valve leaflets will be attempted.

The differential diagnosis includes Uhl's anomaly, a rare condition that involves either focal or complete absence of the right ventricular myocardium, which results in a thin-walled, parchmentlike right ventricle with poor contractability and marked tricuspid insufficiency.

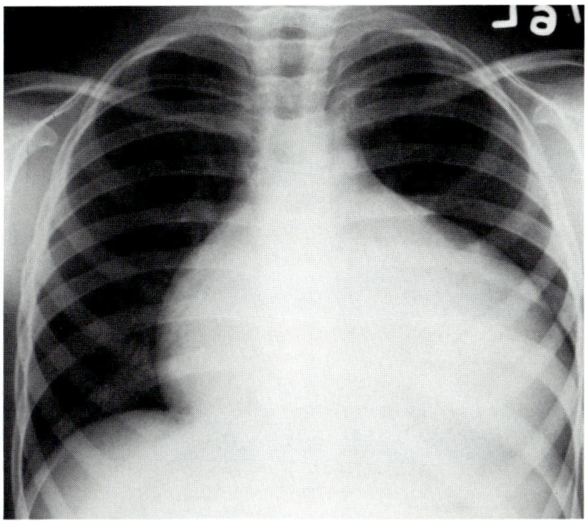

Fig. 4–17 Five-year-old patient with Ebstein's anomaly showing marked cardiomegaly with dilatation of right atrium.

CYANOTIC CONGENITAL HEART DISEASE WITH INCREASED PULMONARY ARTERY FLOW

Transposition of the Great Vessels

D-transposition of the great vessels is the most common congenital heart disease presenting with cyanosis during the first 24 hours of life. Patients with transposition of the great vessels may have normal pulmonary flow, diminished flow if pulmonic stenosis is present, or increased artery flow. In complete transposition of the great vessels, the great vessels are transposed. The atrioventricular connections are concordant (normal) but the ventricular great vessels are discordant. In complete transposition, the aorta still lies slightly to the right of the pulmonary artery; however, it is anterior in relation to the ascending portion of the pulmonary artery. The ventricles are in normal anatomic positions. Hemodynamically, blood flows from the inferior vena cava into the right atrium into the right ventricle with filling of the ascending aorta. Pulmonary venous blood returns to the left atrium and left ventricle with subsequent filling of the pulmonary artery. Separation of the circulation of saturated and unsaturated blood is complete and this lesion is fatal unless communication exists between the two parallel circuits. Frequent sites of communication are an atrial septal defect, ventricular septal defect, or patent ductus arteriosus.

Radiographically the heart is enlarged and the configuration is abnormal (Fig. 4–18). The mediastinum is narrowed and the configuration is described as "egg on a side." The egg-shaped heart is partly related to rotation of the aorta medially, malposition of the pulmonary artery, and the lack of a radiographic thymus. There is also asymmetry of pulmonary artery flow with the right pulmonary artery being slightly higher in position and slightly larger than the left. Infants frequently demonstrate increased pulmonary vascularity. Angiography demonstrates ventricular great vessel discordance (Fig. 4–19). The current surgical approach is summarized below.

In the arterial switch procedure, the great vessels are transsected above the valve leaflets and transferred to the other great vessel. This is a physiologic correction as blood flows from the right atrium to the right ventricle through the aortic valve into the pulmonary artery. Venous blood returns to the left atrium, to the left ventricle, and goes through the pulmonary valve into the aorta. This surgical procedure must be performed early in life for, if there is a delay, the left ventricle will not be able to handle the systemic workload.

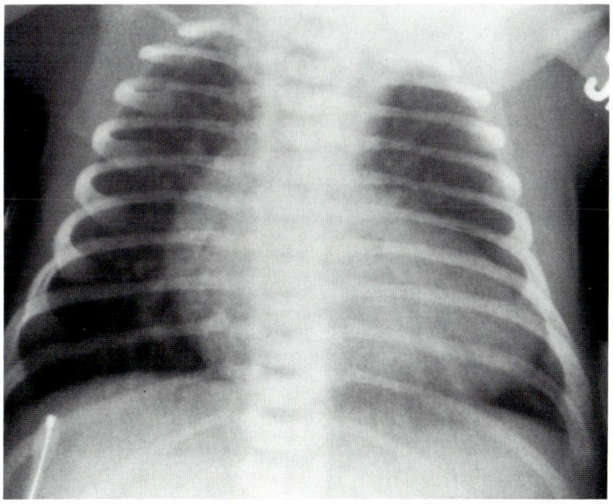

Fig. 4–18 D-transposition of the great vessels. The radiographic findings include a narrow mediastinum, asymmetric pulmonary flow with the right side being more prominent, and lack of visualization of the main pulmonary artery and aorta (due to malposition).

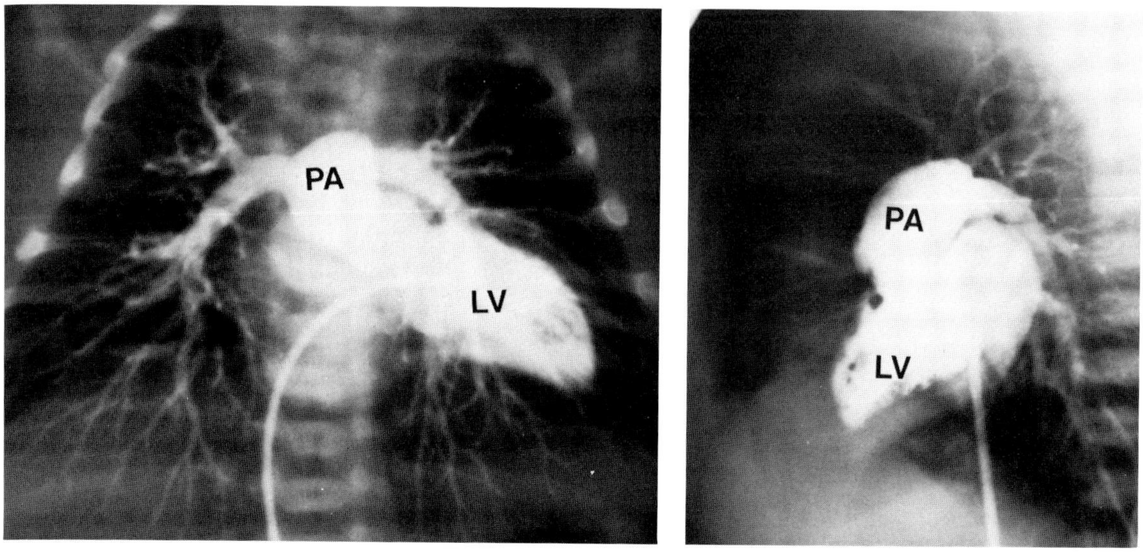

Fig. 4–19 D-transposition of the great vessels. Left ventriculography demonstrating that the left ventricle is related to a posteriorly positioned pulmonary artery (ventricular-arterial discordance). PA, pulmonary artery; LV, left ventricular.

The Mustard and Senning procedures involve repairing the abnormal pathway of blood by creating atrial baffles. The baffle procedure within the atrium redirects systemic venous blood into the right ventricle, which subsequently goes to the pulmonary artery. The difficulty of this procedure is that the right ventricle is the systemic ventricle.

The Rashkind balloon atrial septostomy is performed percutaneously in infants to allow better mixing of the two parallel circuits and to decompress the left atrium.

Persistent Truncus Arteriosus

Truncus arteriosus is characterized by a single trunk arising from the base of the heart and giving origin to the coronary, pulmonary, and systemic arterial circulations. It results from failure of formation of the spiral septum within the truncus in the early embryo. The right ventricle has no infundibulum and a large ventricular septal defect is part of the malformation. The truncal valve has three semilunar cusps, but also may have two, four, or five cusps. Classically, as described by Collett and Edwards, there are four types of truncus (Fig. 4–20). In type I (most common), a short main pulmonary artery arises from the left posterolateral aspect of the truncus and divides into a right and left pulmonary artery. In type II, each pulmonary artery arises independently from the left posterolateral aspect of the truncus. In type III (least common), each pulmonary artery arises independently from the lateral aspect of the truncus. In type IV, the pulmonary arteries arise from the descending aorta. Embryologically, type IV is not a true truncus and is sometimes referred to as a pseudotruncus.

Truncus arteriosus is an admixture lesion as both a right-to-left shunt (from the right ventricle across the ventricular septal defect into the overriding ascending aorta) and a left-to-right shunt (from the aorta to the pulmonary arteries) are present. The degree of cyanosis relates to the amount of pulmonary blood flow and the pulmonary vascular resistance. The pressure in both the right ventricle and left ventricle is identical and the pressure in the initial portion of the ascending aorta and pulmonary arteries is also equal.

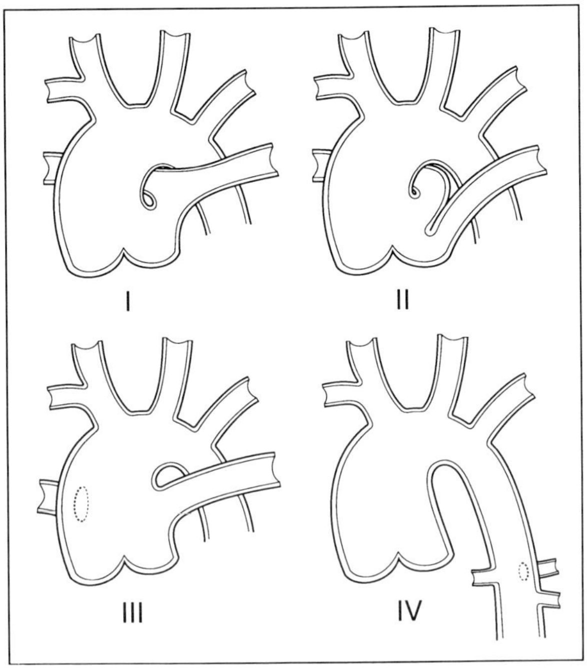

Fig. 4–20 Collett and Edwards' classification of persistent truncus arteriosus. Type I truncus has a single pulmonary trunk. In type II truncus, the right and left pulmonary arteries arise close to each other. In type III truncus, the origins are separate. In type IV truncus, the pulmonary arteries arise from the descending aorta. (Modified from Collett and Edwards,[3] with permission.)

One-third of patients with persistent truncus arteriosus will have a right arch and therefore the presence of a right arch, with cardiomegaly and increased pulmonary arterial flow is strongly suggestive of truncus arteriosus (Fig. 4–21). The "aorta" or truncus is invariably prominent. The main pulmonary artery segment is concave because it is misplaced from its original position. Occasionally the inferior portion of the pulmonary artery can be visualized as it is slightly elevated in position as it emanates from the ascending aorta.

The treatment of truncus arteriosus involves (1) closure of the ventricular septal defect, which commits the left ventricle to empty into the truncus arteriosus; and (2) the pulmonary artery is removed from the truncus and a conduit is placed between the right ventricle and the pulmonary artery. If there is significant truncal insufficiency, an aortic valve prothesis may need to be inserted.

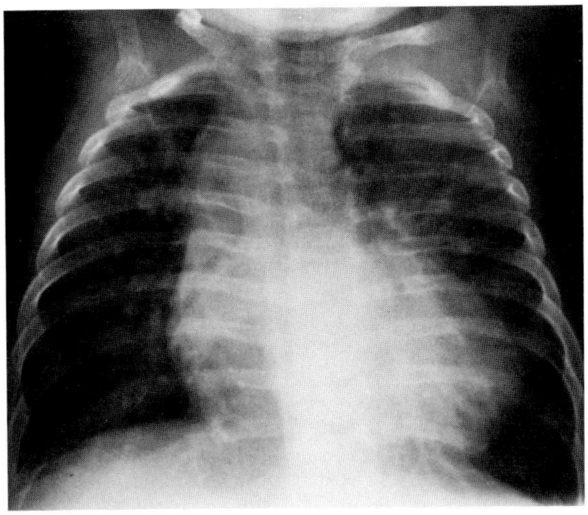

Fig. 4–21 Truncus arteriosus in a 2-month-old infant. The characteristic features include a large right aortic arch and increase in pulmonary arterial flow bilaterally.

Total Anomalous Pulmonary Venous Return

Although total anomalous pulmonary venous return accounts for only 2 percent of congenital cardiac anomalies, it is a lesion that has fascinated many people. In total anomalous pulmonary venous return the pulmonary veins drain anomalously and eventually empty into the right atrium instead of draining into the left atrium. The four types of anomalous return are type I (most common), an anomalous connection at the supercardiac level; type II, an anomalous connection at the cardiac level; type III, an anomalous connection at the infracardiac level; and type IV, an anomalous pulmonary venous connection involving two or more of the above levels. A right-to-left shunt across an atrial septal defect or patent foramen ovale is invariably present. Total anomalous pulmonary venous return can either be obstructive or nonobstructive. The infradiaphragmatic type is almost invariably obstructed. Each of the categories is discussed separately as the physiology and the radiographic appearance of each is somewhat distinct.

In type I total anomalous pulmonary venous return, the pulmonary veins from both lungs form a conflu-

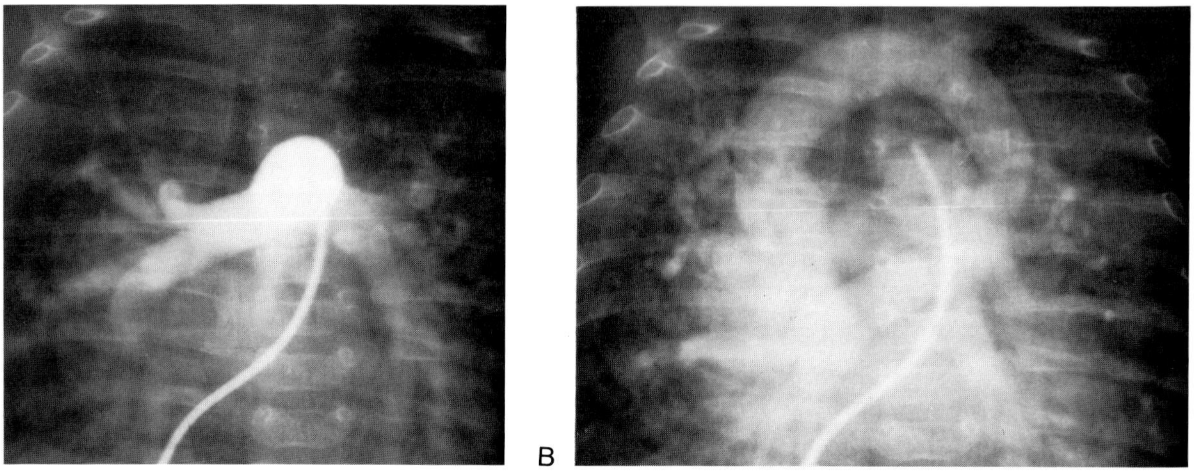

A B

Fig. 4–22 (A) Pulmonary arteriogram demonstrating an injection into the main pulmonary artery. **(B)** On the levophase of the study, the pulmonary veins are seen draining into a left vertical vein that connects to the innominate vein and the superior vena cava with flow into the right atrium.

ence immediately posterior to the left atrium. A venous trunk or vertical vein originates from the left portion of the confluence and passes anterior to the left pulmonary artery and main stem bronchus, and ascends into the superior mediastinum, joining the left innominate vein. The left innominate vein subsequently joins the superior vena cava in a normal fashion (Fig. 4–22). Cardiomegaly is frequently present because of increased volume with dilatation of the right atrium, right ventricle, and main pulmonary artery segments. On chest x-rays, a prominent left vertical vein and a widened upper mediastinum producing a characteristic "snowman" is suggestive of the diagnosis (Fig. 4–23).

In type II total anomalous pulmonary venous return, the veins drain abnormally to the coronary sinus or to the right atrium. The physiology of this lesion is similar to a large left-to-right shunt at the atrial level. The radiographic appearance of type II total anomalous pulmonary venous return simulates the radiographic appearance of patients with large left-to-right shunts.

In type III total anomalous pulmonary venous return, obstruction invariably occurs. A common pulmonary vein is usually present that drains infradiaphragmatically through a long, narrow channel and subsequently drains into the portal or vitelline remnants. Blood then must flow through the portal vein into the hepatic veins and right atrium. Patients with pulmonary venous obstruction clinically present within the first few days of life with cyanosis and heart failure. The radiographic pattern is quite suggestive as the heart is usually normal in size and a fine reticular

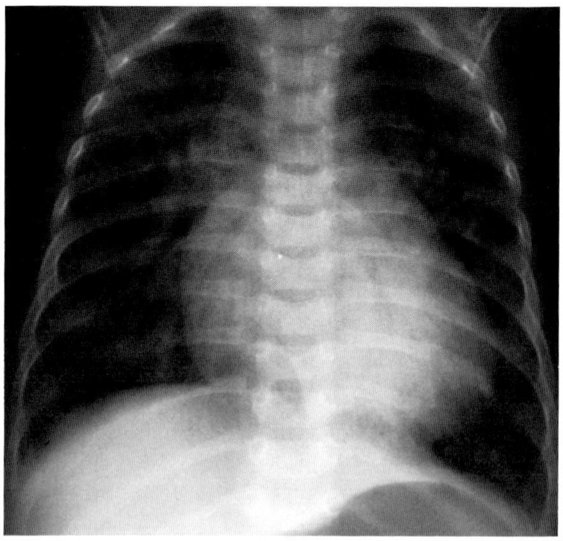

Fig. 4–23 Total anomalous pulmonary venous return. Moderate cardiomegaly with prominence of the superior mediastinum and increase in pulmonary arterial flow.

pattern of pulmonary edema throughout both lungs is seen (see Fig. 4–5).

In type IV total anomalous pulmonary venous return, the venous return from both lungs or from all lobes does not follow the same pathway and there is a variety of patterns of venous return.

The prognosis in total anomalous pulmonary venous connection is determined by the site of the anomaly. Patients with best prognosis have type I or type II. In type I total anomalous pulmonary venous return, the common pulmonary vein posterior to the left atrium can be anastomosed directly to the left atrium. In some surveys of total anomalous pulmonary venous return of all types, 50 percent were dead at 3 months and 80 percent had died in the first year of life. When obstruction exists, the prognosis is poor.

Atresia of the common pulmonary vein is a rare anomaly in which there is no communication between the normally formed pulmonary veins and the left atrium. Severe obstruction of the pulmonary veins is present and is associated with severe pulmonary hypertension.

CONGENITAL HEART DISEASE WITH NORMAL PULMONARY FLOW

Patients in this category have obstruction and the heart reacts by hypertrophy. Included in this category are pulmonic stenosis, aortic stenosis, and coarctation of the aorta.

Pulmonic Stenosis

The majority of patients with pulmonic stenosis have a thickening of the pulmonic valve with a reduction in the size of the central orifice, which is related to fusion of the commissures. Stenosis across the pulmonary valve causes the right ventricular to hypertrophy, which increases right ventricular pressure. Pulmonary valvar stenosis is associated with normal pulmonary flow as no other exit exists out of the right ventricle except forward through the pulmonic valve. Most patients with pulmonary valve stenosis are asymptomatic. In young children with pulmonic stenosis, the radiographic appearance may be entirely normal. In older patients with severe stenosis, the transverse diameter of the heart is of normal size. Dilatation of the main pulmonary artery is present, resulting from poststenotic dilatation secondary to the jet of blood through the orifice to the stenotic valve (Fig. 4–24). The left pulmonary artery is frequently larger than the right due to the jet that is frequently directed into the left lung (Fig. 4–25). On the lateral view, evidence of right ventricular hypertrophy is frequently seen with filling in of the retrosternal clear space.

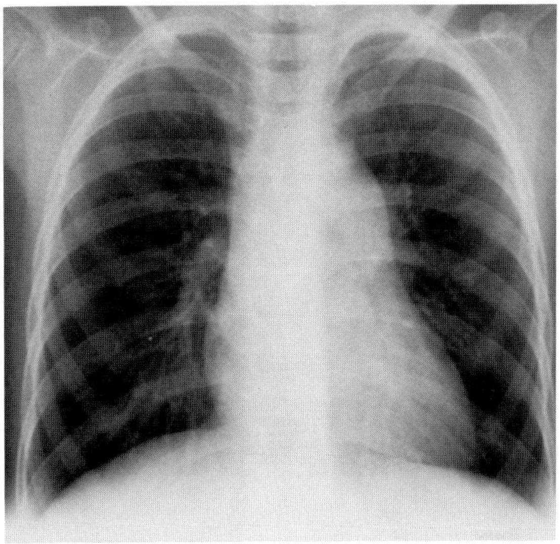

Fig. 4–24 Pulmonary valvar stenosis. Plain radiograph demonstrates enlargement of the main pulmonary artery. The left pulmonary artery appears slightly larger than the right.

The treatment for pulmonary valvar stenosis is currently percutaneous valvotomy. The balloon insufflation ruptures the commissural fusion and significantly decreases the gradient between right ventricle and pulmonary arteries. Mild pulmonary insufficiency may occur following percutaneous pulmonary valvotomy. However, mild pulmonary insufficiency appears to be well tolerated.

In approximately 5 percent of patients, the pulmonary valve is dysplastic. In this type, the commissures are not fused but stenosis occurs because of marked thick-

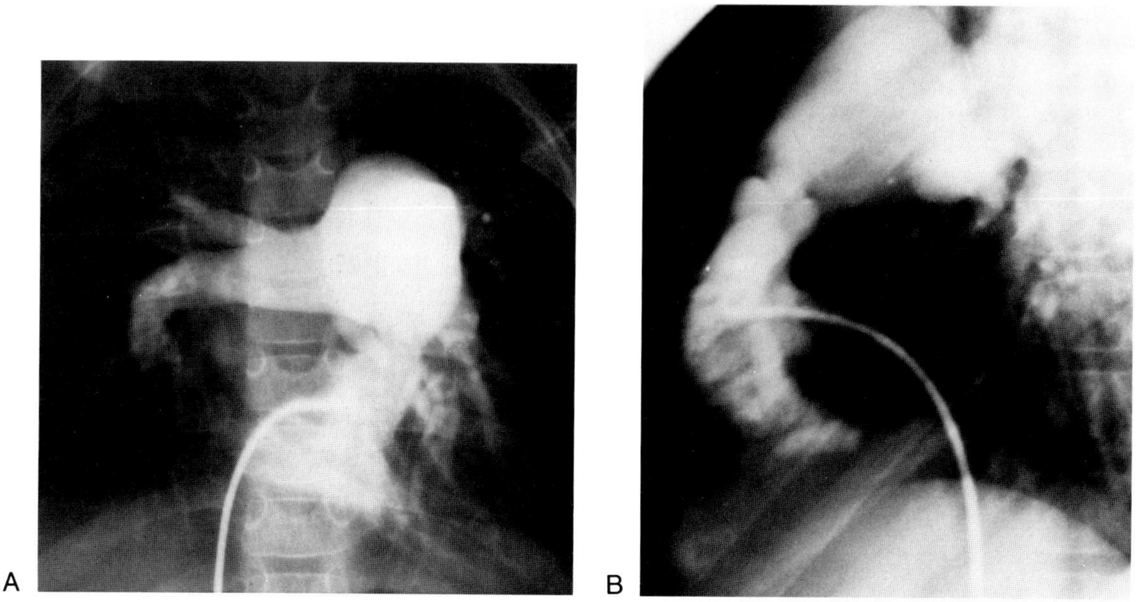

Fig. 4–25 (A) Anteroposterior right ventriculogram injection demonstrating marked dilatation of the main pulmonary artery. **(B)** Lateral right ventriculography shows thickening of the valve cusps, a narrowed orifice, and poststenotic dilatation of the pulmonary artery.

ening and redundancy of the pulmonary valve leaflets. The dysplastic form may be associated with Noonan's syndrome, characterized by peculiar facies and a friendly demeanor. If obstruction is moderately severe, surgery is indicated.

Aortic Stenosis

Aortic stenosis may be supravalvar, valvular (most common), or subvalvular. A bicuspid aortic valve is the most common congenital heart lesion although it certainly is not the most symptomatic congenital lesion. Because the bicuspid aortic valve may become stenotic with time, it may become clinically significant only in adult life. Fused commissures in a centrally placed orifice are frequent in aortic stenosis. The hemodynamic abnormality produced by obstruction to left ventricular outflow is a pressure gradient between the left ventricle and aorta during systolic ejection. Most children react by concentric hypertrophy of the left ventricular wall. Aortic stenosis may present in infancy in which case it is called *critical aortic stenosis* due to severe left ventricular outflow tract obstruction. Most children with aortic stenosis are asymptomatic and grow normally.

The radiographic features include a normal sized heart with poststenotic dilatation of the ascending aorta. In infants with severe obstruction, the radiographs demonstrate cardiomegaly and signs of congestive heart failure. Treatment varies according to the age of the patient and the degree of obstruction. The malformed aortic valve may be associated with endocarditis and prophylactic antibiotic therapy is suggested. Percutaneous balloon aortic valvuloplasty has recently been shown to be of value. Surgery includes direct inspection of the aortic valve leaflets with commissural incision, which enlarges the valve orifice after valvotomy. The patient may have aortic insufficiency or restenosis. Prosthetic valve replacement is required in approximately 35 percent of patients within 15 to 20 years of the original surgery. Aortic valve replacement is difficult in children because the children outgrow their value orifices and also because of the use of anticoagulants.

Discrete subaortic stenosis is less common and more difficult to diagnose. The fibrous ring encircles the subaortic area and causes left ventricular outflow tract obstruction just beneath the base of the aortic valve. Echocardiography is useful in the distinction of valvar and subvalvar stenosis.

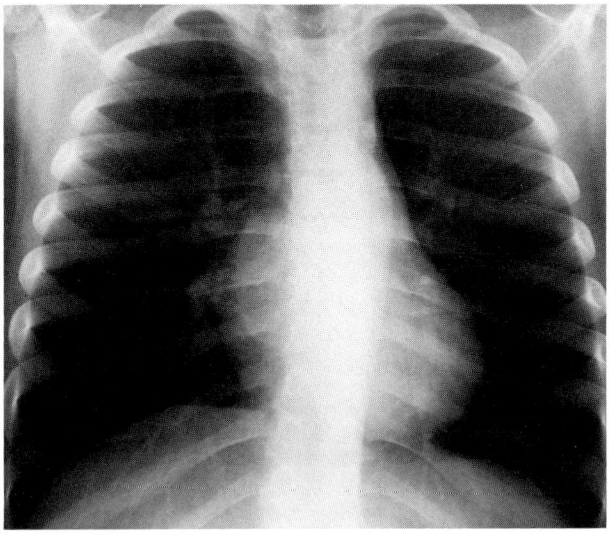

Fig. 4–26 This patient has coarctation, visualized as a discrete narrowing of the descending aorta.

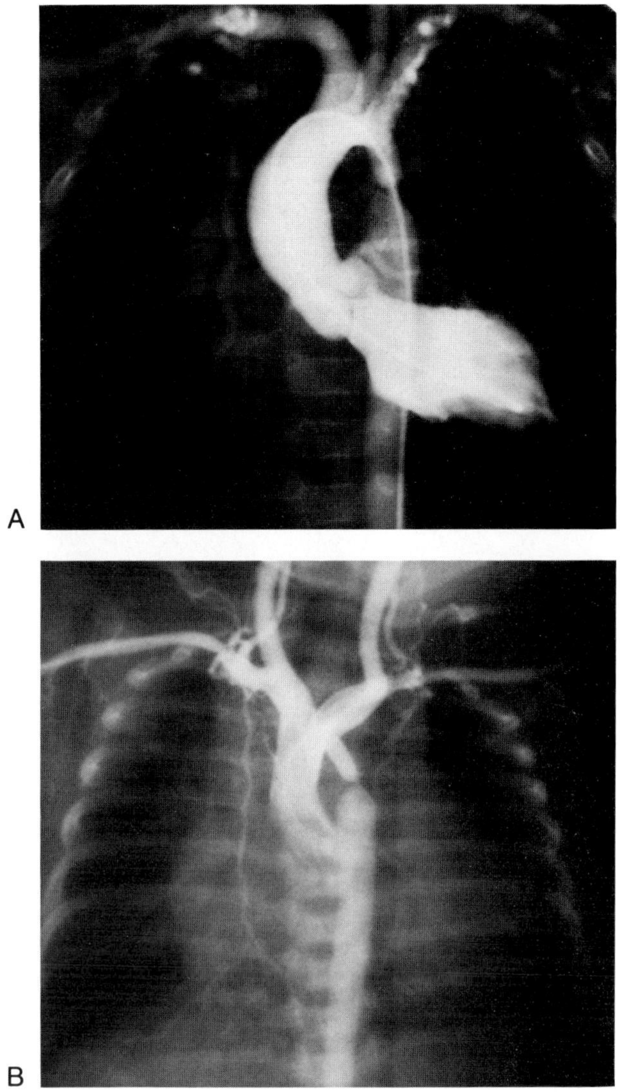

Fig. 4–27 (A) Left ventriculography demonstrating discrete narrowing in descending aorta. **(B)** A 3-day-old infant with diffuse hypoplasia of the aorta in addition to a discrete coarctation.

Supravalvar aortic stenosis is a congenital narrowing of the ascending aorta above the coronary arteries. The area of narrowing is not localized but tends to be diffuse, involving several centimeters. The supravalvar aortic stenosis has been termed *William's syndrome* as these patients have cardiac and multisystem disorder. The anomaly may be familial and is transmitted as an autosomal dominant trait.

Coarctation of the Aorta

Coarctation of the aorta is a congenital narrowing of the aorta. The most common type is a localized narrowing of the proximal descending aorta, which is seen in older patients and termed the *adult type*. In this type, the area of coarctation is just beyond the origin of the left subclavian artery at the level of the ductus arteriosus (Fig. 4–26). The narrowing is short and discrete (Fig. 4–27). The second type involves isthmic narrowing and is occasionally called the *infantile* or *diffuse type* (Fig. 4–27A). This type has a long segment of narrowed aorta that extends from just distal to the left carotid artery at the level of the ductus arteriosus (Fig. 4–27B). Also a localized constriction is present. In the diffuse type of coarctation, a patent ductus arteriosus is almost always present and there is a high association with intracardiac defects including ventricular septal defect, atrial septal defect, and deformed mitral valve.

Clinical symptoms relate to the age of the patient and the type of lesion. Typically, the diffuse type of coarctation occurs in a neonate. The radiograph demonstrates cardiomegaly with evidence of congestive heart failure or shunt vascularity. The isolated coarctation in older patients is more common in males

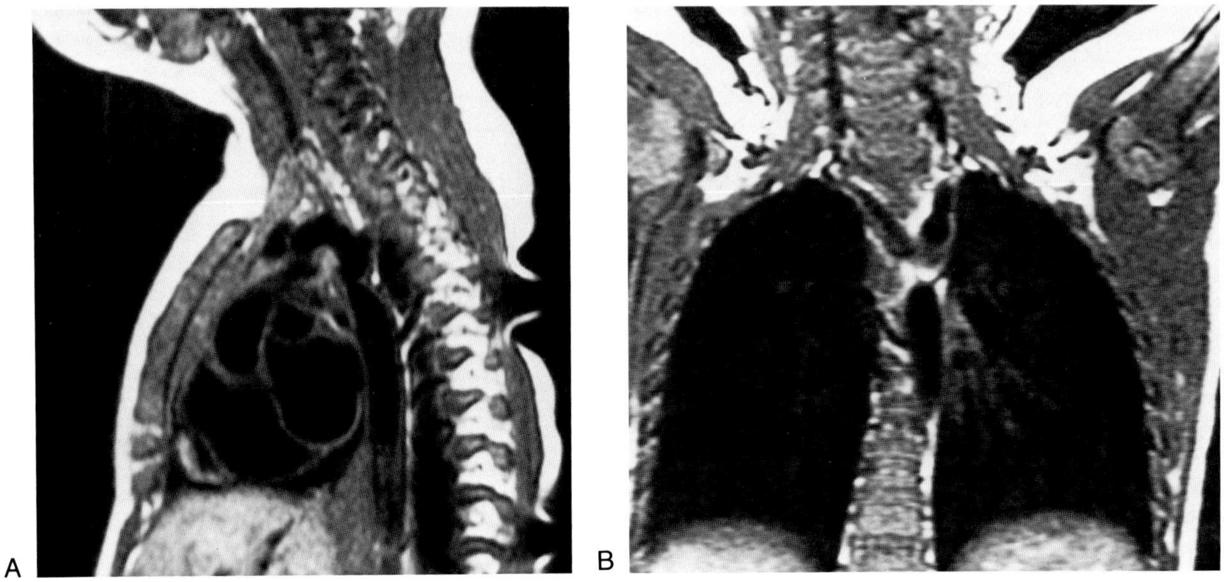

Fig. 4–28 Sagittal **(A)** and coronal **(B)** MRI demonstrating site of coarctation and the presence of collaterals filling the descending aorta.

and may be associated with syndromes such as Turner's syndrome. A bicuspid aortic valve is the most frequently encountered associated malformation, occurring in 85 percent of patients in some series.

In older patients, coarctation of the aorta is usually asymptomatic. Physical examination demonstrates differential blood pressures between the upper and lower extremities. Chest x-ray may show a normal-sized heart with prominence of the aorta. The proximal descending aorta may be notched to resemble the number three (Fig. 4–26). A portion of the "three" is due to a dilated aorta or proximal left subclavian artery; the middle portion of the "three" is due to the actual coarctation of the aorta; and the lower portion of the "three" is due to poststenotic dilatation of the descending aorta. Rib notching involves the inferior portions of the posterior aspects of the third or fourth to eighth or ninth ribs and is due to pressure erosion by the dilated intercostal arteries, which serve as collateral vessels between the internal mammary arteries and the descending aorta. MRI has been shown to demonstrate adequately the site of coarctation and associated anomalies and angiography is rarely indicated (Fig. 4–28).

Surgical techniques involve either a direct end anastomosis, dacryon graft, or subclavian flap. Percutaneous balloon angioplasty has been used for the treatment of restenosis coarctation.

NEONATAL RADIOLOGY

In the past, great emphasis has been placed on diagnosing a specific congenital lesion in the neonate on the basis of the plain radiograph. With marked improvements in echocardiography, this approach is no longer mandatory. However, the radiologist is frequently helpful in suggesting the presence of congenital cardiovascular anomalies or in excluding pulmonary or thoracic causes of cyanosis and/or dyspnea. The overall number of cardiac catheterizations in the first week of life has continued to decrease as refinements in making specific diagnoses based on echocardiography has increased. Common clinical entities occurring in the first week of life are discussed below.

In the first few days of life, congestive heart failure is exceedingly uncommon and, in addition to structural anomalies of the heart, heart failure may be secondary to arrythmia, respiratory diseases, severe anemia, polycythemia, hypoglycemia, septicemia, and peripheral arteriovenous malformations. Massive sepsis with cardiogenic shock may simulate structural anomalies.

The term *hypoplastic left heart syndrome* is a spectrum of cardiac anomalies that are characterized by underdevelopment at the aorta, aortic valve, left ventricle, and mitral valve. Most of these infants present within the first week of life. There is no forward flow from the left ventricle into the ascending aorta. Survival necessitates a large intra-atrial communication and a large patent ductus arteriosus with right-to-left shunting. However, once the ductus closes, the patients have severe metabolic acidosis, shock, and hypovolemia. Infants diagnosed with hypoplastic left heart syndrome have been considered inoperable although some surgical centers are performing the Norwood procedure. The chest x-ray demonstrates mild cardiomegaly, pulmonary edema, and increased pulmonary arterial flow. Echocardiography can accurately assess the size of the mitral valve, left ventricle, and ascending aorta. Angiography is not usually performed.

There are two congenital heart lesions causing marked cardiomegaly in the newborn. Massive cardiac enlargement is usually attributed to right atrial enlargement and is seen in patients that have pulmonary atresia with an intact septum or Ebstein's anomaly. Massive cardiomegaly can also be attributed to herniation of the liver into the pericardial sac, massive pericardial effusion in a neonate, and other more unusual entities.

The term *persistent fetal circulation* is used in neonates who have severe pulmonary hypertension and right-to-left shunting through a persistent patent ductus arteriosus. Severe pulmonary hypertension in neonates may be primary with no underlying cause or secondary to conditions such as severe meconium aspiration, diaphragmatic hernia, and other lesions that lead to anoxemia and increased pulmonary vascular resistance. Persistent fetal circulation may cause severe anoxemia and a relentless cycle of pulmonary

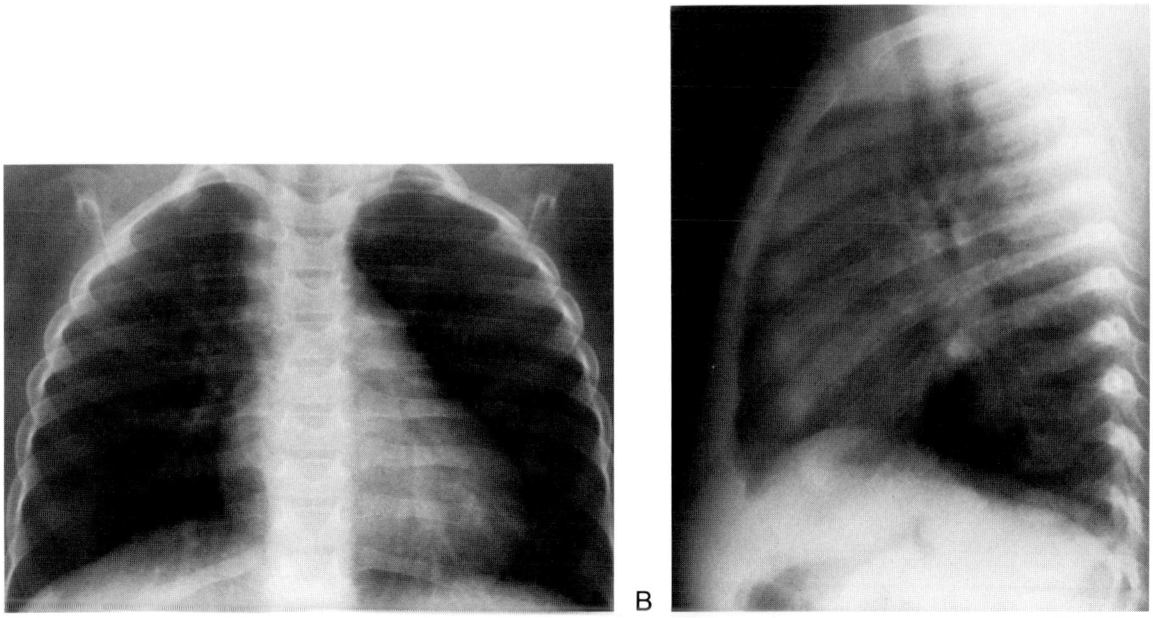

A B

Fig. 4–29 (A) This patient has a right aortic arch. **(B)** The lateral view demonstrates anterior bowing of the trachea suggesting a vascular ring.

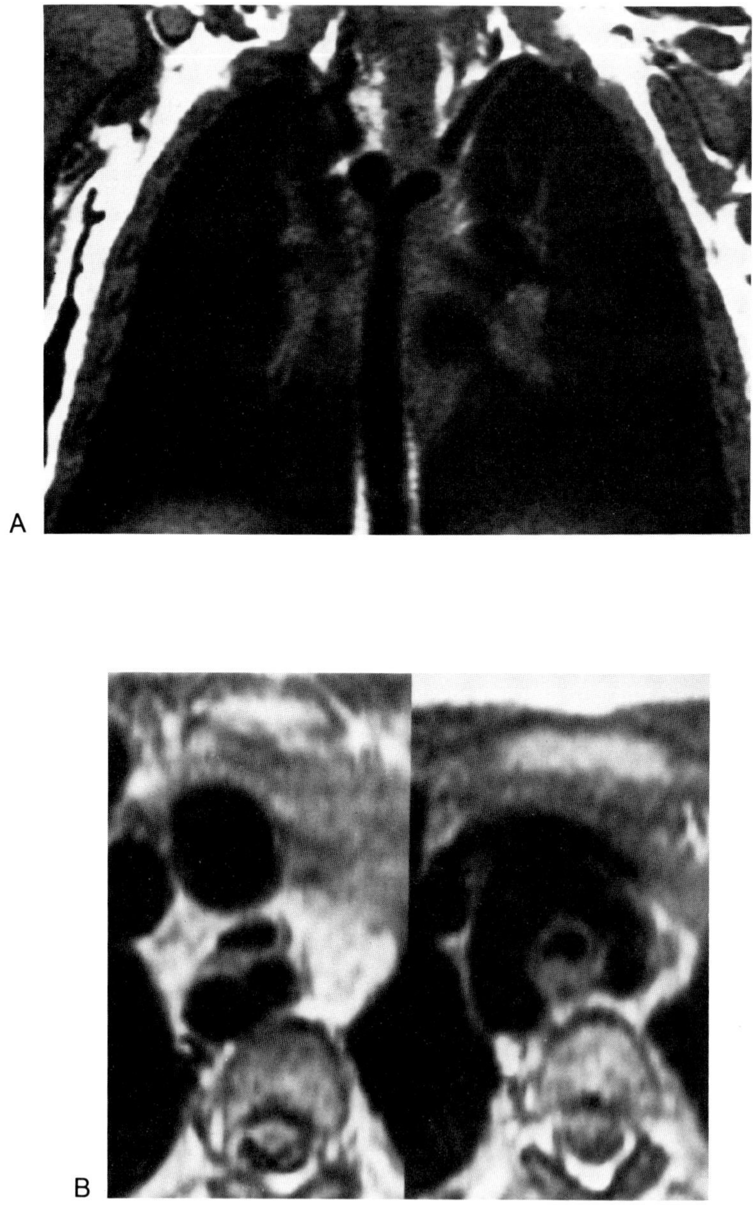

Fig. 4–30 (A) Coronal MRI showing double aortic arch as it joins to form the descending aorta. **(B)** Axial MRI demonstrating encirclement of the trachea, with tracheal compression by a double aortic arch.

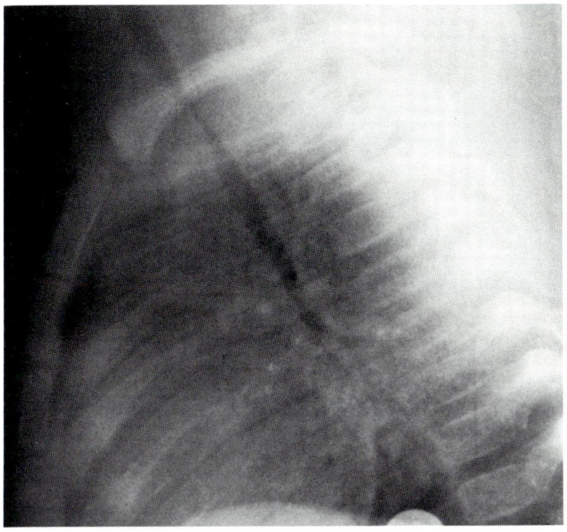

Fig. 4–31 The localized anterior indentation of the trachea is due to the innominate artery. This can be seen normally in one-third of young children.

vasoconstriction as a response to anoxemia may cause more right-to-left shunting across the ductus arteriosus. The development of ECMO has been of primary usefulness in treating these patients while their pulmonary arterial pressure slowly decreases or their underlying cause of severe pulmonary artery hypertension is addressed and treated.

VASCULAR RINGS

Vascular rings are embryologic anomalies of the aortic arch or its branches in which there is tracheobronchial compression. The patients may either present with symptoms of tracheomalacia secondary to tracheal abnormalities or with swallowing difficulties relating to the esophageal compression. The most common anomaly early in life is the double aortic arch. The chest x-ray is the single best clue to the diagnosis of a vascular ring. The presence of a right aortic arch and anterior bowing of the trachea on lateral view suggests the presence of a vascular ring (Fig. 4–29). A right aortic arch and anomalous left subclavian with a diverticulum and a left patent ductus arteriosus simulate the barium swallow findings of a double aortic arch. MRI using the coronal and axial planes is ideal in depicting the vascular anomaly and the degree of tracheal compression (Fig. 4–30). Occasionally, coarctation will be associated with a vascular ring.

Innominate artery compression is one of the most common tracheal compressions. In infants and children, the innominate artery normally has an origin to the left of the trachea and imprints the trachea as it ascends into the superior mediastinum to bifurcate into the right subclavian and right carotid vessels. Localized anterior narrowing just at the thoracic inlet can be seen on lateral chest x-rays in one-third of normal patients under the age of 2 and is not necessarily indicative of disease (Fig. 4–31). In the symptomatic infant, MRI and/or endoscopy may be necessary to evaluate the degree of tracheal compression.

SUGGESTED READINGS

1. Adams FH, Emmanouilides GC, Riemenschneider TA: Moss' Heart Disease in Infants, Children, and Adolescents. 4th Ed. Williams & Wilkins, Baltimore, 1989

2. Bisset GS III: Cardiovascular system. In Cohen MD, Edwards MK (eds): Magnetic Resonance Imaging of Children. BC Decker, Philadelphia, 1990
3. Collett RW, Edwards JE: Persistent truncus arteriosus: Classification according to anatomic types. Surg Clin North Am 29:1245, 1949
4. Condon VR: The heart and great vessels. In Essentials of Caffey's Pediatric X-ray Diagnosis. Year Book Medical Publishers, Chicago, 1990
5. Freedom RM, Culham JAG, Moes CAF: Angiocardiography of Congenital Heart Disease. Macmillan, New York, 1984
6. Gedgaudas E, Moller JH, Castaneda-Quniga WR, Amplatz K: Cardiovascular Radiology. WB Saunders, Philadelphia, 1985
7. Keith JD, Rowe RD, Vlad P: Heart Disease in Infancy and Childhood. 3rd Ed. Macmillan, New York, 1978
8. Kirks DR: Practical pediatric imaging. In Diagnostic Radiology of Infants and Children. Little Brown, Boston, 1984
9. Swischuk LE, Sapire DW: Basic Imaging in Congenital Heart Disease. 3rd Ed. Williams & Wilkins, Baltimore, 1986

5

Gastrointestinal System

Susan D. Stansberry

PLAIN RADIOGRAPHS

The plain radiograph of the abdomen continues to be a valuable tool in the initial evaluation of abdominal pathology in children. One can obtain many diagnostic clues to the etiology of abdominal pain or distension, fever, vomiting, diarrhea, constipation, hematochezia, melena, or palpable masses from supine and erect views of the abdomen. Because of the complex variety of shadows present on these radiographs, an organized approach to their interpretation is essential. This approach should include evaluation of the individual organs, the bowel gas pattern, the retroperitoneum (e.g., psoas shadow, paravertebral stripe), the soft tissues and fat, the bones, the lung bases, and abnormal findings such as calcifications, masses, pneumoperitoneum, and ascites.

Organs and Masses

The liver is generally well seen on the plain radiograph of the abdomen and its size is easily estimated. Liver size and shape are quite variable from patient to patient and at various ages. The liver in neonates occupies a relatively larger portion of the abdomen than in older children and adults. A generalized abnormal radiolucency of the liver can sometimes be seen when a large amount of fatty replacement has occurred. In children, this is most commonly caused by severe protein malnutrition in cystic fibrosis or kwashiorkor, acute hepatic necrosis, diabetes mellitus, Reye's syndrome, or steroid therapy. The increased radiolucency may be more easily seen on the chest x-ray. Increased density in the liver is most often due to diffuse deposition of iron following multiple transfusions (hemochromatosis).

The borders of the spleen are also often fairly well seen on the plain radiographs. Enlargement may cause medial displacement of the stomach, downward displacement of the splenic flexure, and elevation of the left hemidiaphragm. The most common causes of splenomegaly include infection (sepsis, infectious mononucleosis, malaria), hematopoetic disorders, portal hypertension, and infiltrative diseases (histiocytosis X, lymphoma). The kidneys are often difficult to identify on the plain radiographs without the administration of intravenous (IV) contrast. When visible they should be inspected for size, position, and contour (Fig. 5–1).

Plain radiographs are often obtained in children because of an abdominal mass palpated during a physical examination. If large enough, the mass may appear as an area of increased soft tissue density displacing adjacent organs (e.g., bowel, kidneys). The most likely origin of the mass can often be inferred by noting its position within the abdomen. Abdominal masses in infants and children most commonly arise from the kidneys or other retroperitoneal structures. The most common abdominal mass in the neonate is hydronephrosis, usually due to ureteropelvic junc-

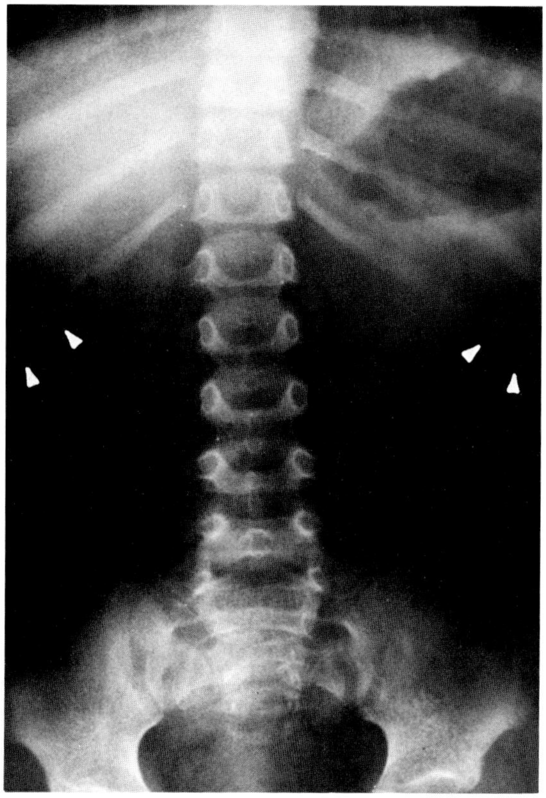

Fig. 5–1 Normal abdominal organs. The absence of gas in this patient's abdomen permits visualization of the edges of the liver and spleen as well as clear delineation of the contours of the normal kidneys.

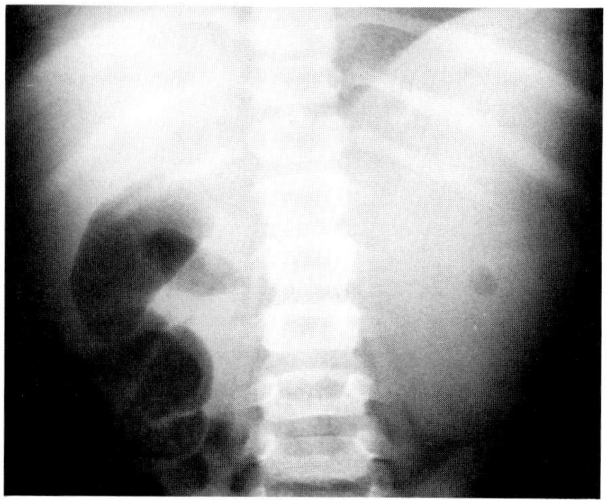

A

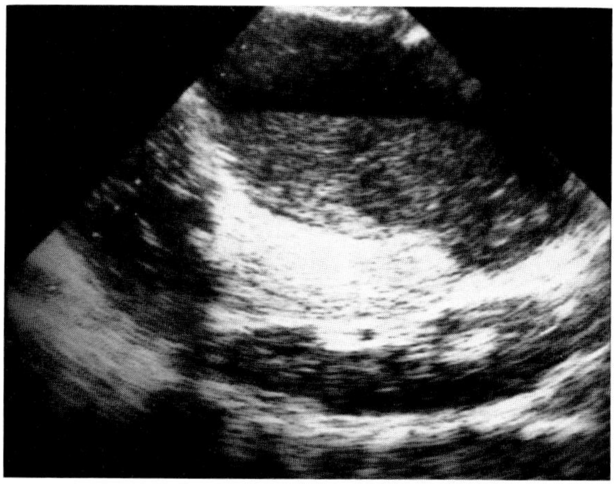

B

Fig. 5–2 Postoperative abscess. **(A)** The abdominal radiograph shows a large soft tissue density mass in the left abdomen displacing the bowel. Note several small collections of gas within this mass. **(B)** Longitudinal ultrasound shows the mass to be a cystic structure containing a large amount of debris, consistent with an abscess.

tion obstruction, posterior urethral valves, or ectopic ureteroceles. Cystic renal disease is also a fairly common cause, especially multicystic dysplastic kidney. In older infants and children, tumors make up a larger percentage of the renal and retroperitoneal abdominal masses. Wilms' tumor and neuroblastoma are the most common of these neoplasms, and these are discussed in more detail in Chapter 6. Other common neonatal abdominal masses include hydrometrocolpos, ovarian cysts, gastrointestinal cysts (duplication cysts, mesenteric cysts), adrenal hemorrhage, and hepatobiliary cysts or neoplasms. Appendiceal abscess is a common cause of a mass after the neonatal period and, after plain radiographs, ultrasonography is the next best step in the evaluation of any abdominal mass (Fig. 5–2).

Bowel Gas Patterns

MECHANICAL OBSTRUCTION

When a significant degree of obstruction is present in a portion of the gastrointestinal tract, the approximate level of obstruction can usually be ascertained on plain radiographs since gas is present in the dilated portions of bowel proximal to the obstruction. The following patterns may be seen.

Dilated Stomach

Many normal infants will swallow a large amount of gas while crying, leading to a large, gas-distended stomach. However, if distension is persistent, gastric outlet obstruction should be suggested, particularly if little gas is present in the distal portions of the gastrointestinal tract. The most common causes of gastric outlet obstruction in early childhood are marked pylorospasm or hypertrophic pyloric stenosis. These two entities may have a similar appearance on an upper gastrointestinal series but usually can be easily differentiated by ultrasonography (see pp. 173–174). Severe spasm or a stricture due to ulcer disease of the gastric antrum or the duodenal bulb may also cause obstruction. Other causes of gastric outlet obstruction are relatively rare in children and include gastrointestinal duplication cysts, gastric polyps or neoplasms, and ectopic pancreatic tissue. Isolated gastric dilatation may be seen without mechanical obstruction in cases of gastroenteritis or adynamic ileus. A large tracheoesophageal fistula also might permit a large amount of gas to enter and distend the stomach acutely. Inadvertent esophageal placement of an endotracheal tube can produce a similar picture.

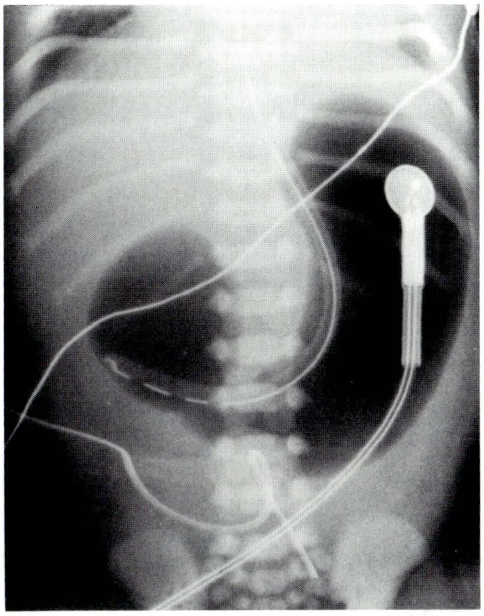

Fig. 5–3 Duodenal atresia. A gas-distended stomach and a dilated, gas-filled proximal duodenum with no gas in the distal bowel comprise the classic double bubble appearance of proximal duodenal obstruction in the newborn.

"Double Bubble" Pattern

The appearance of a gas-distended stomach and duodenal bulb with little or no gas in the remaining bowel is termed the *double bubble sign*. (Fig. 5–3). When seen, this pattern is diagnostic of a duodenal obstruction, usually in the second portion. Air may be present to begin with but also can be introduced into the stomach through a nasogastric tube and usually no other contrast medium is needed. The most common cause of this pattern of obstruction is duodenal atresia with or without associated annular pancreas, but duodenal diaphragms occurring in the descending duodenum also may cause this picture. A rare cause of high duodenal obstruction is anomalous development of the portal vein so that it lies anterior to the duodenum and causes compression. Ladd's bands and the superior mesenteric artery syndrome may cause duodenal obstruction, but this more often lies at the level of the distal second, third, or fourth portions of the duodenum. Midgut volvulus also causes obstruction in this portion of the duodenum.

Small Bowel

When complete or partial small bowel obstruction is present, the level of the obstruction can often be approximated by observing the number of gas-distended small bowel loops on the supine view and the number of air/fluid levels within the small bowel on an erect view. In neonates, the pattern of a low small bowel obstruction should suggest the possibility of meconium ileus, particularly if multiple air-filled loops are seen with few air/fluid levels. A characteristic soap-bubble appearance is sometimes seen, due to air mixed with the meconium (see Fig. 5–44). Congenital atresia or stenosis may occur at any level in the small bowel. Multiple air/fluid levels are usually present and no gas will be seen distal to the obstruction. Incarcerated inguinal hernias most commonly occur from 6 months to 1½ years of age. After the age of 1½ years, the most common causes of low small bowel obstruction are intussusception and perforated appendicitis. The latter occurs in older infants and children and obstruction is probably due to a

SMALL BOWEL OBSTRUCTION

Congenital/developmental
- Congenital atresia or stenosis of jejunum or ileum
- Small bowel volvulus/peritoneal bands
- Incarcerated hernia (inguinal, paraduodenal, umbilical)
- Gastrointestinal duplication

Inflammation
- Perforated appendicitis
- Crohn's disease
- Gastroenteritis (pseudo-obstruction)

Neoplasm
- Small bowel neoplasm/polyp

Trauma/surgery
- Adhesions
- Postradiation

Miscellaneous
- Intussusception
- Meconium ileus (cystic fibrosis)

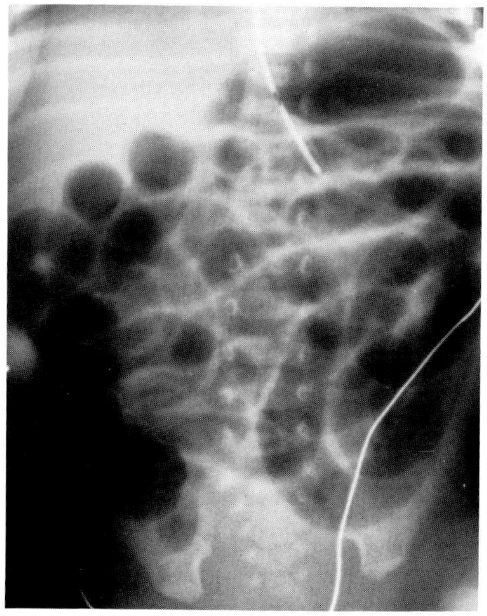

Fig. 5–4 Meconium plug syndrome. Note the numerous gas distended, dilated loops of bowel indicating a distal bowel obstruction. In this patient, the obstruction was due to functional immaturity of the distal colon.

combination of edema and adhesions in the region of the inflammed appendix and the terminal ileum. Intussusception most commonly occurs in children less than 2 years of age and usually is ileocolic in nature. It is most commonly idiopathic, except in children over the age of 5 years, in whom it is usually associated with a lead point. Typical lead points include Meckel's diverticulum, polyps, tumor such as lymphosarcoma, and fecal material in patients with cystic fibrosis. Other less common causes of low small bowel obstruction in children include incarcerated inguinal hernias, postsurgical adhesions, regional enteritis, Meckel's diverticulum, cysts, and small bowel tumors.

Dilated Colon and Small Bowel

In the neonate, the most common cause of colonic obstruction is functional colon obstruction seen with the meconium plug syndrome, small left colon syndrome, and colon immaturity (Fig. 5–4). All these conditions are most likely interrelated, or even the same, and represent inability of the patient to adequately clear the colon of meconium due to incomplete maturation of the ganglion cells of the distal colon. They all must be differentiated from Hirschsprung's disease (aganglionosis of a portion of the colon, usually the rectosigmoid colon). All these conditions present with problems during the first 24 hours of life but when colon obstruction presents in an older child, functional megacolon is the most common cause. This is an acquired obstruction, the cause of which is unknown. It may be due to suppression of the normal urge to defecate or to severe muscle spasm associated with anal fissures. Other causes of colon obstruction in children are rare, but include volvulus, colonic or presacral tumors, aberrant fibrous bands, or postinflammatory strictures.

ADYNAMIC ILEUS

A patient with adynamic ileus presents with multiple distended loops of both large and small bowel (Fig. 5–5). This usually can be differentiated from a low colonic obstruction because the loops will not have an organized appearance (Fig. 5–6). The air/fluid levels on the erect view will be quite long in adynamic ileus, as opposed to the numerous short air/fluid levels at different levels in the obstructed bowel loops (Fig. 5–7). In adynamic ileus, the large and small bowel will be distended to a proportionately similar degree. Adynamic ileus can accompany many conditions, including electrolyte disturbances, dehydration, inflammatory conditions such as gastroenteritis or peritonitis, drugs, autonomic nervous system disorders, and the postoperative state. In neonates, adynamic ileus can be the initial finding in necrotizing enterocolitis and sepsis. Paralytic ileus in necrotizing enterocolitis may be followed by bowel wall thickening and the pathognomonic finding of pneumatosis cystoides intestinalis.

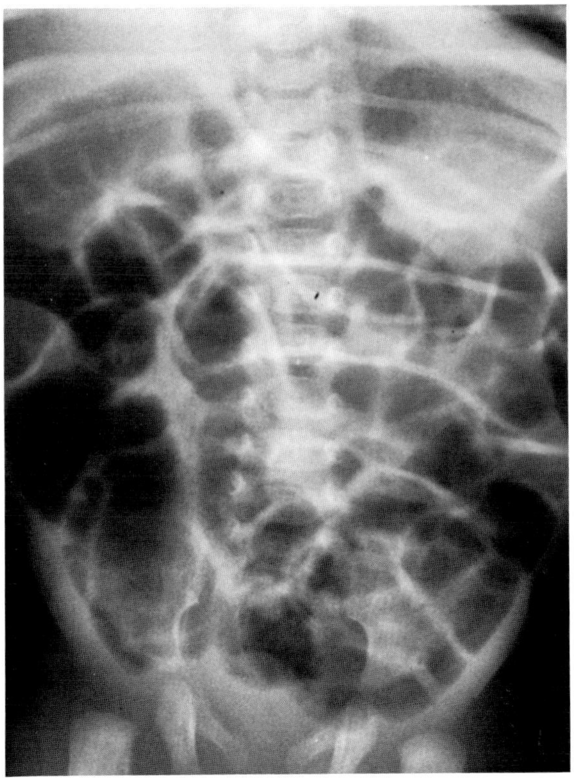

Fig. 5–5 Gastroenteritis. Generalized, symmetrical gaseous distension of both the large and small bowel is consistent with adynamic ileus.

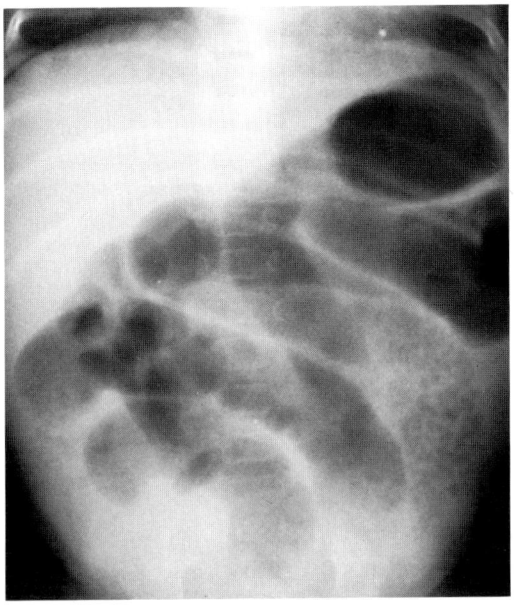

Fig. 5–6 Obstruction due to an incarcerated inguinal hernia. A supine view of the abdomen showing multiple gas-distended, dilated loops of bowel in an organized pattern.

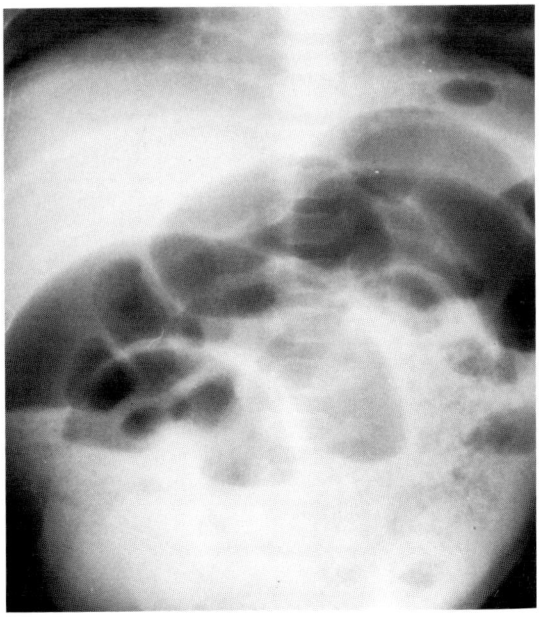

Fig. 5–7 The erect abdominal view of the patient in Fig. 5–6 reveals multiple air-fluid levels at varying levels. This is a classic picture of bowel obstruction.

THE GASLESS ABDOMEN

In normal infants, gas usually enters the gastrointestinal tract almost immediately after birth. Studies have shown that air is found within the stomach within a few minutes after birth, in the small intestine by at least 30 minutes, and in the transverse and descending colon by 5 to 6 hours following birth. Most infants and young children have a generous amount of gas scattered throughout the gastrointestinal tract. The absence of gas in the abdomen should therefore be considered abnormal. The most common reason for this appearance is severe vomiting, often due to gastroenteritis, appendicitis, or neurologic disease (Fig. 5–8). The patient who is obtunded or has decreased ability to swallow may also show little air within the gastrointestinal tract. In a neonate, esophageal atresia without a tracheoesophageal fistula should always be considered if gas does not appear in the abdomen in a timely manner. Other high gastrointestinal obstructions can also present with a paucity of intestinal gas.

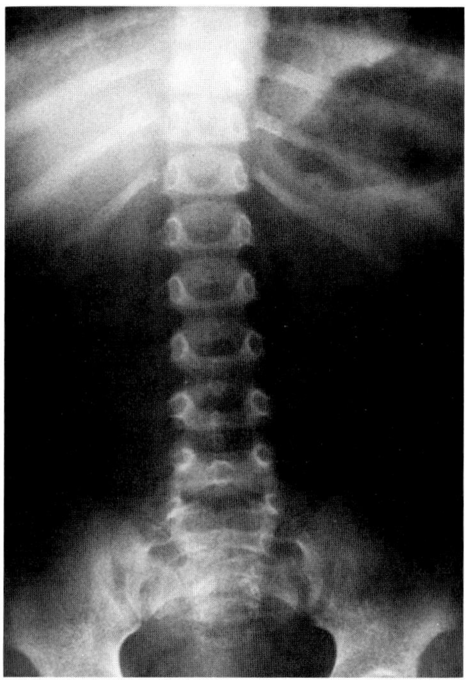

Fig. 5–8 Gasless abdomen. Only a small amount of air is present in the stomach of this patient, who has gastroenteritis due to vomiting.

SENTINEL LOOPS

Focally distended loops of intestine are sometimes referred to as sentinel loops because their presence may alert the radiologist to a nearby pathologic process. They are most often signals of an inflammatory process, usually in a nearby abdominal organ such as appendicitis, pancreatitis, cholecystitis, or an abdominal abscess (Fig. 5–9). Focally dilated loops may also be seen with an early bowel obstruction or closed loop obstruction. In neonates, a sentinel loop may be an indication of bowel ischemia if necrotizing enterocolitis is clinically suspected. Other causes of bowel ischemia in children are rare.

SEPARATED LOOPS

Increased soft tissue density between the gas-filled lumen of adjacent bowel loops may be caused either by bowel wall thickening or a disease process outside of the bowel causing separation of adjacent loops. Bowel wall thickening commonly occurs in inflammatory bowel disease or in diseases in which the bowel wall may be infiltrated, such as Whipple's disease, amyloidosis, or lymphoma. Intestinal hemor-

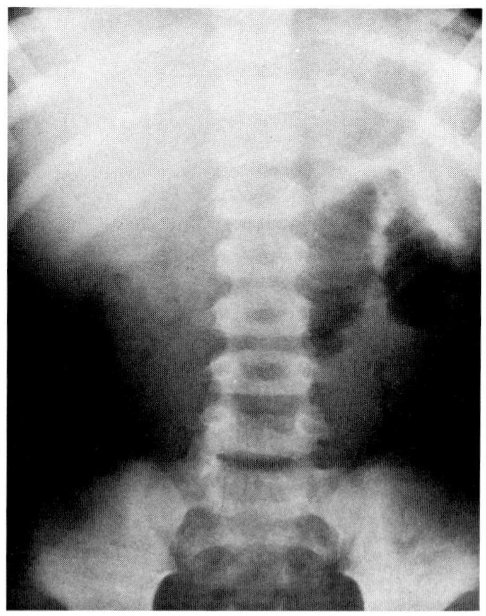

Fig. 5–9 Sentinel loop. Note the paucity of intestinal gas except for a single dilated loop of small bowel in this patient with gastroenteritis.

rhage may also thicken the bowel wall, as in Henoch-Schönlein purpura. Generalized separation of bowel loops may be seen in the presence of ascites or peritonitis. A focal area of separation may be caused by an abdominal abscess, cyst, neoplasm, or focal inflammation.

Calcifications

Many causes of calcifications within the abdomen are known. The appearance and location of calcifications are sometimes characteristic or even pathognomonic for certain disease processes. Intra-abdominal calcifications can be classified according to their appearance.

STONELIKE

A round or oval calcification within the abdomen is most likely to represent some type of a stone. A fecalith within the appendix is the most common stone seen in childhood (Fig. 5–10). In a symptomatic patient, it is diagnostic of appendicitis. Urinary tract calculi and gallstones are probably more common in children than is often realized. Gallstones are fairly common in children with hemolytic anemias such as sickle cell anemia, but idiopathic stones may also occur. Most urinary tract calculi in children are associated with hypercalcemic states or urinary tract obstruction with or without infection. Thrombus within the abdominal vessels, such as the portal vein or the inferior vena cava, may calcify and have a stonelike appearance. Calcified phleboliths, commonly seen in the adult pelvis, are rare in children. When seen they should suggest the presence of an hemangioma or an arteriovenous malformation. Hepatic or splenic granulomas may become densely calcified and look like stones. Ingested materials may also have a stonelike appearance and indeed may be stones or pebbles.

AMORPHOUS CALCIFICATIONS

In the neonate, amorphous calcifications within the abdomen are usually a sign of meconium peritonitis (Fig. 5–11). Such calcifications may be focal or widespread and are due to calcification of meconium that has leaked into the peritoneal cavity from a bowel perforation in utero. These patients may have signs and symptoms of peritonitis or obstruction, but in some cases the perforation will spontaneously seal-off in utero and the patient will be asymptomatic after birth. A common cause of meconium peritonitis is obstruction due to meconium ileus in a patient with cystic fibrosis.

In slightly older infants, irregular calcifications may be noted within the adrenal glands due to previous

ABDOMINAL CALCIFICATIONS

- Stonelike
  - Fecalith of appendix or Meckel's diverticulum
  - Urinary tract calculi
  - Gallstones
  - Calcified intravascular thrombus
  - Hepatic or splenic granulomas
  - Ingested foreign body
- Amorphous
  - Meconium peritonitis
  - Previous adrenal hemorrhage
  - Tumors
    - Neuroblastoma
    - Ganglioneuroma
    - Wilms' tumor
    - Hepatoblastoma
    - Hemangioma
    - Hamartoma
  - Nephrocalcinosis
  - Postinflammatory
  - Ingested materials
- Curvilinear
  - Meconium peritonitis
  - Cyst walls
    - Multicystic dysplastic kidney
    - Cystic tumors (adrenal cortical carcinoma)
  - Adrenal hemorrhage (resolved)
  - Bladder wall
    - Hemorrhagic cystitis
    - Schistosomiasis
- Formed
  - Teratoma
  - Fetus-in-fetu
  - Staghorn calculi
  - Adrenal glands (Wolman's disease)

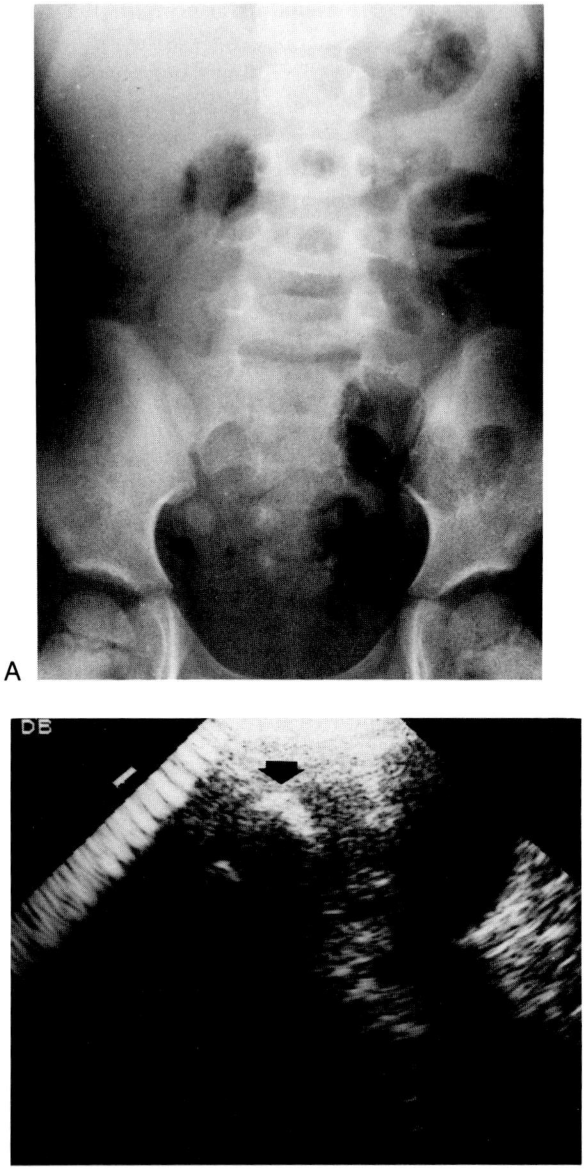

Fig. 5–10 Acute appendicitis. **(A)** The abdominal radiograph on this 13-year-old patient shows mild lumbar scoliosis with concavity to the right, indistinctness of the right psoas margin, and a large fecalith in the right pelvis (*arrow*). **(B)** The calcified fecalith was also identified by sonography of the right lower quadrant (*arrow*).

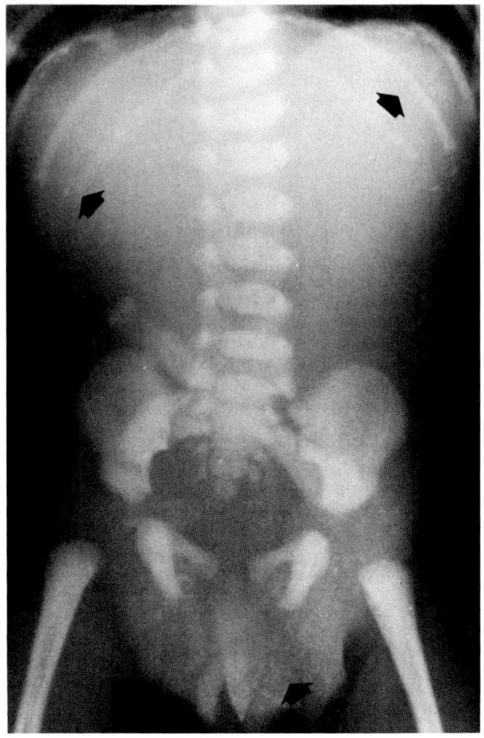

Fig. 5–11 Meconium peritonitis. Note the amorphous, stippled calcifications throughout the peritoneal cavity. Calcifications were also present in the scrotum due to bilateral inguinal hernias (*arrows*).

adrenal hemorrhage (Fig. 5–12). These calcifications also may be rimlike. Amorphous calcifications also commonly occur within intra-abdominal tumors in children. Most often this occurs in neuroblastoma or ganglioneuroma (Fig. 5–13). Less commonly, such calcification occurs within Wilms' tumor, hepatoblastoma, hepatic hemangioma, or hamartoma. Irregular calcifications in the kidneys may be due to renal tubular acidosis, renal papillary necrosis, or secondary to a variety of hypercalcemic states. Diffuse fine calcifications can be seen in the renal parenchyma with oxalosis, while irregular postinflammatory calcifications can be seen within lymph nodes, the liver, spleen, or kidney. Rarely they can be seen within the pancreas or the prostate gland. Pancreatic calcifications usually occur only in the chronic forms of pancreatitis, which are uncommon in children. Nevertheless, calcifications have been noted in association with cystic fibrosis (Fig. 5–14). A hereditary form of pancreatitis develops large, rounded calcifications in the pancreatic head.

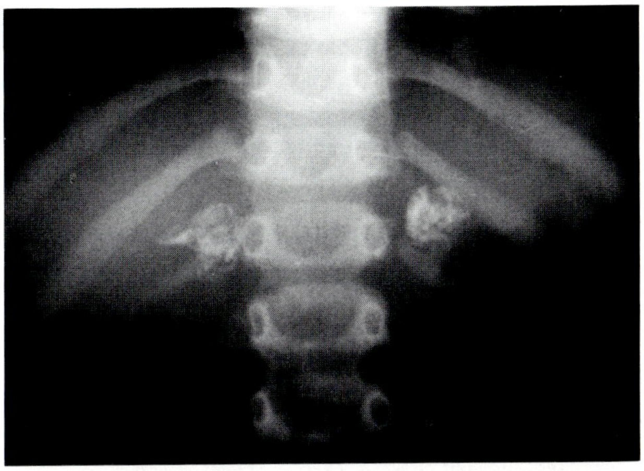

Fig. 5–12 Adrenal calcifications. The calcified adrenal glands due to previous adrenal hemorrhages were an incidental finding in this asymptomatic 1-year-old patient.

Infarction in such organs as the ovaries, intra-abdominal testes, liver, spleen, kidney, or intestine may result in the formation of focal irregular calcifications. Certain ingested materials appear as irregular radiodensities in the abdomen. This is most commonly seen with the ingestion of dirt, lead or other heavy metals, and medications containing bismuth.

CURVILINEAR CALCIFICATIONS

Curvilinear calcifications are quite uncommon in children. In neonates, they are most commonly seen as a manifestation of meconium peritonitis in which the curvilinear calcification may outline a soft tissue mass referred to as *cystic* or *pseudocystic meconium peritonitis*. Other intra-abdominal cysts that are known to calcify in a curvilinear pattern include multicystic dysplastic kidneys and cystic abdominal tumors, particularly adrenal cortical carcinoma. A calcific rim around the adrenal gland may also be seen with the resolution of an adrenal hemorrhage. Bladder wall calcification has been noted following hemorrhagic cystitis due to cyclophosphamide (Cytoxan) therapy and in schistosomiasis; however, these conditions are both quite rare.

FORMED CALCIFICATIONS

Formed calcifications or ossifications, commonly appearing as teeth, are seen in two-thirds of patients

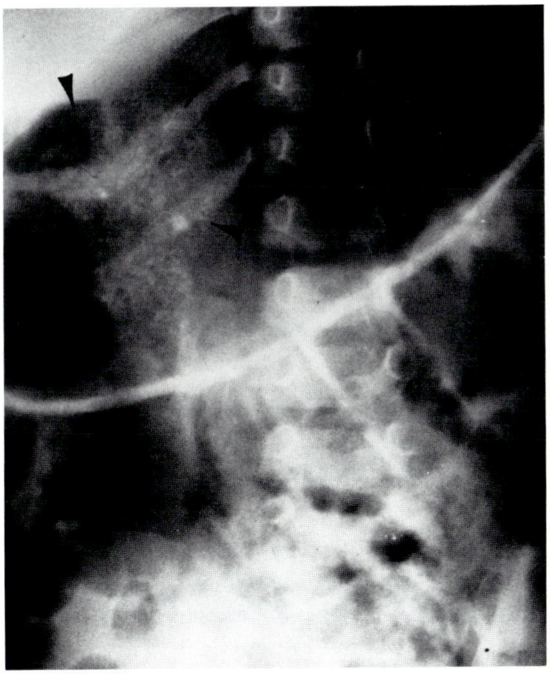

Fig. 5–13 Ganglioneuroma of the right adrenal. Note the large right suprarenal mass containing multiple stippled calcifications and displacing the right kidney inferiorly (*arrows*).

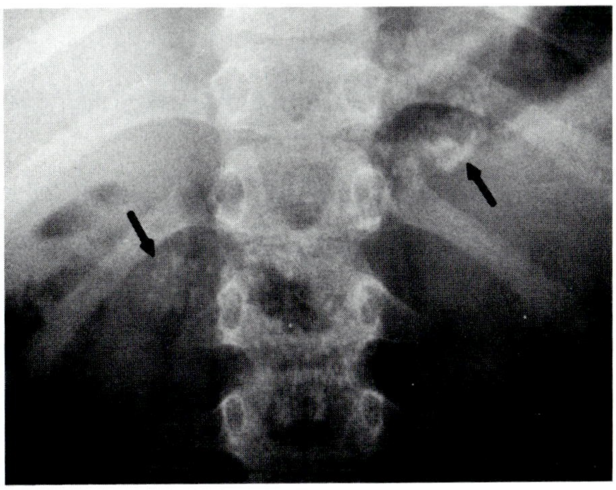

Fig. 5–14 Pancreatic calcifications. Multiple stippled calcifications in the pancreas (*arrows*) of a 9-year-old patient with cystic fibrosis.

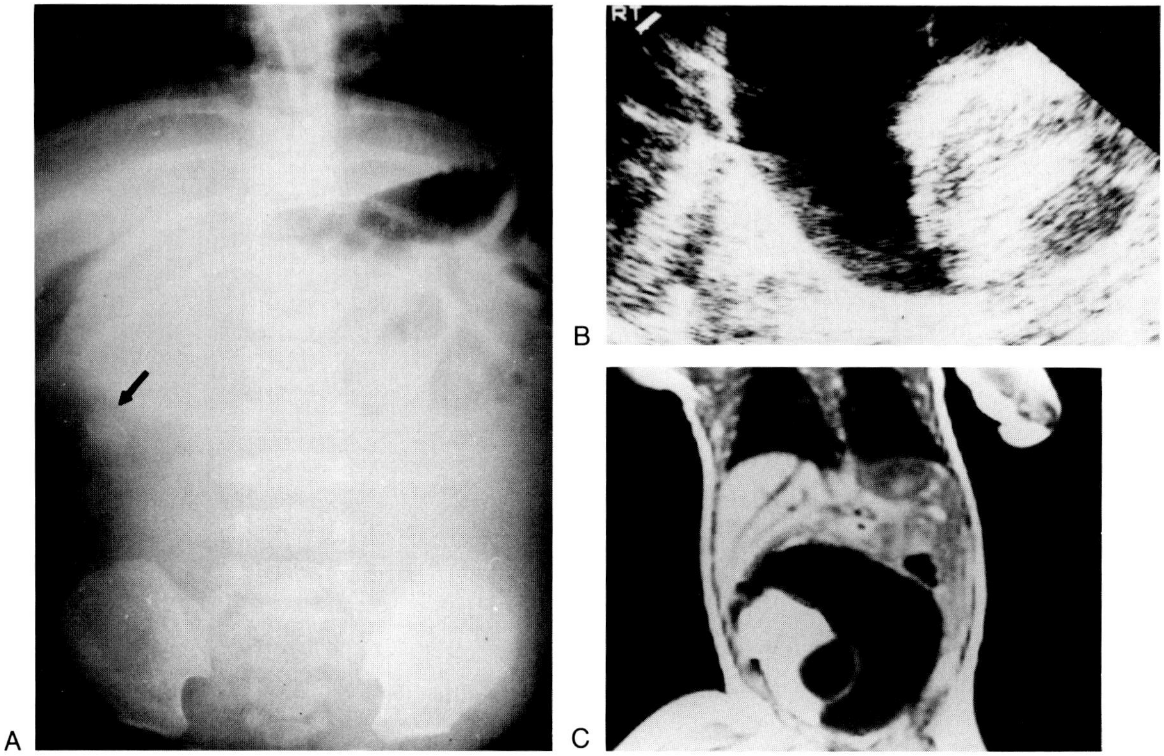

Fig. 5–15 Retroperitoneal teratoma in a 5-month-old patient. **(A)** The plain radiograph shows a large abdominal mass containing a tooth-shaped calcification (*arrow*). Areas of radiolucency noted around the calcification suggest the presence of fat. **(B)** Longitudinal ultrasound of the mass showed it to be predominantly cystic with a large internal area of echogenicity. **(C)** Sagittal MRI verified the complex nature of the mass, which contained septations and a large area of fat (*arrow*).

with ovarian teratomas (Fig. 5–15). Similar calcifications are also seen in the less common presacral and retroperitoneal teratomas. Bonelike calcifications also occur in these entities. In the rare condition known as fetus-in-fetu, a fairly well-formed aborted fetus is present within the infant's abdomen. On plain radiographs, body parts usually containing recognizable bones and surrounding fat differentiate it from the teeth and less formed ossifications of the teratoma. Stag-horn renal calculi are rarely seen in children. Densely calcified, enlarged adrenal glands are a sign of Wolman's disease, an unusual lipidosis.

Extraintestinal Air

PNEUMOPERITONEUM

Previous surgery is probably the most common cause of air within the peritoneal cavity, but this cause will be easy to diagnose. A perforation somewhere in the gastrointestinal tract should be the next consideration and in the neonate, it is usually the result of necrotizing enterocolitis or idiopathic perforation of the stomach. Iatrogenic perforations are also common, usually due to thermometer or catheter perforations of the colon. In addition, because of the common use of mechanically assisted ventilation in premature neonates, pneumoperitoneum due to dissection of mediastinal air into the peritoneal cavity has become increasingly common (Fig. 5–16). In older infants and children, bowel perforations are more commonly due to perforated ulcers or Meckel's diverticulum.

The detection of pneumoperitoneum is sometimes difficult on the supine radiographs usually obtained on infants and children. If a large amount of free air is present, it may appear as an oval radiolucency of the entire abdomen (Fig. 5–17), which overlies the liver and outlines a central linear opacity represent-

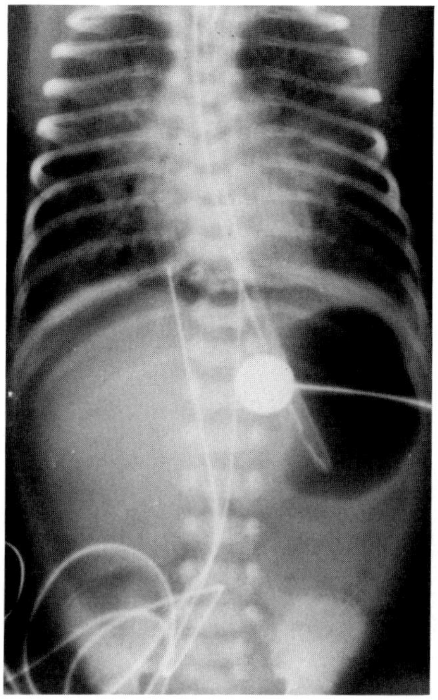

Fig. 5–16 Iatrogenic pneumoperitoneum. This premature newborn infant with bronchopulmonary dysplasia developed pneumoperitoneum secondary to the high pressures generated during mechanically assisted ventilation. Note the radiolucent air surrounding the liver.

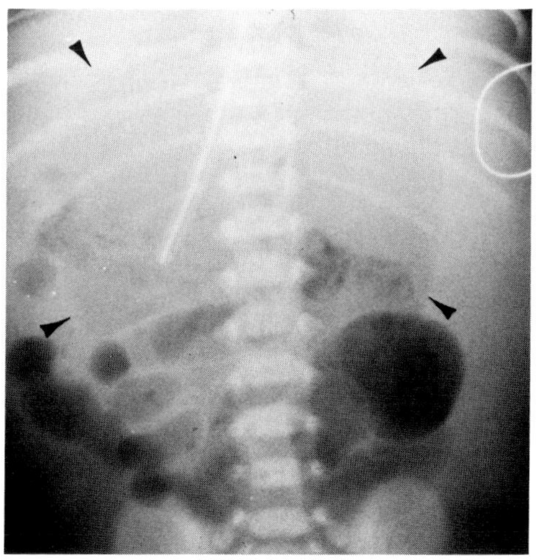

Fig. 5–17 Pneumoperitoneum in a newborn with necrotizing enterocolitis. On supine abdominal views, free intraperitoneal air often lies anteriorly and appears as an oval shaped radiolucency over the abdomen (*arrows*).

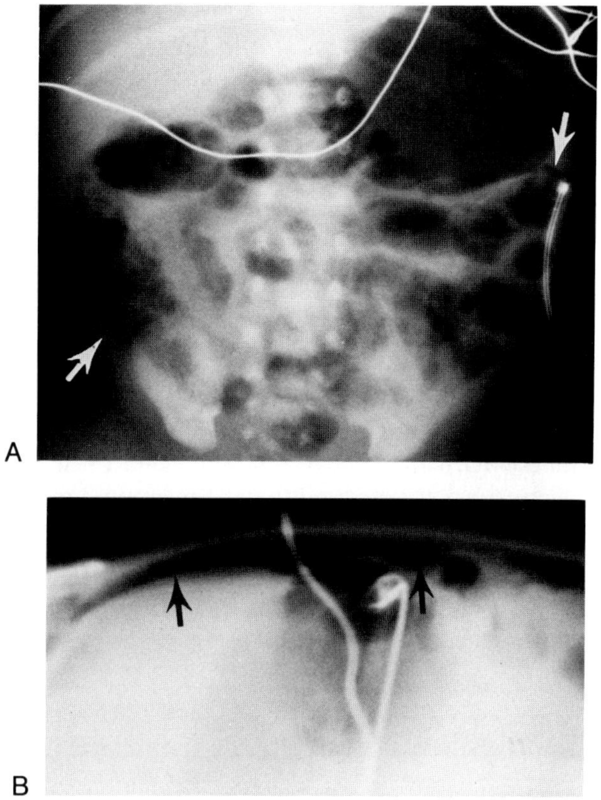

Fig. 5–18 Pneumoperitoneum secondary to necrotizing enterocolitis. **(A)** The bubbly and curvilinear air collections (*arrows*) represent pneumatosis cystoides intestinalis in this premature infant with necrotizing enterocolitis. **(B)** Later, a cross-table lateral view shows a large amount of free intraperitoneal air layered anteriorly beneath the abdominal wall (*arrows*).

ing the falciform ligament. This appearance has been termed the *football sign*. The urachus and umbilical arteries may produce similar linear densities in the lower abdomen. The walls of the bowel loops may appear unusually well defined due to the presence of air along both the inner and outer borders. Lateral decubitus and cross-table lateral views may be useful for detecting smaller amounts of intraperitoneal air. A triangular lucency just below the liver edge on the cross-table lateral view is a clue to an early pneumoperitoneum (Fig. 5–18).

PNEUMATOSIS CYSTOIDES INTESTINALIS

Unlike adults, the presence of linear or bubbly collections of gas within the bowel wall is almost always a sign of significant pathology. In the neonate, pneumatosis intestinalis most commonly suggests the presence of necrotizing enterocolitis (Fig. 5–19). The presence of the gas is thought to be mainly due to bacterial overgrowth within the bowel wall. Bowel ischemia can present with a similar picture. Beyond the neonatal period, pneumatosis intestinalis is uncommon. It can be seen in children with cystic fibrosis, collagen-vascular diseases, leukemia, milk intolerance, or immunosuppressive therapy and immunodeficiencies (Fig. 5–20). The exact cause of the pneumatosis in these conditions is uncertain. Overdistention of the bowel can lead to mucosal tears, which permit the entrance of air into the bowel wall. This is termed *benign pneumatosis* as it is not associated with compromised bowel.

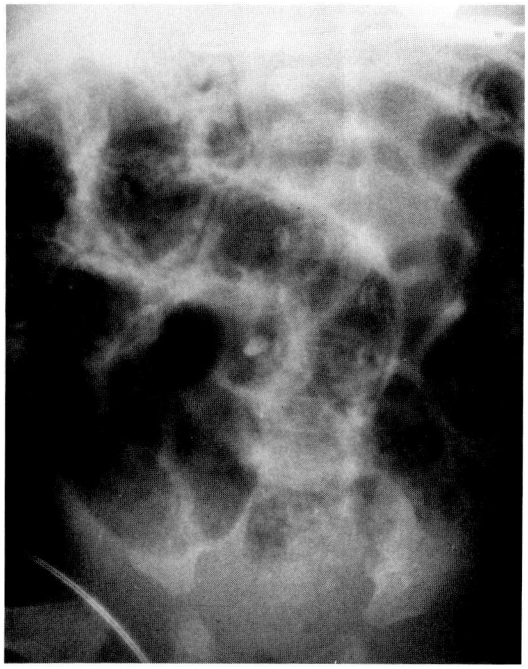

Fig. 5–19 Necrotizing enterocolitis. Notice the bubbly and curvilinear pattern of pneumatosis cystoides intestinalis.

PORTAL VEIN AND BILIARY TRACT GAS

Linear radiolucency seen extending through the liver in a branching pattern may be due to either gas within the portal venous system or the biliary tract. Gas within the portal veins is carried by flow into the fine peripheral radicles. This results in fine linear radiolucencies that extend to the edge of the liver and usually can be differentiated from the more central distribution of gas within the biliary tract. Classically, portal venous gas has been associated with pneumatosis cystoides intestinalis due to necrotizing enterocolitis. At one time this was considered an indicator of a very grave prognosis; but now the treatment of necrotizing enterocolitis has greatly improved. Mesenteric artery occlusion leading to bowel infarction can also be a cause of portal vein gas (Fig. 5–21). Introduction of gas into the portal venous system through umbilical catheters has become increasingly common in neonatal intensive care units and may be incidentally noted on abdominal ultrasound examination.

Air within the biliary tract is uncommon in children. It is predominantly the result of obstruction of the duodenum past the ampulla of Vater but may be due to previous biliary surgery.

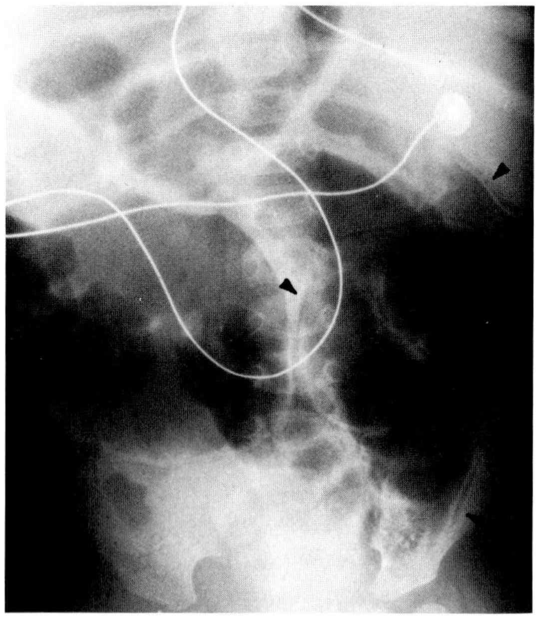

Fig. 5–20 Pneumatosis intestinalis in an older infant with short gut syndrome. The abdominal radiograph shows markedly dilated loops of bowel with extensive pneumatosis (*arrowheads*) of the bowel wall.

PNEUMATOSIS INTESTINALIS

Inflammation
- Necrotizing enterocolitis
- Hirschsprung's disease
- Toxic megacolon
- Milk intolerance

Neoplasm
- Leukemia

Trauma/surgery
- Prolonged overdistention due to obstruction
- Pneumomediastinum due to positive-pressure respirator-assisted ventilation

Systemic/metabolic
- Cystic fibrosis
- Collagen-vascular diseases
- Immunodeficiencies

Miscellaneous
- Bone marrow transplantation
- Steroids

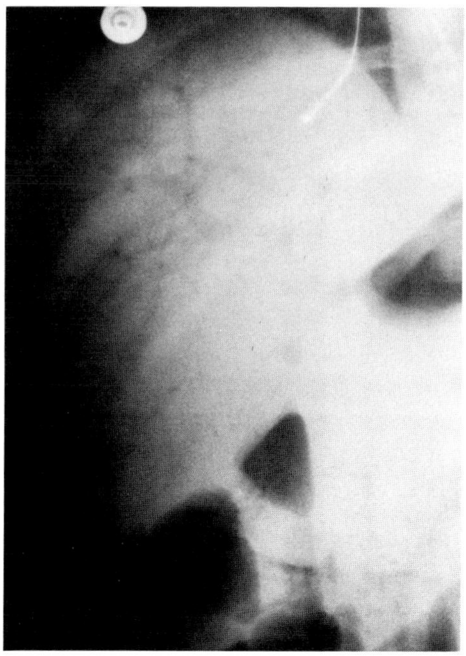

Fig. 5–21 Portal venous gas due to bowel ischemia. Note extensive gas within the portal vein branches of the liver in this 2-year-old patient with bowel ischemia secondary to severe dehydration.

Intraperitoneal Fluid

When a large amount of fluid of various types is present within the peritoneal cavity, it may be seen on plain radiographs as an overall increase in the density of the abdomen. The bowel loops may "float" in the fluid, causing them to cluster centrally within the abdomen (Fig. 5–22). The most sensitive method for identifying intraperitoneal fluid, however, is ultrasound (Fig. 5–23).

In the neonate, urine is the most common fluid found in the peritoneal cavity. This is usually due to urinary tract obstruction secondary to posterior urethral valves in male infants. Chylous ascites can be seen in neonates and is most likely due to hypoplasia or obstruction of the lymphatic system. Chylous ascites has also been reported in association with volvulus causing mesenteric vein obstruction.

In older children, ascites is often due to renal disease (e.g., nephrotic syndrome) or cirrhotic liver disease. Other less common causes of ascites include portal vein obstruction, intestinal lymphangiectasia, hypo-

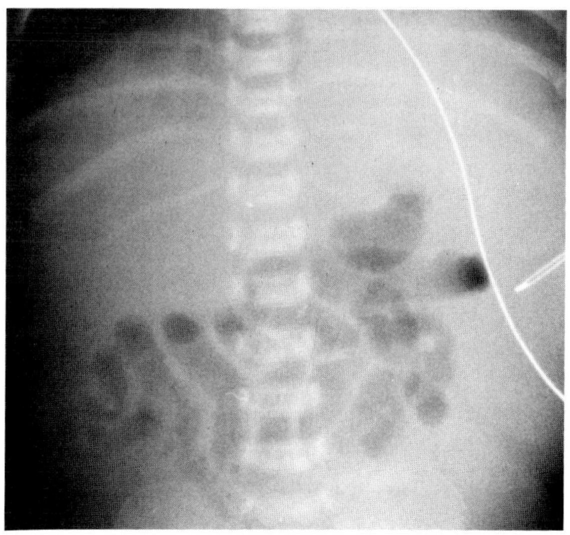

Fig. 5–22 Newborn with ascites of unknown origin. Note the centrally located bowel loops within the fluid-distended abdomen.

A

B

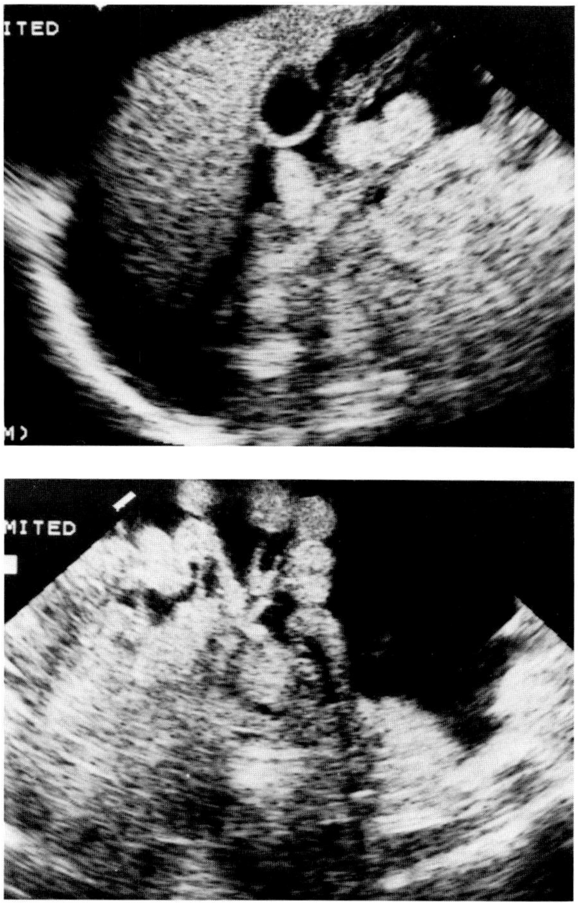

Fig. 5–23 Ascites in a patient with an immunodeficiency syndrome. **(A)** Sagittal and **(B)** transverse ultrasound images of the abdomen show the large amount of ascites surrounding the liver and bowel.

ASCITES

- Types of Fluid
  - Transudate
    - Renal failure
    - Liver disease
    - Erythroblastosis fetalis
    - Portal vein obstruction
    - Intestinal lymphangiectasia
    - Hypoproteinemia
    - Pancreatitis
    - Cardiac disease
    - Peritoneal metastasis
  - Urine
    - Urinary tract obstruction
    - Bladder abnormalities
  - Pus or bowel contents
    - Bacterial peritonitis
    - Meconium peritonitis
    - Perforation
  - Chyle
    - Neonatal chylous ascites
    - Volvulus
    - Lymphangiectasia
  - Bile
    - Biliary tract perforation
  - Blood
    - Trauma
    - Bleeding disorders
  - Cyst fluid
    - Ruptured ovarian, mesenteric, omental cysts

proteinemia, pancreatitis, and ruptured ovarian cysts. Bile ascites is rare in children. It is usually the result of a perforation of the biliary tract, which is often idiopathic. Blood within the peritoneal cavity is usually a result of trauma, although bleeding disorders may also result in hemoperitoneum.

Bacterial peritonitis is an additional important cause of intraperitoneal fluid and may be the result of a perforation of the gastrointestinal tract or may accompany generalized sepsis. Spontaneous bacterial peritonitis can also occur in older children and is a common complication of the nephrotic syndrome. The appearance of the intraperitoneal fluid is nonspecific and cannot be differentiated from other causes of intraperitoneal fluid.

ESOPHAGUS

Esophageal Atresia and Tracheoesophageal Fistula

Esophageal atresia and tracheoesophageal fistula are components of a group of congenital anomalies thought to be due to abnormal separation of the primitive trachea and esophagus leading to faulty formation of the esophagus and an abnormal communication between the trachea and esophagus. The basic forms of this malformation include isolated esophageal atresia with no fistula, isolated tracheoesophageal fistula with no esophageal atresia, or esophageal atresia with

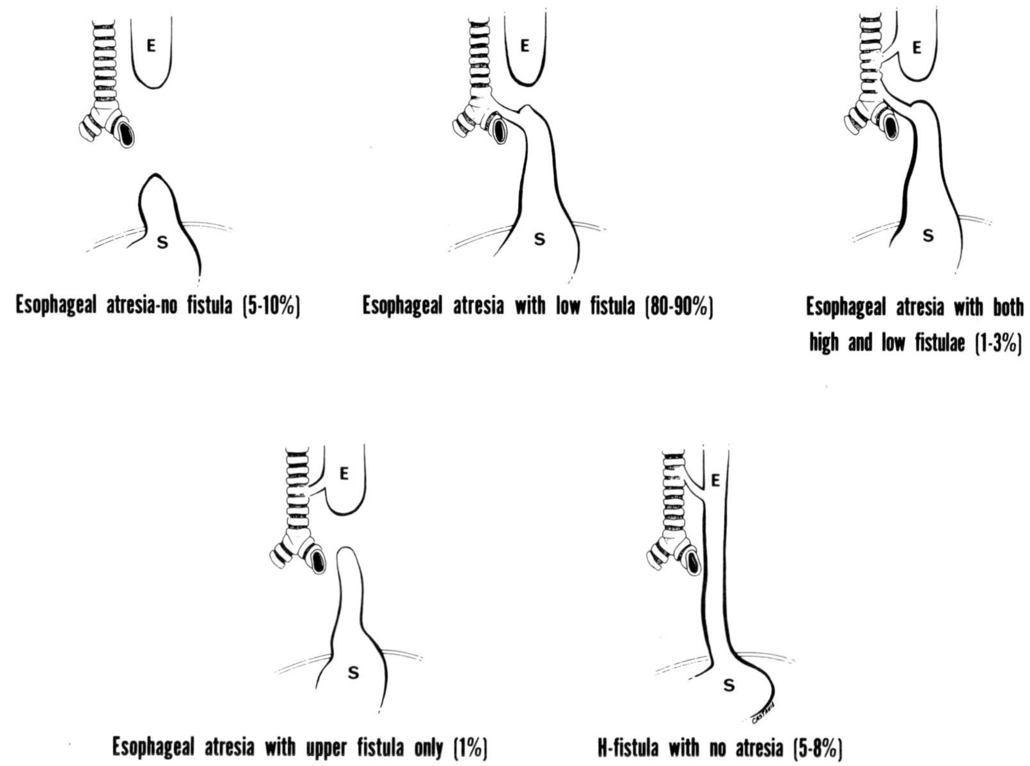

Fig. 5–24 Esophageal atresia and tracheoesophageal fistula. Diagrammatic representation and relative frequency of the various types of tracheoesophageal anomalies. (From Swishuk LE, Imaging of the Newborn, Infant, and Young Child. 3rd Ed. Williams & Wilkins, Baltimore, 1989, with permission.)

tracheoesophageal fistula (Fig. 5–24). The most common form consists of esophageal atresia with a fistula connecting the trachea to the distal portion of remaining esophagus. This comprises 80 to 90 percent of the cases. The size of the atretic portion of the esophagus is variable and is an important factor in determining the prognosis and type of repair. Esophageal atresia with a fistula to the proximal esophageal pouch or to both the proximal and distal esophageal segments is the least common form of this anomaly.

Esophageal atresia with no tracheoesophageal fistula is the second most common anomaly within this group of esophageal anomalies. Isolated tracheoesophageal fistula with no esophageal atresia is the third most common anomaly. This has been termed the *H-fistula,* although the fistula actually takes an upwardly oblique course from the esophagus to the trachea giving it more of an N-type appearance (Fig. 5–25).

Patients with any type of esophageal atresia present clinically with difficulty in handling secretions and severe choking, vomiting, and aspiration upon feeding. When tracheoesophageal fistula is present without esophageal atresia, the presentation may be more insidious, particularly if the fistula is small. In such cases the diagnosis may be delayed until later in childhood.

The radiographic findings can be quite different in the various types of these abnormalities. When esophageal atresia with no tracheoesophageal fistula or a fistula connecting the trachea only to the proximal pouch is present, no gas will be able to enter the gastrointestinal tract. These abnormalities should be strongly suspected in a neonate with a gasless abdomen and the former is much more common. The proximal esophageal segment in esophageal atresia is often well seen on the plain radiograph, appearing as an oval-shaped radiolucency in the neck or upper

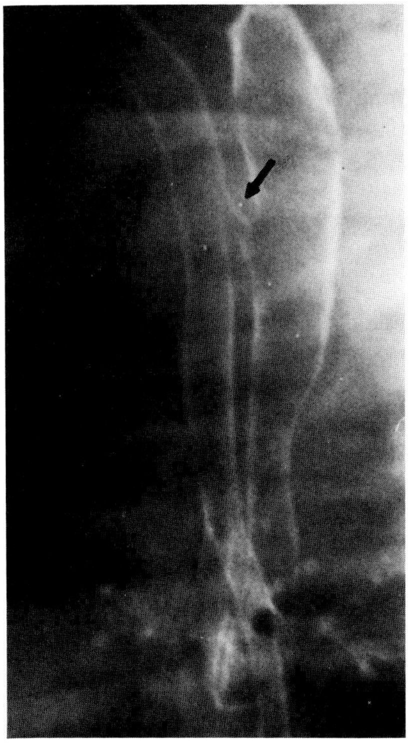

Fig. 5–25 Tracheoesophageal fistula without esophageal atresia. Note the small fistulous tract extending caudally from the trachea to the esophagus (*arrow*) on the lateral esophogram.

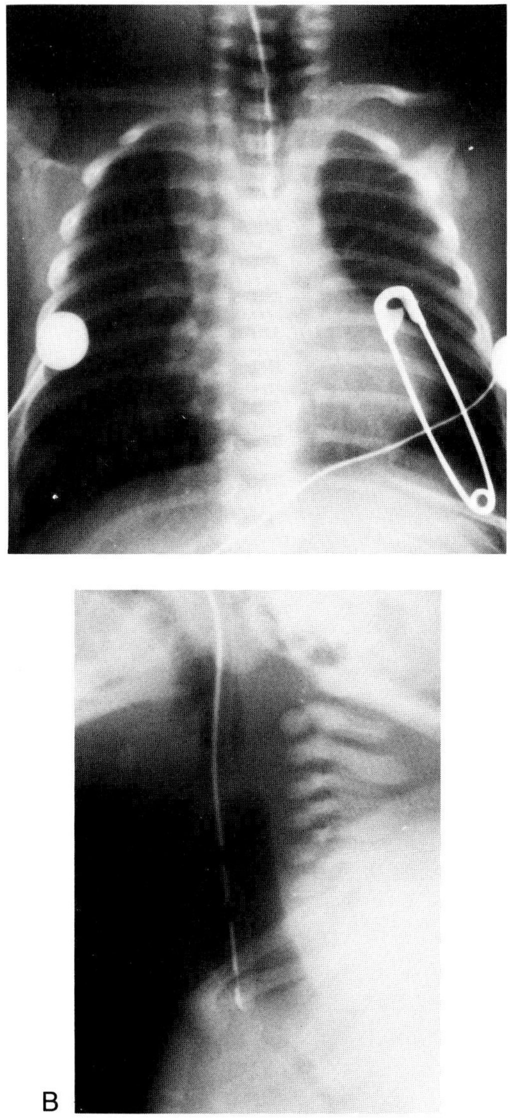

Fig. 5–26 Esophageal atresia. The blind-ending proximal esophageal pouch, when distended with gas, is clearly identifiable on the posteroanterior **(A)** and lateral **(B)** views.

thorax (Fig. 5–26). Air within the suprasternal fossa can sometimes give a similar appearance, however a lateral view will quickly differentiate the two. On the lateral view, the dilated, air-filled proximal esophageal segment will be seen clearly, often anteriorly displacing and compressing the trachea (Fig. 5–26). Aspiration pneumonia is also often present in these patients, commonly involving the right upper lobe.

Contrast studies usually are necessary only to identify the presence of a tracheoesophageal fistula when no esophageal atresia is present. A small amount of thin barium may be used safely and is injected through a nasogastric tube. The patient should be imaged in lateral and prone positions, since the fistulae extend from the ventral aspect of the esophagus. If the fistula is small, it may be difficult to delineate. Excessive air within the distal esophagus may be a clue to a fistulous connection between the trachea and esophagus. When esophageal atresia is present, the distal esophageal segment can usually be studied by refluxing barium from the stomach into the esophagus after placement of a gastrostomy tube.

Occasionally, traumatic perforation of the proximal esophagus with a nasogastric tube or a finger in the oropharynx can occur, creating a pharyngeal pseudodiverticulum. This abnormality usually can be differentiated from esophageal atresia by its paraesophageal location. In other cases contrast may actually drain into the mediastinum.

Postoperatively, contrast studies may be performed to rule out leaks or strictures at the site of anastomosis that may complicate the repair. A small amount of narrowing at the anastomosis can normally be expected. Other postoperative complications that may occur include recurrent fistulae and sinus tracts, abnormal motility in the distal portion of the esophagus, shortening of the esophagus leading to a hiatal hernia and gastroesophageal reflux, and focal tracheomalacia due to chronic compression of the trachea by the dilated proximal esophageal pouch in utero.

Esophageal atresia is often associated with other congenital atresias in the gastrointestinal tract, predominately duodenal atresia or stenosis and imperforate or ectopic anus. When duodenal atresia occurs in conjunction with isolated esophageal atresia, the gastric secretions become trapped within the stomach causing it to become markedly distended. The distal esophageal segment will also distend with fluid and may be seen as a mass behind the heart on the chest x-ray. Cardiac anomalies are commonly associated with esophageal atresia and tracheoesophageal fistula or isolated tracheoesophageal fistula, especially patent ductus arteriosus and ventricular septal defects. A right aortic arch occurs in 5 percent of the patients, an important observation for surgical planning. Tracheoesophageal fistula and esophageal atresia are also a well-known part of the VATER syndrome.

Hiatal Hernia and Gastroesophageal Reflux

Gastroesophageal reflux is quite common in young infants up to 7 or 8 weeks of age due to functional immaturity and abnormal tone of the lower esophageal sphincter. Generally this is a minor problem that spontaneously resolves as the infant matures. In a few cases, reflux may be severe, leading to complications such as esophagitis and stricture. The entity of partial intrathoracic stomach (congenital short esophagus) is now most often thought to be an acquired lesion due to severe reflux esophagitis leading to shortening of the esophagus in utero. A fixed hiatal hernia will also be present in these patients. The incidence of hiatal hernia in infants and children is probably similar to that of adults. Paraesophageal hernias can occur in childhood, although they are much less common and are not associated with an incompetent lower esophageal sphincter. The term *chalasia* refers to a condition in which the lower esophageal sphincter fails to contract properly in the resting phase, leading to gross gastroesophageal reflux. This is generally diagnosed in young infants and often resolves with age.

The appropriate imaging sequence for evaluating a patient with gastroesophageal reflux is quite controversial. The most sensitive imaging method for detecting the presence of gastroesophageal reflux is gastroesophageal scintigraphy, although it gives no information about the anatomy of the esophagus and stomach. The gastric emptying time also can be reasonably well assessed by nuclear medicine studies, but a prolonged gastric emptying time cannot determine the precise underlying cause. When gastroesophageal reflux has been diagnosed either clinically or with an imaging modality, it is particularly important to evaluate the gastric antrum for any obstructing lesions. Both ultrasonography and contrast upper gastrointestinal studies have been used but, more and more, ultrasonography is favored (Fig. 5–27).

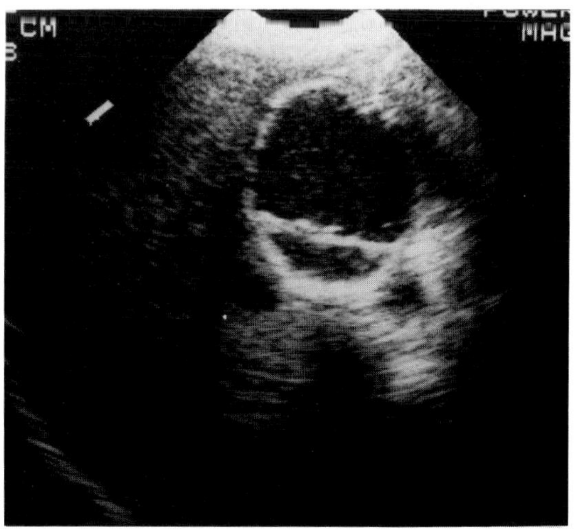

Fig. 5–27 Congenital diaphragm of the gastric antrum. Transverse ultrasound clearly identifies the thin diaphragm extending across the distal gastric antrum in this patient with gastroesophageal reflux.

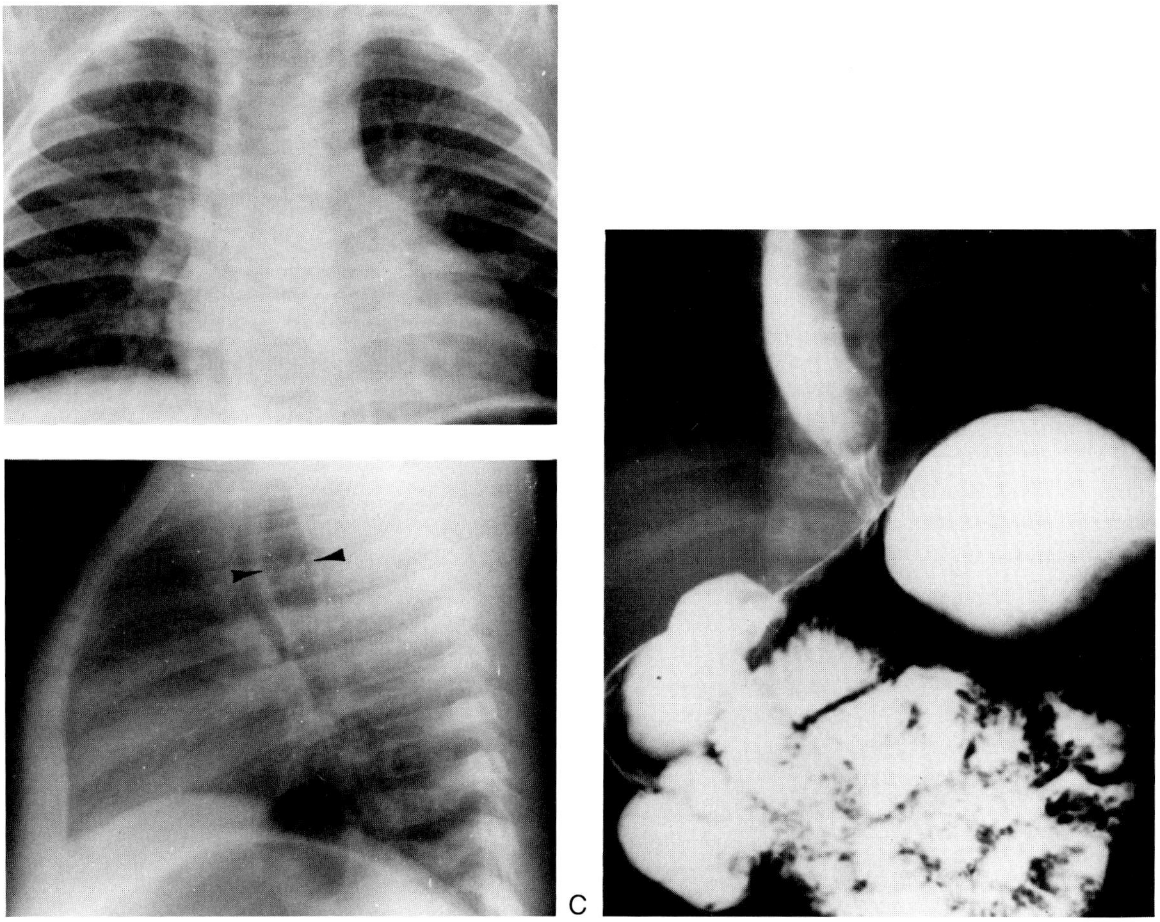

A

B

C

Fig. 5–28 Gastroesophageal reflux. **(A & B)** A dilated, air-filled esophagus (*arrowheads*) is visible on the posteroanterior and lateral chest views, suggesting the presence of gastroesophageal reflux. **(C)** A contrast study confirms the presence of marked reflux.

A dilated, air-filled esophagus (mega-aeroesophagus) may be seen on chest x-rays in patients with chronic gastroesophageal reflux (Fig. 5–28) and hiatal hernias are also commonly demonstrated with contrast studies. Many special maneuvers have been advocated by various authors to facilitate the detection of gastroesophageal reflux during an upper gastrointestinal series, but their use is variable from radiologist to radiologist.

Inflammation

In children, as in adults, chronic gastroesophageal reflux is the most common cause of inflammation of the esophagus. Although gastroesophageal reflux is quite common in pediatric patients, particularly young infants, the incidence of reflux esophagitis is not nearly as high as might be expected. Nevertheless, it is known to occur, and in severe cases it may be complicated by stricture formation. The intrathoracic stomach (short esophagus) syndrome is actually the sequel of peptic esophagitis, leading to shortening of the esophagus, stricture, and development of a fixed hiatal hernia (Fig. 5–29). The earliest finding in peptic esophagitis is abnormal peristalsis in the involved portion of the esophagus. Eventually tiny ulcerations can appear, and these may progress to larger irregular ulcers and a thickened esophageal wall. Severe esophagitis with stricture formation, however, is not common in children, nor is the development of Barrett's esophagus.

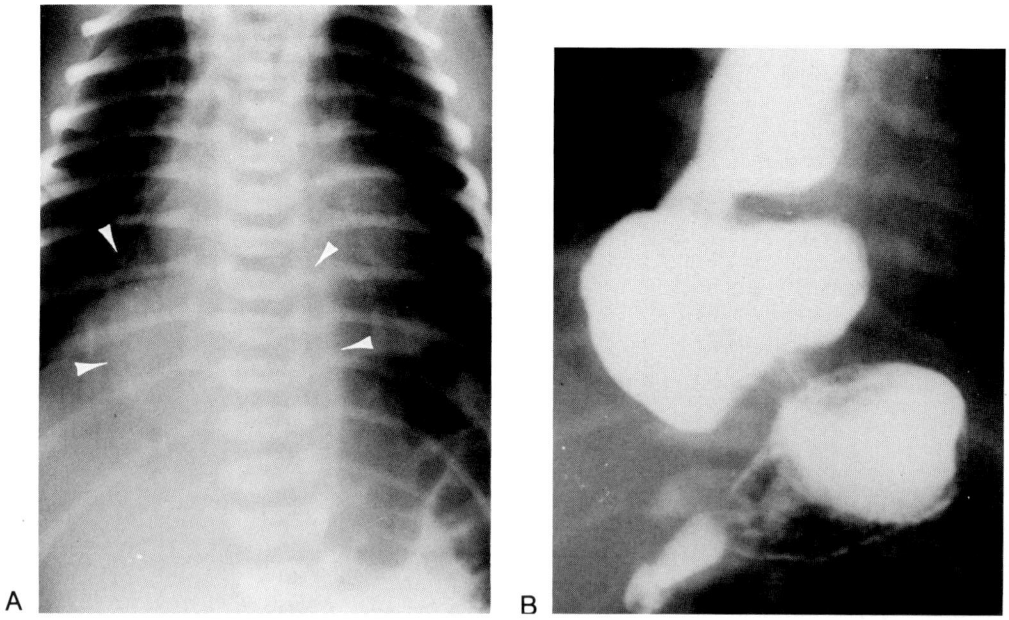

Fig. 5–29 Congenital short esophagus. **(A)** The plain radiograph shows a mass in the upper abdomen extending into the thorax (*arrowheads*). **(B)** Contrast studies showed the mass to consist of a partially intrathoracic stomach due to a shortened esophagus.

Of the infectious forms of esophagitis, *Candida* infections are the most common. These are predominantly a problem in immunocompromised children. Oral thrush may or may not be present. The initial changes may be focal; however, diffuse involvement of the esophagus is often seen. The radiographic findings on a barium swallow study include spasm, impaired peristalsis, thickened mucosal folds, and fine diffuse ulcerations. In more severe infections, characteristic plaquelike defects can be seen, representing actual colonies of *Candida* organisms.

Herpes esophagitis is rare in children. The radiographic changes are similar to those seen in adults and include focal spasm, abnormal motility, and diffuse, fine ulceration.

Corrosive ingestion is an important cause of esophagitis in children. Alkaline corrosive agents, including alkaline disc batteries and Clinitest tablets, cause a penetrating burn that may lead to perforation and later, stricture. Acids cause more superficial necrosis of the esophagus, with more severe burns occurring in the stomach. Tetracycline tablets are also known to cause a focal form of esophagitis.

The acute changes of corrosive esophagitis include lack of peristalsis, rigidity due to edema, and spasm. Mucosal irregularity, ulceration, and frank extravasation due to perforation can be seen in more severe burns (Fig. 5–30). Clues to the presence of perforation on the chest x-ray are mediastinal widening, pleural effusion, and pneumomediastinum. Stricture formation begins 3 to 4 weeks after corrosive ingestion. Intraluminal adhesions and diverticula may also form. As these various scars contract, the esophagus shortens, leading to development of a hiatal hernia.

Although reflux and corrosive esophagitis are by far the most common causes of esophageal strictures in childhood, other causes exist. A stricture sometimes forms at the site of surgical repair of a tracheoesophageal fistula. Congenital stenoses also occur in patients with tracheoesophageal fistulas due to the presence

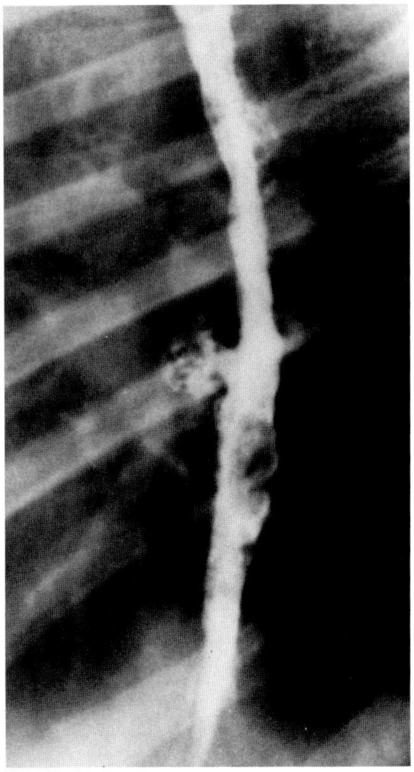

Fig. 5–30 Acute corrosive esophagitis. Note the marked narrowing, mucosal irregularity, and sinus tract formation following the ingestion of lye.

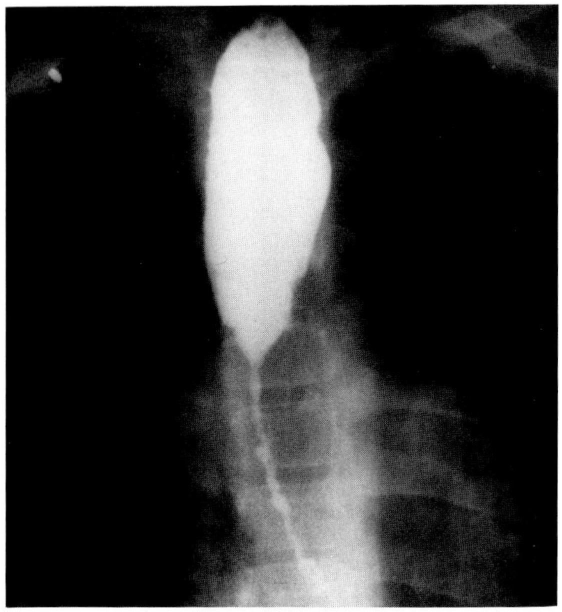

Fig. 5–31 Esophageal stricture due to epidermolysis bullosa. Note the long, distal esophageal stricture.

of cartilaginous or muscular tracheobronchial remnants. On barium swallow examination, these remnants have the appearance of small diverticulum-like structures in the distal esophagus surrounding an area of stenosis. Congenital esophageal webs are also sometimes associated with tracheoesophageal fistulas and have the appearance of a focal stenosis of the esophagus. Webs and strictures have also been described as a complication of epidermolysis bullosa (Fig. 5–31).

Esophageal Foreign Body

It is common knowledge that small children explore their world by tasting everything in sight; therefore almost any small object may be found as an esophageal foreign body. Often these foreign bodies pass without difficulty, but some become lodged, most commonly at the level of the cricopharyngeus muscle, the aortic arch, or the gastroesophageal junction. An esophageal stricture also can become a site for foreign body impaction (Fig. 5–32).

Most children with esophageal foreign bodies are quite symptomatic with pain, gagging, and vomiting; however the symptoms need not be restricted to the esophagus. Pressure on the airway from the foreign body may create the clinical impression of upper airway obstruction or pneumonia rather than an esophageal obstruction. Radiopaque foreign bodies, such as coins, are clearly apparent on plain radiographs, but a barium study may be necessary for identification of nonradiopaque substances such as food.

Removal of foreign bodies that are sharp or irregular and those that have been present for more than 24 to 48 hours requires esophagoscopy with anesthesia. Smooth foreign bodies, usually coins, that have been present for less than 48 hours can usually be easily removed using a Foley catheter under fluoroscopic control. The child should be immobilized and placed in a prone Trendelenburg position. A Foley catheter with the balloon deflated is passed through the mouth or nose past the foreign body. The balloon is inflated using aqueous contrast material under fluoroscopic

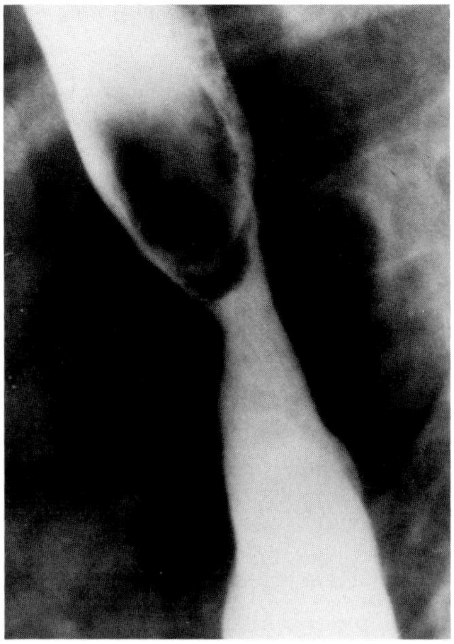

Fig. 5–32 Foreign body impaction due to esophageal stricture. A peach pit became lodged at the site of a stricture due to an old tracheoesophageal fistula repair.

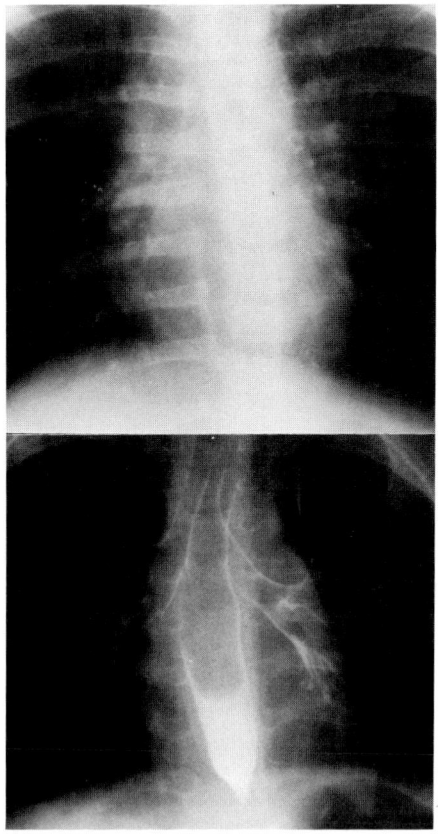

Fig. 5–33 Achalasia. **(A)** Plain radiographs reveal a gas-distended, dilated esophagus. **(B)** A barium esophagram shows the characteristic tapered deformity of the distal esophagus (*arrowheads*). A small amount of contrast was aspirated into the tracheobronchial tree.

control. The catheter is slowly withdrawn and, one hopes, brings the foreign body with it. The foreign body is retrieved from the patient's mouth, and indeed it often will simply fall from the patient's pharynx. Certainly, a pediatric laryngoscope and someone competent to use it should be standing by when this procedure is performed. A follow-up study of the esophagus after removal of the foreign body may be useful to rule out an underlying stricture or traumatic injury to the esophagus.

Achalasia

Achalasia of the esophagus, an abnormality of unknown etiology, consists of failure of relaxation of the lower esophageal sphincter after swallowing. This condition is rare in childhood, with only 4 to 5 percent of patients presenting in childhood. Absence of ganglion cells in the myenteric plexus of the distal esophagus has been noted, but it is thought that this is a secondary change rather than the primary cause of the disease.

The radiographic appearance of achalasia in children is similar to that in adults. The esophagus is dilated and may be seen distended with air or, more commonly, with food and fluid on the plain radiographs. A barium swallow shows the enlarged esophagus with abnormal peristalsis and the distal esophagus tapered into a beak deformity at the point of distal obstruction (Fig. 5–33).

In older children, dilatation of the distal esophagus is often attempted as initial therapy, but surgical esophagomyotomy is usually the treatment of choice in children below the age of 9. Peptic esophagitis with spasm or stricture at the lower esophageal sphincter may have a similar appearance to achalasia, but peristaltic activity of the esophagus is not as severely impaired or bizarre. Chagas disease and esophageal carcinoma are very rare causes of distal esophageal beaklike obstruction in children.

STOMACH

Gastric Dilatation

A large, gas-distended stomach is a common finding on plain radiographs of the abdomen in children, particularly in infants. This is not necessarily pathologic and, in fact, is most often due to air swallowing by a crying infant or child. In older infants and children, however, an overdistended gas-filled stomach is suggestive of possible gastric outlet obstruction, particularly if there is very little gas in the remainder of the gastrointestinal tract. The stomach can also be dilated in association with adynamic ileus. This is a common occurrence in the postoperative period, but can also be seen with any severe illness and in some cases of gastroenteritis. Other causes of excessive air swallowing, such as respiratory distress, fistulas between the tracheobronchial tree and the esophagus, or incorrectly positioned endotracheal tubes, can also introduce large amounts of air into the stomach causing it to appear obstructed.

> **GAS-DISTENDED STOMACH**
>
> Normal air-swallowing infants
>
> Gastric outlet obstruction
> - Pylorospasm
> - Hypertrophic pyloric stenosis
> - Enteric duplication cyst
> - Gastric atresia, antropyloric membranes
> - Postulcer stricture
> - Ectopic pancreas
> - Gastric volvulus
> - Gastric polyps or tumors
>
> Gastroenteritis
>
> Adynamic ileus (postoperative)
>
> Severe illness (adynamic ileus)
>
> Excessive air swallowing (respiratory distress, tracheoesophageal fistula)
>
> Endotracheal tube incorrectly positioned
>
> Duodenal obstruction (fluid-filled duodenum in supine position)

Obstruction of the gastric outlet in children is most often due to either severe pylorospasm or hypertrophic pyloric stenosis. Pylorospasm in infants and young children is most often an isolated phenomenon, but underlying inflammatory or ulcer disease can also be a cause. When pylorospasm is severe enough to cause gastric outlet obstruction, antispasmodic therapy may be necessary. Usually pylorospasm can be easily differentiated from hypertrophic pyloric stenosis on an ultrasound examination, as the pyloric musculature will be of normal thickness in pylorospasm.

Hypertrophic pyloric stenosis is an important cause of gastric outlet obstruction in infants. The obstruction is due to acquired hypertrophy of the circular pyloric musculature. The etiology of the hypertrophy remains uncertain; however it appears that prolonged spasm of the pylorus is a contributing factor. Other possible etiologic factors include elevated gastrin levels and vagal overstimulation.

Most patients with pyloric stenosis develop symptoms at 2 to 8 weeks of age, although presentation during the first week of life or between 2 to 4 months of age is occasionally seen. Boys are affected five times more commonly than girls. Pyloric stenosis is also more common than expected in patients with esophageal atresia and tracheoesophageal fistula. Jaundice may also accompany pyloric stenosis, probably due to liver immaturity and decreased glucuronyl transferase.

The classic case of hypertrophic pyloric stenosis is usually diagnosed clinically by the presence of projectile vomiting, prominent gastric peristalsis, and a palpable antral muscle mass (olive). If the clinical findings are questionable or the examination is difficult, not an uncommon occurrence in infants, ultrasound is invaluable in making the diagnosis. Ultrasonography, as compared to barium studies, has the advantage of being able to visualize directly the hypertrophied muscle mass. In addition, other classic findings can be seen, such as markedly delayed gastric emptying, hyperperistalsis of the gastric antrum, thickened an-

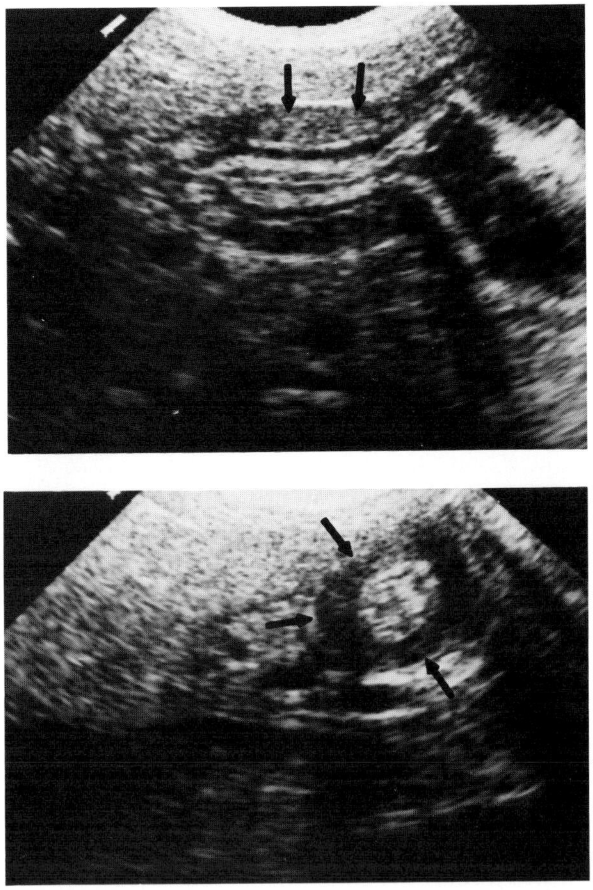

A

B

Fig. 5–34 Hypertrophic pyloric stenosis. **(A)** Sonography along the long axis of the pyloric channel shows elongation of the channel and thickening of the pyloric muscle (*arrows*). **(B)** In cross section, the thickened pyloric musculature forms a hypoechoic "donut" (*arrows*).

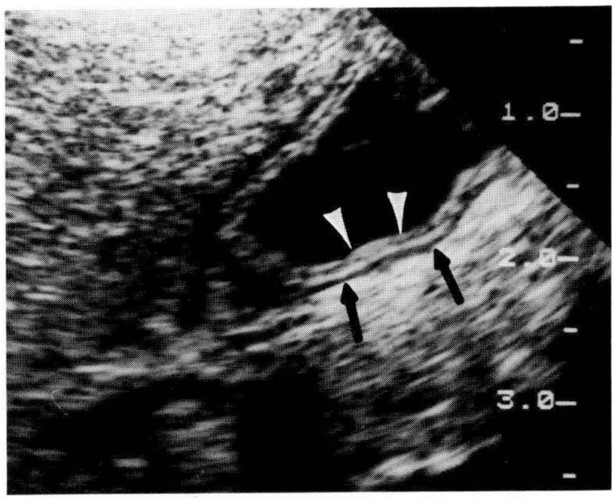

Fig. 5–35 Sonography of the normal gastric antrum. Note the thin hypoechoic rim of circular muscle (*black arrows*) surrounding the echogenic layers of mucosa and submucosa (*white arrowheads*).

tral walls, and deformities of the gastric antrum and duodenal bulb due to the adjacent muscle mass.

The ultrasonographic diagnosis of pyloric stenosis depends on evidence of gastric outlet obstruction associated with an elongated pyloric canal surrounded by thickened pyloric musculature in both longitudinal and cross-sectional images (Fig. 5–34). The pyloric muscle appears hypoechoic in most cases, and in cross-section has the appearance of a hypoechoic donut. The hypoechoic donut may contain areas of increased echogenicity in the twelve o'clock and six o'clock positions, due to the anisotropic effect. Similar echogenicity may be seen in the midsagittal, longitudinal scan.

The normal pyloric muscle should be less than 3 mm thick, and actually in most instances will be only 1 to 1.5 mm thick (Fig. 5–35). Muscle thickness in the classic case of pyloric stenosis usually measures from 3 to 7 mm. The length of the pyloric canal in most cases of pyloric stenosis measures 1.4 cm or greater. Feeding the infant several ounces of sugar water during the ultrasound examination confirms gastric outlet obstruction.

In most cases, the diagnosis will be clear following ultrasonography but if any doubt remains, a barium study may be helpful. A well-formed olive creates a characteristic deformity of the pylorus and gastric antrum: a string sign with an upward curving pyloric canal (Fig. 5–36). A beak sign is present where the contrast enters the narrowed pyloric canal and the tit sign, a small peak along the superior aspect of the antrum where it abuts the muscle mass, also may be present. With less hypertrophied muscle, the pyloric canal will be flattened, creating a double tract sign. Prominent peristaltic waves end abruptly after reaching the hypertrophied pyloric muscle. Less typical patterns with pyloric stenosis include an eccentric lesser curve indentation, a funnel-shaped antrum, spiculated antrum, or a niche in the central portion of the pylorus. Since false positive and false negative exams are possible with both modalities, a repeat examination after several days is useful in questionable cases.

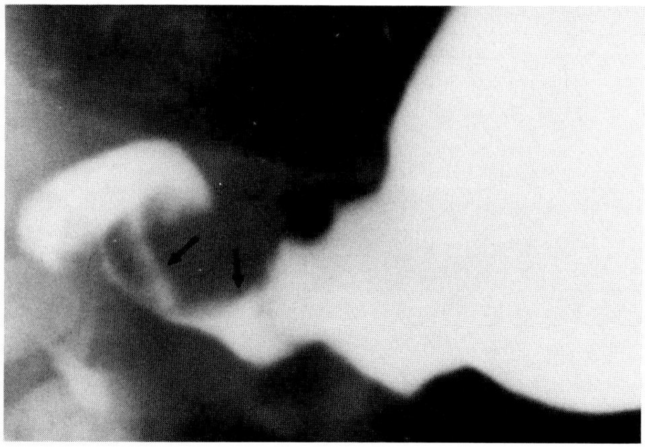

Fig. 5–36 Hypertrophic pyloric stenosis. The classic findings of a narrowed antropyloric canal with an eccentric lesser curvature indentation (*arrows*) are demonstrated.

GASTRIC FILLING DEFECTS

Bezoar

Foreign body

Neoplasm
- Teratoma
- Carcinoma
- Sarcoma
- Lymphoma
- Hamartoma
- Hemangioma

Polyp

Ectopic pancreas

Gastric duplication

Markedly thickened gastric folds (e.g. Ménétrier's disease)

The treatment of choice in the United States for hypertrophic pyloric stenosis is pyloromyotomy. In most cases, normal emptying of the stomach occurs within 2 to 3 days after the procedure. When the question of residual muscle hypertrophy arises, barium studies are usually not helpful as antral deformities persist for weeks and sometimes years. Ultrasound, however, can clearly identify any persistent muscular thickening. The muscle should return to its normal thickness by at least 6 weeks after pyloromyotomy.

Gastric Filling Defects

Because children tend to explore their world by tasting, filling defects encountered in the stomach are often due to an ingested foreign body. Many of these will be radiopaque and most will pass spontaneously. Pointed objects should be removed, as they tend to lead to perforation.

Chronic ingestion of hair or vegetable matter such as citrus pulp may lead to bezoar formation. Currently, a more common cause of bezoars is the lactobezoar which occurs in infants who are fed improperly prepared powdered formula. Bezoars appear as freely mobile, irregular filling defects within the stomach. They sometimes are seen as a solid or granular appearing mass outlined by air in the region of the stomach on the plain radiograph (Fig. 5–37). On ultrasound, air within and around the bezoar causes a fairly characteristic strongly echogenic arc over the bezoar with distal shadowing. If the stomach is filled with fluid, the bezoar may be seen to float freely within the stomach (Fig. 5–37).

Gastric duplications can present as a gastric mass but the stomach is the least common location for a duplication within the gastrointestinal tract. These duplications present as masses in the gastric antrum and often cause gastric outlet obstruction. Barium studies are often inconclusive since these cysts commonly do not communicate with the gastric lumen. Ultrasound will clearly show the mass to be cystic and to be lined by echogenic mucosal and hypoechoic muscular layers. These cysts can undergo ulceration leading to bleeding or even perforation. If obstruction is present, the cysts can mimic hypertrophic pyloric stenosis on barium studies.

Gastric neoplasms are uncommon in children. Primary gastric carcinoma, sarcoma, lymphoma, or leiomyoma occur rarely. Teratoma is the most common neoplasm in infants. They are usually benign and often contain calcifications. Intrathoracic extension can occur. Gastric polyps are also uncommon

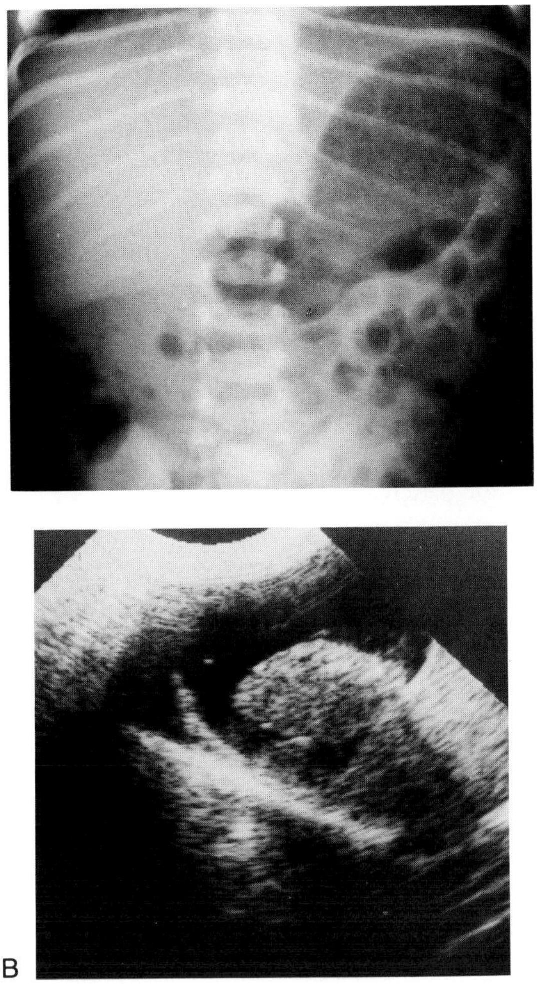

A B

Fig. 5–37 Gastric bezoar in a neonate. **(A)** Note the granular appearance of the gastric fundus in this three-day-old infant. **(B)** Ultrasound revealed a heterogeneous, echogenic mass that floated freely in the fluid-filled stomach. This bezoar resolved with conservative therapy.

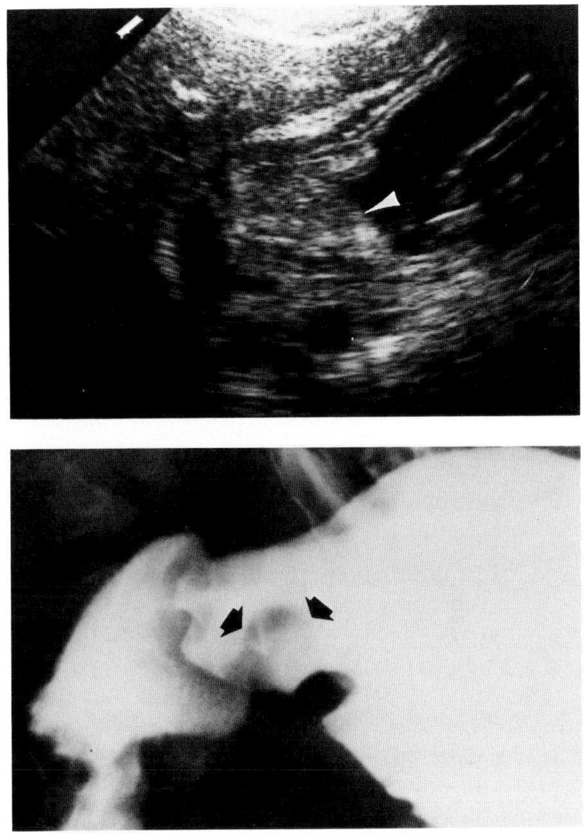

A B

Fig. 5–38 Ectopic pancreas. **(A)** Ultrasound identified a mass affixed to the wall of the distal gastric antrum. **(B)** A contrast study also confirmed the presence of a fixed filling defect in the gastric antrum (*arrows*). Endoscopic biopsy showed this to represent ectopic pancreatic tissue.

in children and, when seen, are often associated with one of the intestinal polyposis syndromes such as Peutz-Jeghers syndrome.

Ectopic pancreatic tissue can occur in the gastric antrum, appearing as a small nodular filling defect, often with a central umbilication representing a draining duct (Fig. 5–38). In rare cases, ectopic pancreatic tissue can lead to gastric outlet obstruction or gastrointestinal bleeding. Occasionally, markedly thickened gastric mucosal folds, as might be seen with Ménétrier's disease, may give the appearance of multiple polypoid filling defects.

DUODENUM AND SMALL BOWEL

Duodenal Obstruction

When a newborn presents with vomiting, the various causes of duodenal obstruction must be considered,

DUODENAL OBSTRUCTION

- Site of obstruction
  - Immediate postbulbar
    - Duodenal atresia
    - Duodenal stenosis
    - Annular pancreas
  - Descending
    - Duodenal diaphragm
    - Duodenal bands
  - Transverse
    - Duodenal bands
    - Midgut volvulus
    - Preduodenal portal vein
    - Superior mesenteric artery syndrome
  - Variable
    - Duplication cyst
    - Intramural hematoma
    - Adhesions (postoperative)

particularly if bile is present in the vomitus. A plain radiograph of the abdomen may help to localize the level of obstruction, thus narrowing the differential diagnostic possibilities.

The classic radiographic presentation of complete duodenal obstruction at or near the ampulla of Vater consists of a dilated, gas-filled stomach and duodenal bulb with no gas in the remainder of the gastrointestinal tract. This appearance is known as the *double bubble sign* and is nearly always due to duodenal atresia with or without annular pancreas (see Fig. 5–3). If the sign is present, no further studies are necessary. Additional air can be introduced through a nasogastric tube if the radiographic findings are inconclusive.

The etiology of duodenal atresia is unknown; however most cases are thought to be due to abnormal embryologic development (failure of recanalization) rather than intrauterine intestinal ischemia. Duodenal atresia and stenosis are more common in patients with Down's syndrome, and both abnormalities are known to be associated with other gastrointestinal and biliary tract anomalies such as malrotation, esophageal atresia, annular pancreas, biliary atresia, and ectopic anus.

A small amount of air occasionally can be seen distal to the obstruction and is due to an anomalous Y-shaped hepatopancreatic duct that has connections both above and below the site of atresia. This appearance is indistinguishable from that seen with severe duodenal stenosis or other forms of incomplete duodenal obstruction. In these cases, some type of contrast study is usually indicated.

The combination of duodenal atresia and esophageal atresia leads to an unusual radiographic pattern. Since the stomach is isolated by the two sites of atresia, the radiograph may show a large opaque upper abdominal mass with no evidence of air within the gastrointestinal tract. Ultrasound will clearly identify this mass as a large fluid-filled stomach and duodenal bulb.

Annular pancreas is the second most common condition to produce the double bubble sign. This condition most likely results from abnormal rotation of embryonic pancreatic tissue causing it to grow in a ring and encircle the descending duodenum. It is invariably associated with some degree of duodenal stenosis or atresia; therefore the radiographic findings will be the same in these conditions.

When the plain radiographs indicate that the obstruction is in the distal descending duodenum, the most likely cause is either a duodenal diaphragm or duodenal band, with or without midgut volvulus. As with duodenal atresia, duodenal diaphragms are thought most likely to be due to failure of recanalization. Variable degrees of obstruction will be present depending on the size of the opening in the diaphragm. If the diaphragm is completely obstructing, the radiographic findings may resemble the double bubble configuration seen with duodenal atresia. Barium studies are usually diagnostic but sometimes the diaphragm is difficult to demonstrate. If obstruction is incomplete and diagnosis is delayed, the diaphragm may become stretched into what has been called an intraluminal or wind-sock diverticulum. It is important to remember that duodenal diaphragms often accompany other obstructing lesions such as duodenal bands, midgut volvulus, or duodenal atresia. Therefore, their presence should always be excluded even though another form of duodenal obstruction is identified.

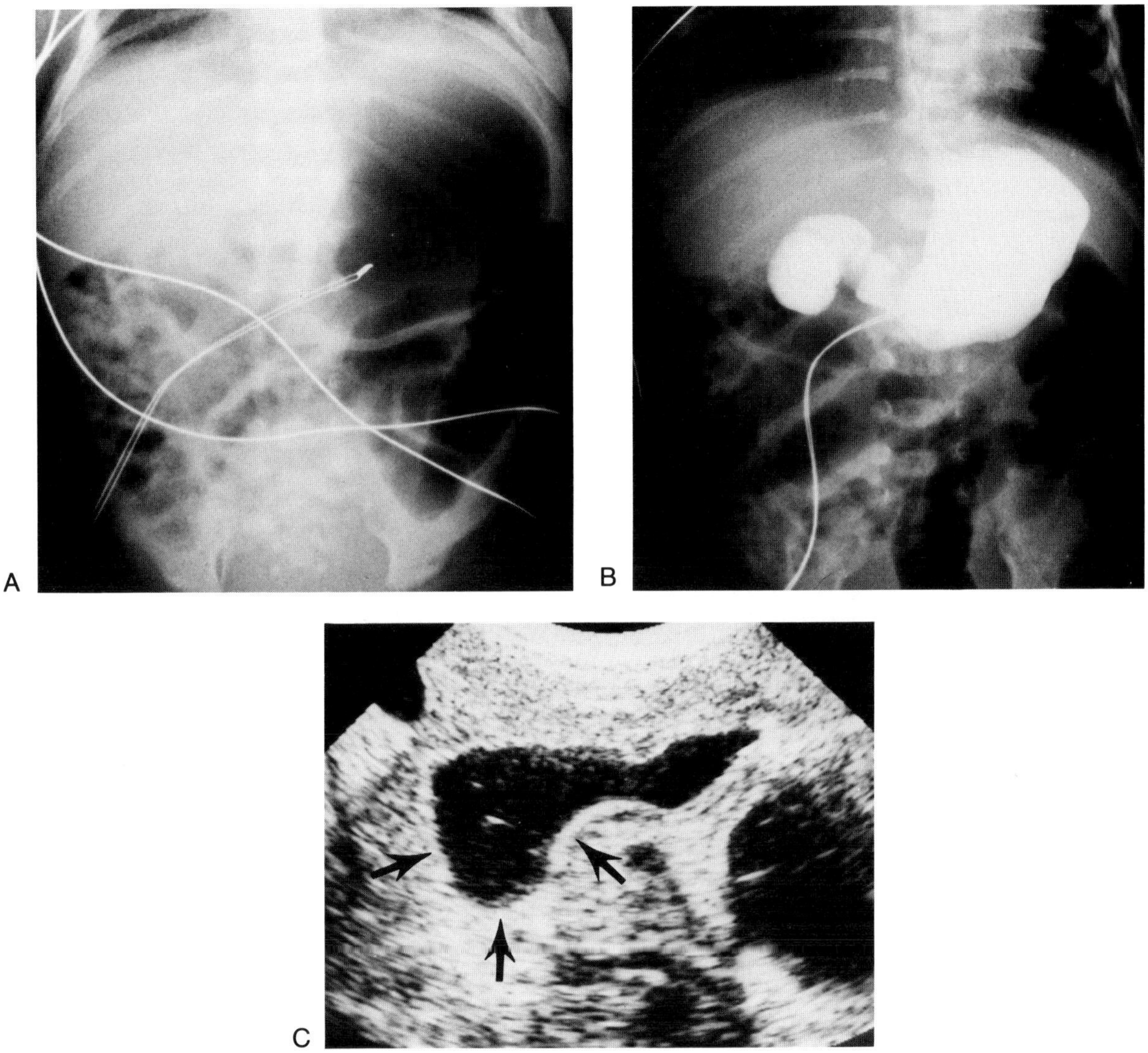

Fig. 5–39 Nonrotation of the bowel with duodenal obstruction. **(A)** The plain abdominal radiograph shows bowel nonrotation, with the small bowel lying entirely on the right and the colon on the left. **(B)** A contrast study reveals complete obstruction of the descending duodenum. At surgery, peritoneal bands were found to be the cause of the obstruction. **(C)** The obstructed, fluid-distended duodenum was also readily identified by transverse sonography (*arrows*).

A variety of anomalies of intestinal rotation occur. Although these rotational abnormalities can be entirely asymptomatic, they are usually accompanied by peritoneal bands (Ladd's bands), which may lead to intestinal obstruction (Fig. 5–39). In addition, defective mesenteric attachment predisposes to midgut volvulus. The bands most likely represent remnants of embryonic peritoneal folds that usually extend from the malplaced cecum across the duodenum to the lateral abdominal wall or the porta hepatis. Although they most commonly produce obstruction in the distal second and third portions of the duode-

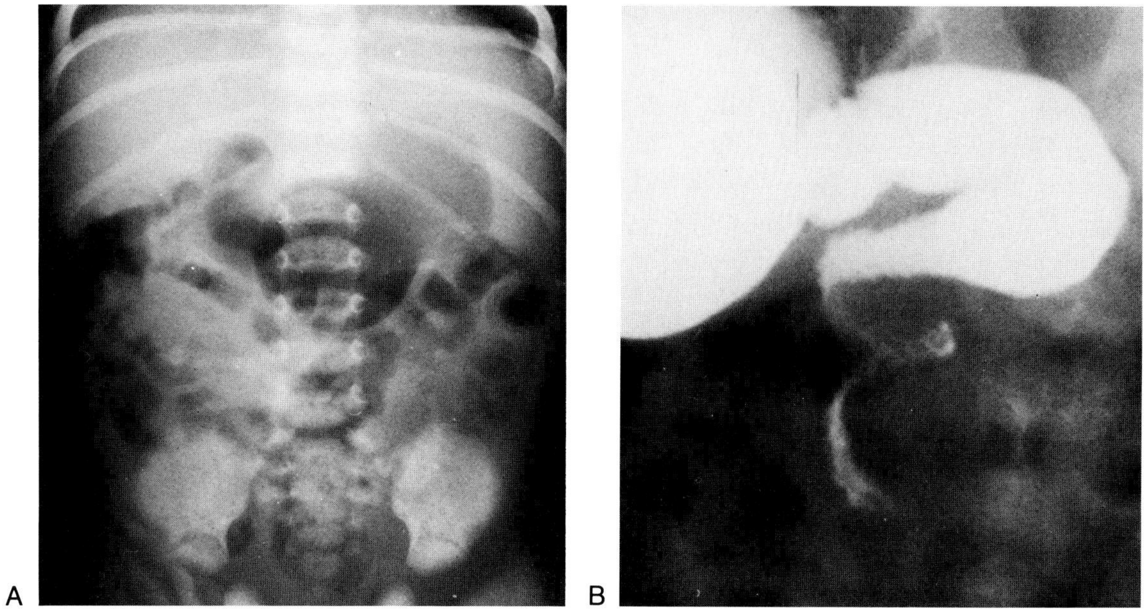

Fig. 5–40 Midgut volvulus. **(A)** The plain radiograph of the abdomen shows only mild distension of the stomach and proximal duodenum. **(B)** A contrast study clearly shows the obstruction of the distal duodenum as it spirals around the superior mesenteric artery.

num, obstruction of the terminal ileum may also occur. Obstruction due to duodenal bands usually occurs in infancy, but may present later in life.

Whenever obstruction occurs with abnormal rotation or fixation of the bowel, midgut volvulus should be a primary consideration. Clinically these patients present with bilious vomiting and, unfortunately, the plain radiographic findings may range from normal to evidence of duodenal or even low small bowel obstruction. The upper gastrointestinal series is usually the best study for diagnosing midgut volvulus. The classic findings consist of beaking at the site of obstruction in the duodenum and, often, associated spiraling of the small bowel as it twists around the superior mesenteric artery (Fig. 5–40). Other supportive findings include absence of the ligament of Treitz and edema of the bowel wall. If the obstruction in the duodenum is complete, the spiraled small bowel will not be visualized. However midgut volvulus must still be considered as a very likely possibility. If further proof of its presence is desired before surgery, a barium enema may be performed. In most cases of midgut volvulus, the cecum is pulled superiorly and medially so that it comes to lie just below the transverse colon (Fig. 5–41). If this confirmatory evidence is found, surgery should not be delayed.

A rare cause of obstruction in the region of the second and third portion of the duodenum is anomalous development of the portal vein so that it comes to lie anterior to the duodenum. Most often this anomaly is associated with other gastrointestinal tract anomalies such as malrotation with duodenal bands, esophageal atresia, biliary atresia, intestinal atresia, and annular pancreas. The preduodenal portal vein may produce indentation and partial or complete obstruction of the duodenum appearing very similar to that seen with duodenal bands. Intestinal duplication cysts and intramural hematomas (trauma, battered child syndrome) may also cause obstruction at variable sites in the duodenum.

Small Bowel Obstruction

The differential diagnosis of obstruction of the small bowel greatly depends on the age of the patient (see list on p. 176). If intestinal obstruction beyond the

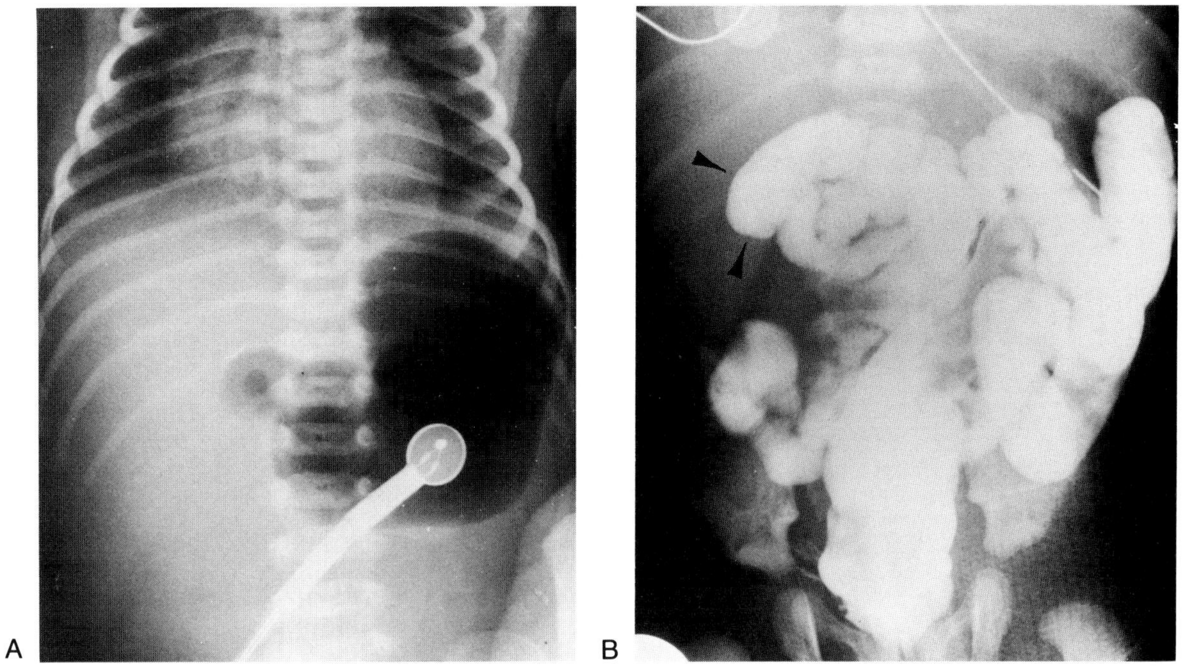

Fig. 5–41 Midgut volvulus. **(A)** The plain radiograph shows a double bubble appearance indicating obstruction in the proximal duodenum. **(B)** A contrast enema shows elevation and medial displacement of the cecum (*arrowheads*) characteristic of midgut volvulus.

duodenum occurs in the neonatal period, atresia or stenosis of the jejunum or ileum should be considered. Congenital atresia in these locations is somewhat more common than in the duodenum and is thought to be due to intrauterine intestinal ischemia rather than failure of recanalization. Atresia may involve any portion of the jejunum or ileum and in some cases multiple sites of atresia are present. The location of the atresia can often be inferred from the number of gas-distended loops seen on the abdominal radiograph. If the obstruction appears to be in the distal ileum, a barium enema may be necessary to exclude a colonic obstruction. Classically, low small bowel obstruction will be accompanied by a microcolon (Fig. 5–42). If atresia involves the more proximal small bowel, the colon has a more normal appearance. The barium enema will also help to exclude any rotational anomalies of the intestine. Intramural calcifications are occasionally seen in conjunction with jejunoileal atresia and peritoneal calcifications may be seen if intestinal perforation has occurred (meconium peritonitis) (Fig. 5–43). This is more commonly seen with meconium ileus than with ileal atresia.

Meconium ileus is the other common cause of low small bowel obstruction in the neonate. It is almost invariably a manifestation of cystic fibrosis, although rarely it can be idiopathic. The obstruction results from impaction of thick meconium in the distal small bowel. Ileal atresia, stenosis, volvulus, and perforation with meconium peritonitis are common complications of the condition. Due to the presence of thick, tenacious meconium in the small bowel, a paucity of air/fluid levels is often seen. Air mixed with meconium may give a soap-bubble appearance to the obstructed loop (Fig. 5–44); however, this can be seen occasionally with other causes of intestinal obstruction.

Once meconium ileus is suspected, a water-soluble contrast enema is necessary to confirm the diagnosis. Typically, the study will demonstrate a microcolon that is empty or contains only a few small pellets of meconium. Reflux into the terminal ileum will demonstrate more, impacted pellets. Once identified, the condition should be treated with a gastrografin enema, for the hyperosmolarity of gastrografin and

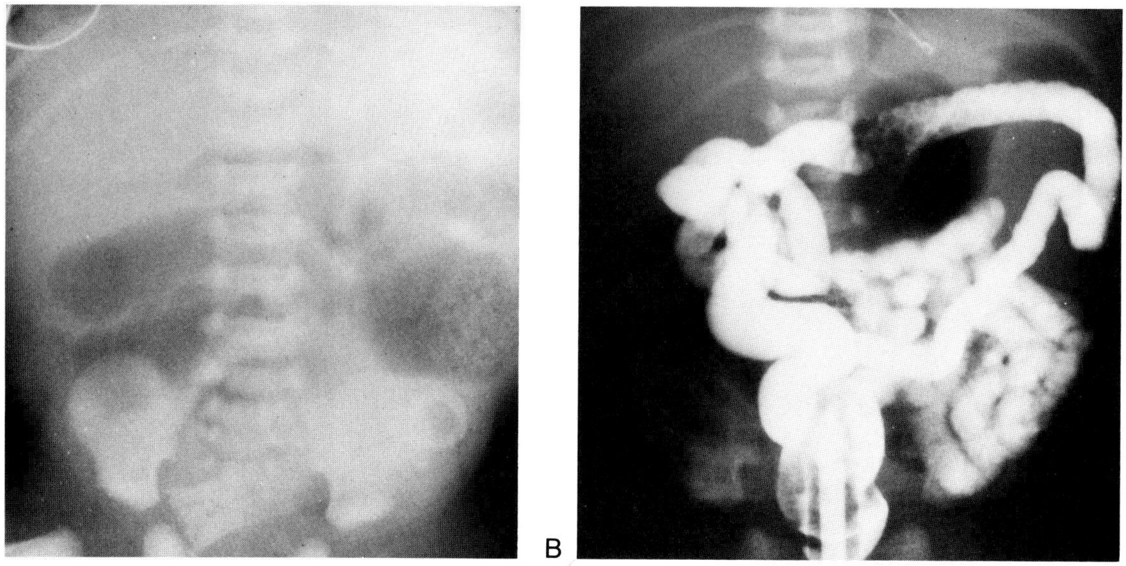

A B

Fig. 5–42 Microcolon secondary to low small bowel atresia. **(A)** Multiple gas-filled dilated loops of bowel on the plain radiograph indicate a small bowel obstruction. **(B)** A contrast enema shows a microcolon. The contrast refluxed into a number of loops of ileum and, at surgery, atresia was discovered in the distal jejunum.

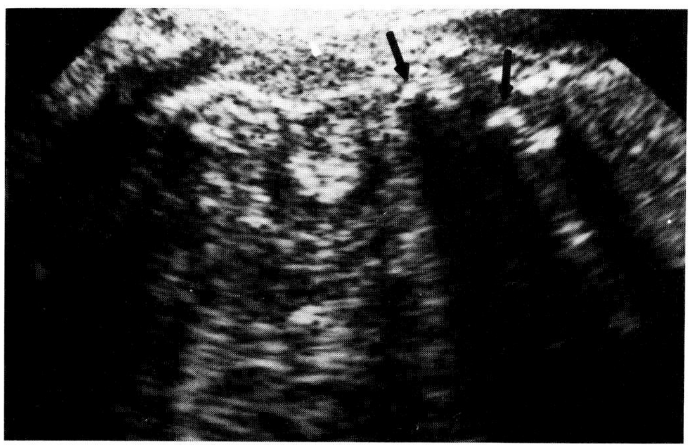

Fig. 5–43 Meconium peritonitis. The intraperitoneal calcifications of meconium peritonitis can be identified by sonography as echogenic structures with sharp acoustical shadowing surrounding the bowel loops (*arrows*).

the presence of an emulsifying agent (Tween 80) often induces the obstructing mass of meconium to be passed without surgical intervention. This procedure should be performed with caution, as fluid and electrolyte imbalances have been known to occur.

Incarcerated hernias, small bowel volvulus, peritoneal bands, and gastrointestinal duplication cysts are less common causes of small bowel obstruction in newborns, but incarcerated inguinal hernia probably is the most common cause of obstruction in boys between the ages of 6 and 18 months.

Beyond early infancy intussusception becomes the

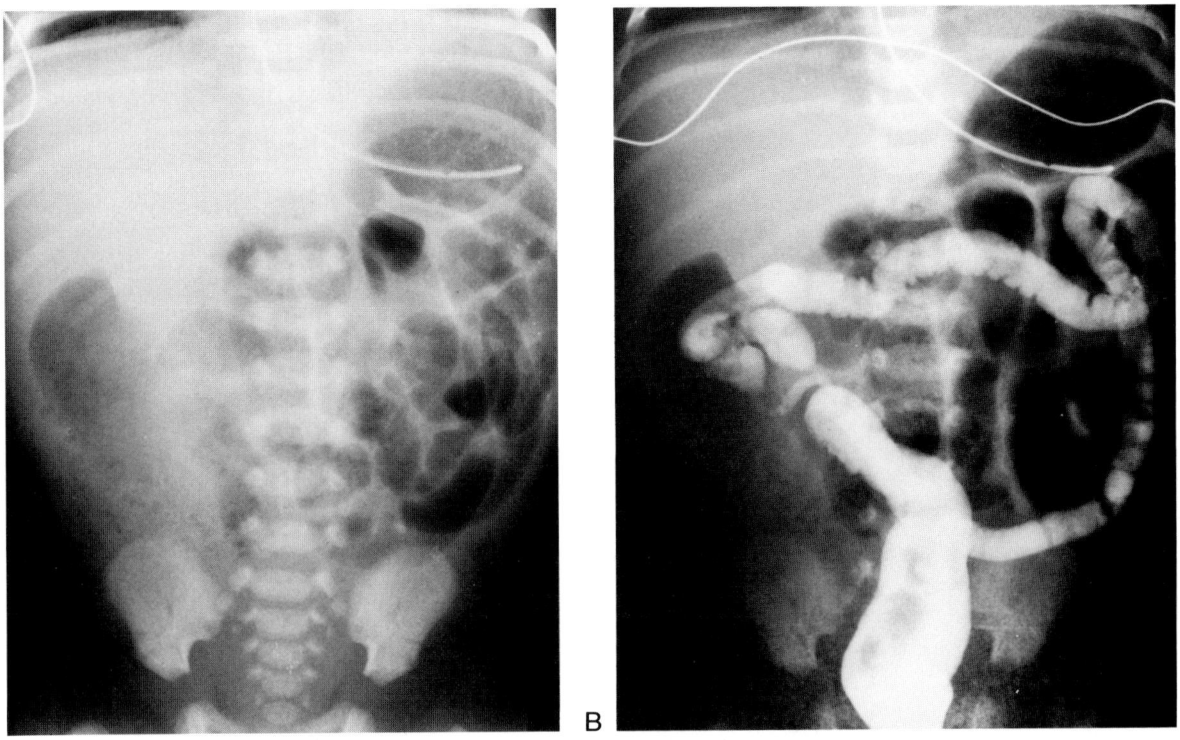

A B

Fig. 5–44 Meconium ileus. **(A)** The plain radiograph shows multiple gas-distended loops of bowel consistent with a low small bowel obstruction. Note the bubbly appearance of air mixed with meconium in the right lower quadrant. **(B)** A contrast enema reveals a microcolon and shows the meconium-filled bowel to be distal ileum.

most common cause of small bowel obstruction. It most commonly occurs between the ages of 6 months and 4 years, but it can occur in older children, particularly if a lead point such as a polyp or a Meckel's diverticulum is present. In most cases, the intussusceptum consists of a portion of ileum that telescopes through the ileocecal valve into the colon. The plain radiograph findings of intussusception are variable; however, eventually some evidence of small bowel obstruction will appear. Often a mass effect is present in the right abdomen and sometimes the intussusceptum can be visualized as a soft tissue density mass within the colon.

If intussusception is suspected clinically, an ultrasound of the abdomen can be very helpful. The intussusception can usually be visualized as a sonolucent ring or oval with bright central echoes (Fig. 5–45). The sonolucency represents the edematous wall of the intussuscepted bowel. Although these findings can occasionally be seen with other causes of edematous bowel, in the proper clinical setting they are very suggestive of intussusception.

Eventually, all patients with suspected intussusception will have some type of contrast enema examination. Classically, a barium enema was performed to identify the characteristic convex and sometimes lobulated filling defect within the colon (Fig. 5–46). Contrast trapped in the folds surrounding the intussusceptum gives the classic "coiled spring" appearance.

Once an intussusception is identified, one may proceed with reduction of the intussusception by an enema under fluoroscopic control. Although barium still may be used, water-soluble contrast and air insufflation have recently been suggested as preferable methods for reduction. The success rate for reduction by hydrostatic pressure now approaches 90 to 95 per-

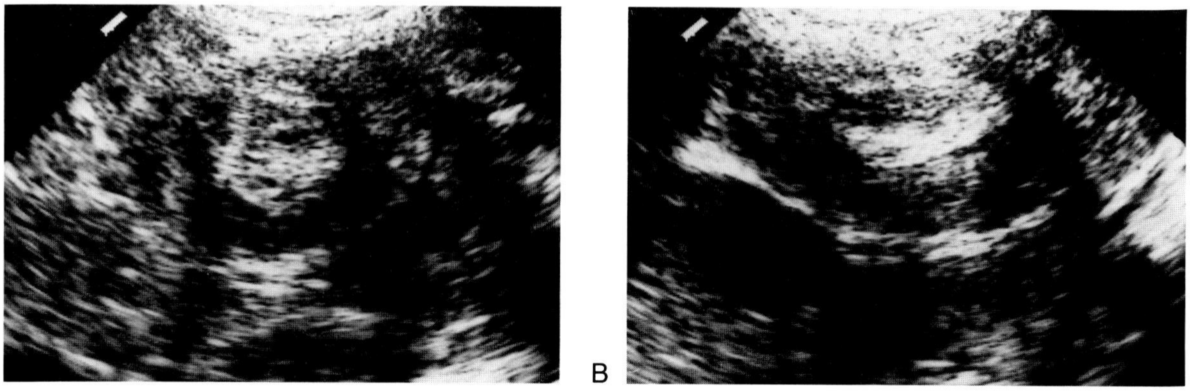

A B

Fig. 5–45 Ileocolic intussusception. **(A)** Ultrasound in the transverse plane through the intussuscepted bowel demonstrates a hypoechoic "donut" with bright central echoes. **(B)** In the longitudinal plane, a more elongated appearance (pseudokidney) is seen.

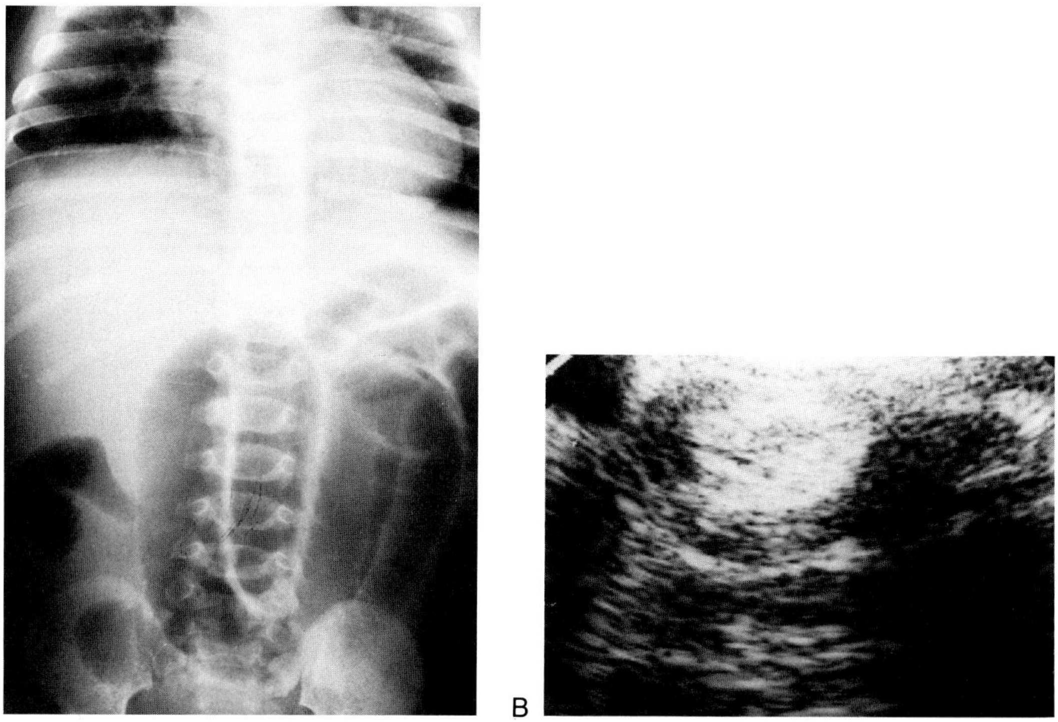

A B

Fig. 5–46 Ileocolic intussusception. **(A)** A 2-year-old child presented with abdominal distension due to multiple dilated loops of small bowel indicating a small bowel obstruction. **(B)** Ultrasound revealed a hypoechoic donut appearance in the right upper quadrant. (*Figure continues.*)

C

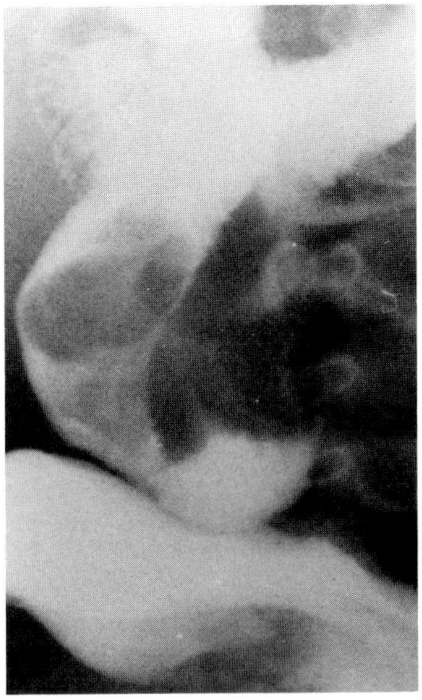

Fig. 5–46 (*Continued*). **(C)** A water-soluble contrast enema verified the presence of an ileocolic intussusception. The intussusception was also reduced by the use of hydrostatic pressure.

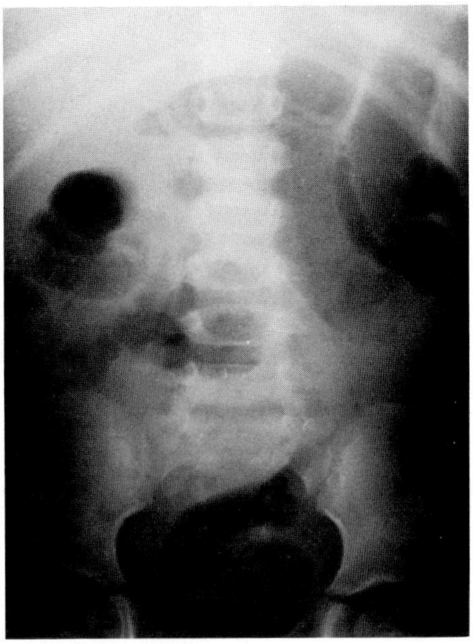

Fig. 5–47 Perforated appendicitis. The suggestive findings on the plain radiograph include a mass effect in the right lower quadrant, indistinctness of the right psoas muscle, and evidence of a small bowel obstruction.

cent at many centers. The acceptable height of the column of contrast and the length and number of fillings varies from radiologist to radiologist. The only absolute contraindications to hydrostatic pressure reduction include evidence of perforation, peritonitis, or dead bowel. Once complete reduction is attained, most cases of intussusception do not recur. Nevertheless, postreduction and 24 hour follow-up radiographs should be obtained as recurrence can occur in up to 10 percent of cases.

In children older than 4 to 5 years of age, perforated appendicitis is the most common cause of a pattern of small bowel obstruction. Although appendicitis often presents with classic clinical findings, these are often more difficult to assess in children and imaging may be requested. The plain abdominal radiograph often provides important clues to the presence of perforated appendicitis. Multiple gas-distended, dilated loops of small bowel are frequently present, most likely due to a combination of partial obstruction in the region of the ileocecal valve and localized paralytic ileus due to inflammation (Fig. 5–47). Other supportive evidence includes scoliosis with concavity

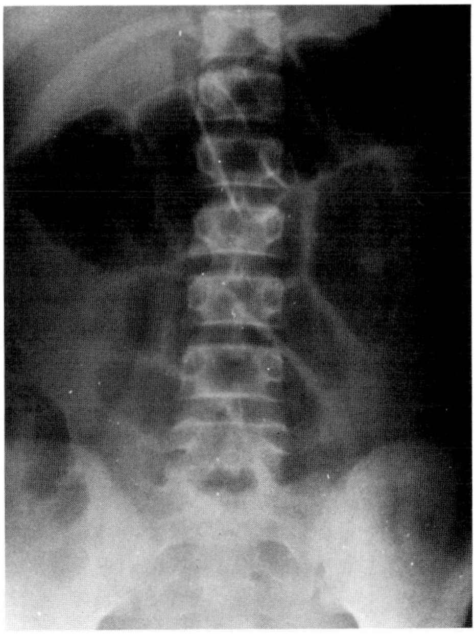

Fig. 5–48 Perforated appendicitis. Dilatation of the transverse colon with abrupt cut-off at the hepatic flexure constitutes the colon cut-off sign, probably due to spasm of the ascending colon. Also note multiple loops of dilated small bowel in the mid-abdomen.

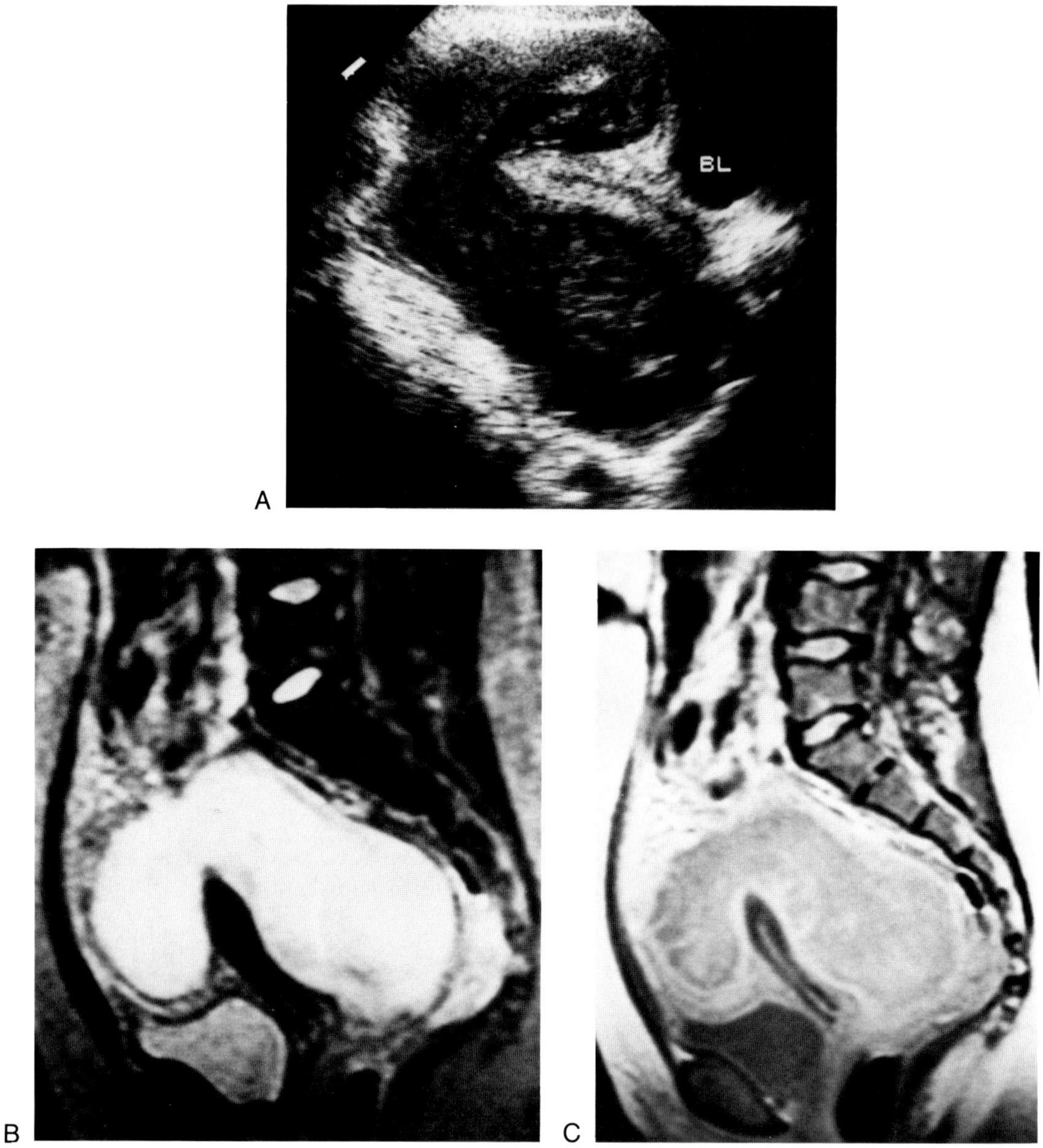

Fig. 5–49 Large appendiceal abscess. This 12-year-old girl presented for evaluation of a pelvic mass. The patient had only mild lower abdominal tenderness and no fever. **(A)** Longitudinal ultrasound revealed a heterogeneous U-shaped mass that was draped over the fundus of the uterus. MRI confirmed the presence of a sausage-shaped mass surrounding the uterus. The signal intensity on **(B)** the sagittal T_2-weighted image and **(C)** the sagittal T_1-weighted images is consistent with proteinaceous fluid. At surgery, a large abscess secondary to perforated appendicitis was found.

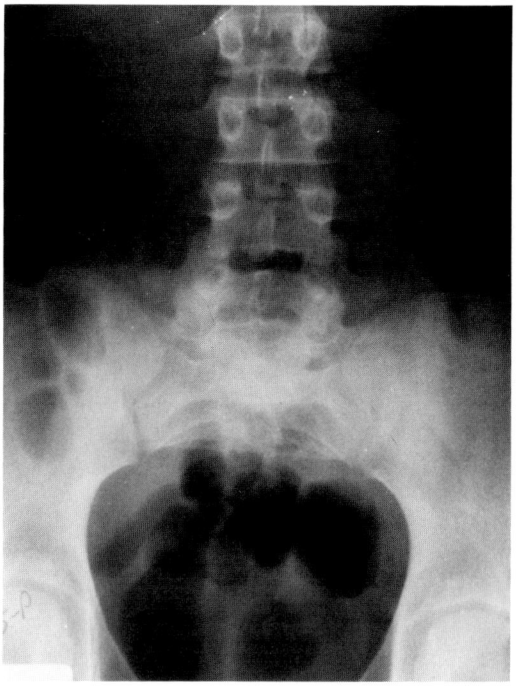

Fig. 5–50 Acute nonperforated appendicitis. Little gas is present within the bowel except for a few localized loops in the right lower quadrant and pelvis. Also note the scoliosis with concavity to the right.

to the side of the appendix, a soft tissue mass in the right lower quadrant, obliteration of the right properitoneal fat line, medial displacement of the bowel from the right lateral abdominal wall, a colon cut-off sign (Fig. 5–48), and occasionally a calcified fecalith. Ultrasound may reveal a localized fluid collection in the region of the appendix. In a few cases, the patient may present for evaluation of an abdominal or pelvic mass with little, if any, evidence of an inflammatory process (Fig. 5–49).

The abdominal radiograph can also be helpful in nonperforated appendicitis, although the appearance is quite different from that following perforation. Most children with acute nonperforated appendicitis demonstrate diminished air in the gastrointestinal tract due to nausea, vomiting, and diarrhea (Fig. 5–50). Other helpful radiographic findings include scoliosis with concavity to the right, poor visualization of the right psoas margin, localized gas-distended loops in the right lower quadrant, air in the appendix, and a calcified fecalith.

The development of high resolution ultrasound now permits direct visualization of the inflamed appendix in some cases. With compression techniques over the right lower quadrant, the thickened, hypoechoic wall of the appendix can be clearly identified (Fig. 5–51).

In cases in which clinical uncertainty remains and the above techniques do not provide sufficient supportive evidence, a barium enema can be quite helpful. A completely filled, fully distended appendix on the barium enema essentially excludes the possibility of acute appendicitis. Nevertheless, it should be noted that 10 to 15 percent of normal appendices do not fill on barium examination. The presence of a pointed beak of barium at the base of the appendix, mucosal edema or irregularity within the appendix, and spasm, irregularity, or deformity of the cecum in the region of the appendix suggests the presence of appendicitis (Fig. 5–52).

Intestinal Filling Defects

Lymphoid hyperplasia usually presents as multiple small, uniform nodules that are seen predominantly in the colon of normal children. Often, characteristic central umbilications are seen (Fig. 5–53). When the nodules of lymphoid hyperplasia are slightly larger or involve the small bowel, they may be associated with such conditions as immunodeficiency, food allergy, or infections. An unusual form of lymphoid hyperplasia, known as *giant lymphoid hyperplasia,* takes the form of large polypoid lesions, which can lead to bleeding and intussusception. This condition may be the result of *Yersinia* ileocolitis.

Polypoid lesions in the colon are quite common in childhood and usually represent juvenile inflamma-

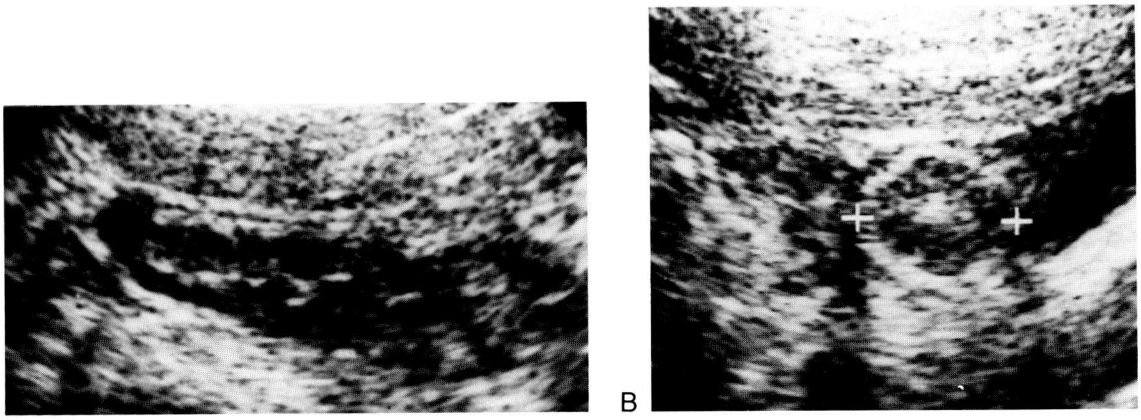

A B

Fig. 5–51 Acute appendicitis. Ultrasound in the **(A)** longitudinal and **(B)** transverse planes clearly demonstrates the thickened, hypoechoic wall of the inflamed appendix.

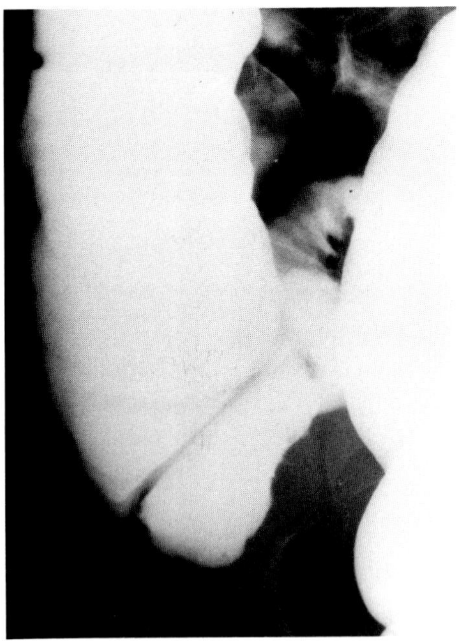

Fig. 5–52 Barium enema diagnosis of acute appendicitis. Note the lack of filling of a normal appendix and the concave deformity of the cecum in the region of the edematous appendix.

INTESTINAL FILLING DEFECTS

Congenital/developmental
- Polyposis syndromes
  - Small bowel—Peutz-Jehgers syndrome
  - Colon—Familial polyposis, Gardner's syndrome, Canada-Cronkhite syndrome, Turcot syndrome
- Neurofibromatosis
- Tuberous sclerosis

Inflammatory
- Lymphoid hyperplasia
- Juvenile polyps
- Pseudopolyps (ulcerative colitis, Crohn's disease)

Neoplasm
- Metastatic
- Primary
  - Carcinoma
  - Leiomyoma
  - Sarcoma
  - Lymphosarcoma

Trauma/surgery
- Hematoma
- Foreign body

Miscellaneous
- Meconium plugs
- Enterolith

tory polyps. These are benign, nonadenomatous polyps that may be sessile or pedunculated and solitary or multiple (Fig. 5–54). Occasionally they may also be present within the small bowel. Although 95 percent of these polyps are accompanied by gastrointestinal bleeding, they are usually treated conservatively. Endoscopic removal is indicated if possible. It is generally agreed that these polyps are not premalignant lesions.

Multiple intestinal polyps are the hallmark of the various hereditary polyposis syndromes. Most commonly polyps are colonic, except in the Peutz-Jeghers syndrome where they are predominantly found in the small bowel (Fig. 5–55). The polyps of Peutz-Jeghers syndrome are hamartomas, without malignant potential. Nevertheless, a slightly increased incidence of bowel cancer occurs in these patients. Adenomatous polyps are present in the other polyposis syndromes, the best known of which is familial polyposis of the colon. Characteristically, in this syndrome, the colon is carpeted by numerous polyps

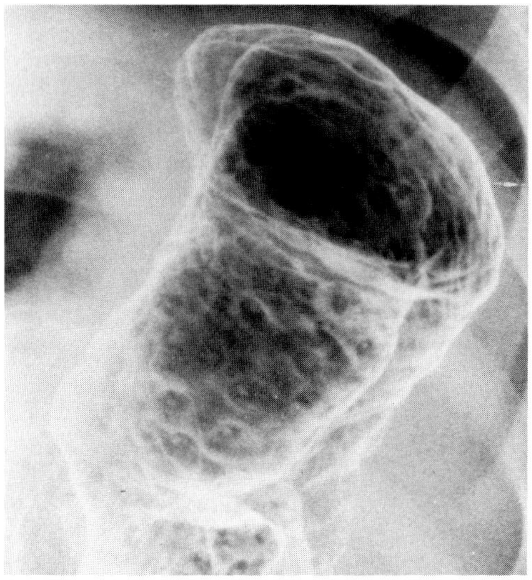

Fig. 5–53 Lymphoid hyperplasia of the colon. Note the multiple sessile nodules of uniform size scattered diffusely along the splenic flexure of the colon. The central umbilications are characteristic of this condition.

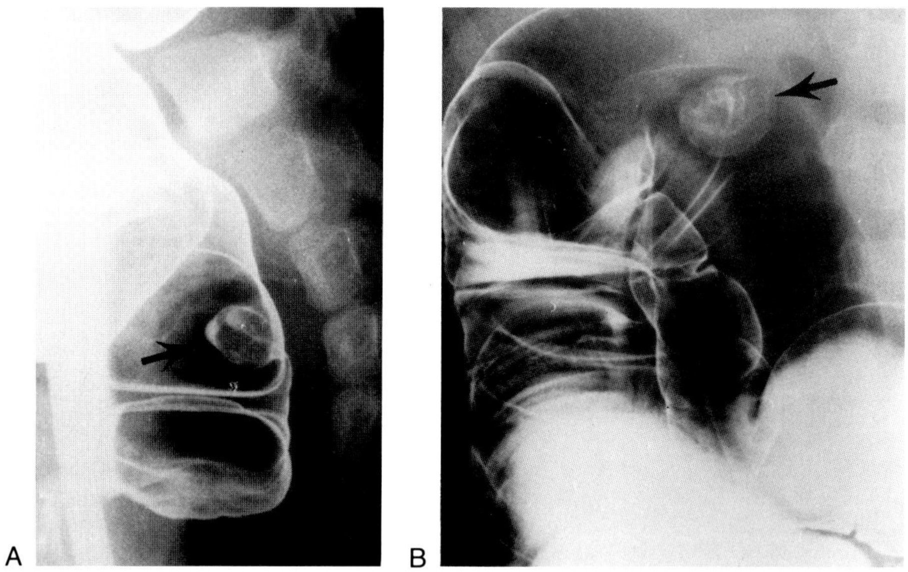

Fig. 5–54 Benign juvenile polyps. **(A & B)** An air-contrast barium enema reveals two juvenile inflammatory polyps (*arrows*) in the rectum and the hepatic flexure in this child who presented with rectal bleeding.

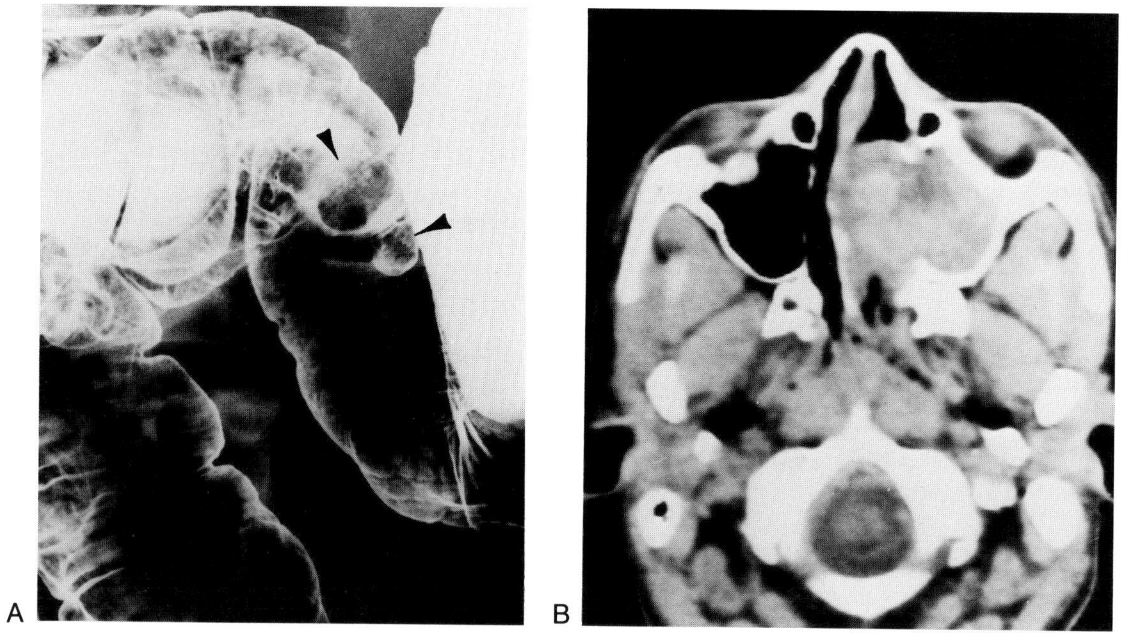

Fig. 5–55 Peutz-Jeghers syndrome. Hamartomatous small bowel and **(A)** colonic (*arrowheads*) and **(B)** nasal polyps were found in this patient.

of variable sizes, both sessile and pedunculated (Fig. 5–56). Due to the nearly 100 percent incidence of eventual malignant transformation of one of the polyps, the usual treatment is total colectomy by 8 years of age. The adenomatous polyps of Gardner's syndrome are usually less numerous but are also premalignant. Osteomas of the skeleton and multiple soft tissue tumors (hemangiomas) are also seen with this syndrome. Canada-Cronkhite syndrome (alopecia, skin pigmentation, and adenomatous polyps) and Turcot syndrome (adenomatous polyposis and central nervous system tumors) are uncommon in children.

Thickened Mucosal Folds in the Small Bowel

Thickening of the small bowel mucosal folds is generally due to some type of inflammatory or infiltrating disease affecting the bowel. The pattern of the fold thickening may be helpful to narrow the differential diagnosis. Straight thickened folds tend to be the result of intestinal hemorrhage or edema. Edema resulting from hypoproteinemia is the most common cause of thickened small bowel folds and nephrotic

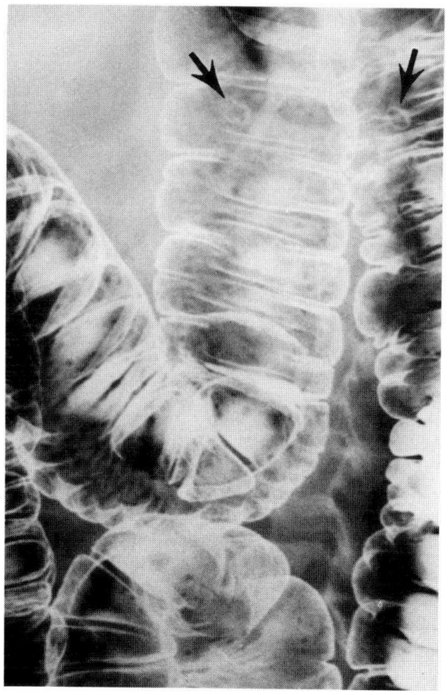

Fig. 5–56 Familial polyposis. Note the multiple small polypoid defects carpeting the colon that mimic lymphoid hyperplasia. In addition, larger polyps were also noted (arrows).

THICKENED MUCOSAL FOLDS—SMALL BOWEL

Congenital/developmental
- Lymphangiectasia**

Inflammation
- Crohn's disease**
- Pseudomembranous enterocolitis*
- Giardiasis**
- Eosinophilic gastroenteritis*
- Zollinger-Ellison syndrome*
- Allergic enteritis*
- Gastroenteritis*
- Celiac disease*

Trauma/surgery
- Intramural hemorrhage—secondary to trauma, hemorrhagic diathesis, anticoagulant therapy*,**

Systemic/metabolic
- Edema
  - Nephrotic syndrome*
  - Hypoproteinemia*
  - Portal vein obstruction*
  - Portal hypertension*
- Cystic fibrosis**
- Whipple's disease*

* Straight.
** Tortuous.

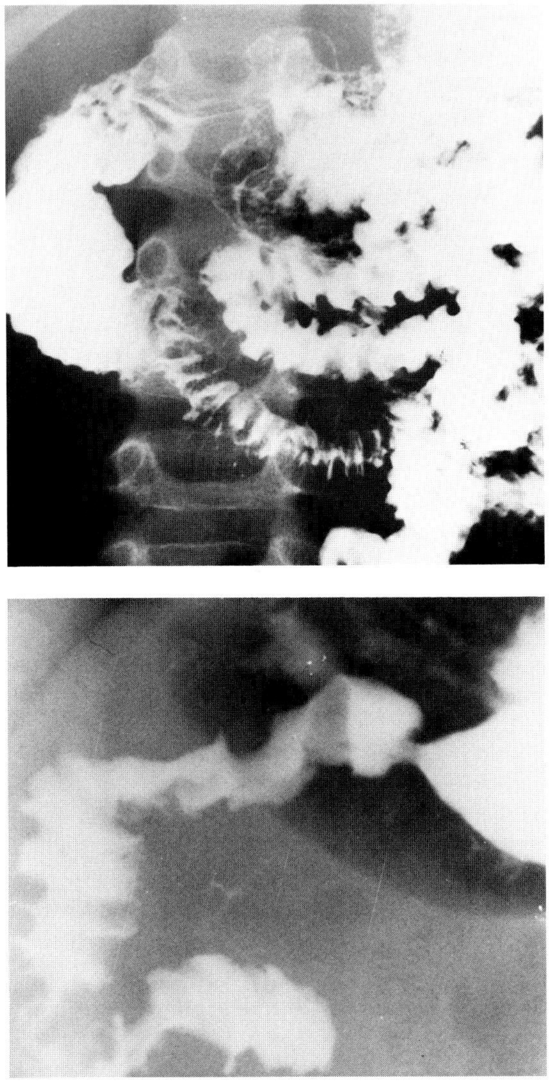

A

B

Fig. 5–57 Thickened small bowel folds. **(A)** Straight, thickened small bowel mucosal folds due to eosinophilic gastroenteritis. **(B)** Irregular duodenal and small bowel fold thickening in a patient with cystic fibrosis.

syndrome is the most common cause of hyperproteinemia in childhood. Edema may also result from liver disease or protein-losing enteropathy such as that seen with intestinal lymphangiectasia. The fold thickening associated with lymphangiectasia is due to a combination of intestinal edema and dilated, obstructed lymphatics and the dilated lymphatics may cause the fold pattern to appear more nodular. The most common inflammatory condition to thicken the small bowel folds is viral gastroenteritis, but eosinophilic enteritis (Fig. 5–57), allergic enteritis, and the Zollinger-Ellison syndrome can also lead to straight, thickened mucosal folds.

A more tortuous, nodular pattern of thickened small bowel folds is typical of parasitic infestations such as giardiasis, intestinal lymphangiectasia, and cystic fibrosis. Whipple's disease can also have this appearance, although it is rare in childhood.

If the small bowel fold thickening is segmental rather than generalized, intramural hemorrhage, infarction, or inflammation should be considered. For example, regional enteritis classically presents with such a pic-

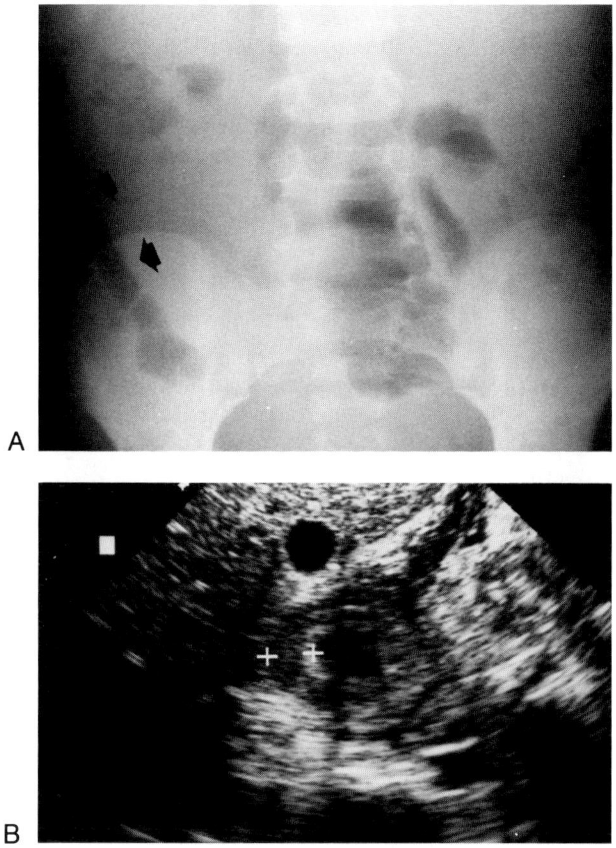

Fig. 5–58 Henoch-Schonlein purpura. **(A)** The plain radiograph of the abdomen suggests thumb printing of the bowel in the right abdomen (*arrows*). **(B)** Ultrasound confirmed thickening of the bowel wall.

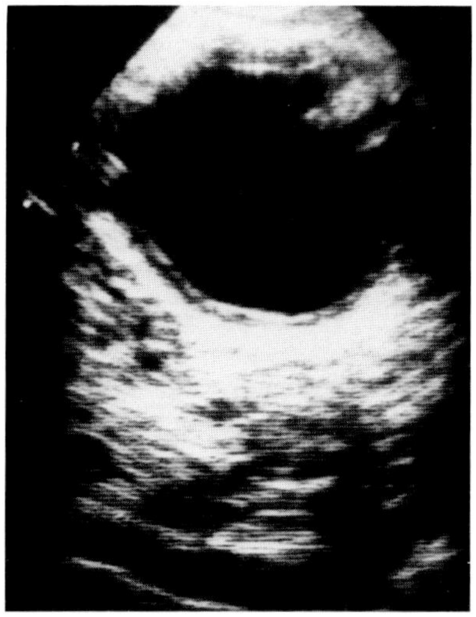

Fig. 5–59 Small bowel duplication cyst. Ultrasound demonstrates a cystic mass surrounded by a rim of thin hypoechoic muscle and overlying echogenic mucosa, a characteristic appearance of a gastrointestinal duplication.

ture. Henoch-Schönlein purpura, an acute arteritis leading to hemorrhage within the bowel wall, also can cause segmental areas of thickened, straight small bowel mucosal folds (Fig. 5–58). This syndrome is usually characterized by other signs of arteritis such as nephritis, joint pain, and purpura of the skin.

Duplication Cysts

The small bowel is the most common location for gastrointestinal duplication cysts. They typically are located in the terminal ileum near the ileocecal valve; however, duplications of the esophagus, stomach, duodenum, or any other portion of the gastrointestinal tract can occur. These cysts generally present as an abdominal mass. Contrast studies of the gastrointestinal tract are usually not diagnostic, since most of these cysts do not communicate with the bowel lumen.

Ultrasound is extremely helpful in evaluation of duplication cysts. They usually are unilocular and are filled with anechoic fluid. Occasionally duplication cysts may contain ectopic gastric mucosa, which can ulcerate and bleed, creating echoes within the cyst fluid. Often a thin hypoechoic muscular rim can be identified around the periphery of the cyst, accompanied by the inner, irregular, echogenic mucosal lining (Fig. 5–59). These are useful findings to help distinguish duplication cysts from other cystic abdominal masses. Vertebral anomalies may be associated with these duplications, which occasionally extend into the spinal cord, and therefore are sometimes referred to as *neurenteric* cysts.

Meckel's Diverticulum

Meckel's diverticulum represents a remnant of the omphalomesenteric duct extending from the terminal ileum near the ileocecal valve. Some important char-

CYSTIC ABDOMINAL MASSES

Congenital/developmental
- Multicystic dysplastic kidney
- Hydronephrosis (ureteropelvic junction obstruction)
- Gastrointestinal duplication
- Omental or mesenteric cysts
- Ovarian cyst
- Choledochal cyst
- Urachal cyst
- Teratoma/dermoid cyst

Inflammation
- Pancreatic pseudocyst
- Echinococcal cyst
- Abscess

Neoplasm
- Necrotic tumors
- Retroperitoneal cyst
- Lymphangioma

Miscellaneous
- Resolving adrenal hemorrhage

acteristics of this diverticulum follow the "rule of two's": it occurs in 2 percent of the population, it usually occurs within 2 feet of the ileocecal valve, and most symptoms occur prior to 2 years of age. The most common complication of a Meckel's diverticulum is gastrointestinal bleeding due to the presence of gastric mucosa within the diverticulum. Occasionally these diverticula become inflamed or act as a lead point for intussusception.

Meckel's diverticula are difficult to demonstrate radiographically, since they usually do not fill on barium enema or small bowel examinations. Those diverticula that contain ectopic gastric mucosa may be detected on a ^{99m}Tc pertechnetate study (Fig. 5–60). This radioisotope accumulates in the parietal cells of the gastric mucosa, and visualization may be enhanced by premedication of the patient with pentagastrin or cimetidine. False-positive radioisotope studies have occurred with intussusception, urinary tract obstruction, inflammatory bowel disease, and intestinal duplication cysts.

Perforation is another recognized complication of Meckel's diverticula. When this occurs, the radiographic findings may mimic those of perforated ap-

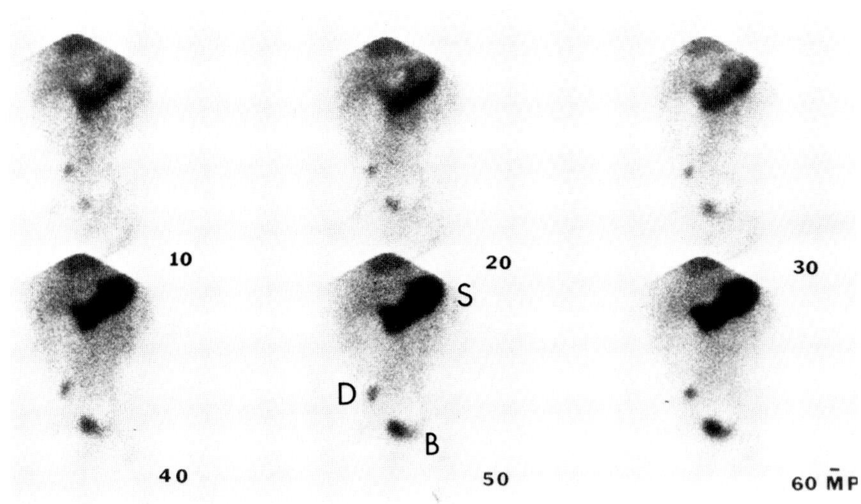

Fig. 5–60 Meckel's diverticulum. Scintigraphy using ^{99m}Tc pertechnetate demonstrates an abnormal collection of radiotracer activity in the right lower quadrant. This represents the presence of gastric mucosa within this Meckel's diverticulum. S, stomach; B, bladder; D, Meckel's diverticulum.

pendicitis, including scoliosis with concavity to the right, absence of the psoas margin, and an abnormal bowel gas pattern in the right lower quadrant. Rarely, a radiopaque stone may form within the diverticulum.

Meckel's diverticula can occasionally be very large, the so-called giant Meckel's diverticulum. In such cases, a large area of air mixed with feces may be seen, and intestinal obstruction can occur.

COLON

Megacolon

When a gas-distended, dilated colon is encountered in a neonate, Hirschsprung's disease, ectopic (imperforate) anus, and congenital atresia or stenosis of the colon must be excluded. Four types of colonic atresia have been described: membranous atresia, atresia with a residual thin fibrous band, atresia with no connecting band, and multiple atresias. The atresia may occur at any point in the colon and is generally considered to be the result of an intrauterine vascular insult. The portion of colon proximal to the atresia is usually massively dilated (Fig. 5–61) and often contains meconium mixed with air, leading to a granular appearance. If membranous atresia is present, the membrane may bulge outward producing a wind sock sign. The colon distal to the area of atresia is often very small (Fig. 5–62).

Hirschsprung's disease (aganglionosis of the colon) results in colonic obstruction due to hypertonicity of the aganglionic segment. Usually this segment involves the distal colon, specifically the rectum and rectosigmoid. Nevertheless, the length of the aganglionic segment is variable, and cases of total colonic aganglionosis, as well as small bowel involvement, have been reported. The exact etiology of Hirschsprung's disease is unknown, but it is suspected to be the result of incomplete craniocaudal migration of the primitive intestinal neuroblasts in the fetus. The absence of ganglion cells in the myenteric and submucosal plexus leads to a lack of organized peristaltic activity in the segment, and subsequent constipation. Hirschsprung's disease often presents in the neonate and young infant. The infant may present with obstruction and vomiting or sometimes diar-

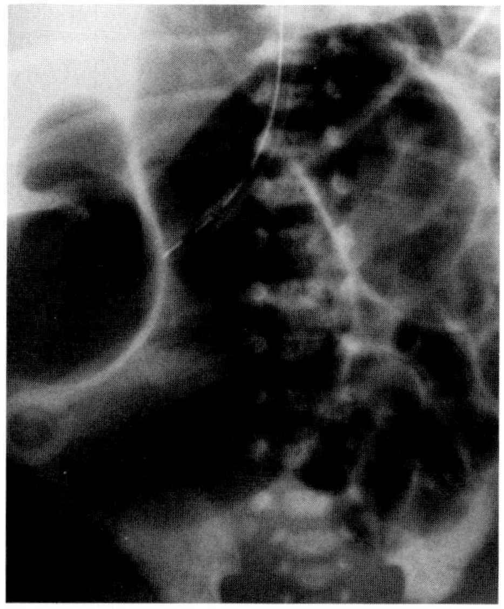

Fig. 5–61 A plain radiograph shows massive distension of the colon proximal to its site of atresia near the splenic flexure.

MEGACOLON

Congenital/developmental
- Atresia or stenosis
- Hirschsprung's disease
- Anorectal anomalies
- Segmental dilatation of colon
- Neuronal colonic dysplasia

Inflammation
- Neonatal sepsis
- Toxic megacolon
- Chagas disease

Neoplasm
- Neurofibromatosis

Trauma/surgery
- Adhesions

Metabolic/systemic
- Medication
- Hypothyroidism

Miscellaneous
- Meconium plug syndrome
- Small left colon syndrome
- Volvulus
- Idiopathic megacolon

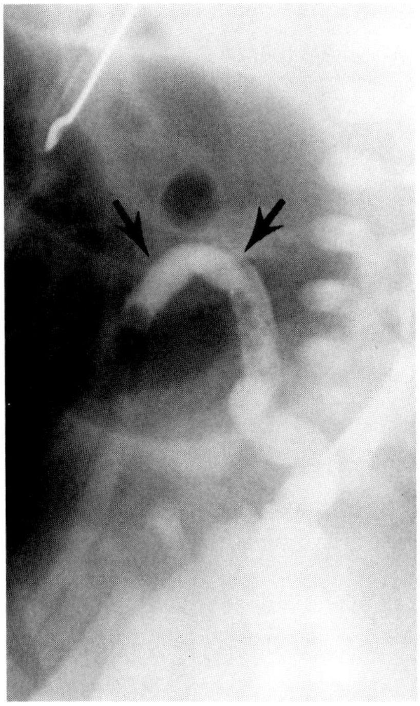

Fig. 5–62 Colon atresia. A contrast study demonstrates the small distal colon with a characteristic hook (*arrows*).

rhea. Failure to pass meconium within the first 24 hours should be regarded as highly suspicious of underlying Hirschsprung's disease.

The plain radiograph of the abdomen in a patient with Hirschsprung's disease typically shows numerous gas-distended loops of bowel suggesting low small bowel or colonic obstruction (Fig. 5–63), although the exact level of obstruction often is difficult to ascertain. As a result, a barium enema is required to establish definitely the diagnosis and to determine the length of the aganglionic segment. The examination should be performed on an unprepared colon, since removal of the retained feces from the colon can make identification of the transition zone more difficult. The barium contrast medium should be prepared with isotonic saline rather than tap water to prevent the possible complication of water intoxication.

The characteristic barium enema findings consist of a sharp transition zone between the slightly narrowed, distal aganglionic segment of colon and the dilated proximal colon containing normal ganglion cells (Fig. 5–64). This transition zone most commonly lies in

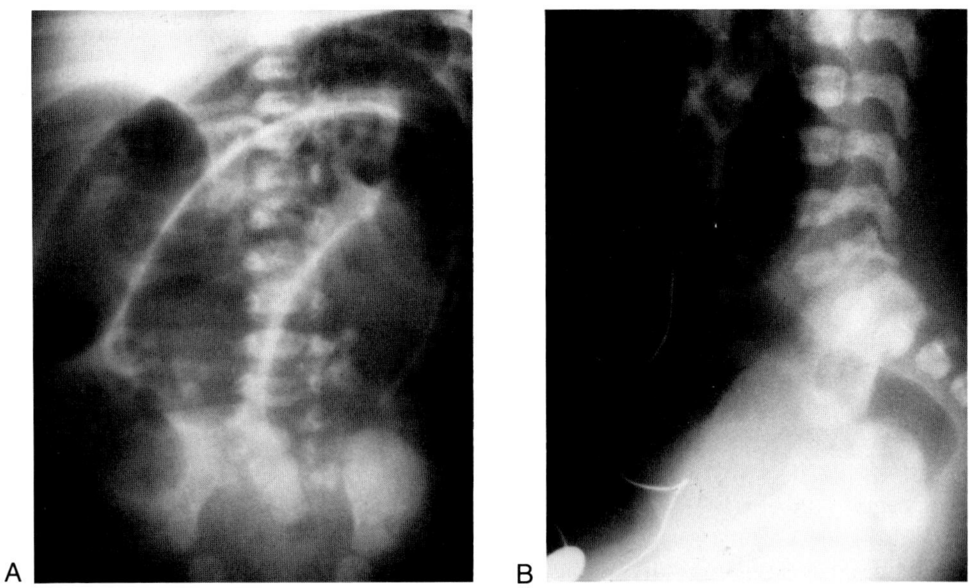

Fig. 5–63 Hirschsprung's disease. **(A)** The plain abdominal radiograph shows multiple dilated loops of bowel characteristic of a low small bowel or colonic obstruction. **(B)** The lateral view clearly shows narrowing of the aganglionic rectum as compared to the more proximal dilated bowel.

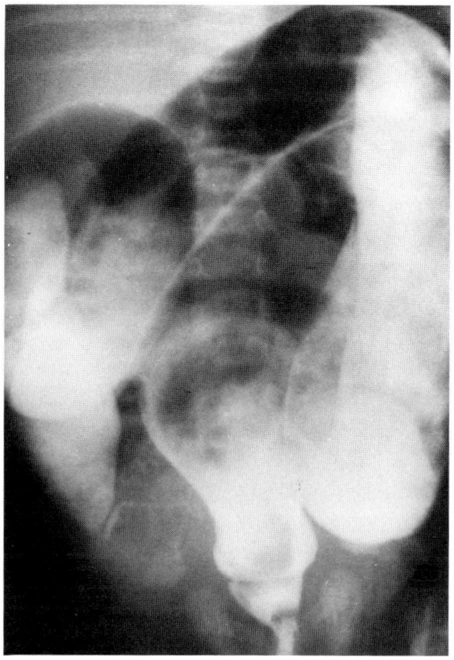

Fig. 5–64 Hirschsprung's disease. Barium enema clearly delineates the transition zone in the rectosigmoid colon.

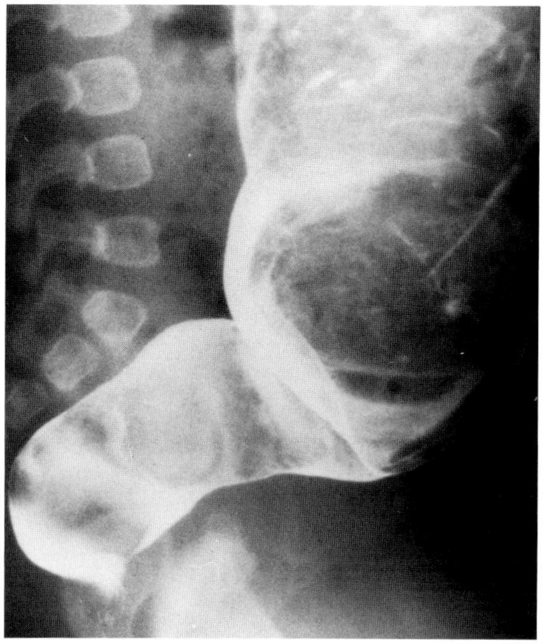

Fig. 5–65 Hirschsprung's disease. Barium enema clearly demonstrates the transition zone with a reversed rectosigmoid index.

the region of the rectosigmoid, although it is not uncommon for it to be slightly more proximal. Unfortunately, the transition zone is not always clearly demarcated, possibly because of some hypoganglionosis of the bowel immediately proximal to the aganglionic segment. The transition zone is particularly difficult to identify in the neonate and in patients with total colonic involvement. A fairly large percentage (perhaps as many as 30 percent) of patients with Hirschsprung's disease may show a completely normal colon at barium enema. Rectal biopsy is necessary to confirm or make the definitive diagnosis of Hirschsprung's disease in all suspected cases.

Another useful finding in Hirschsprung's disease is a decrease in the so-called rectosigmoid index. Normally, comparison of the diameters of the rectum and the sigmoid colon yields a 1:1 or greater ratio. If at any time the rectal diameter is less than that of the sigmoid, Hirschsprung's disease should be suspected (Fig. 5–65). This finding is more easily appreciated in older infants and children.

In some cases of Hirschsprung's disease the aganglionic segment appears corrugated due to peculiar irregular contractions (Fig. 5–66). Simple intermittent spasm is an uncommon occurrence in the neonatal rectum, and therefore its presence should be regarded as highly suspicious of Hirschsprung's disease. Occasionally, long segments of colon proximal to the transition zone may also demonstrate considerable spasm, the etiology of which is uncertain. Other findings that may seen include thickening and nodularity of the mucosa proximal to the transition zone. This is sometimes associated with protein-losing enteropathy. Occasionally Hirschsprung's disease may be complicated by enterocolitis of the proximal colon. In such cases, spasm, edematous mucosal folds, cobblestoning, ulcerations, and even pneumatosis intestinalis can be seen (Fig. 5–67). This complication is probably the result of stasis in the obstructed colon leading to pressure on the mucosa and subsequent mucosal ischemia.

In the typical case of Hirschsprung's disease, treatment consists of colostomy and subsequent colonic pull through. Myomectomy of the anorectal sphincter may be sufficient if the aganglionic segment is ex-

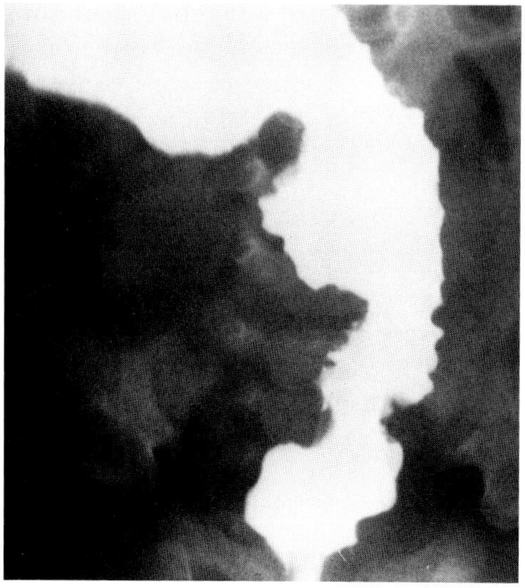

Fig. 5–66 Hirschsprung's disease. Note the peculiar, irregular contractions of the aganglionic segment.

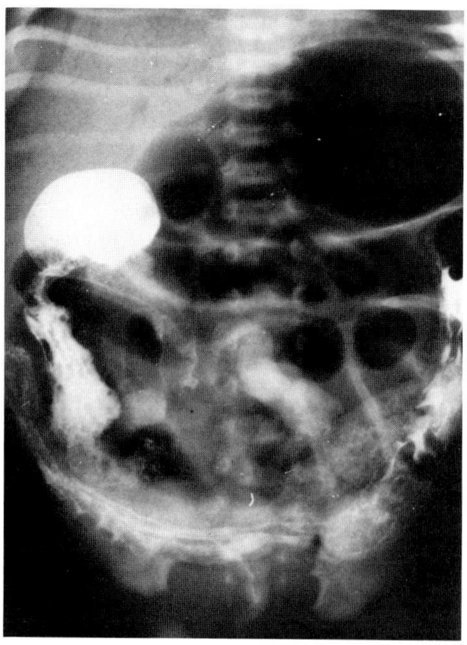

Fig. 5–67 Hirschsprung's disease presenting as necrotizing enterocolitis. This full-term infant developed pneumatosis cystoides intestinalis indicating necrotizing enterocolitis. Later Hirschsprung's disease was revealed.

tremely short. Total aganglionosis requires an ileostomy.

The meconium plug syndrome and small left colon syndromes are probably the same entities, as both are manifestations of functional immaturity of the colon leading to colonic obstruction. The findings may mimick those of Hirschsprung's disease. Because the problem is one of colonic immaturity, it is easy to understand why it is more commonly seen in both premature infants and in infants of diabetic mothers. Other implicated contributing factors include hypermagnesemia, excess glucagon production, and delayed oral feedings failing to induce the gastrocolic reflex. Usually infants with obstruction due to colon inertia present within the first 24 to 36 hours of life with abdominal distension, bilious vomiting, and failure to pass meconium.

Plain radiographs generally show evidence of some type of low small bowel obstruction. Erect views tend to show a paucity of air/fluid levels and little or no gas within the colon. Occasionally air mixed with the meconium may give a granular appearance, which could be mistaken for early pneumatosis intestinalis. The barium enema examination is diagnostic and often therapeutic in infants with meconium plug syndrome. The colon is filled with inspissated meconium which, when surrounded by barium, gives the appearance of a double contrast barium enema (Fig. 5–68). The bowel is often of normal caliber, however if some of the meconium has passed, the emptied portion of colon may appear narrowed, thus the term *small left colon syndrome* (Fig. 5–69).

Generally, irritation of the rectum and colon will lead to evacuation of the meconium plugs and cure of the condition. Often the barium enema examination provides adequate irritation, but more persistent cases may require the use of dilute gastrografin (2:1) or other water-soluble contrast agents. If intestinal problems recur following the complete evacuation of the meconium, a rectal biopsy to exclude Hirschsprung's disease is indicated.

A wide variety of congenital abnormalities of the anus and rectum may present with colonic obstruction early in the neonatal period. These anomalies include imperforate anus, ectopic anus, and anorectal atresia

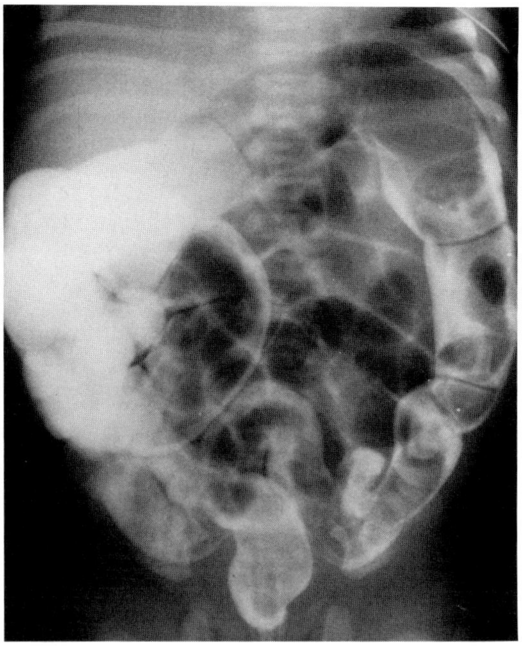

Fig. 5–68 Meconium plug syndrome (colon inertia). Contrast surrounding the retained meconium in the colon gives an appearance not unlike a double contrast barium enema.

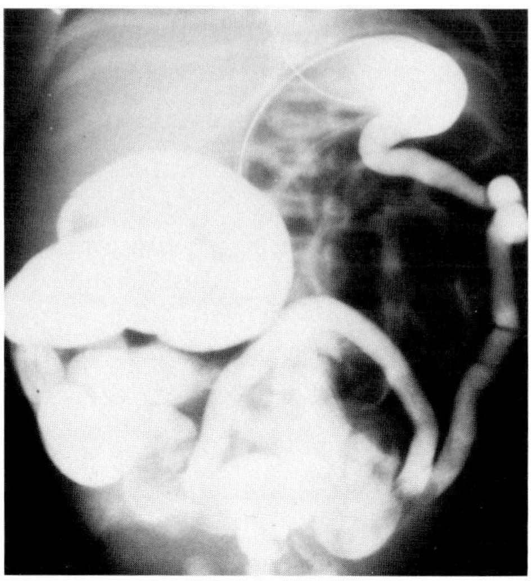

Fig. 5–69 Newborn with small left colon syndrome. Note the narrowed left colon compared to the more normal caliber of the remaining colon.

or stenosis. Most commonly, some communication between the distal colon and the perineum or genitourinary tract exists. Ectopic anus probably is the result of failure of the normal descent of the hindgut through the puborectalis sling. Multiple other visceral and skeletal anomalies are often associated with anorectal malformations. Sacral abnormalities ranging from dysplasia to agenesis are frequently present. Genitourinary tract anomalies are present in 25 to 40 percent of cases. Vaginal atresia with hydrometrocolpos and gastrointestinal abnormalities such as duodenal or esophageal atresia are also quite common. Ectopic anus is a constant feature of the VATER syndrome.

The most important information the radiologist can provide when presented with a patient with an anorectal malformation is the relationship of the rectal pouch to the puborectalis sling. In addition, the presence and location of fistulas and the presence of any associated malformations are important to identify. The presence of a high obstruction or fistula above the puborectalis sling suggests that the anal sphincter is most likely underdeveloped. An abdominal-perineal surgical approach is necessary in such cases and rectal continence will be difficult to achieve. If a low atresia or fistula is present, that is below the puborectalis sling, a perineal approach is usually preferable. The level of termination of the hindgut can generally be inferred from the physical examination. If a fistula is noted in the perineum, the pouch is most likely located below the puborectalis sling. If the opening of the fistula is not readily visible, it is fair to assume that the hindgut most likely terminates above the puborectalis sling.

The plain abdominal radiograph will usually show a gas pattern consistent with a low colonic obstruction. Occasionally, bubbles of gas may be noted in the bladder or the vagina of a female infant, giving clues to the location of the ectopic opening. Upside-down views have classically been used to distend the rectal pouch with gas in an attempt to determine its location but prone, cross-table lateral views also provide the same information with less manipulation of the patient (Fig. 5–70). The level of the puborectalis muscle approximately corresponds to a line drawn through the junction of the upper two-thirds and the lower one-third of the ischia ("M" line). The

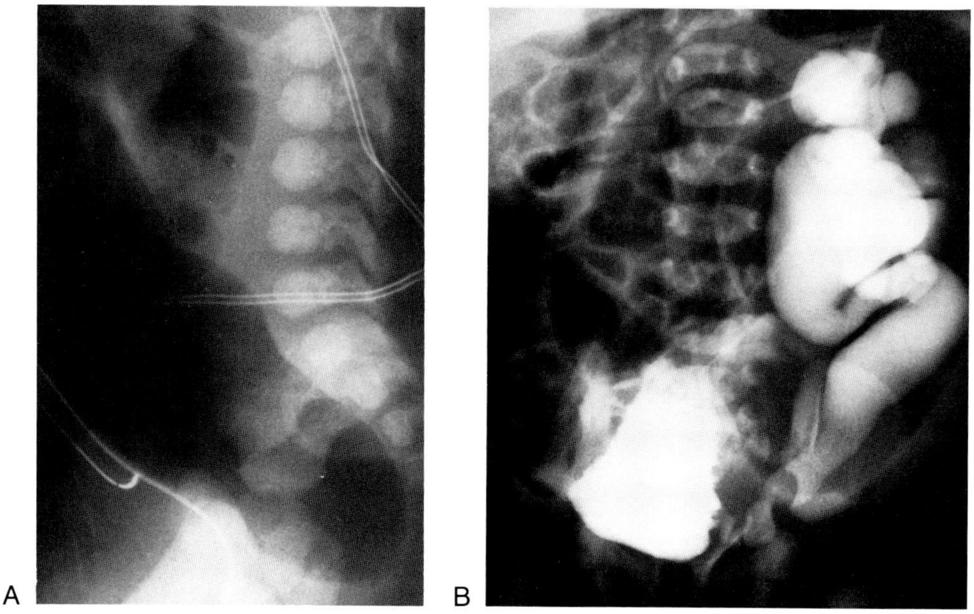

Fig. 5–70 Anal atresia. **(A)** A prone cross-table lateral view clearly shows the rectal pouch to extend well below the imaginary "M" line, indicating a low pouch. **(B)** A cystogram shows an irregular bladder with marked vesicoureteral reflux on the left.

level of termination of the gas-distended rectal pouch as related to this line can sometimes aid in determining the type of anomaly present. Ultrasonography has also been utilized to locate the level of the blind-ending pouch. With the transducer at the anal dimple, the distance measured from the skin's surface to the end of the rectal pouch should measure less than 1.5 cm in a low lesion. Also, direct puncture through the anal plate to inject contrast material directly into the rectal pouch can be performed, although it is not usually necessary. CT and MRI may be useful for evaluating the size and location of the puborectalis muscle and to evaluate the success of a pull-through procedure.

Microcolon

The term *microcolon* is used to describe a narrowed, unused colon, which is seen in newborns with complete distal small bowel and colonic obstructions (i.e., meconium ileus, ileal atresia, colonic atresia). The volume of intestinal secretions and amniotic fluid that passes through the colon in fetal life determines the size of the colon; therefore, with distal small bowel obstruction, the colon will be very small and contain only a few mucous strands and sloughed mucosa (Fig. 5–71). If the obstruction lies in the more proximal small bowel, the colon will be more normal in size.

The megacystis-microcolon-intestinal hypoperistalsis syndrome is an uncommon condition, characterized by a massively distended bladder and a microcolon.

MICROCOLON

Congenital/developmental
- Colonic atresia
- Ileal atresia
- Total aganglionosis
- Megacystitis-microcolon-intestinal hypoperistalsis syndrome

Miscellaneous
- Meconium ileus
- Small left colon syndrome*
- Functional obstruction of newborn*

* Partial.

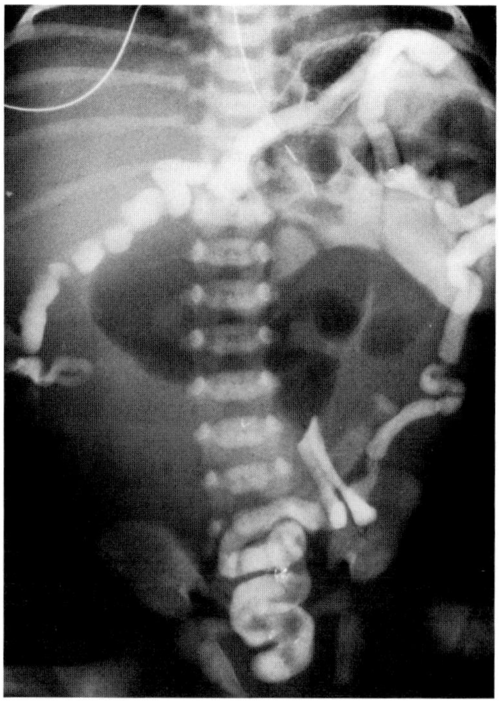

Fig. 5–71 Microcolon in a patient with ileal atresia. Note the small caliber of the entire colon secondary to distal small bowel obstruction.

Abnormal peristalsis is demonstrated throughout the gastrointestinal tract. The reason for the greatly distended bladder is uncertain, as there is no bladder neck or urethral obstruction. The kidneys may be hydronephrotic, although ureteral reflux usually does not occur. This condition is generally refractory to any form of therapy. Other causes of a small colon include the occasional cases of total aganglionosis (Hirschsprung's disease) and functional obstruction of newborn. Distal colonic microcolon is seen with colonic atresia and in the small left colon syndrome.

Inflammatory Disease

In the neonate, inflammation of the colon is most commonly due to necrotizing enterocolitis. This serious condition is most often seen in premature infants, although it can occur in a full-term neonate. Although the exact etiology is unknown, it is believed to be due to intestinal ischemia or hypoperfusion resulting from a combination of prematurity, hypoxia, and perinatal stress. Bacterial overgrowth and irritation of the bowel by oral feedings are also thought to be contributing factors. Conditions that predispose the patient to hypoperfusion of the gastrointestinal tract include hypothermia, hyperviscosity, hypovolemia, congenital heart disease with large left-to-right shunts or decreased left ventricular output, sepsis, and shock. This disease is most commonly sporadic, however epidemic forms sometimes occur.

Early diagnosis of necrotizing enterocolitis is critical, for mild disease is completely cureable with medical management. Sometimes the course of the disease can be quite fulminant, and delay of diagnosis and therapy significantly increases the risk of complications. The earliest radiographic finding consists of generalized intestinal dilatation due to adynamic ileus. Occasionally focal distension of loops in the right lower quadrant may be seen in early disease. The intestinal dilatation may be followed by thickening and indistinctness of the bowel wall. The pathognomonic finding of necrotizing enterocolitis consists of pneumatosis cystoides intestinalis. Pneumatosis represents gas within the intestinal wall due to loss of the mucosal integrity. This bowel wall gas may appear as bubbly, linear, or curvilinear collections of gas (Fig. 5–72). Pneumatosis is generally best visualized in the colon, although it can involve almost

INFLAMMATORY DISEASE OF THE COLON

- Neonates
  - Necrotizing enterocolitis
  - Hirschsprung's disease
  - Cow's milk allergy
- Older infants and children
  - Infections
    - *Shigella*
    - Rotavirus
    - Amebiasis
    - *Yersinia*
  - Ulcerative colitis
  - Regional enteritis
  - Hemolytic-uremic syndrome
  - Pseudomembranous enterocolitis
  - Postirradiation
  - Appendicitis
  - Typhilitis

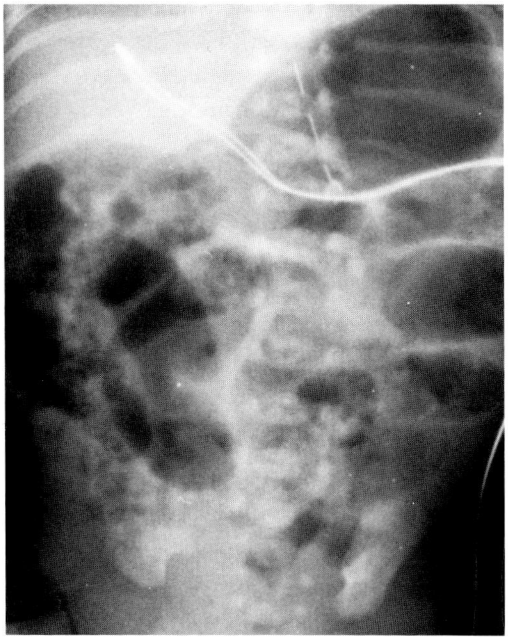

Fig. 5–72 Necrotizing enterocolitis. This radiograph of a preterm infant demonstrates the characteristic bubbly pattern of pneumatosis cystoides intestinalis.

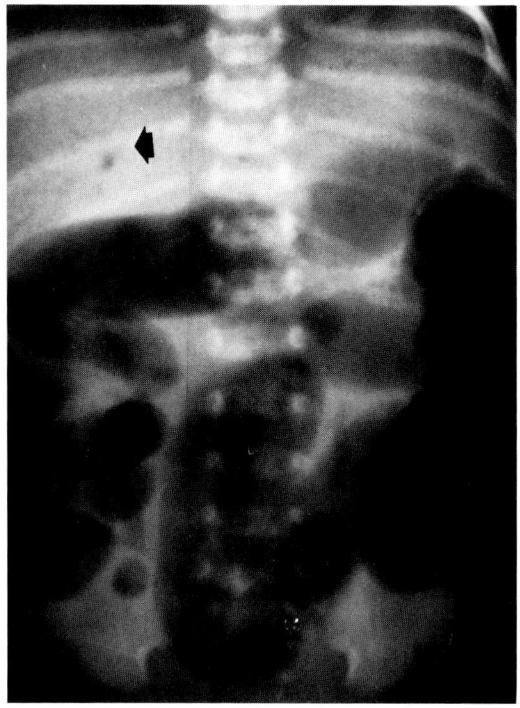

Fig. 5–73 Necrotizing enterocolitis. The presence of gas within the portal veins, seen as radiolucent branching structures in the liver (*arrow*), indicates severe disease.

any portion of the gastrointestinal tract. The differential diagnosis of pneumatosis has been discussed earlier (see list on p. 185).

The presence of gas within the portal veins indicates advanced disease (Fig. 5–73). Although the prognosis remains guarded in the face of this finding, portal vein gas is no longer considered a sign of certain demise and indeed presence of the gas can be quite transient. Gas within the portal veins may be visualized ultrasonographically as echogenic, intravascular foci within the portal vein or liver, which may actually move on a real-time examination. Ultrasound may also demonstrate the edematous wall of the affected bowel.

Once the diagnosis is established, the radiologist must be alert for the development of complications. In this regard, the presence of pneumoperitoneum indicates bowel perforation and is a clear indication for surgical intervention. However, the amount of free intraperitoneal air is often small and decubitus and cross-table lateral views are helpful to detect such air. In addition, in many cases of perforation, no detectable free air will be present but a decrease in the amount of intestinal bowel gas and a generalized increase in the density of the abdomen due to intraperitoneal fluid should suggest peritonitis and perforation. Another ominous finding is the presence of focally dilated loops of intestine that persist unchanged on several examinations. This suggests bowel necrosis and surgery is mandatory.

Complications that may occur during the convalescent period of necrotizing enterocolitis include transient malabsorption, persistent low-grade bleeding, and recurrence of the disease due to premature resumption of oral feeding. Persistence of blood in the stools suggests subacute enterocolitis, which is commonly accompanied by inflammatory stenosis of the bowel (Fig. 5–74). Often these stenoses are reversible and resolve with appropriate medical therapy. Some strictures, however, become fibrotic and require surgical correction or balloon dilatation. Less common

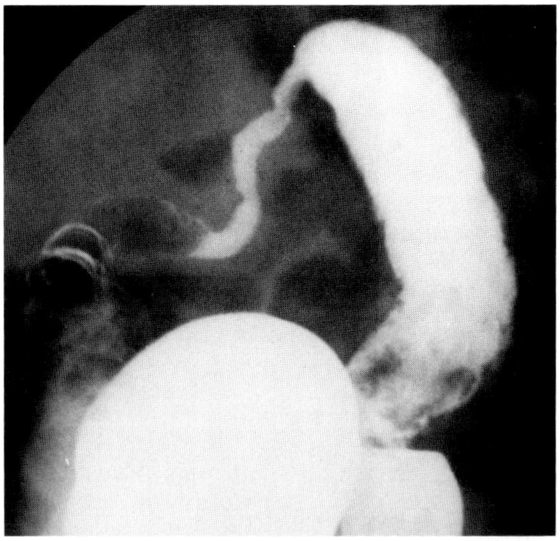

Fig. 5–74 Colonic stricture following necrotizing enterocolitis. This long stricture of the transverse colon occurred as a complication of necrotizing enterocolitis.

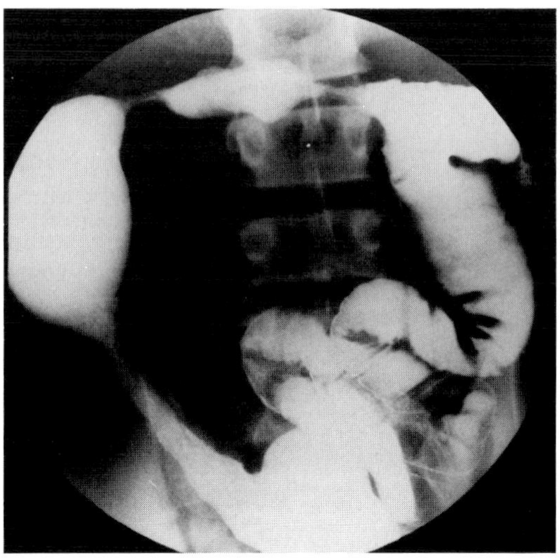

Fig. 5–75 Advanced regional enteritis. Note the multiple areas of narrowing with loss of the normal mucosal markings, characteristic of the skip lesions of regional enteritis.

complications include enterocolic fistulas and enterocysts.

Colitis in the neonate can also be a sequel of Hirschsprung's disease. The inflammation involves the colon proximal to the aganglionic segment and is most likely due to stasis of bowel contents. Findings on barium enema examination include spasm, mucosal edema, cobblestoning, ulcerations, and even pneumatosis cystoides intestinalis. A segmental form of colitis has also been noted in neonates thought to have cow's milk allergy. Other causes of colitis are rare in the newborn period.

Infectious colitis can be seen in older infants and children and is most commonly due to *Shigella,* rotavirus, or amebiasis. The first two conditions seldom are investigated beyond plain radiographs. On barium enema examination, the findings of amebiasis usually consist of diffuse mucosal ulceration, followed by the development of a cone-shaped cecum.

Ulcerative colitis may occur in infants as well as in older children, however regional enteritis (Crohn's disease) is much more common in older children. Ulcerative colitis that occurs in early infancy seems to have a more rapidly progressive and severe course than that encountered in older children. The barium enema findings of these two conditions is the same in children as in adults (Fig. 5–75). The thickened, edematous loops of intestine may also be demonstrated by ultrasound (Fig. 5–76). A nonspecific colitis has also been described in association with the hemolytic uremic syndrome, occurring mainly in older children.

LIVER AND BILIARY TRACT

Neonatal Cholestasis

Cholestasis in the neonate may be caused by a wide variety of abnormalities, however the vast majority of cases are due to either neonatal hepatitis or biliary atresia. It has been suggested that these two entities may in fact be related and many authors now believe that biliary atresia is the result of a chronic cholangiohepatitis. Balistreri[7] suggests that the neonatal hepatitis syndrome should be divided into three groups:

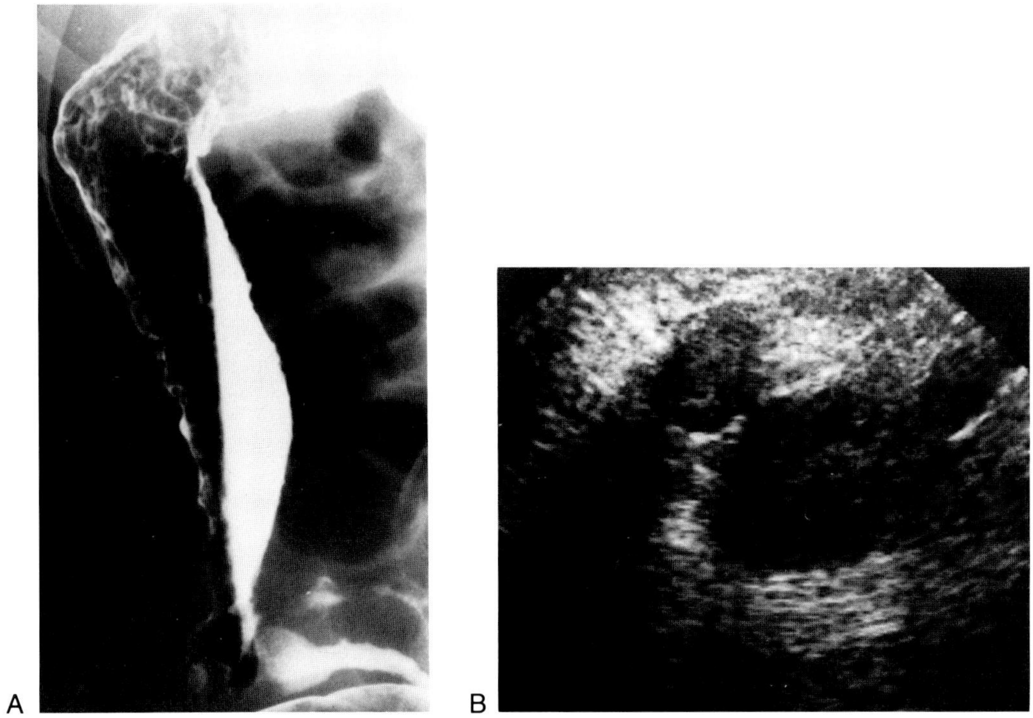

Fig. 5–76 Regional enteritis. **(A)** Note pseudopolyp formation in the right colon of this patient with regional enteritis. **(B)** Some bowel wall thickening was also evident by ultrasound examination.

hepatitis due to a specific virus such as hepatitis B virus or cytomegalovirus; intrahepatic cholestasis, which occurs with diseases such as alpha[1]-antitrypsin deficiency, Byler's disease, and arteriohepatic dysplasia; and neonatal hepatitis. The third group, an idiopathic process in which the cause of cholestasis is undetermined, accounts for the majority of cases of cholestasis in the neonatal period.

Biliary atresia has also been divided into three types: focal atresia of the biliary ducts, presumably due to an intrauterine vascular insult; intrahepatic ductal atresia; and extrahepatic ductal atresia. Extrahepatic atresia is the most common form and presents very early in life. The other types of atresia are quite uncommon.

Despite the similarities between neonatal hepatitis and biliary atresia, it is important to differentiate the two entities because treatment is quite different. Cholestatic jaundice due to infectious hepatitis, metabolic diseases, or idiopathic neonatal hepatitis is usually managed conservatively. On the other hand, biliary atresia requires prompt surgical intervention. Biliary atresia seems to be a progressive postnatal obstructive process and, therefore, is more likely to be successfully treated in its earlier stages. It has been noted that hepatic portoenterostomy leads to successful bile drainage in more than 90 percent of patients who undergo surgery prior to 2 months of age, but successful drainage drops to less than 20 percent when the surgery is delayed beyond 3 months of age.

The initial radiologic evaluation of neonatal cholestasis should include ultrasonography for the evaluation of the biliary tract. Although ultrasound can be useful in excluding such abnormalities as focal extrahepatic biliary atresia, choledochal cysts, and spontaneous perforation of the bile duct, it is much less helpful in differentiating neonatal hepatitis from extrahepatic biliary atresia. The sonographic findings are nonspecific; the liver may be normal or increased in size with normal or increased echogenicity. The intrahepatic bile ducts may not appear dilated and the ex-

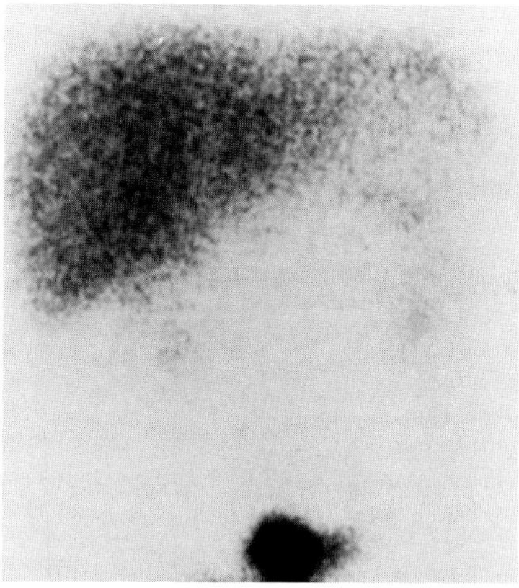

Fig. 5–77 Biliary atresia. Hepatobiliary scintigraphy reveals normal hepatic radiotracer uptake with no excretion into the biliary tract or intestine.

trahepatic ducts are often quite difficult to visualize in infants. The gallbladder may be large, normal, small or not visible. Later in the course of biliary atresia, increasing fibrosis in the liver may lead to irregularly increased echogenicity or marked periportal echogenicity.

Hepatobiliary scintigraphy using ^{99m}Tc-IDA analogs has been shown to be a more useful examination in differentiating extrahepatic biliary atresia from neonatal hepatitis. Early in the course of biliary atresia, the hepatocytes function normally and take up the radiotracer, but excretion into the biliary tract and intestine is absent (Fig. 5–77). On the other hand, hepatocyte uptake of the radiotracer may be more sluggish in neonatal hepatitis, but eventually some of the radiotracer should reach the intestinal tract (Fig. 5–78). Pretreatment of the patient with phenobarbital for 5 days prior to the examination has been utilized to enhance biliary excretion of the radioisotope.

The definitive diagnosis of biliary atresia is usually made with intraoperative cholangiography and liver biopsy. In biliary atresia, the cholangiogram generally will demonstrate a small gallbladder and nonfilling of the hepatic radicles. In neonatal hepatitis, the gallbladder tends to be near normal in size. Unfortunately, poor filling of the hepatic radicles may also occur, but usually at least minimal duct filling can be demonstrated.

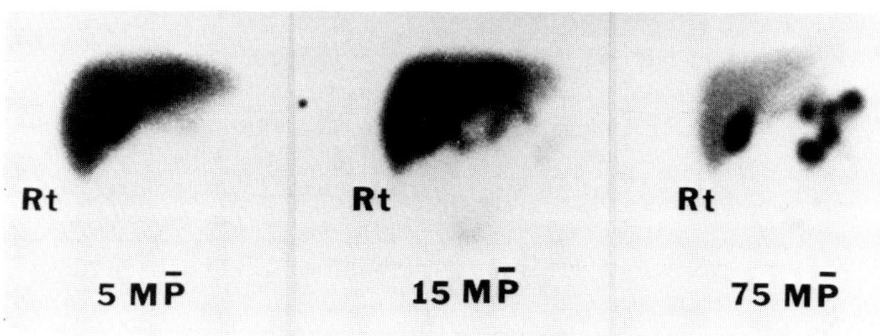

Fig. 5–78 Normal hepatobiliary scintigraphy. In this newborn with neonatal hepatitis, normal excretion of the radiotracer into the gallbladder and small intestine was present.

Cysts and Cystic Structures

Choledochal cysts include several different types of localized dilatation of the biliary tract. A rather complex system of five types of choledochal cysts has been described, but the most common form (80 to 90 percent of cases) results in fusiform dilatation of a portion of the biliary tract. The dilatation tends to involve either the common bile duct below the cystic duct or both the common bile and hepatic ducts. Choledochal diverticulum and choledochocele (dilatation of the distal intramural portion of the common bile duct) are sometimes included as types of choledochal cysts. Caroli's disease (saccular dilatation of the intrahepatic bile ducts) is sometimes included in this classification.

Barlow et al.[3] suggested two categories of choledochal cysts: (1) those secondary to stenosis or atresia of a portion of the biliary tract, associated with cirrhosis and portal hypertension and (2) those due to anomalous development of the common bile and pancreatic ducts, which allows reflux of pancreatic secretions into the bile ducts with resultant cholangitis. The former type is usually seen in the jaundiced newborn, whereas the second type presents later in life and is often accompanied by pancreatitis and common duct stones.

The classic presentation of a choledochal cyst includes the triad of jaundice, pain, and a right upper quadrant mass. However, this triad is found in less than 20 percent of patients with the disease. Females seem to be more commonly affected and the more severe cases seem to involve infants.

The diagnosis of choledochal cyst can usually be made with a combination of ultrasound and hepatobiliary scintigraphy. Ultrasonographically, the cyst appears as a fluid-containing structure in the right upper quadrant separate from the gallbladder (Fig. 5–79). Usually some dilatation of the bile ducts is evident. These findings are usually confirmed by scintigraphy using ^{99m}Tc-IDA analogs. Typically, hepatic excretion of

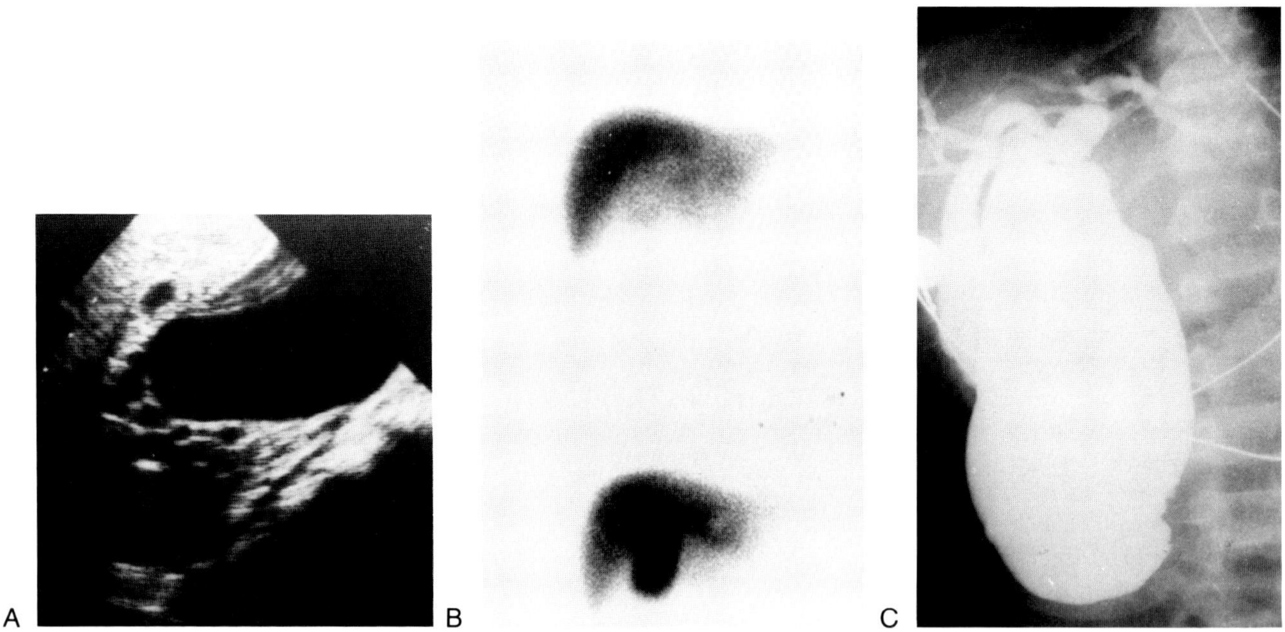

Fig. 5–79 Choledochal cyst. **(A)** Sonography revealed a large cystic mass in the right upper quadrant surrounded by multiple dilated tubular structures. **(B)** Hepatobiliary scintigraphy demonstrated radiotracer concentration within the large cystic mass, indicating that it was connected with the biliary tract. **(C)** Cholangiography verified the massive dilatation of the common bile duct with milder dilatation of the hepatic ducts.

the radiotracer is normal and accumulation within the cyst can be identified. This study helps to differentiate choledochal cyst from other cystic structures, such as hydrops of the gallbladder or duplication cysts.

Hepatic cysts are uncommon lesions that may be either congenital or acquired. Solitary congenital cysts of the liver are usually incidental in children, although occasionally some are massive. Multiple hepatic cysts are usually associated with a more generalized disease process, the most common of which is autosomal dominant (adult-type) polycystic kidney disease. However, only a small percentage of patients with adult polycystic renal disease have multiple hepatic cysts.

Acquired cystic lesions in the liver are usually the result of infection, such as abscess or echinococcal cyst or resolving hematomas. Necrotic primary or metastatic tumors of the liver are an uncommon cause of cystic lesions in the liver of children. Most cases of hepatic abscess in children are secondary to bacterial sepsis, which in the older child may be the result of an immune disorder (e.g., chronic granulomatous disease or malignancy). Perforated appendicitis associated with pyelophlebitis now seems to be a less common cause of pyogenic hepatic abscesses. In the neonate, these abscesses are usually due to neonatal sepsis or umbilical vein catheterization. In certain areas of the United States, where amebiasis is endemic, amebic abscess is not uncommon in children. Usually this occurs before the age of 5 years.

The radiographic findings of hepatic abscess are nonspecific and consist of hepatomegaly, elevation of the right hemidiaphragm, and pleural effusion. Ultrasonography is considered by many to be the best method for evaluating hepatic abscesses. The ultrasound appearance of an abscess in the liver can be quite variable, often appearing as a purely anechoic mass with a rim of variable thickness, but other abscesses may contain debris, leading to a more echogenic appearance. If gas is present within the abscess, the lesion may appear intensely echogenic.

Amebic hepatic abscesses also tend to have a variable sonographic appearance. The presence of a peripheral, round or oval, predominantly sonolucent mass that is moderately well-defined and contains fine, low level echoes has been described as a specific appearance for hepatic abscess. Nevertheless, amebic abscesses may also appear as more complex masses that are difficult to differentiate from other types of hepatic abscess (Fig. 5–80).

CYSTIC LIVER LESIONS

Congenital/developmental
- Simple congenital cyst
- Choledochal cyst

Inflammation
- Abscess
- Parasitic cyst

Neoplasm
- Cystic hepatoblastoma
- Mesenchymal hamartoma
- Embryonal sarcoma
- Necrotic metastasis

Trauma/surgery
- Hematoma
- Biloma

Miscellaneous
- Biloma due to spontaneous perforation of bile duct

CT and MRI may also be used to identify and localize hepatic abscesses, and ultrasound and CT may be useful for the guidance of percutaneous aspiration or drainage of hepatic abscesses. Percutaneous drainage is more commonly used with pyogenic hepatic abscesses, although it has been used to treat amebic abscesses when medical management has failed or there is suspicion of superimposed bacterial infection or imminent rupture. Hepatic amebic abscesses have been noted to have a tendency to rupture through the diaphragm into the pleural space. Rupture into the pericardium is a dreaded complication with a very high mortality rate.

Echinococcal cysts may also occur in childhood, particularly in the endemic areas of the United States such as central California, Utah, and Arizona. Sonographically, these cysts usually appear as simple fluid-filled cysts in children, occasionally containing internal membranes.

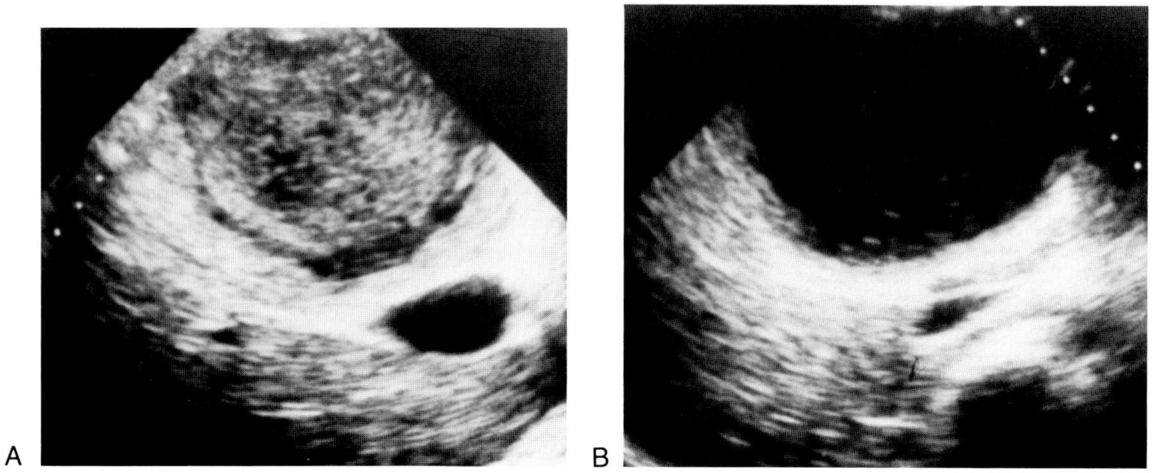

Fig. 5–80 Amebic abscess of the liver. **(A)** Initially, ultrasound showed a complex mass containing both fluid and echogenic material. **(B)** Shortly after therapy was instituted, this abscess appeared as a predominantly cystic mass with multiple fine echoes.

Hepatic Neoplasms

The majority of primary liver tumors in neonates and infants are benign, however malignant primary liver tumors are more common in older children. In infancy, the most common benign liver tumor is the hemangioma or hemangioendothelioma, a tumor composed of masses of immature endothelial cells interspersed with vascular channels. These tumors usually occur in infants before the age of 6 months and may be single or multiple. Forty-five percent of the cases are associated with cutaneous hemangiomas. Hemangiomas may be complicated by high output cardiac failure due to extensive arteriovenous shunting (Fig. 5–81), microangiopathic hemolytic anemia, thrombocytopenia, or intraperitoneal hemorrhage.

Ultrasonography is the procedure of choice for the initial evaluation of hepatic tumors. Hemangioendotheliomas classically appear on ultrasound as a complex liver mass containing multiple sonolucencies, which represent the vascular channels. Large draining veins and a dilated aorta proximal to the tumor may also be seen. The sonographic appearance can be quite variable, however, and other studies may be necessary. Radionuclide blood pool imaging may be helpful in demonstrating persistent radiotracer activity on delayed images in the region of the tumor. On CT, these tumors appear as hypodense lesions that enhance peripherally or diffusely following contrast. Doppler ultrasound can demonstrate increased blood flow through these tumors. The role of MRI is as yet uncertain for the diagnosis of hemangiomas in children but may prove useful as high signal intensity on heavily T_2-weighted images is characteristic of hemangiomas in general (Fig. 5–82). With arteriography, the enlarged feeding arteries are evident, as well as early filling of the hepatic veins. Arteriovenous shunting in the tumor is also demonstrable on Doppler ultrasound studies.

Many methods of treatment of hemangioendothelioma have been used, including lobectomy, steroids, radiation therapy, embolization, and hepatic artery ligation. Generally the choice of treatment depends on the size of the lesion and the degree of arteriovenous shunting involved.

The next most common benign liver tumor in infants and young children is the mesenchymal hamartoma.

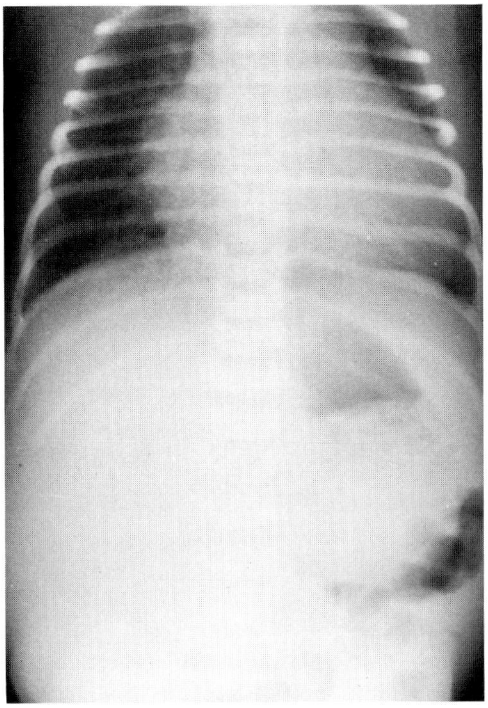

Fig. 5–81 Hemangioendothelioma of the liver with congestive heart failure. This infant presented with hepatomegaly, cardiomegaly, and pulmonary vascular congestion due to high output cardiac failure secondary to arteriovenous shunting within a large hemangioendothelioma.

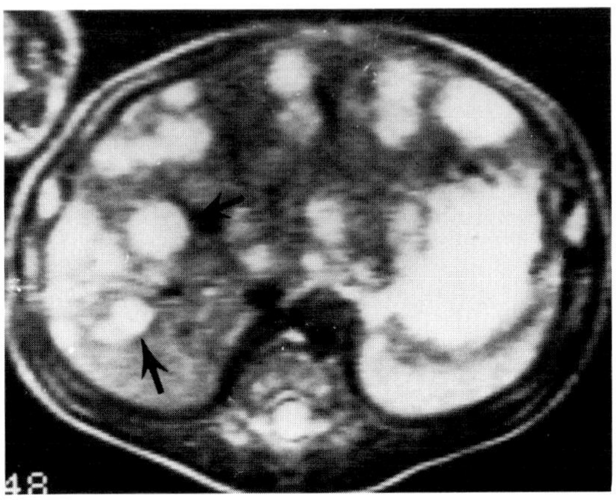

Fig. 5–82 Hemangioendotheliomatosis of the liver. Note the high signal intensity of the multiple hepatic nodules (*arrows*) on the axial T_2-weighted MRI.

Sonographically, this tumor usually appears as a multiloculated, septated cystic mass with scattered solid components. The mass on CT appears as multiple hypodense, ill-defined lesions, and MRI also shows the cystic nature of the lesion. The arteriographic appearance is quite variable and can be confused with that of hemangioma or malignancy. Malignant mesenchymomas have been reported in older children.

Hepatic adenoma is uncommon in children and when seen is almost always associated with glycogen storage disease. These tumors are hyperechoic on ultrasound, however the appearance may vary if the surrounding liver parenchyma demonstrates increased echogenicity. Nuclear scintigraphy usually shows areas of photon deficiency corresponding to these lesions.

Focal nodular hyperplasia is a condition that is sometimes confused with hepatic adenoma. On ultrasound, this condition may appear as single or multiple well-defined lesions of variable echogenicity. The true nature of these lesions is evident on scintigraphy using ^{99m}Tc sulfur colloid, because they are composed of normal hepatic tissue containing Kupffer cells, which demonstrate normal or increased concentration of the radiotracer. On CT, this lesion usually appears as a hypodense lesion that becomes hyperdense following contrast administration. A hypervascular mass with a spoke wheel appearance is typically seen on angiography.

Cystic hepatoblastoma is a rare tumor thought to arise from aberrant biliary ducts. On ultrasound it appears as a septated cystic lesion that often resembles mesenchymal hamartoma. Although it is a benign tumor, it does have malignant potential.

Malignant primary liver tumors are more common than benign tumors in children overall. Hepatoblastoma is the most common primary malignant tumor in children, occurring predominantly in children younger than 3 years of age. Hepatocellular carcinoma is the next most common malignant tumor and occurs more often in older infants and children. The ultrasound appearance of these tumors is rather nonspecific. They both may present as heterogenously echogenic masses with poorly defined margins (Fig. 5–83). Occasionally, the tumor may be surrounded by

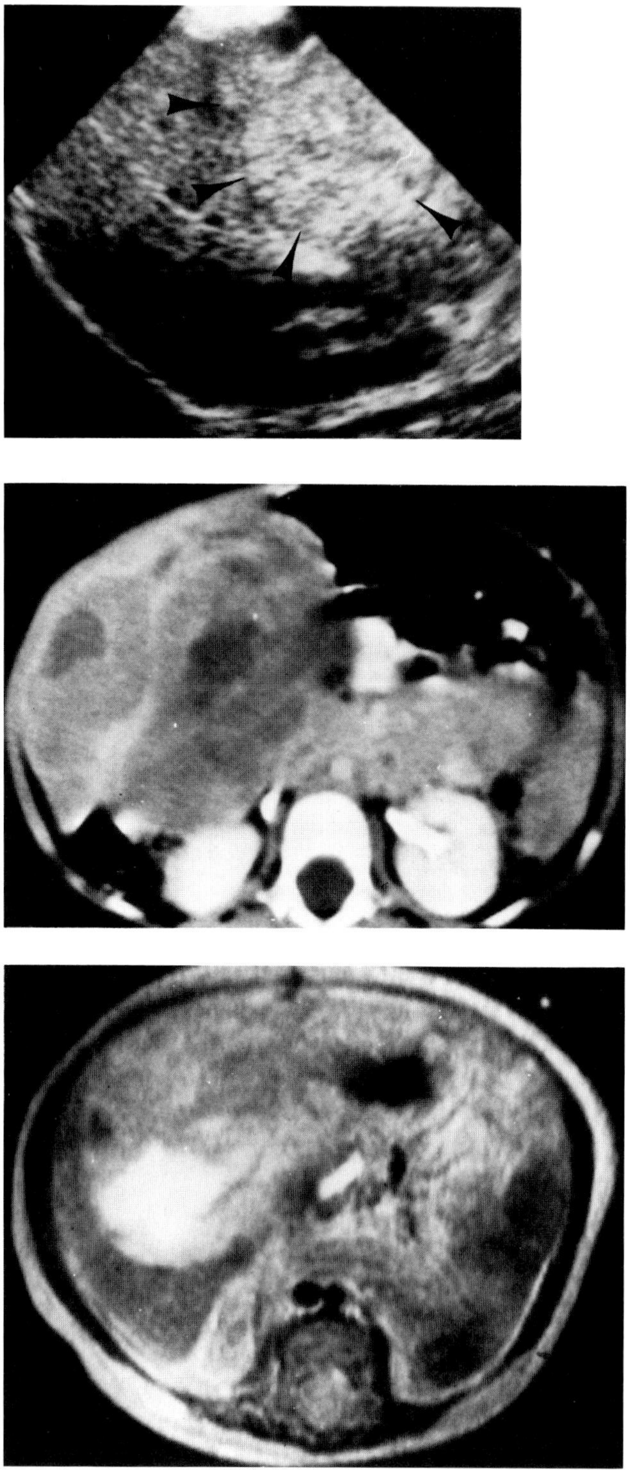

A

B

C

Fig. 5–83 Hepatoblastoma. **(A)** Longitudinal ultrasound shows a primarily echogenic mass extending from the inferior aspect of the liver (*arrowheads*). **(B)** Contrast-enhanced axial CT reveals involvement of most of the liver by a heterogeneous, nonenhancing mass. Multiple, low density areas indicating necrosis are present. **(C)** Axial T_2-weighted MRI also shows diffuse involvement of the liver by the high intensity tumor. Only a small portion of the posterior right lobe is spared.

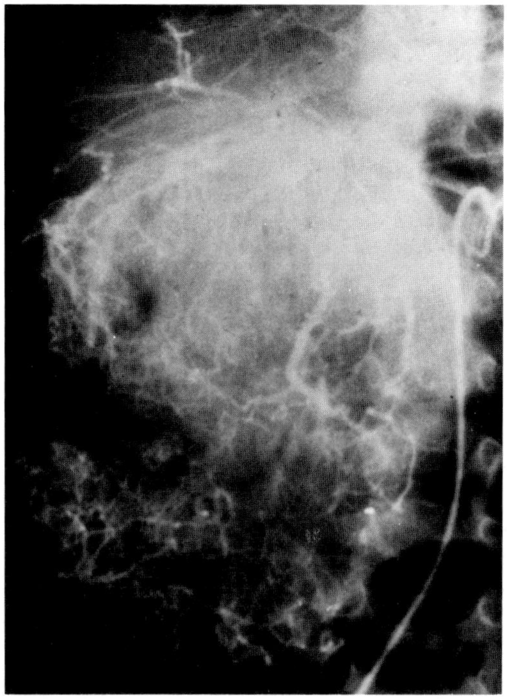

Fig. 5–84 Hepatoblastoma. Arteriography with selective injection of the hepatic artery demonstrates stretched vessels, neovascularity, and tumor blush.

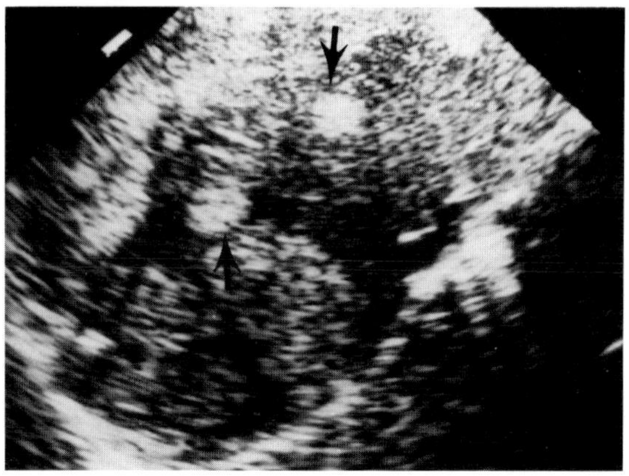

Fig. 5–85 Neuroblastoma metastatic to liver. These metastatic lesions appeared hyperechoic on longitudinal ultrasound (*arrows*).

a hypoechoic rim. On CT, these tumors are hypodense with variable degrees of contrast enhancement. This correlates with the angiographic findings that show them sometimes to be hypovascular and other times to be quite vascular. On angiography, both types of malignant tumors demonstrate neovascularity and diffuse tumor blush (Fig. 5–84). The evaluation of the hepatic vessels either by ultrasound or angiography is desirable, as invasion of the portal or hepatic veins is quite common and may affect subsequent therapy.

Neuroblastoma and Wilms' tumor are the most common neoplasms to metastasize to the liver in children. Lymphoma also is known to involve the liver. Although these tumors are usually hypoechoic sonographically, they occasionally may appear hyperechoic (Fig. 5–85). CT and MRI also are commonly used for evaluating the extent of these tumors.

Parenchymal Disease

Diffuse hepatic parenchymal disease in children may

FATTY LIVER

Inflammation
- Hepatitis

Systemic/metabolic
- Chronic protein malnutrition
- Cystic fibrosis
- Glycogen storage diseases
- Wilson's disease
- Galactosemia
- Tyrosinosis
- Fructose intolerance
- Alpha$_1$-antitrypsin deficiency

Miscellaneous
- Reye's syndrome
- Hyperalimentation
- Steroid therapy

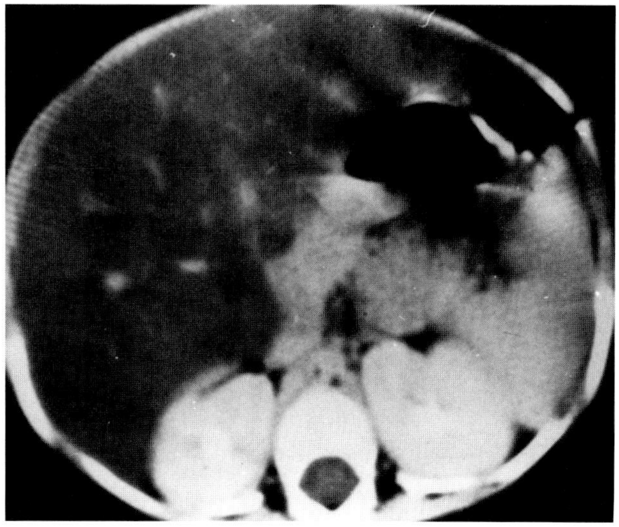

Fig. 5–86 Fatty infiltration of the liver. Note the diffusely decreased density of the liver by contrast-enhanced CT.

be due to a wide variety of conditions, including hepatitis and a variety of developmental and metabolic abnormalities. The radiologist plays a relatively minor role in the evaluation of most types of hepatitis, except in neonatal hepatitis. Nevertheless, when evidence of hepatic dysfunction is present in a child, some type of liver imaging is usually sought. Ultrasound is now the most common modality used for the initial evaluation of hepatic parenchymal abnormalities. A diffuse hyperechoic hepatic parenchymal pattern is often seen in pediatric patients with fatty infiltration, fibrosis, or cirrhosis of the liver.

In children a diffusely echogenic liver on ultrasound is most commonly due to fatty infiltration. Increased fat within the hepatocytes may be the result of hepatitis, metabolic or nutritional disorders, or exposure to certain toxins or drugs. If the fatty change is severe, increased radiolucency of the liver may be detectable on plain radiographs. Although diffusely increased echogenicity is a very common sonographic finding, it is somewhat subjective and may be difficult to detect in less severe cases. The change in liver density with fatty infiltration is probably most dramatic on CT (Fig. 5–86).

Chronic protein malnutrition is the most common cause of fatty infiltration of the liver in children. This is also the main cause for the development of hepatic fatty change in children with cystic fibrosis. Other metabolic diseases associated with fatty infiltration of the liver include glycogen storage diseases, Wilson's disease, galactosemia, tyrosinosis, fructose intolerance, and alpha$_1$-antitrypsin deficiency. Reye's syndrome, hyperalimentation, and steroid therapy may also lead to the accumulation of fat within the hepatocytes.

Sonographically, hyperechogenicity of the liver with fatty infiltration cannot be differentiated from that due to fibrosis or cirrhosis. This is not surprising since fatty infiltration precedes the development of cirrhosis in many of these diseases. The most common causes of cirrhosis in children are hepatitis and long-standing biliary tract obstruction (eg., biliary atresia, choledochal cysts). Many metabolic disorders such as Wilson's disease or alpha$_1$-antitrypsin deficiency also result in cirrhosis. Byler's disease is a hereditary form of intrahepatic cholestasis associated with abnormal bile acid transport, which eventually results in portal fibrosis, cirrhosis, and death.

Congenital hepatic fibrosis is a part of a group of diseases that include variable degrees of renal tubular ectasia with hepatic fibrosis and bile duct dilatation. If the cystic renal disease is the predominant abnormality, minor degrees of hepatic fibrosis occur and the condition presents in infancy as infantile polycystic kidney disease. If the condition presents in older children, hepatic fibrosis tends to be the predominant abnormality with less severe renal involvement. Children with the latter form of this disease tend to present in adolescence with evidence of portal hypertension and bleeding gastroesophageal varices.

Portal hypertension is a common result of any of the causes of hepatic fibrosis and cirrhosis. In children, however, it is more commonly due to extrahepatic portal vein obstruction due to thrombosis. The cause of this thrombosis is often idiopathic, although sepsis, umbilical vein catheterization, omphalitis, and intra-abdominal infections such as perforated appendicitis have all been implicated. Uncommonly portal venous pressure may also be elevated by increased flow through the portal system (eg., arteriovenous malformations of the bowel) or by hepatic vein thrombosis or increased right atrial pressure.

Classically, the evaluation of portal hypertension requires invasive studies such as splenoportography or selective visceral arteriography (Fig. 5–87). These studies are essential for the evaluation of the vascular anatomy and collateral circulation prior to surgery. Nevertheless, initial use of ultrasound can provide important information, such as thickening of the lesser omentum in the presence of esophageal varices. Collateral vessels also may be identified, and Doppler studies may demonstrate abnormal direction of flow in the portal vessels. In cases of portal vein thrombosis, the portal vein may not be visible with only an area of increased echogenicity in its expected location (Fig. 5–88). Occasionally the thrombus itself may be visible within the portal vein. The development of cavernous transformation of the portal vein may appear as a reticulated subhepatic mass. Dynamic CT and MRI can also be quite useful for identifying the thrombosed vessels, collaterals, varices, and cavernous transformation.

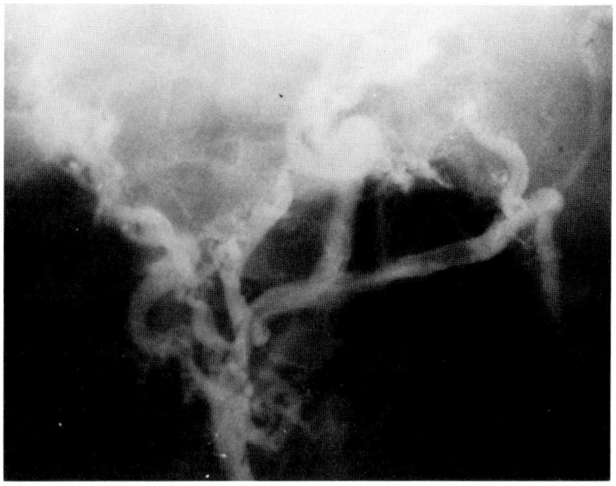

Fig. 5–87 Portal vein thrombosis. An intraoperative splenoportogram revealed nonfilling of the normal portal vein with cavernous transformation due to multiple collaterals from the splenic and superior mesenteric veins. Collaterals are also noted in the region of the gastric fundus.

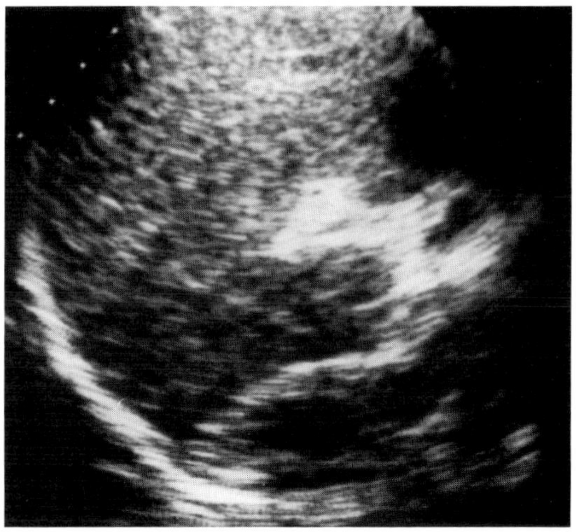

Fig. 5–88 Portal vein thrombosis. Longitudinal ultrasound shows an area of increased echogenicity in the expected location of the portal vein.

Miscellaneous Biliary Tract Abnormalities

Cholelithiasis and cholecystitis are not as common in children as in adults, however now that ultrasound is available, gallstones are discovered more commonly than was previously suspected. Not only do gallstones occur in patients with hematologic disorders such as sickle cell disease, they also commonly are found in patients with no known hemolytic disorder. Cholecystitis is usually associated with cholelithiasis, but occasionally acalculous cholecystitis occurs in childhood, especially in infants with neonatal sepsis.

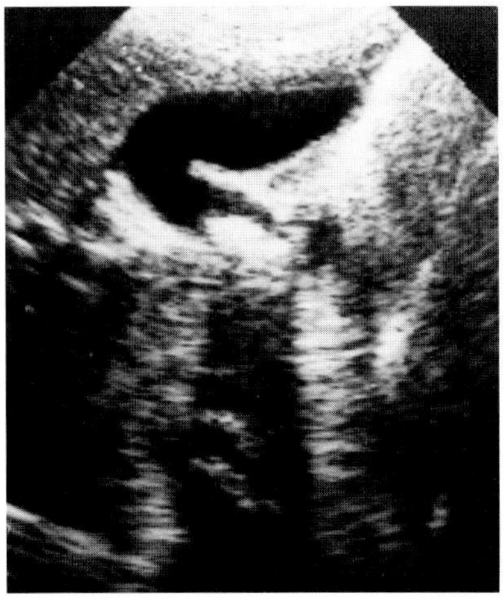

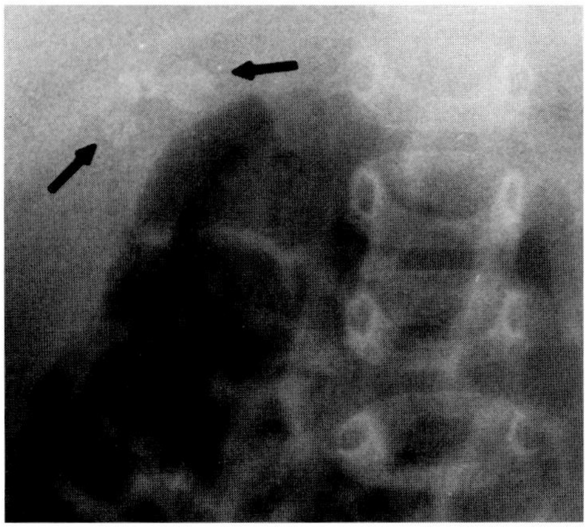

Fig. 5–89 Cholelithiasis. **(A)** Echogenic gallstones with sharp acoustical shadowing are identified by transverse sonography near the gallbladder neck. **(B)** Calcified gallstones in the right upper quadrant (*arrows*) on an abdominal radiograph.

Ultrasonography and hepatobiliary scintigraphy are the most useful studies for evaluating possible gallbladder disease. Ultrasound easily identifies the echogenic gallstones with sharp acoustical shadowing (Fig. 5–89) and helps to exclude bile duct obstruction by the stones. The gallbladder wall may be thickened in cholecystitis; however, this is a nonspecific finding that can also be seen with ascites, hypoalbuminemia, and systemic venous hypertension. Because the cystic duct is obstructed in acute cholecystitis, hepatobiliary scintigraphy will demonstrate nonfilling of the gallbladder.

In some infants, a layer of debris or sludge may be seen in the gallbladder (Fig. 5–90). Sludge and gallstones are more common in infants receiving total parenteral nutrition and possibly in those receiving diuretics. Any cause of ileal dysfunction leading to abnormal bile salt metabolism can also lead to gallstones.

Hydrops of the gallbladder is not common in children, although it has been associated with the mucocutaneous lymph node syndrome. More commonly the cystic duct obstruction will be due to gallbladder sludge in the bile ducts or other causes of mechanical obstruction. The gallbladder can become quite large in this condition and may be palpable as a right upper quadrant mass.

Spontaneous bile duct perforation is an uncommon cause of ascites in infancy. The exact etiology of this condition is unknown, although it has been postulated that congenital weakness of the bile duct wall, bile duct obstruction due to congenital stenosis or stones, or trauma may be involved. The site of leakage is usually at the junction of the cystic and common bile ducts. The bile may leak into a loculated collection below the liver or may be widely distributed in the peritoneal cavity or cause peritonitis. Ultrasound will show either diffuse or loculated areas of intraperito-

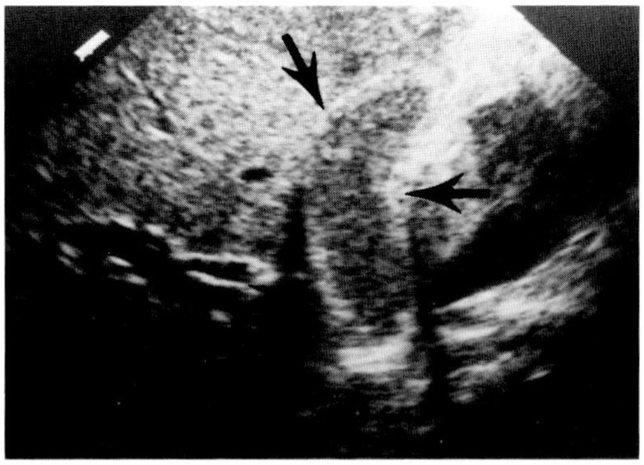

Fig. 5–90 Acalculous cholecystitis in a child with sickle cell disease. Transverse sonography revealed a large amount of sludge filling the gallbladder (*arrows*). No echogenic calculi were identified.

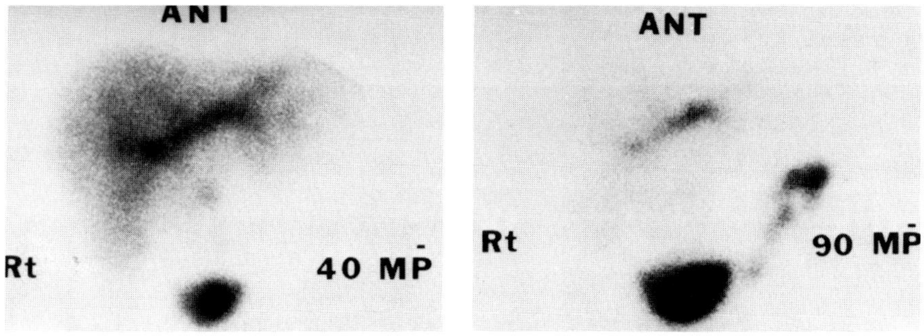

Fig. 5–91 Spontaneous bile duct perforation. Hepatobiliary scintigraphy reveals leakage of the radiotracer from the biliary tract into a loculated infrahepatic collection. At surgery, the site of leakage was at the junction of the cystic and common bile duct.

neal fluid, which can be verified by hepatobiliary scintigraphy. The latter study will clearly show excretion of the radiotracer into the areas of abnormal fluid seen on the ultrasound (Fig. 5–91).

PANCREAS

Pancreatitis

Although less common than in adults, pancreatitis is not an uncommon condition in children. The most common cause of pancreatitis in childhood is blunt abdominal trauma, often secondary to child abuse. Other causes include viral infection and drugs (eg., steroids, L-asparaginase). Many cases are idiopathic. An hereditary form of chronic relapsing pancreatitis has also been described.

Ultrasound is an excellent modality for evaluating the pancreas in pediatric patients. As opposed to adults, a child's pancreas can usually be visualized in its entirety, due to a lack of fat and the relatively large size of the left lobe of the liver in children. Unfortunately, acute pancreatitis produces a variable sonographic appearance. Although some authors have noted enlargement or decreased echogenicity in such cases, more commonly the pancreas is normal in size and echogenicity. Ultrasound can readily identify pancreatic or extrapancreatic fluid collections and is a useful means of diagnosing the development of a pancreatic pseudocyst. Occasionally, acute pancreatitis is accompanied by the development of increased echogenicity in the pararenal space (Fig. 5–92). This is presumably due to the liberation of pancreatic enzymes, leading to lipolysis and edema of the perinephric tissues. In chronic pancreatitis, the pancreas becomes small and contracted with areas of increased echogenicity corresponding to fatty infiltration and calcification.

Pancreatitis may also be a complication of cystic fibrosis, in which the thick secretions become impacted in the small pancreatic duct leading to dilatation of the ducts and eventually cyst formation. If pancreatitis is present, the pancreas may enlarge but more often the pancreas appears normal in size and echogenicity sonographically.

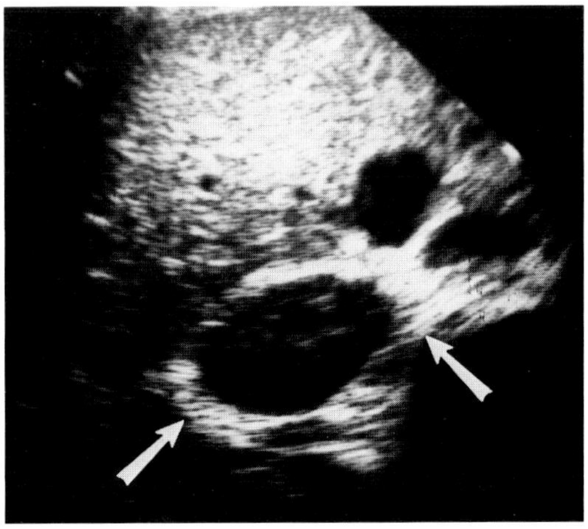

Fig. 5–92 Acute pancreatitis. Note the increased perinephric echogenicity (*arrows*) by transverse ultrasound.

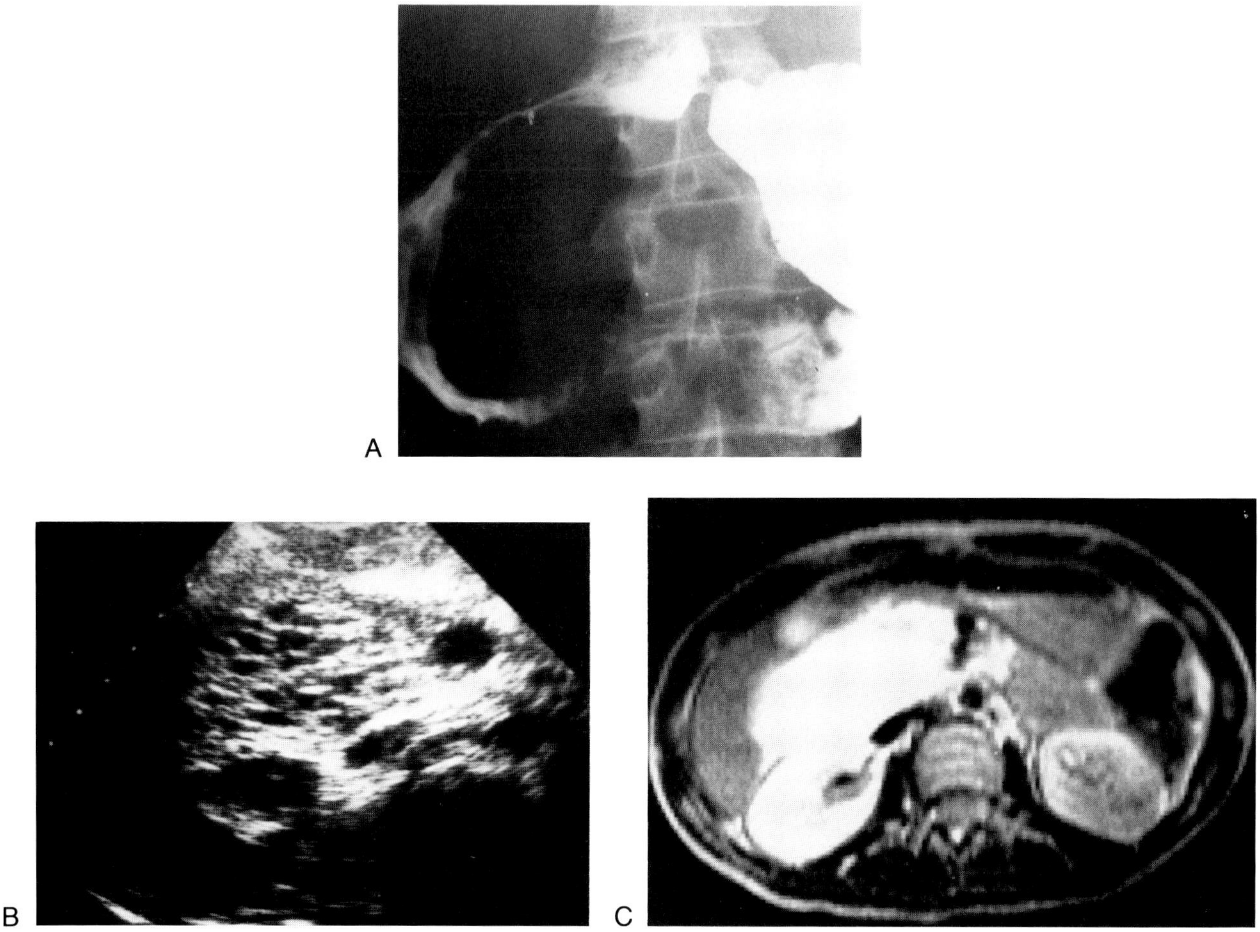

Fig. 5–93 Lymphangioma of the pancreas. **(A)** An upper GI series on this child with chronic pancreatitis shows widening and effacement of the duodenal C-loop. **(B)** Transverse ultrasound revealed a mass containing multiple tubular cystic structures in the region of the head of the pancreas. **(C)** T_2-weighted MRI showed the pancreatic head mass to be of high signal intensity.

Pancreatic Tumors

All tumors of the pancreas are rare in infants and children. The majority of cystic lesions of the pancreas represent pancreatic pseudocysts, usually due to pancreatic trauma. True congenital cysts of the pancreas are very rare. The most significant of the benign pancreatic tumors is the beta islet cell tumor or insulinoma. These tumors may result in profound neonatal hypoglycemia due to their production of insulin. The diffuse form of this tumor is referred to as *nesidioblastosis*. The insulinoma is very difficult to identify on imaging studies and even at surgery; the ultrasound appearance of nesidioblastosis has not been reported. Other benign pancreatic tumors include cystadenoma, hamartoma, lipoma, lymphangioma (Fig. 5–93) and hemangioma.

Primary malignant tumors of the pancreas are also quite rare in children. Pancreatic carcinoma does occur and, as in adults, is usually quite large at the time of discovery, often with distant metastases.

SUGGESTED READINGS

1. Babcock DS: Neonatal and Pediatric Ultrasonography. Churchill Livingstone, New York, 1989
2. Balistreri WF: Neonatal cholestasis. J Pediatr 106:171, 1985
3. Barlow B, Tabor E, Blanc WA, Santolli TV, Harris RC: Choledochal cyst: A review of 19 cases. J Pediatr 89:934, 1976.
4. Bass EM, Cremin BJ: Choledochal cysts: a clinical and radiological evaluation of 21 cases. Pediatr Radiol 5:81, 1976
5. Bisset GS III, Kirks DR: Intussusception in infants and children: diagnosis and therapy. Radiology 168:141, 1988
6. Campbell JB, Quattromani FL, Foley LCL: Foley catheter removal of blunt esophageal foreign bodies. Experience with 100 consecutive children. Pediatr Radiol 13:116, 1983
7. Daneman A, Woodward S, de Silva M: The radiology of neonatal necrotizing enterocolitis (NEC). A review of 47 cases and the literature. Pediatr Radiol 7:70, 1978
8. Franken EA Jr, Kao SCS, Smith WL, Sato Y: Imaging of the acute abdomen in infants and children. AJR 153:921, 1989
9. Hayden CK Jr, Swischuk LE: Pediatric Ultrasonography. Williams & Wilkins, Baltimore, 1987
10. Hayden CK Jr, Swischuk LE, Lobe TE, et al: Ultrasound: the definitive imaging modality in pyloric stenosis. RadioGraphics 4:517, 1984
11. Kirks DR, Coleman RE, Filston HC, et al: An imaging approach to persistent neonatal jaundice. AJR 142:461, 1984
12. Laurin S, Kaude JV: Diagnosis of liver-spleen abscesses in children—with emphasis on ultrasound for the initial and follow-up examinations. Pediatr Radiol 14:198, 1984
13. Leonidas JC, Berdon WE, Baker DH, Santulli TV: Meconium ileus and its complications: a reappraisal of plain film roentgen diagnostic criteria. AJR 108:598, 1970
14. LeQuesne GW, Reilly BJ: Functional immaturity of the large bowel in the newborn infant. Radiol Clin North Am 13:331, 1975
15. Merten DF, Kirks DR: Amebic liver abscess in children: the role of diagnostic imaging. AJR 143:1325, 1984
16. Miller JH, Greenspan BS: Integrated imaging of hepatic tumors in childhood. Part I. Malignant lesions (primary and metastatic). Radiology 154:83, 1985
17. Miller JH, Greenspan BS: Integrated imaging of hepatic tumors of childhood. Part II. Benign lesions (congenital, reparative, and inflammatory). Radiology 154:91, 1985
18. Rosenfield NS, Ablow RC, Markowitz RI, et al: Hirschsprung's disease: accuracy of the barium enema examination. Radiology 150:393, 1984
19. Swischuk LE, Fawcett HD, Hayden CK Jr: Gastroesophagal reflux: how much imaging is required? RadioGraphics 8:1137, 1988

6
Genitourinary System

Lori L. Barr

The pediatric genitourinary system helps illustrate the complimentary roles of diagnostic imaging modalities. Recent refinements in real-time ultrasound equipment have improved image quality to the point that ultrasound is now the screening modality of choice, with very few exceptions, for evaluating a child's abdomen. Retroperitoneal structures and pelvic organs can be readily identified and measured. Blood flow to the organ of interest may be evaluated using duplex Doppler analysis. Although ultrasound provides excellent anatomic detail, it provides little information about organ function and is quite nonspecific in certain pathologic conditions.

Renal scintigraphy using technetium 99m-diethylenetriamine-pentacetic acid (^{99m}Tc-DTPA) allows anatomic visualization and an accurate evaluation of renal function. The clearance rate of DTPA correlates well with creatinine clearance and thus provides useful information about glomerular filtration. Bolus administration permits cortical imaging, evaluation of renal perfusion, and excretion. Computer analysis allows differential evaluation of each kidney in all phases of excretion. Two other radionuclides, technetium 99m-2,3 dimercaptosuccinic acid (^{99m}Tc-DMSA) and technetium 99m-glucoheptonate (^{99m}Tc-GH) are utilized for dedicated cortical imaging. These agents are reserved for differentiation of specific parenchymal conditions, including inflammatory defects, cortical pseudotumors, and neoplasms.

Information about structure and function may be provided by excretory urography. While children demonstrate the fewest side effects from administration of intravenous contrast material, the use of low osmolality, nonionic contrast agents, in a dose of 2 mg/kg, lowers the incidence of contrast reactions even further. Excretory urography provides optimal visualization of nondilated ureters and may be helpful in delineating uncomplicated congenital anomalies difficult to detect with other modalities. In the neonate, diminished parenchymal concentration of contrast material results in suboptimal visualization of the urinary tract. The value of excretory urography in this age group is limited.

Low osmolality, nonionic contrast agents may also be used for contrast-enhanced CT, arteriography, and venography. Contrast-enhanced CT is the imaging modality of choice for pediatric blunt abdominal trauma evaluation. It is more sensitive in detecting renal parenchymal contusions than any other modality. Associated injuries are also readily detected. Contiguous, dynamic, 5-mm thick CT scans obtained after IV injection of contrast material allow thorough evaluation of both kidneys. Delayed images may be useful in documenting contrast extravasation. If renal calculi are suspected, noncontrast images are obtained prior to dynamic contrast bolus scanning.

While MRI does not provide much additional information in the staging of renal and pararenal neoplasms, its use has several advantages. The option to image in both the coronal and parasagittal planes allows excellent visualization of the retroperitoneal vasculature and the reproductive organs. It is especially useful for evaluation of inferior vena cava thrombus. Complex congenital anomalies of the female reproductive system are readily classified using multiplanar MRI. Evaluation of intersex anomalies and staging of testicular neoplasms may be achieved with MRI as well.

Evaluation of the pelvocaliceal collecting structures and ureters is best accomplished by opacification of the system with contrast material. This may be achieved through excretory urography, retrograde ureterography, and antegrade pyelography. None of the cross-sectional imaging modalities add significant information to that obtained with use of the excretory urogram, except in cases of extrinsic ureteral displacement or compression.

Bladder form and function are best evaluated with retrograde studies. In girls, conventional voiding cystourethrography or radionuclide cystography provides equal information about vesiculoureteral reflux. In boys, it is useful to perform at least one conventional cystogram early in the course of the patient's care to evaluate the anatomy of the male urethra and bladder outlet.

KIDNEY ABNORMALITIES

Normal

In fetal life, the renal cortex is formed by the development of renal lobes, the number is determined by the number of calyces. The size is determined by the number of ducts draining into each calyx. The cortex of the renal lobe is divided into the septal cortex (columns of Bertin), which encircles the sides of the medulla, and the central lobar cortex at the base of the lobe. In fetal life, the septal cortex extends down to the level of the papillae. Central extension is usually not as pronounced in adult life. Occasionally, a prominent column of Bertin extending to the level of the papilla may be mistaken for a renal neoplasm on either ultrasound or excretory urography.

KIDNEY ABNORMALITIES

- Normal
  - Parenchymal shape, contour, echotexture
  - Ptosis
  - Compensatory hypertrophy
- Congenital
  - Position anomalies
  - Fusion anomalies
  - Duplication
  - Hypoplasia/agenesis
  - Cysts/dysplasia
  - Vascular anomalies
- Infection/inflammation
  - Acute/chronic pyelonephritis
  - Reflux nephropathy
  - Tubulointerstitial nephritis
  - Glomerular diseases
- Vascular
  - Hemolytic uremic syndrome
  - Renal artery thrombosis
  - Renal vein thrombosis
  - Cortical/papillary necrosis
  - Acute tubular necrosis
  - Hypertension
- Neoplasm
  - Angiomyolipoma
  - Metanephric ridge tumors
  - Renal cell carcinoma
  - Neuroblastoma
  - Lymphoma
- Generalized/systemic
  - Nephrocalcinosis/urolithiasis
- Trauma/iatrogenic
  - Catastrophic injury
  - Major injury
  - Minor injury
  - Urinoma
  - Transplantation
  - Arteriovenous fistula

^{99m}Tc-DTPA imaging rapidly delineates normally functioning cortex from neoplasm.

The fetal kidney consists of seven anterior and seven posterior lobes separated by a fibrous longitudinal groove. Later in fetal life fusion of the anterior and posterior renal masses occurs. Often, the fibrous band separating the two masses remains visible on ultrasound as the inter-renicular septum (Fig. 6–1). Visible in the medial parasagittal plane, this should not be confused with scarring. When incomplete fusion of the anterior and posterior lobules occurs, the junctional parenchymal defect is visible as a wedge of increased echogenicity in the longitudinal plane (Fig. 6–2).

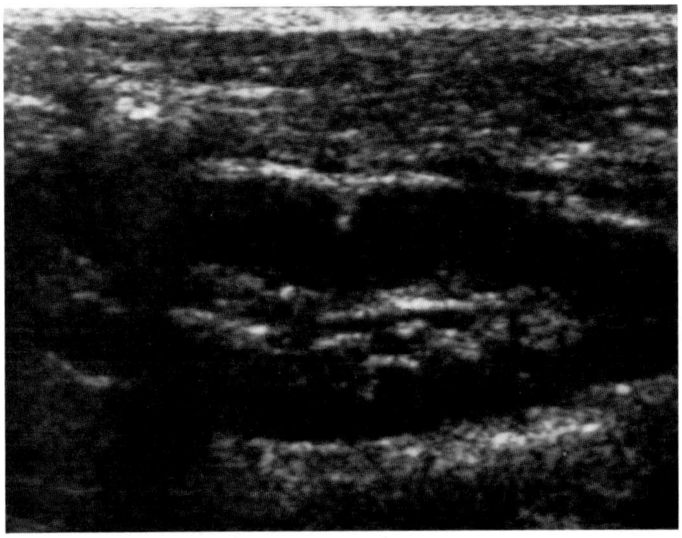

Fig. 6–1 Inter-renicular septum. Longitudinal scan of the right kidney demonstrates an echogenic line representing a normal variant rather than focal scarring in the midportion of the right kidney.

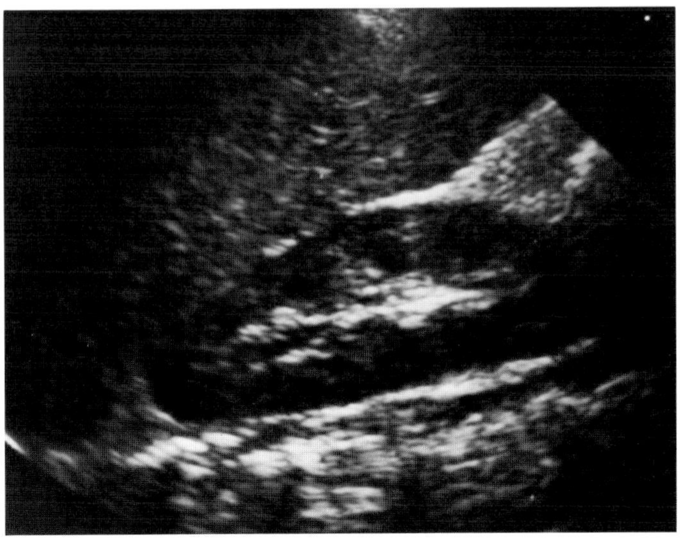

Fig. 6–2 Junctional parenchymal defect. Longitudinal scan of the right kidney demonstrates a wedge-shaped area of increased echogenicity in the midportion of the kidney. Note no decrease in the thickness of the cortex to indicate scarring is present.

The fetal kidney is much more lobulated than the adult kidney; smoothing occurs as one approaches adulthood. However, fetal lobulation may persist throughout life and is a normal variant. The lobulation of the cortex should correspond with the contour of the interpapillary line on excretory urograms and ultrasound examination (Fig. 6–3). If the thickness of the parenchyma is uneven, a pathologic cause of parenchymal thinning should be considered.

In all age groups it is useful to compare the echogenicity of the renal parenchyma with that of adjacent liver or splenic parenchyma. Premature infants may normally demonstrate increased echogenicity of the renal parenchyma as compared with the liver (Fig. 6–4). Neonates should demonstrate equal echogenicity of the two organs. Factors contributing to increased renal parenchymal echogenicity in the neonatal period include a greater proportional volume of the glomeruli to surrounding tissue in the renal cortex and a greater proportion of the cellular components in the glomerular tuft. Also, a greater number of loops of Henle are located within the cortex during early infancy. After infancy, the renal parenchyma

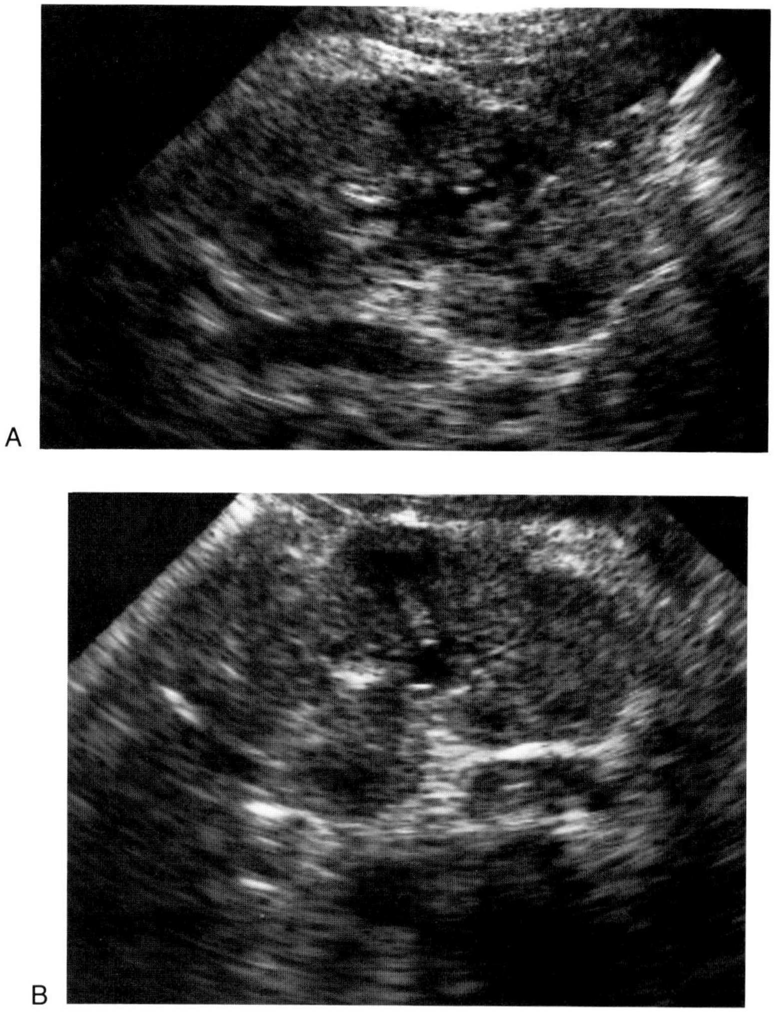

Fig. 6–3 Fetal lobulation. **(A)** Longitudinal ultrasound examination of the right kidney demonstrates a lobulated cortical margin. The parenchymal thickness and corticomedullary differentiation are normal. **(B)** Longitudinal ultrasound of the left kidney demonstrates a "dromedary hump," a normal fetal lobulation.

usually appears less echogenic than that of the liver or spleen. As the child ages, the corticomedullary junction should remain easily discernible with ultrasound. The medullary pyramids become slightly more echogenic. The renal sinus should always have bright echoes caused by the combination of sinus fat, collecting structures, and blood vessels.

The number of calices present varies between patients and between kidneys. Incomplete division of the calyces results in dysmorphism and megacalyces. These variations are more common at the poles than in the midportion of the kidney.

Diaphragmatic motion is responsible for movement

A

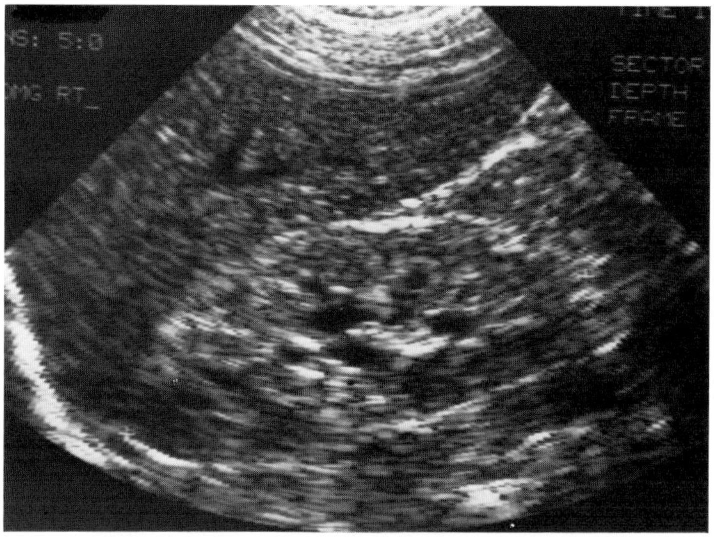

B

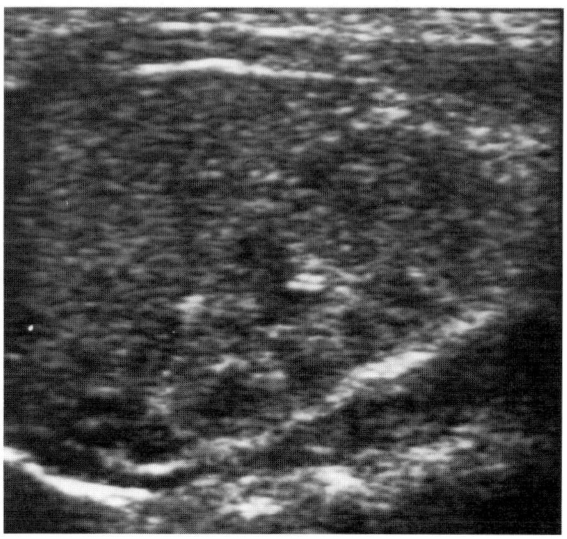

Fig. 6–4 Normal neonatal renal echogenicity. **(A)** Longitudinal scan of the right kidney demonstrates an increase in the echogenicity of the parenchyma as compared with the adjacent liver in a premature infant. **(B)** Longitudinal scan of the right kidney in a full-term neonate demonstrates that the renal parenchymal echogenicity is equal to that of the liver.

of the kidney, which occasionally will be hypermobile or ptotic. Excess mobility is of no clinical significance, although patients may rarely present with abdominal pain. The diagnosis is confirmed with the use of ^{99m}Tc-DTPA scintigraphy when the kidney moves more than 1.5 vertebral body lengths in the crainocaudad direction or across the midline. Ptosis is more common in females than males and usually occurs on the right.

If a 75 percent loss of renal function occurs, the kidney has the ability to hypertrophy in response. Most of the increase in renal size is due to nephron dilatation although a minor increase in the number of cells in the kidney also occurs. Either congenital agenesis of the contralateral kidney or acquired loss of function during childhood will result in compensatory hypertrophy. The hypertrophied kidney is greater than two standard deviations in size as compared with normal size for the patient's age, height, or weight. The average kidney in the neonate is approximately 4 cm in size. Growth of the kidneys is linear throughout childhood. The average kidney at age 18 is 10 cm in craniocaudal length.

Congenital

Ectopic kidneys are the result of abnormal migration of the metanephros from its original location in the pelvis (Fig. 6–5). Ectopia is more common in males than females. Simple ectopia describes a kidney that has either failed to migrate (pelvic kidney) or has migrated too far (thoracic kidney). Crossed ectopia results when one of the kidneys migrates along the

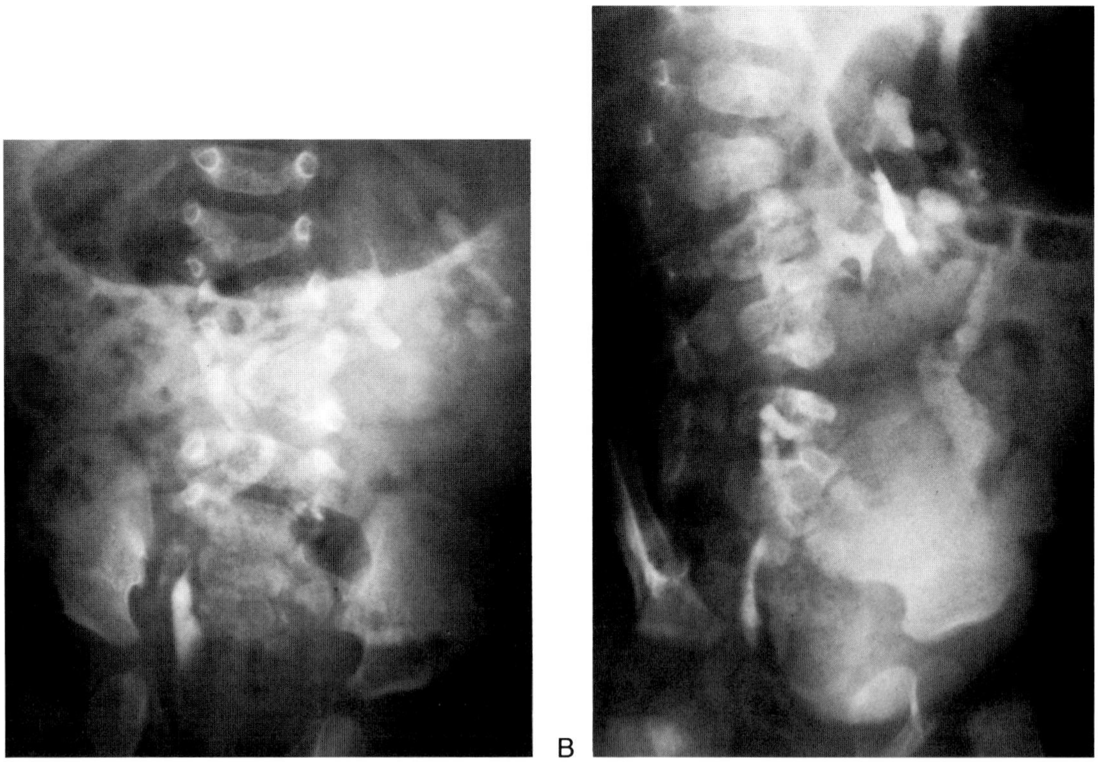

A B

Fig. 6–5 Ectopic kidney. **(A)** Frontal view from an excretory urogram demonstrates conspicuous absence of the right kidney in the right renal fossa. Two renal masses and two collecting structures are identified on the left, although the right ureter inserts normally. Note the segmentation fusion anomalies of the lumbar spine. **(B)** Oblique view better demonstrates the abnormal low orientation of the crossed, fused, right ectopic kidney.

opposite side of the body so that both kidneys lie along the same psoas muscle margin. The ureter from the ectopic kidney crosses the midline and enters the trigone in the usual location. Occasionally both kidneys may be crossed. Crossed ectopia most commonly occurs with fusion of the two kidneys and occasionally is associated with absence of a kidney. Ten to fifteen percent of pelvic kidneys also demonstrate crossed ectopia.

One of the most common renal anomalies is the horseshoe kidney, which occurs in approximately 1 out of every 350 to 600 people, and may be associated with Turner's syndrome. Males are affected more often than females. Patients may present with abdominal pain or a palpable mass may be detected. Other congenital malformations occur in up to one-third of patients. Midline fusion of the two renal masses is most likely to occur at the lower poles anterior to the aorta and inferior vena cava. Frequently, malrotation, vascular anomalies, and caudal displacement are associated with the horseshoe kidney. The renal pelvis often arises from the superior aspect of the renal mass and the ureters course anterolaterally (Fig. 6–6). The abnormal positioning of the pelvocalyceal collecting structures predisposes the patient to stone formation and obstruction.

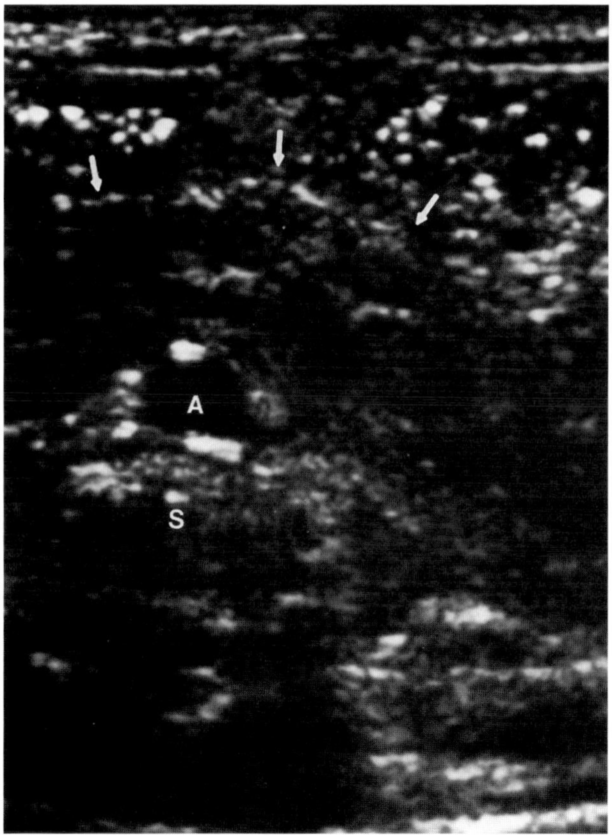

Fig. 6–6 Horseshoe kidney. Transverse scan of the midabdomen demonstrates the aorta (*A*) and spine (*S*) in the midline. Anterior to the aorta is the renal mass, demonstrating normal corticomedullary differentiation (*arrows*).

Other less common fusion anomalies include lump, disk, and pancake kidneys. Like the horseshoe kidney, these are solitary renal masses usually located low in the pelvis. The radiologist's role in fusion anomalies is to decide whether the abdominal mass is functioning renal tissue either by radionuclide scanning or CT. Failure to recognize the presence of a fused renal anomaly before surgery for an abdominal mass will lead to increased mortality if no other functioning renal tissue is present.

Duplication of the kidney describes the presence of two renal pelves draining the same kidney (Fig. 6–7). The surrounding renal parenchyma may be uniform in size or a cleft may be seen at the junction of the renal masses. The latter may be confused with the diagnosis of supernumerary kidneys. The two renal pelves may share a common ureter or have two separate ureters. In the latter case, the upper pole is drained by a ureter inserting ectopically into the bladder, reproductive organs, or perineum. The lower pole ureter inserts into the bladder trigone as usual. The upper pole moiety is predisposed to ureterovesicular reflux only if drained by an ectopic ureter inserting outside of the bladder. The lower pole moiety is commonly damaged secondary to ureterovesicular reflux. Hydronephrosis may occur if the upper pole ureter is obstructed (Weigert-Meyer rule).

Three forms of renal hypoplasia are recognized pathologically: unilateral, simple bilateral, and oligomeganephronie. Unilateral hypoplasia is exceedingly rare and is a diagnosis of exclusion. Other causes of a unilateral small kidney such as dysplasia and reflux nephropathy must be ruled out. Bilateral simple hypoplasia is perhaps the rarest of renal anomalies. Ten percent of bilateral simple hypoplasia cases are famil-

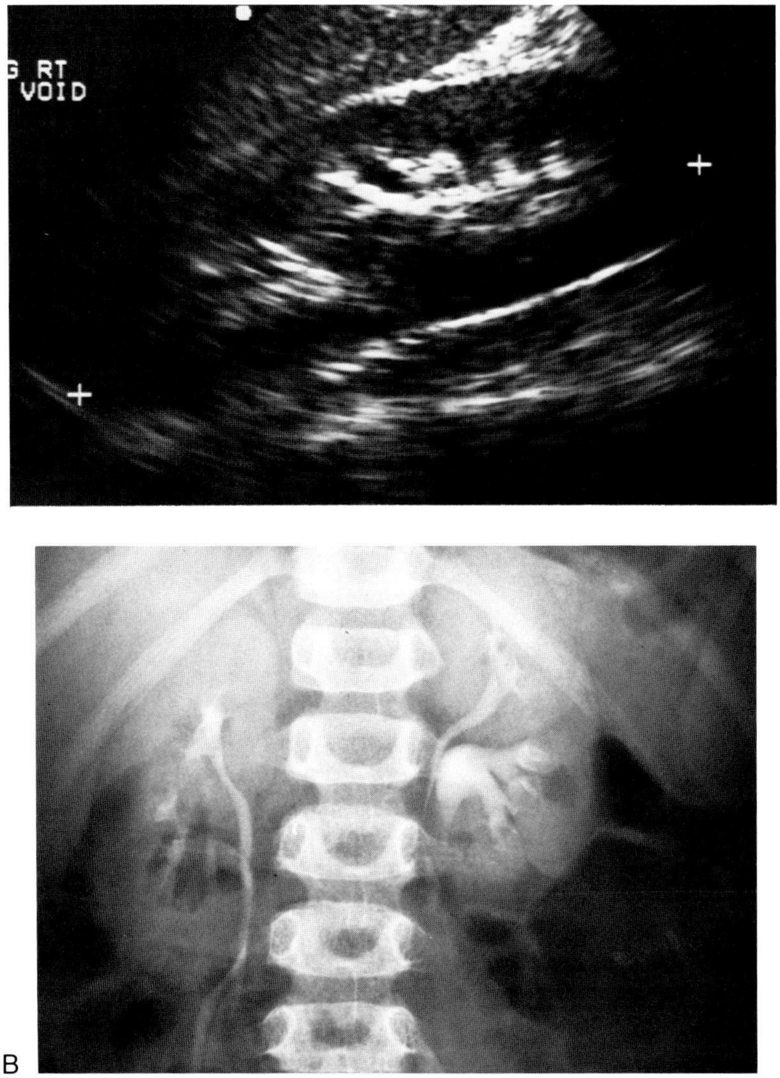

A

B

Fig. 6–7 Duplex kidney. **(A)** Longitudinal ultrasound image demonstrates a cortical bar extending through the middle of the elongated right kidney. **(B)** Excretory urogram demonstrates bilateral renal duplications with slight prominence of the left lower pole moiety collecting structures. On a voiding cystourethrogram, reflux was seen into the left lower pole moiety.

ial. The diagnosis is made when the pathologist identifies normal histology rather than dysplasia after biopsy. If untreated, patients develop hypertension and progressive renal tubular acidosis; therefore, transplant is the treatment of choice. Oligomeganephronie describes the condition of small kidneys due to a decreased number of glomeruli that are larger than normal in size. Patients present with symptoms of polydypsia and polyuria because the ability to concentrate the urine has been lost. Renal insufficiency leads to progressive renal failure and the child may die during the second decade of life.

Unilateral agenesis of the kidney occurs in approximately 1 in 500 live births and is frequently associated with other anomalies of the genitourinary tract and cardiovascular system. Resultant compensatory hypertrophy of the remaining kidney occurs. Bilateral renal agenesis is incompatible with life.

A 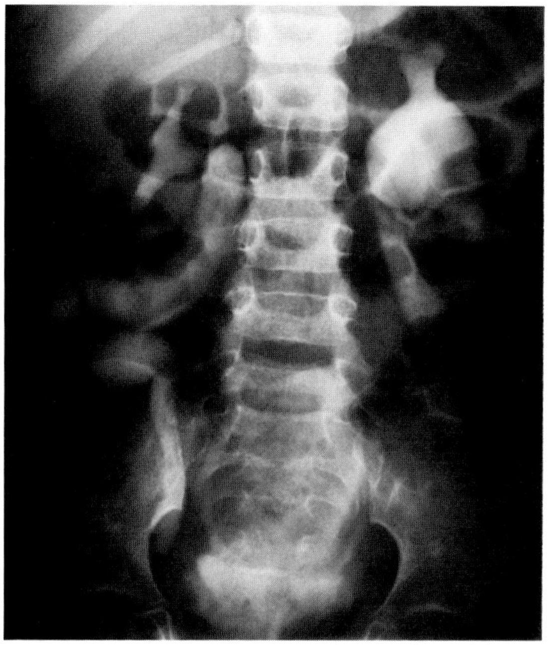 B 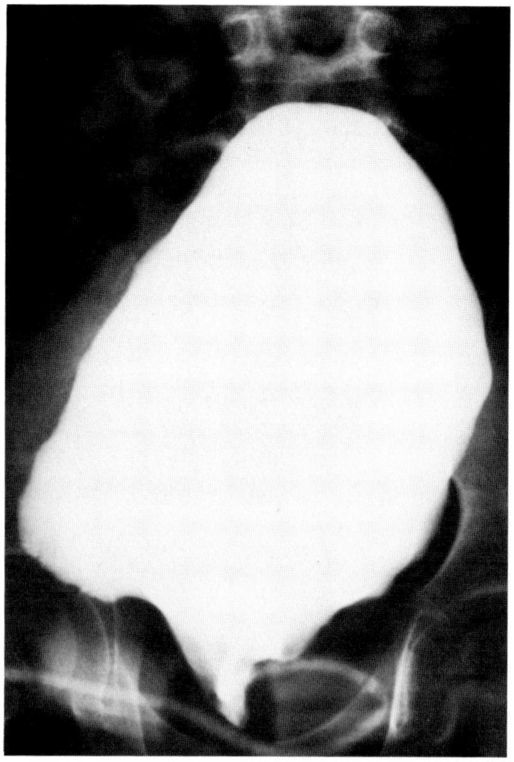

Fig. 6–8 Prune-belly syndrome. **(A)** Excretory urogram from a patient with absent abdominal musculature, cryptorchidism, and symptoms of bladder outlet obstruction. Note the global parenchymal loss of the left kidney and bilateral megacalyces and megaureters. **(B)** Megacystis is demonstrated on the filled bladder radiograph during voiding cystourethrography. All of the findings are consistent with the diagnosis of prune-belly syndrome.

Potter's syndrome describes the association of ascites, oligohydramnios, and pulmonary hypoplasia. This syndrome may be the first indication that a child has prune-belly syndrome (Eagle-Barrett syndrome). Prune-belly syndrome is the association of absent or hypoplastic abdominal muscles, cryptorchidism, and cystic dysplasia of the kidneys. The type of dysplasia present with this disease varies considerably. Other associated anomalies are megaureter, megacystis, and urethral obstruction (Fig. 6–8).

One of the rarest renal anomalies is supernumerary kidneys. The supernumerary kidney is usually smaller than the ipsilateral kidney and drains to the bladder by either a common distal ureter or through an ectopic ureterocele. It may be difficult to distinguish supernumerary kidneys from renal duplication. These patients usually present with recurrent urinary tract infections. Since the supernumerary kidney has an increased rate of infection, surgical removal may be necessary.

Renal cystic/dysplastic disease encompasses a spectrum of clinical and pathologic entities. The classification of these diseases continues to generate controversy throughout the medical literature. The first reliable classification was published by Osathanondh and Potter in 1964. Much of the radiologic literature centers around the Potter classification. Potter's classification of polycystic kidneys has questionable clinicopathologic application today since many factors such as lower urinary tract obstruction and infection have been shown to cause cystic kidney disease. Variations on the Elkin-Bernstein classification published in 1969 take into consideration the clinical and radiographic features of the patient (Table 6–1). Ultrasound has increased our ability to differentiate some of the

Table 6–1 Renal Cystic/Dysplastic Disease

Name	Heredity	Age	Symptoms	Laterality
Renal dysplasia				
Multicystic dysplasia (Potter type II)	None	Infancy	Asymptomatic, usually bilateral renal failure	Unilateral or bilateral
Aplastic dysplasia	None	Infancy	Asymptomatic usually	Unilateral or bilateral
Segmental dysplasia	None	Childhood through adulthood	+/− (Related to duplex kidney)	Usually unilateral
Focal dysplasia	Acquired	Any age	Symptomatic	Unilateral
Peripheral cortical cystic dysplasia with lower urinary tract obstruction (Potter type IV)	None	Birth to childhood	Related to lower urinary tract obstruction	Bilateral
Familial cystic dysplasia	Autosomal recessive	Birth	Related to associated syndrome	Bilateral
Polycystic kidney disease				
Infantile polycystic kidney disease (Potter type I)	Autosomal recessive	Neonate through childhood	Inverse relationship between severity of renal disease and age of presentation	Bilateral
Congential hepatic fibrosis	Autosomal recessive	Adolescence to adulthood	Related to portal hypertension	Bilateral
Adult polycystic kidney disease (Potter type III)	Autosomal dominant	Usually adulthood; occasionally in infancy	Asymptomatic in childhood; mass, hypertension, renal failure	Bilateral
Medullary cysts				
Medullary cystic disease, childhood type	Autosomal recessive	Infancy to adolescence	Azotemia, polydipsia, polyuria	Bilateral
Medullary cystic disease, adulthood type	Autosomal dominant	Late adolescence through adulthood	Same as childhood type	Bilateral
Medullary sponge kidney (precaliceal cannicular ectasia)	None	Any	Related to infection or calcium deposition	Unilateral or bilateral
Renal cortical cysts				
Glomerulocystic kidney disease	None	Neonate through childhood	Proteinuria, hematuria, and bilateral abdominal masses	Bilateral
Simple cysts	None	Adulthood	None	Bilateral

Table 6–1 Renal Cystic/Dysplastic Disease (*Continued*)

Radiology	Pathology	Associated Malformations: Genitourinary	Associated Malformations: Other
US: Multiple cysts of varying sizes with no identifiable parenchyma or renal pelvis EU/scintigraphy: Usually no function	Large nonreniform mass with disorganized tubules and multiple cysts	Ureteropelvic junction obstruction or other lower urinary tract obstruction in almost all cases	Cardiovascular, gastrointestinal, and central nervous system
US: No identifiable renal tissue EU/scintigraphy: No function	Small solid mass with disorganized tubules	Ureteral atresia or other lower urinary tract obstruction	Cardiovascular, gastrointestinal, central nervous system
US: Duplex kidney with small scarred upper pole that demonstrates increased echogenicity of parenchyma	Disorganized tubules, appearance of chronic pyelonephritic scarring	Renal duplication with ectopic ureterocele or other ureteric anomaly	None
Focal parenchymal scarring	Dysplasia	Vesicoureteral reflux	None
US: Small cortical cysts, small kidneys, hydronephrosis	Hydronephrosis, hydroureter, microcysts	Posterior urethral valves or other lower urinary tract obstruction	None
US: Multiple small cortical cysts—variable kidney size	Cystic dysplasia, peripheral cortical cysts, other histologic abnormalities	Cryptorchidism, hypospadias, epididymal cysts	Jeune's thoracic dystrophy, Ivemark's syndrome, Meckel's syndrome, Zellweger syndrome
US: Enlarged kidneys with increased echogenicity of cortex and medulla, possible sonolucency along parenchymal margins, cortical striations EU: "puddling" of contrast, splayed calices, radiating dilated collecting tubules	3-mm cylindrical cysts in cortex and medulla	None	Cerebral aneurysm, hepatomegaly present in later age of onset group
Same as infantile polycystic kidney disease although less severe	Same as IPKD although less severe	None	Cerebral aneurysm, marked portal hypertension, hepatic fibrosis, gastrointestinal bleeding
US: Infants—large kidneys with echogenic parenchyma without a sonolucent rim; older patients—cysts of varying sizes	Spherical cysts up to 5 cm in size arising from all nephron elements	None	Cerebral aneurysm, liver, pancreas, spleen cysts
US: Normal or small kidneys with less than 1-cm cysts at corticomedullary junction EU: Normal or small kidneys with little excretion	Cysts at corticomedullary junction, tubular atrophy, periglomerular fibrosis	None	Hepatic fibrosis, retinal dysplasia
Indistinguishable from childhood type	Indistinguishable from childhood type	None	None
US: Normal or nephrocalcinosis EU: Normal or linear areas of increased density in region of the papillae	Calculi in papillary tips, tubular ectasia, and cysts	None	None
Indistinguishable from IPKD	Distinguishable from IPKD only by histology	None	Hepatic cysts, hepatic adenomas
US: Anechoic fluid collection with smooth wall and good through transmission	Solitary or multiple simple cysts	None	None

Table 6–1 Renal Cystic/Dysplastic Disease (*Continued*)

Name	Heredity	Age	Symptoms	Laterality
Syndromes associated with cysts or dysplasia				
Potter's syndrome	—	Birth	Respiratory distress, ascites, oligohydramnios	Bilateral
Tuberous sclerosis	Autosomal dominant	Any	Pain, hypertension	Bilateral
von Hippel-Lindau syndrome	Autosomal dominant	Usually adulthood	Visual field defects or related to CNS	Bilateral
Neoplastic Cysts				
Cystic nephroma	None	Birth to adulthood	Palpable mass, hypertension	Unilateral

Abbreviations: US, ultrasound; EU, excretory urography, IPKD, infantile polycystic kidney disease; APKD, adult polycystic kidney disease; CNS; central nervous system.

conditions. However, many of the conditions appear identical even with high resolution scanning. Often the final diagnosis is made only with microscopic examination.

The most common form of renal dysplasia is multicystic dysplasia. Usually detected in infancy, it is associated with a ureteropelvic junction obstruction or other lower urinary tract obstruction in greater than 98 percent of cases. It is thought that the lower tract obstruction occurs in utero. When unilateral, the entity may go undetected until late childhood. Bilateral multicystic dysplasia is the most common type of bilateral cystic kidney disease in the neonate. The infant presents with symptoms of renal failure. Lower urinary tract obstruction is present in virtually all cases. Ultrasound examination reveals a large mass of multiple cysts that vary in size with no identifiable renal parenchyma or renal pelvis (Fig. 6–9). Renal scintigraphy reveals no function. While the appear-

A

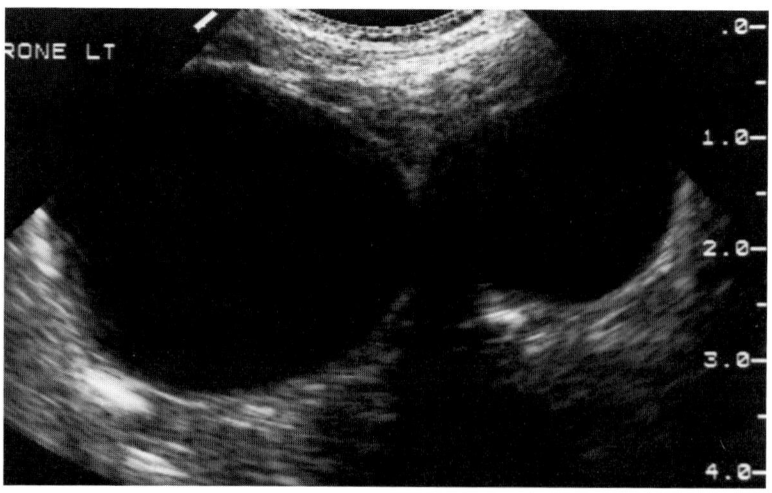

Fig. 6–9 Multicystic dysplastic kidney. **(A)** Transverse scan of the left renal fossa fails to demonstrate a normal kidney. Instead, multiple large cysts with no interposed renal parenchyma are identified. (*Figure continues.*)

Table 6–1 Renal Cystic/Dysplastic Disease (*Continued*)

Radiology	Pathology	Associated Malformations: Genitourinary	Associated Malformations: Other
US: Small kidneys	Variable types of dysplasia	Eagle-Barrett syndrome	Pulmonary hypoplasia
US: Multiple cortical cysts of varying sizes	Simple cysts less than 2 cm in size with hypertrophic eosinophilic lining	None	Renal angiomyolipomas, calcifying CNS tubers, glial neoplasms, cardiac rhabdomyomas, and adenoma sebaceum
Indistinguishable from APKD	Cortical cysts of varying sizes, which may be precursors of multifocal cystic adenocarcinoma	Adenoma, hemangioma, renal cell carcinoma, epididymal cysts, tumor	Hemangioblastoma, spinal cord arteriovenous malformation, syrinx, meningioma, cysts, benign tumors of pancreas, liver, adrenal gland, spleen, lung, peritoneal cavity
US: Multicystic complex mass	Multiloculated cysts with intercystic neoplasm	None	None

ance described represents classic multicystic dysplasia, occasionally function is detected in the dysplastic kidney during ^{99m}Tc-DTPA scintigraphy and a hydronephrotic renal pelvis is identified. Follow-up ultrasound examinations may reveal involution and shrinkage of the dysplastic kidney. Occasionally, the dysplastic kidney will shrink to the point where it is not identifiable by ultrasound examination; preoperative differentiation from aplastic dysplasia then becomes difficult.

The autosomal recessive form of polycystic kidney disease (Potter type I) is most likely to present in early infancy and childhood. Affected patients also have a variable amount of hepatic fibrosis present. The younger the child the less severe the liver disease and the more severe the renal disease. The opposite is true as the child ages. Those children presenting during the second decade often have severe portal hypertension and very little evidence of renal disease. In the infant, the kidneys appear large on ultrasound

B

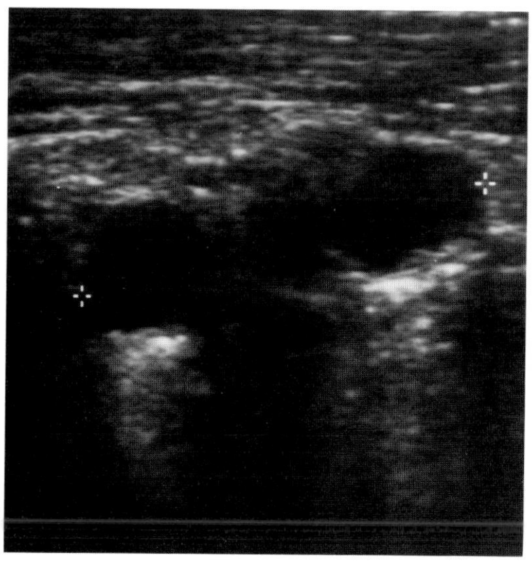

Fig. 6–9 (*Continued*). **(B)** Longitudinal scan obtained 2 years later demonstrates interval shrinkage of the cysts consistent with an involuting multicystic dysplastic kidney.

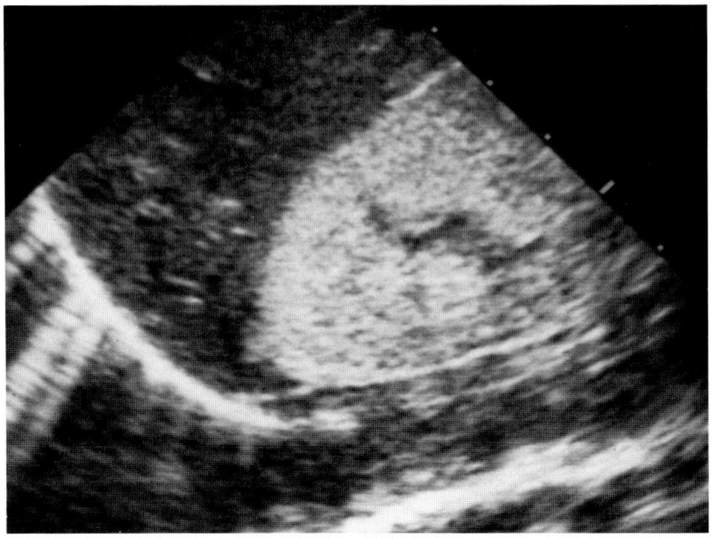

Fig. 6–10 Autosomal recessive polycystic kidney disease. Longitudinal ultrasound of an infant's right kidney demonstrates a marked increase in the echogenicity as compared with the adjacent liver. The left kidney was equally affected. Both kidneys were large with loss of the corticomedullary differentiation. No concomitant liver disease was detected in this patient.

examination and have an echogenic parenchyma (Fig. 6–10). Using a high resolution transducer (7.5 MHz) striations may be seen in the region of the renal papillae representing dilated distal collecting tubules. On excretory urography the kidneys appear large and demonstrate poor contrast excretion. Delayed radiographs demonstrate radiating dilated distal collecting tubules. The calyces are not dilated but are splayed due to the increased size of the renal parenchyma. The same findings are seen in older children but may be more subtle. Hepatomegaly and reversal of the portal venous flow is often seen on duplex doppler examination in the older patient.

The autosomal dominant form (Potter type III) is the most common polycystic kidney disease. Most cases present in adulthood. However, some patients present in the perinatal period or during infancy. The patients demonstrate large kidneys with a homogeneous increase in the echogenicity of the parenchyma (Fig. 6–11). The findings of multiple cysts of varying sizes throughout the renal cortex is usually only detected in the fourth and fifth decades of life, although pathologically the parenchyma is abnormal from birth. Excretory urography demonstrates good renal function but nodular puddling of contrast material is seen in the parenchyma.

Two cystic diseases specifically involve the renal medulla: medullary cystic disease complex and medullary sponge kidney. Medullary cystic disease complex is comprised of a group of renal cystic diseases with similar clinical, radiographic, and pathologic features but which differ in the mode of genetic transmission. Both the infantile form of medullary cystic disease complex and renal retinal dysplasia are inherited as autosomal recessive traits. The adult form of medullary cystic disease complex is transmitted as an autosomal dominant trait. Patients present with azotemia, polydipsia, and polyuria. On ultrasound examination the kidneys are small to normal in size and may demonstrate medullary or corticomedullary cysts. A loss of the corticomedullary differentiation and an increase in the parenchymal echogenicity is seen. On excretory urography the kidneys are small to normal in size and very little excretion of contrast material is seen.

Medullary sponge kidney (precalyceal canalicular ectasia) may present in infancy but is more common in adulthood. The patients may have flank pain or hematuria due to renal stones. Other symptoms may relate to recurrent urinary tract infection or nephrocalcinosis; either unilateral or bilateral involvement may occur. On ultrasound examination the kidneys may

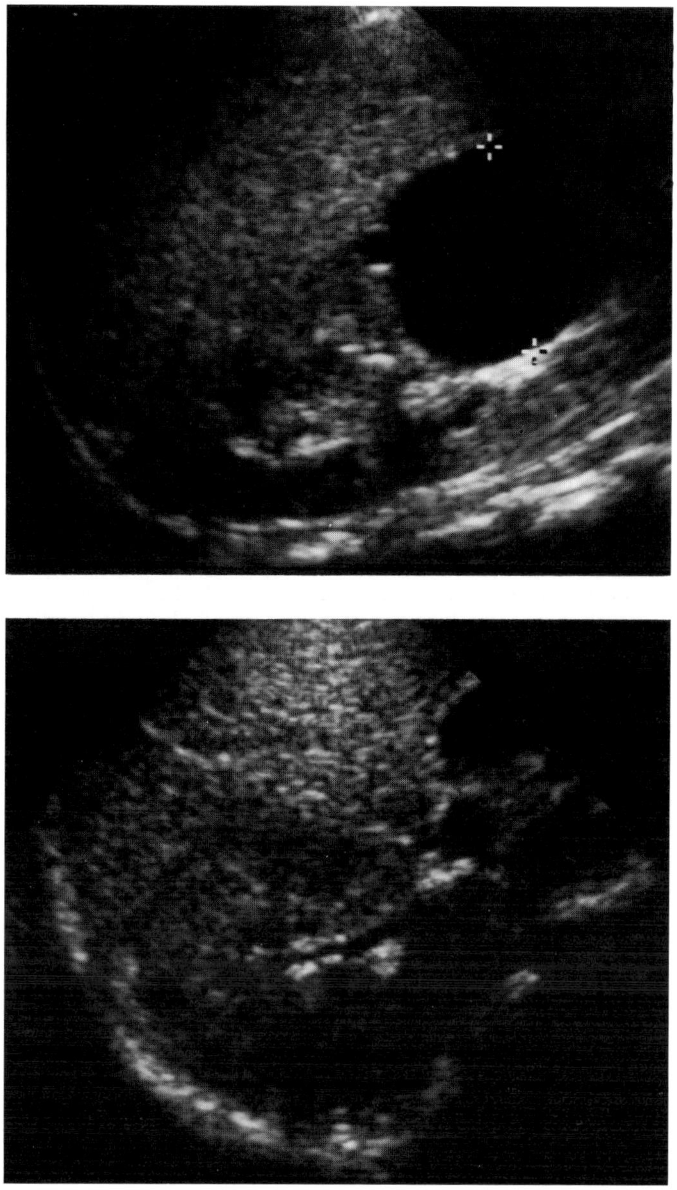

A

B

Fig. 6–11 Autosomal dominant polycystic kidney disease. **(A)** Longitudinal ultrasound of a child whose father has polycystic kidney disease demonstrates multiple cysts of varying sizes in the echogenic cortex of the left kidney. **(B)** Transverse scan of an infant sibling demonstrates a tiny cortical cyst consistent with adult type polycystic kidney disease.

appear normal. Increased echogenicity may be seen in the renal pyramids due to nephrocalcinosis. Renal stones may be incidentally noted within the collecting structures. Excretory urography is usually normal, although ectatic medullary tubules may lead to a papillary contrast blush. Histologically, the medullary collecting tubules are dilated and cystic communicatons are noted.

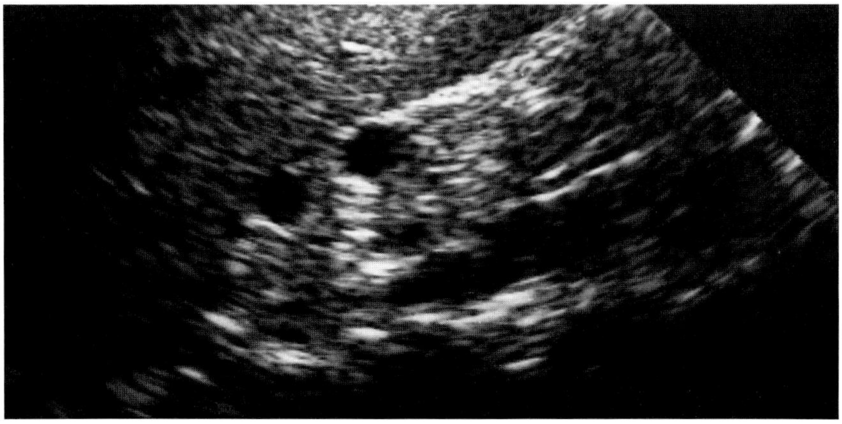

Fig. 6–12 Cortical cysts. Longitudinal scan, right upper abdomen. Note the two cysts located in the cortex of the small echogenic right kidney, which functioned poorly. Both kidneys are equally affected, indicating end-stage renal dysplasia.

Ultrasound examination in patients with symptoms of diminished renal function may reveal cysts localized to the renal cortex (Fig. 6–12). Congenital cortical cysts may be asymptomatic and have been associated with a variety of hereditary syndromes. Acquired cysts also occur.

Glomerulocystic disease is a congenital disorder with symptoms of hematuria, proteinuria, and bilateral abdominal masses presenting during infancy. On ultrasound examination enlarged kidneys with increased parenchymal echogenicity are seen. Occasionally, associated hepatic adenomas or subcapsular cysts may be detected. The condition is difficult to differentiate from infantile polycystic disease using radiographic examinations. On excretory urography puddling of the contrast material is seen in poorly functioning kidneys. Pathologic examination reveals cysts up to 2 cm in size and tubular ectasia. Microscopically, the cysts appear irregular, thus differentiating glomerulocystic disease from infantile polycystic kidney disease.

Simple cysts of the renal cortex occur much more commonly in adults than in children. On ultrasound examination a solitary anechoic fluid collection with a well-circumscribed smooth margin is identified. Decreased acoustic impedance due to fluid in these cysts results in back wall enhancement. While cyst aspiration is a common diagnostic tool in adults, the medical management of a simple-appearing cyst of childhood remains controversial. A child presenting with a renal lesion that does not meet all of the criteria for a simple cyst usually undergoes surgical resection.

The most common vascular anomaly involving the kidneys is the presence of multiple renal arteries. Since renal vascular anomalies are usually asymptomatic, the necessity to document the site of origin rarely occurs in childhood. Their origin may be the abdominal aorta, iliac artery, or the mesenteric arteries. Unilateral involvement is common. The incidence of arterial anomalies associated with fusion anomalies and malrotated kidneys is increased. The aberrant arteries may enter the kidneys directly through the capsule and are most common in the lower pole. Multiple renal arteries are difficult to detect on ultrasound examination. The spatial resolution of both scintigraphy and MRI limit the utility of these modalities in identifying the anomalies as well. If it is necessary to see the vessels, angiography is the only useful imaging technique.

Infection/Inflammation

Pyelonephritis refers to infection of the kidney. This condition, whether acute or chronic, is recognized less often in infancy and childhood than in adulthood. In infancy, the incidence of acute pyelonephritis is

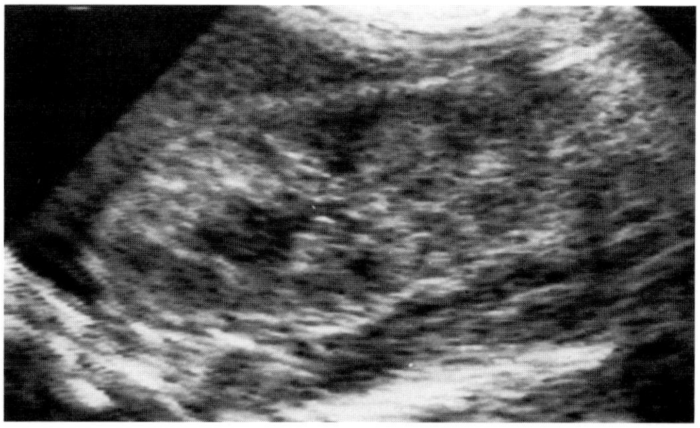

Fig. 6–13 Fungal pyelonephritis. Longitudinal right kidney ultrasound reveals plumpness of the kidney with loss of the corticomedullary differentiation. Diffuse inhomogeneous areas of increased echogenicity distort the parenchyma. Blood cultures revealed fungal sepsis.

equal between the sexes. After infancy, the incidence increases in females. In the older child, the route of contamination may be blood-borne or, more commonly, due to ascension of organisms from the lower urinary tract. The blood-borne form is usually related to skin or bone infection and gram-positive organisms (*Staphylococcus aureus* is most common) are isolated. *Escherichia coli* is the most common organism isolated in cases of ascending lower urinary tract infection and is responsible for 70 percent of cases of pyelonephritis. Other coliforms may be isolated as well. While not common in the United States, hematogenous spread of tuberculosis may lead to renal parenchymal involvement. Fungi are not uncommon in premature infants, neonates, or the immunosuppressed host. *Candida albicans* and *Aspergillus* species are common organisms. Patients with chronic fungal infections usually present with symptoms of renal failure. Ultrasound examination of these cases demonstrates a nonspecific loss of corticomedullary differentiation, indicating infiltrating parenchymal disease associated with either cavitary lesions or areas of increased echogenicity (Fig. 6–13).

Both ultrasonography and excretory urography are usually normal in patients with bacterial pyelonephritis. In less than one-half of cases a size difference between the infected kidney and the normal kidney is detectable (Fig. 6–14). Ultrasound examination may reveal a subjective fullness in the anteroposterior diameter suggesting swelling. When the kidney size is plotted against normograms, a slight enlargement will be noted. Often, no finding is noted until a repeat examination is done after the patient has been adequately treated. On the repeat examination the involved kidney will decrease in size, especially in the anteroposterior diameter. Other reported findings include loss of the differentiation between the renal cortex and medulla and paralytic ileus of the ureter. Acutely, excretory urography may reveal compression and thinning of the calyces. Chronically, fullness of the involved renal pelvis and blunt calyces may be noted with ultrasonography or excretory urography. The most sensitive method for detecting renal parenchymal involvement in urinary tract infection is radionuclide imaging with either ^{99m}Tc-DMSA or ^{99m}Tc-GH. While both radionuclides provide excellent parenchymal visualization, the radiation dose with ^{aam}Tc-GH is lower. ^{aam}Tc-DMSA offers superior visualization of the collecting structures. While the sensitivity for parenchymal defects is high, the specificity is low. Coordination of the scintigram with either an excretory urogram or ultrasound examination is useful in the differentiation of scars, cysts, and neoplasms.

Sequelae of pyelonephritis include carbuncle, abscess formation, and lobar nephronia. *Staphylococcus aureus* sepsis is the usual cause of abscesses and renal carbuncles. Both complications are uncommon in child-

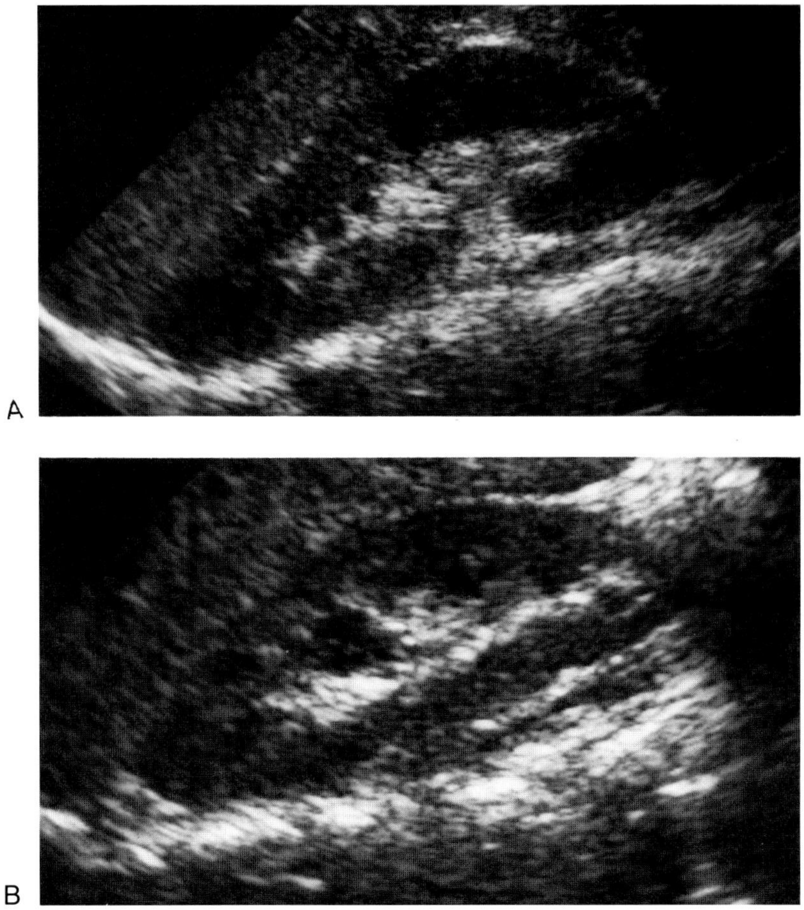

Fig. 6–14 Pyelonephritis. **(A)** Longitudinal ultrasound of the left kidney demonstrates diffuse enlargement with loss of the corticomedullary differentiation. The patient had left flank pain. **(B)** Longitudinal scan of the normal right kidney, which is 2 cm shorter, for comparison.

hood. If untreated, an abscess may rupture into the renal capsule and rapidly spread through the subcapsular space (perirenal abscess). Ultrasound examination is useful in identifying the echogenic collection of pus within Gerota's fascia along with secondary signs of perinephric spread such as displacement of the kidney, ipsilateral elevation of the diaphragm, and sympathetic pleural effusion. Excretory urography only shows displacement of the kidney and is nonspecific in cases of suspected extrarenal involvement. Ultrasound, fluoroscopy, or CT guidance may be employed for placement of percutaneous drainage catheters. Lobar nephronia refers to the acute tubulointerstitial inflammatory reaction following reflux of infected urine into the collecting ducts of an individual renal lobe.

The terms *chronic atrophic pyelonephritis* and *reflux nephropathy* are sometimes used interchangeably. Reflux nephropathy is a radiographic term used to describe cortical thinning associated with widening of corresponding calyx and papillary retraction (Fig. 6–15). Pathologically this results from replacement of inflammatory infiltrates in the involved lobe because of reflux of infected urine into the collecting ducts (lobar nephronia) by fibroblasts and fibrosis. Repeated insult to the kidney from vesicoureteral reflux and ascending infection results in two patterns of

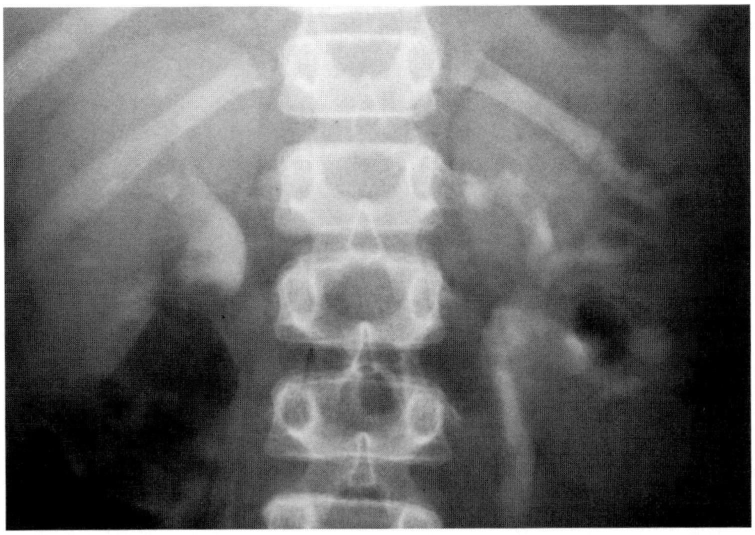

Fig. 6–15 Reflux nephropathy. Seven-minute radiograph from an excretory urogram in a patient with documented bilateral vesicoureteral reflux. Note the dilated calyces bilaterally. Thinning of the cortex is especially notable in the right upper pole and in the midportions of both kidneys.

scarring. The first is focal scarring at both poles with a decrease in the size of the kidney (Ask-Upmark kidney). The second pattern is an overall decrease in the thickness of the renal parenchyma with flattening of the papillae. These patterns are easily recognizable on either ultrasonography or excretory urography (Fig. 6–16).

Repeating ultrasound examinations in a patient with known vesicoureteral reflux and recurrent urinary tract infections allows for changes in clinical management. If there is lack of growth or interval scarring after the patient has taken prophylactic antibiotics, re-implantation of the involved ureter may be therapeutic. Low-grade vesicoureteral reflux unassociated with recurrent urinary tract infection is unlikely to lead to a clinically significant decrease in the involved kidney's function. In these cases, normal growth will be evident on follow-up examination. Vesicoureteral reflux may spontaneously resolve.

An unusual form of chronic pyelonephritis that occurs most frequently in older females is xanthogranulomatous pyelonephritis. This entity is associated with repeated urinary tract infections from either *E. coli* or *Proteus vulgaris*. Segmental involvement of the kidney is more common in childhood than in adults. The involved segment is enlarged and demonstrates a pattern of mixed echogenicity that may extend beyond the renal capsule. Since differentiation from a renal neoplasm may be difficult, CT is useful for further evaluation. The treatment of choice is nephrectomy, since differentiation from Wilms' tumor is difficult with any imaging modality.

The currently used imaging modalities are unable to differentiate various causes of medical renal parenchymal disease. While ultrasonography is the most sensitive indicator of early parenchymal disease, the specificity is poor. Disease is indicated by an increase in the echogenicity of the renal parenchyma as compared with the patient's liver parenchyma. The greater the echogenicity of the parenchyma, the greater the extent of renal involvement demonstrated at pathologic examination (Fig. 6–17).

The majority of patients with glomerular disease present clinically with either acute nephritic syndrome or nephrotic syndrome.

Acute nephritic syndrome is characterized by abrupt onset of hypertension, oliguria, azotemia, hematuria, and proteinuria; and usually develops from poststreptococcal glomerulonephritis. This entity is the most

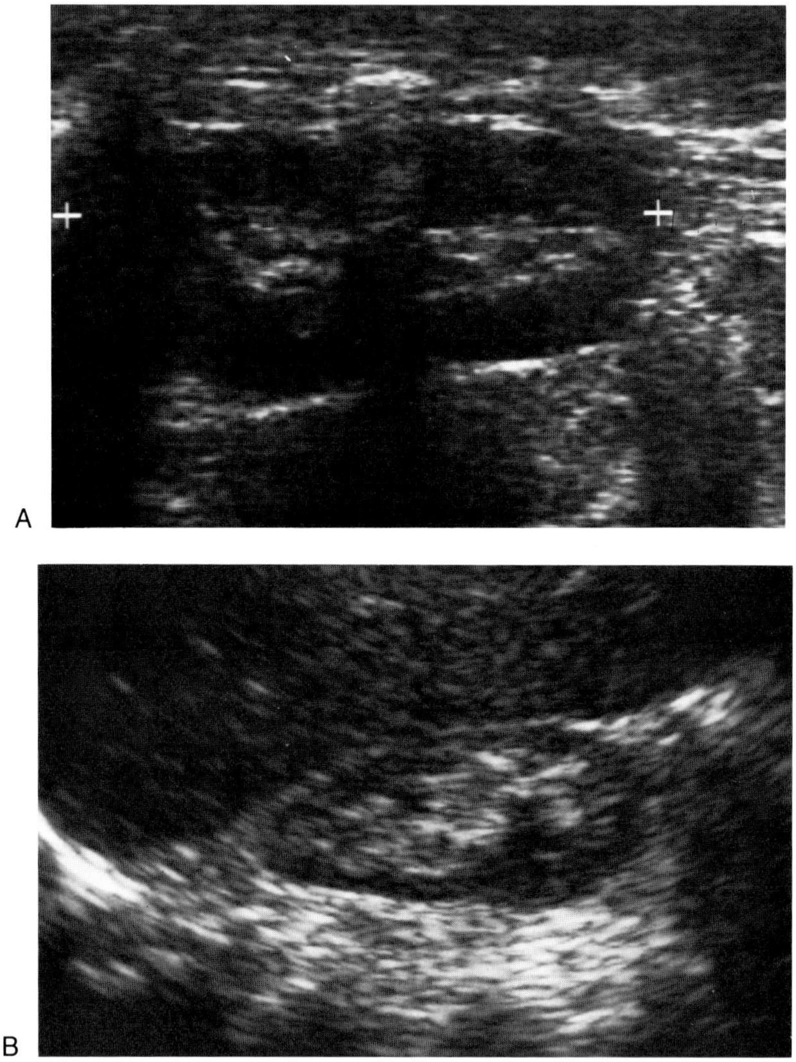

Fig. 6–16 (A) Prone longitudinal scan of the left kidney demonstrates focal lower pole scarring with extension of the hyperechoic renal sinus fat toward the periphery. **(B)** Longitudinal ultrasound of the right kidney demonstrates global thinning of the renal parenchyma following an acute episode of pyelonephritis 6 years earlier.

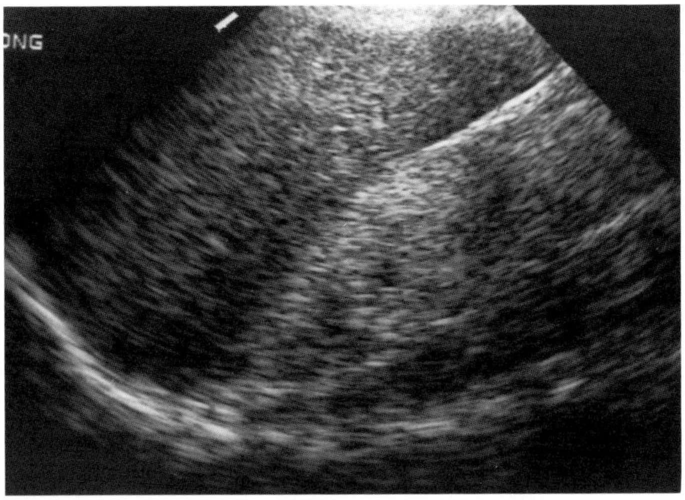

Fig. 6–17 Medical renal disease. The small echogenic kidney is difficult to visualize adjacent to the inferior liver edge on the longitudinal scan of the upper abdomen. The loss of corticomedullary differentiation and increased echogenicity are consistent with severe parenchymal disease.

common form of immune complex renal disease encountered in childhood. In most cases, the child has a history of a group A beta-hemolytic streptococcal infection of either the pharynx or the skin. The peripheral infection occurs about 2 weeks before the onset of renal symptoms. Boys are affected more often than girls and the peak incidence is between 3 and 7 years of age. Ninety-five percent of children recover completely from the first episode of acute glomerulonephritis. Approximately 2 percent of children will have a second episode and in 3 percent the disease will become chronic. If symptoms do not resolve within 2 weeks or if there is a recurrence, the kidney should be biopsied. The mechanism of injury is deposition of streptococcal antigen-antibody complexes along the basement membrane at the glomerulus. Other causes of postinfectious glomerulonephritis include indwelling catheters, bacterial endocarditis, visceral abscesses, viral infection, and hepatosplenic schistosomiasis. Acute nephritic syndrome has been associated with a variety of other conditions unassociated with infection. These include Goodpasture's syndrome, Henoch-Schönlein purpura, hereditary nephropathies, systemic lupus erythematosis, and Wegener's granulomatosis. In all cases, the mechanism of injury is immune complex mediated.

The nephrotic syndrome is characterized by hypoproteinemia, proteinuria, and hypercholesterolemia. The hypoproteinemia causes serous fluid to seep into the interstitial spaces. Radiographically the patient usually presents with large bilateral pleural effusions and a normal-sized heart (Fig. 6–18). Two glomerular disease groups characteristically present in this manner: steroid-responsive nephrotic syndrome and steroid-resistant nephrotic syndrome. Steroid-responsive nephrotic syndrome (minimal change nephrotic syndrome) is responsible for more than one-half of the cases of childhood nephrotic syndrome. The most frequent malignancy associated with childhood nephrotic syndrome is Hodgkin's lymphoma.

Vascular

The most common cause of acute renal failure in infants is hemolytic uremic syndrome. An episode of diarrhea, vomiting, and/or respiratory distress is followed by acute renal failure, hypertension, hemolytic anemia, and gastrointestinal tract hemorrhages. The kidneys are affected in 90 percent of cases. Infarction leads to acute cortical necrosis characterized by increased echogenicity of the parenchyma in a normal-sized or slightly enlarged kidney (Fig. 6–19). Fifty percent of patients recover with no evidence of residual renal disease. However, hypertension, chronic renal failure, brain damage, and gastrointestinal strictures are reported long-term consequences.

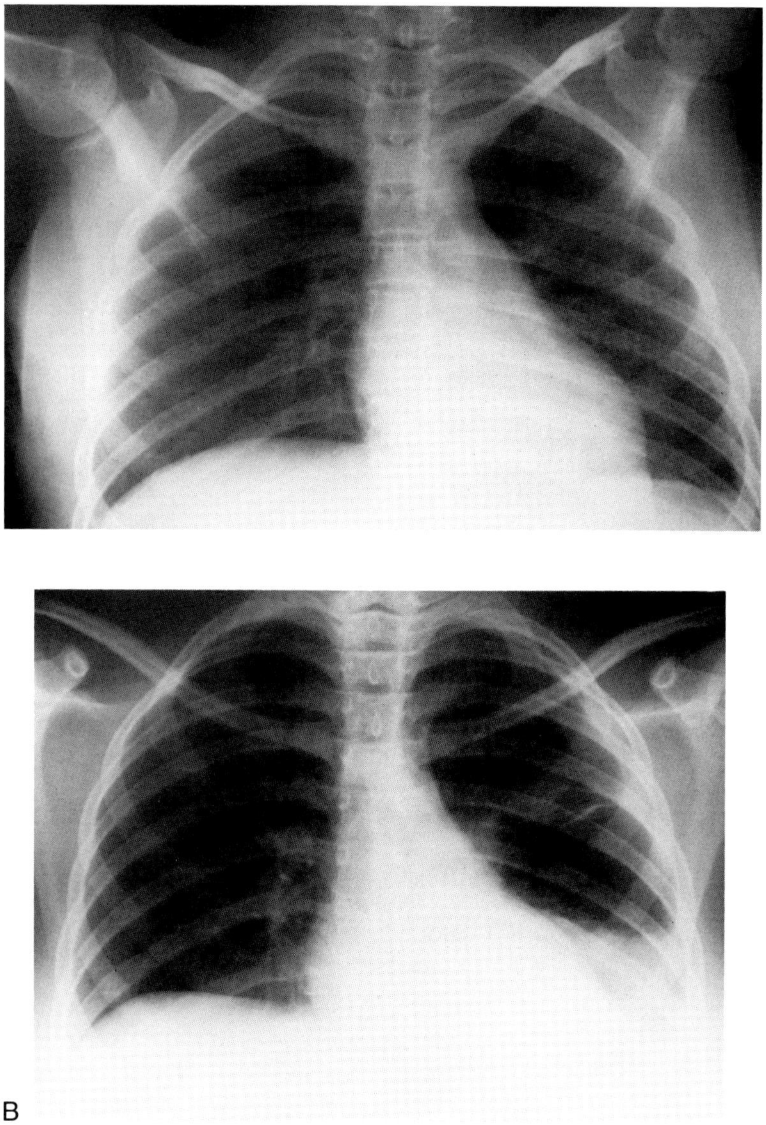

A

B

Fig. 6–18 Nephrotic syndrome. **(A)** This child presented with acute respiratory distress. The posteroanterior chest x-ray demonstrates small bilateral pleural effusions. **(B)** On a radiograph 1 week later, the left pleural effusion has increased in size. The right pleural effusion is unchanged. The heart size remains normal. Ultrasound revealed bilateral renal parenchymal disease.

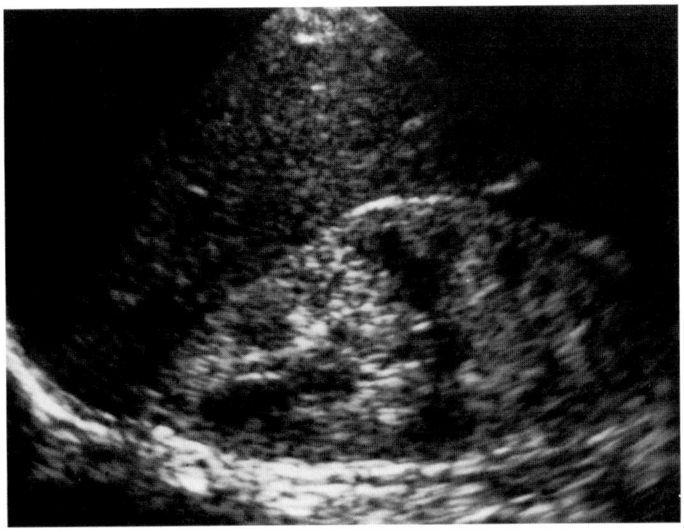

Fig. 6–19 Hemolytic uremic syndrome. After an acute episode of respiratory distress in this patient, a longitudinal ultrasound scan reveals an enlarged echogenic right kidney. The left kidney appeared similar. After the diagnosis of hemolytic uremic syndrome, acute cortical necrosis led to nonfunction. The patient eventually underwent renal transplantation.

The most common cause of hypertension during the neonatal period is renal artery thrombosis. Most cases are secondary to emboli from abnormally positioned umbilical arterial catheters. The position of the arterial catheter tip should be in the thoracic aorta (approximately T8 level) or below the third lumbar vertebra. Other predisposing factors include dehydration, blood loss, and sepsis hemoconcentration states. Ultrasound examination should be performed using duplex scanning to evaluate the flow through both renal arteries and the abdominal aorta, especially if an arterial catheter is in place. Although thrombus may appear echogenic, resolving thrombus becomes hypoechoic and may be difficult to detect on B-mode scanning. Absence of an arterial flow pattern will be demonstrated on both color flow and spectral analysis. Slight enlargement of the kidney may be seen. The contralateral kidney usually appears normal.

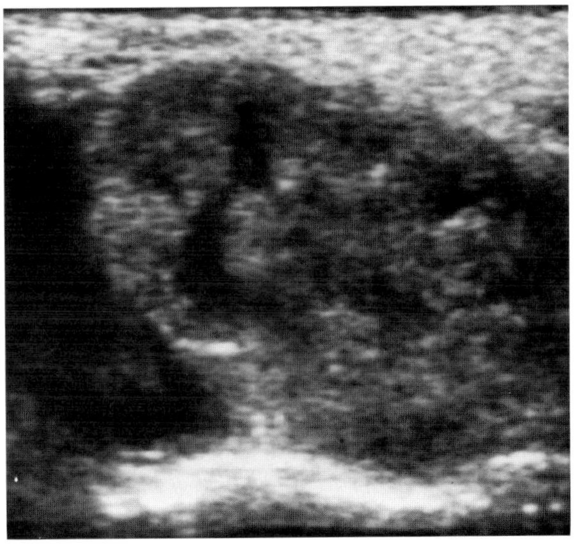

Fig. 6–20 Renal vein thrombosis. Prone longitudinal scan of the left kidney of a dehydrated infant demonstrates a plump kidney with coarse, mottled internal architecture. The corticomedullary differentiation is lost. These findings may indicate acute renal artery or renal vein thrombosis. In this case, Doppler examination revealed renal vein thrombosis.

The most common renal vascular abnormality during the neonatal period is renal vein thrombosis. Most cases occur in children less than 1 year of age with a peak incidence at 2 weeks of age. Predisposing factors include nephrotic syndrome, sepsis, dehydration, and hemoconcentration states (polycythemia, infants of diabetic mothers). Thrombus is most likely to begin in the arcuate veins. Venous congestion causes the kidney to enlarge. If ultrasound is performed in the acute phase of thrombosis, the enlarged kidney demonstrates a coarse, mottled distortion of the parenchymal architecture and may appear hypoechoic (Fig. 6–20). Duplex examination reveals absence of the venous flow pattern in the renal vein; clot may

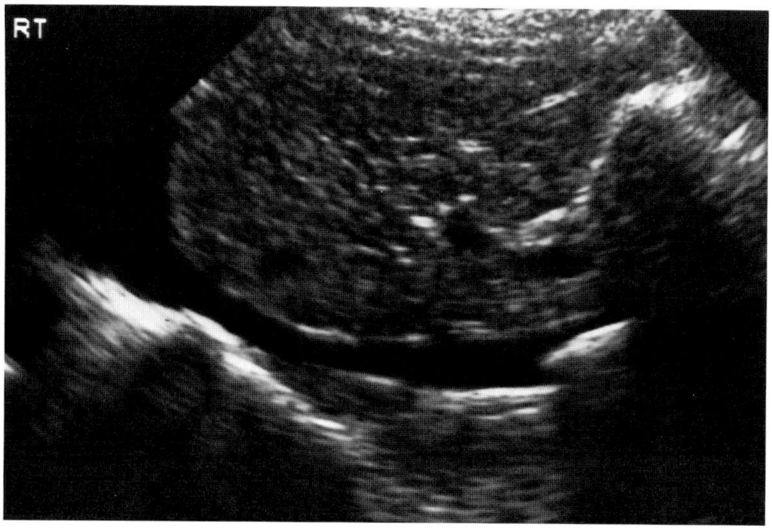

Fig. 6–21 Inferior vena cava thrombus. Longitudinal scan of the inferior vena cava demonstrates an echogenic focus with posterior shadowing representing a calcified thrombus that extended cephalad from a right renal vein thrombosis.

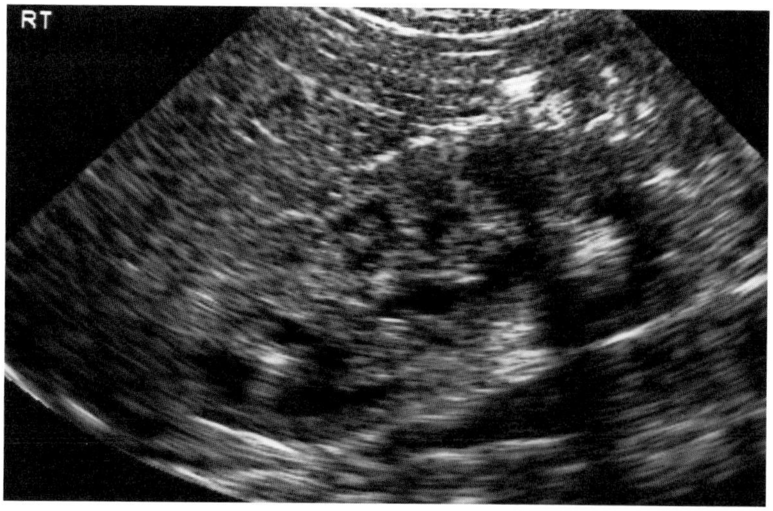

A

Fig. 6–22 Papillary necrosis. **(A)** Longitudinal scan of the right kidney demonstrates multiple foci of increased echogenicity in the regions of the papillae. (*Figure continues.*)

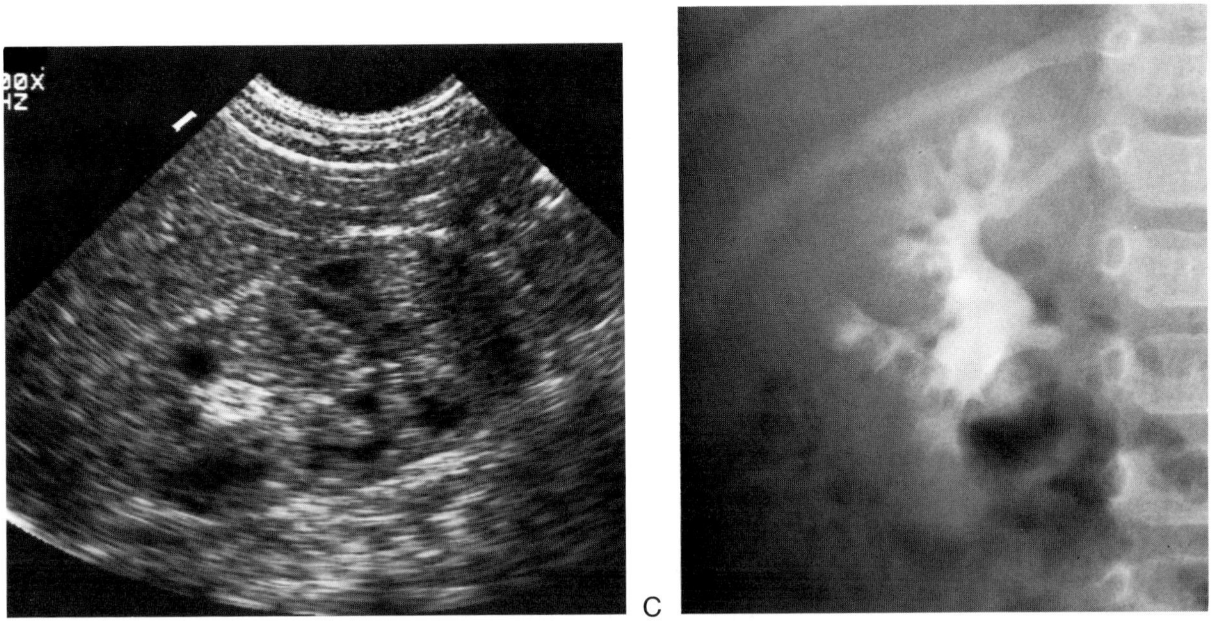

B C

Fig. 6–22 (*Continued*). **(B)** Slightly obliqued view better demonstrates an upper pole echogenic focus. **(C)** Radiograph of the right kidney during an excretory urogram demonstrates irregularity of the papillae and widening of the calyces consistent with papillary necrosis.

be present in the inferior vena cava as well (Fig. 6–21). Both excretory urography and renal scintigraphy reveal an enlarged kidney with poor function. After the acute phase, the kidney returns to normal size. CT demonstrates similar findings in cortical necrosis, renal artery thrombosis, and renal vein thrombosis. After intravenous contrast administration, the kidneys demonstrate no central concentration of contrast material, but an enhancing subcapsular rim of parenchyma due to increased flow through capsular perforating arteries is present. The incidence of associated ipsilateral adrenal hemorrhage is increased.

Predisposing factors that lead to cortical and papillary necrosis are often the same as those conditions leading to renal arterial and venous thrombosis. Parenchymal necrosis usually occurs in patients under 1 month of age with asphyxia, dehydration, gastroenteritis, hemolytic uremic syndrome, hypotension, or septicemia. After infancy, conditions such as thrombotic thrombocytopenic purpura, sickle cell anemia, and all forms of allograft rejection are causes. Cortical and papillary necrosis may occur in the same kidney and both kidneys are usually involved. The sonographic findings are nonspecific in both the acute and chronic phases (Fig. 6–22). Acutely, the kidneys appear normal in size or slightly enlarged and may demonstrate increased echogenicity. In the chronic phase focal parenchymal scarring is seen appearing as a localized area of parenchymal thinning.

The pathogenesis of acute tubular necrosis is similar to that of cortical and papillary necrosis. Dehydration from any cause is the most common predisposing factor in the infant. In later childhood, severe infection, aminoglycocide toxicity, poisoning, and surgery are predisposing factors. Acute tubular necrosis has followed the use of iodinated contrast agents for various imaging studies. Clinically, the child demonstrates polyuria in the face of dehydration. During this time ultrasound examination demonstrates a large kidney with increased echogenicity of the cortex and/or renal pyramids and enlargement of the pyramids (Fig. 6–23). The classic findings on the excretory urogram are dense, persistent nephrograms and small kidneys with poor visualization of the pelvocalyceal collecting structures and ureters. Because of the risk of precipitation of Tamm-Horsfall proteins, excre-

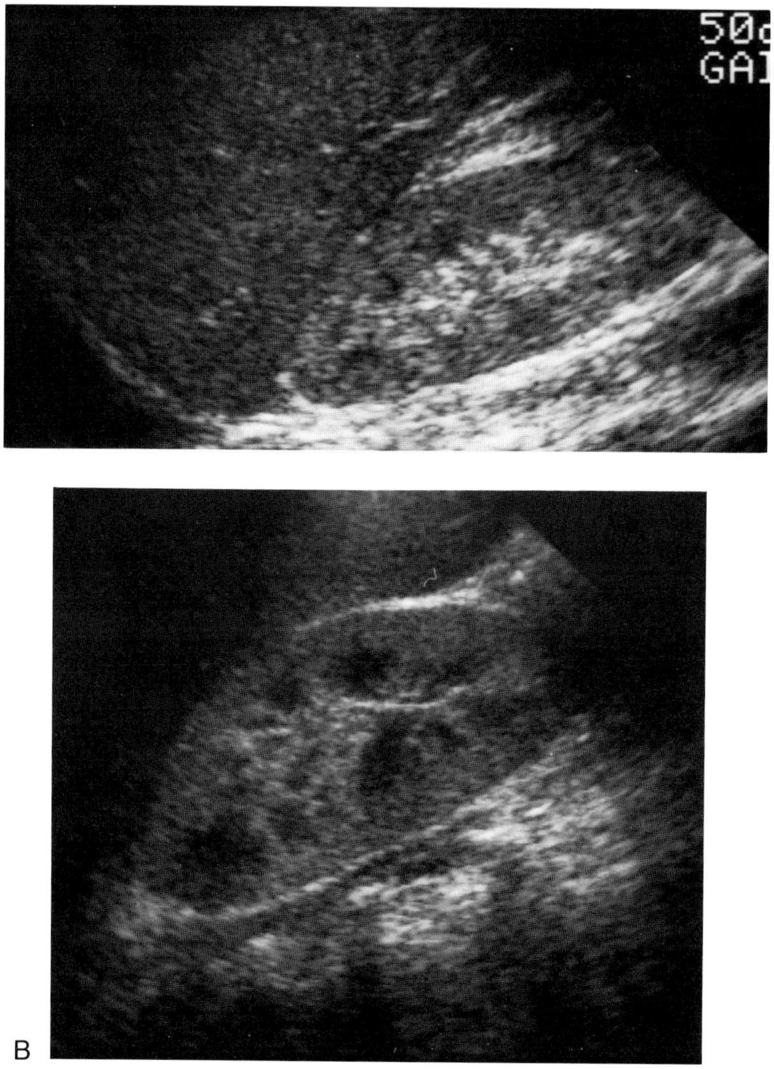

A

B

Fig. 6–23 Acute tubular necrosis. **(A)** Longitudinal scan of the right kidney demonstrates diffuse enlargement with a loss of the corticomedullary differentiation. The medullary pyramids are increased in echogenicity. **(B)** Repeat scan 1 month later shows resolution of the acute tubular necrosis with a return of the normal corticomedullary differentiation. Note that the parenchymal echogenicity remains increased when compared with the liver.

tory urography is not recommended in severely dehydrated infants. Follow-up ultrasound examinations or excretory urograms may reveal findings consistent with papillary necrosis such as the "ball-in-cup" deformity.

One of the more common presenting problems requiring radiologic evaluation in childhood is hypertension. Primary hypertension is diagnosed in only about 10 percent of patients. In the remainder, hypertension is secondary to other disease processes, 60 percent are due to renal parenchymal disease. Bilateral parenchymal disorders such as glomerulonephritis, cystic-dysplastic disease, and hemolytic uremic syndrome are best treated with medical management or renal transplantation. Unilateral changes of chronic pyelonephritis account for approximately 15 percent of hypertensive patients who are potentially curable by nephrectomy. Other entities implicated in hypertension that are detectable on ultrasound examination include Wilms' tumor, coarctation of the aorta, obstructive uropathy, and adrenal abnormalities. Renovascular diseases account for less than 10 percent of cases of childhood hypertension and include congenital anomalies, fibromuscular dysplasia, neurofibromatosis, arteriovenous fistula, aneurysm, and thrombotic phenomenon. Any unilateral cause of hypertension will usually present with a small shrunken kidney on one side and a normal or hypertrophied kidney on the opposite side. If renal ultrasound examination demonstrates a greater than 1 cm size difference between the two kidneys, differential renal function studies, such as ^{99m}Tc-DTPA scintigraphy, are helpful in determining if the size difference is significant. Captopril may increase the sensitivity of scintigraphy but controlled studies in the pediatric population have not been performed. Arteriography remains the "gold standard" by which renal artery stenosis is diagnosed in childhood. Results from attempts at transluminal angioplasty in children are variable.

Neoplasms

The kidney is a common site of origin for childhood renal neoplasms. The metanephric ridge tumors, including mesoblastic nephroma and Wilms' tumor, are the most common renal tumors of children. Mesoblastic nephroma is most common in the neonate and Wilms' tumor is most common in children over 1 year of age. Benign epithelial and mesenchymal tumors occur much less commonly than Wilms' tumor during childhood.

Angiomyolipoma is a benign renal tumor that may occur as a solitary mass. However, about 40 percent of individuals presenting with angiomyolipomas have multiple and/or bilateral lesions associated with tuberous sclerosis. The hallmarks of tuberous sclerosis are adenoma sebaceum, mental retardation, and epilepsy. If the renal mass is incidentally noted in an asymptomatic individual with tuberous sclerosis, it may be followed conservatively with cross-sectional imaging studies such as CT or MRI. However, if massive hemorrhage develops or if there is a doubt in differentiation from Wilms' tumor, nephrectomy is recommended. The angiomyolipoma is a hamartomatous lesion with primary constituents of either fibrous tissue or fat. If adipose tissue predominates, an echogenic mass will be detected with ultrasonography. Wilms' tumor may also appear echogenic, so diagnosis must not rely on ultrasound evaluation alone. CT demonstrates a distinctive appearance of angiomyolipoma in most cases (Fig. 6–24). The Hounsfield unit density differences within the mass range from fat

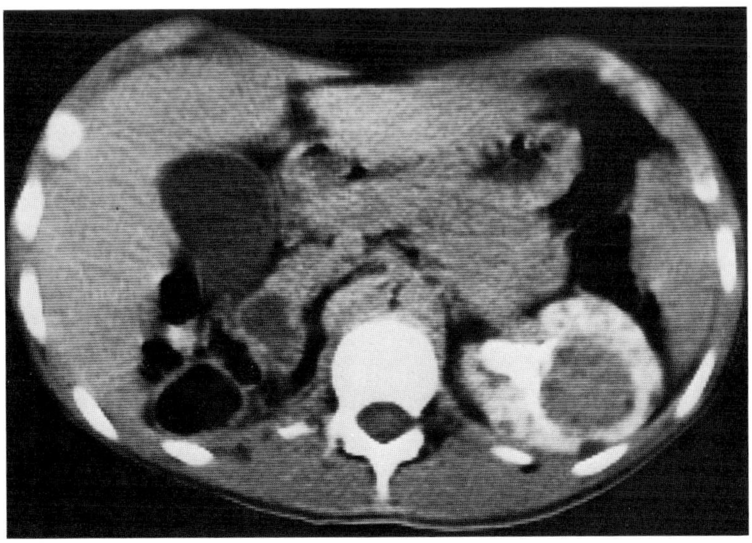

Fig. 6–24 Angiomyolipoma. Enhanced axial CT demonstrates a fat density mass within the solitary left kidney of this patient with documented tuberous sclerosis.

to calcium. The fibrous components enhance after contrast administration, while the fat remains low density. The identification of fat within the mass is specific for angiomyolipoma. It is only when the fat is not identified that the examination is ambiguous and differentiation from Wilms' tumor impossible. About 20 percent of angiomyolipomas are locally invasive. Extension into the inferior vena cava has been reported. Other benign tumors that rarely occur in childhood include adenomas, juxtaglomerular cell tumor, fibromas, and intrarenal teratoma.

The most common tumors of the kidney arise from the embryonic metanephric ridge. This is the site of the metanephric blastema that has the ability to differentiate into both epithelial and mesenchymal tissues. Neoplasms arising from this area range from benign to malignant. Wilms' tumor (nephroblastoma) is the most common tumor from this site of origin. The other four neoplastic derivatives are the cystic nephroma, mesoblastic nephroma (fetal renal hamartoma), nodular renal blastema-nephroblastomatosis complex, and rhabdomyosarcoma.

Wilms' tumor is the fourth most common solid malignancy of childhood and occurs at a frequency of approximately 5 cases per 1,000,000 children. It is more common in boys than in girls and is usually diagnosed in the first 5 years of life. It is uncommon to encounter a Wilms' tumor in a child younger than 1 year of age. An asymptomatic abdominal mass is usually detected by the patient's family or primary physician. Wilms' tumor occurs in about one-third of patients with aniridia. Other anomalies associated with Wilms' tumor include other genitourinary tract anomalies, hemihypertrophy, and Beckwith-Wiedemann syndrome. Drash syndrome is the association of gonadal dysgenesis, glomerulonephritis, and Wilms' tumor. Ultrasound examination reveals a well-circumscribed echogenic mass in the majority of cases (Fig. 6–25). Other ultrasound findings that have been reported are irregular anechoic areas, mixed echogenicity, distortion of the remaining renal tissue, and extension into the inferior vena cava. Calcification occurs in less than 10 percent of cases. Preoperative staging includes either CT or MRI, which will demonstrate a large complex intrarenal mass (Fig. 6–

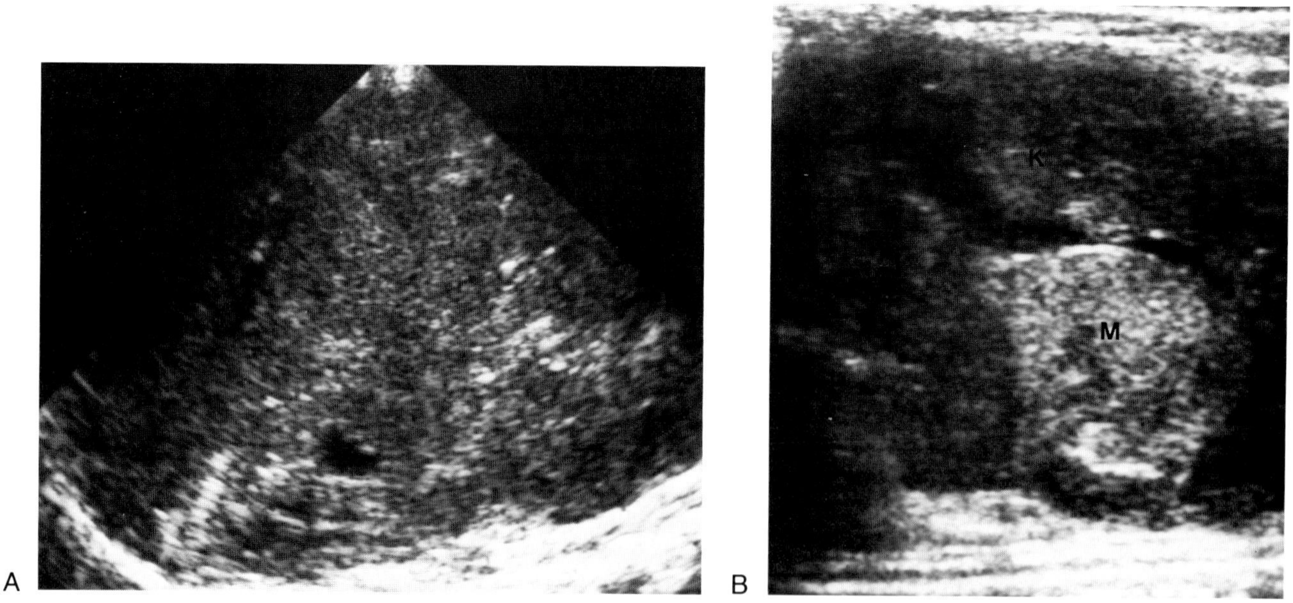

Fig. 6–25 Wilms' tumor. **(A)** The longitudinal ultrasound of the left renal fossa demonstrates no identifiable kidney. An echogenic mass abuts the inferior aspect of the spleen. **(B)** A transverse scan lower in the left abdomen demonstrates the distorted collecting system of the left kidney (K). The inferior margin of the echogenic mass (M) is well defined, consistent with the diagnosis of Wilms' tumor.

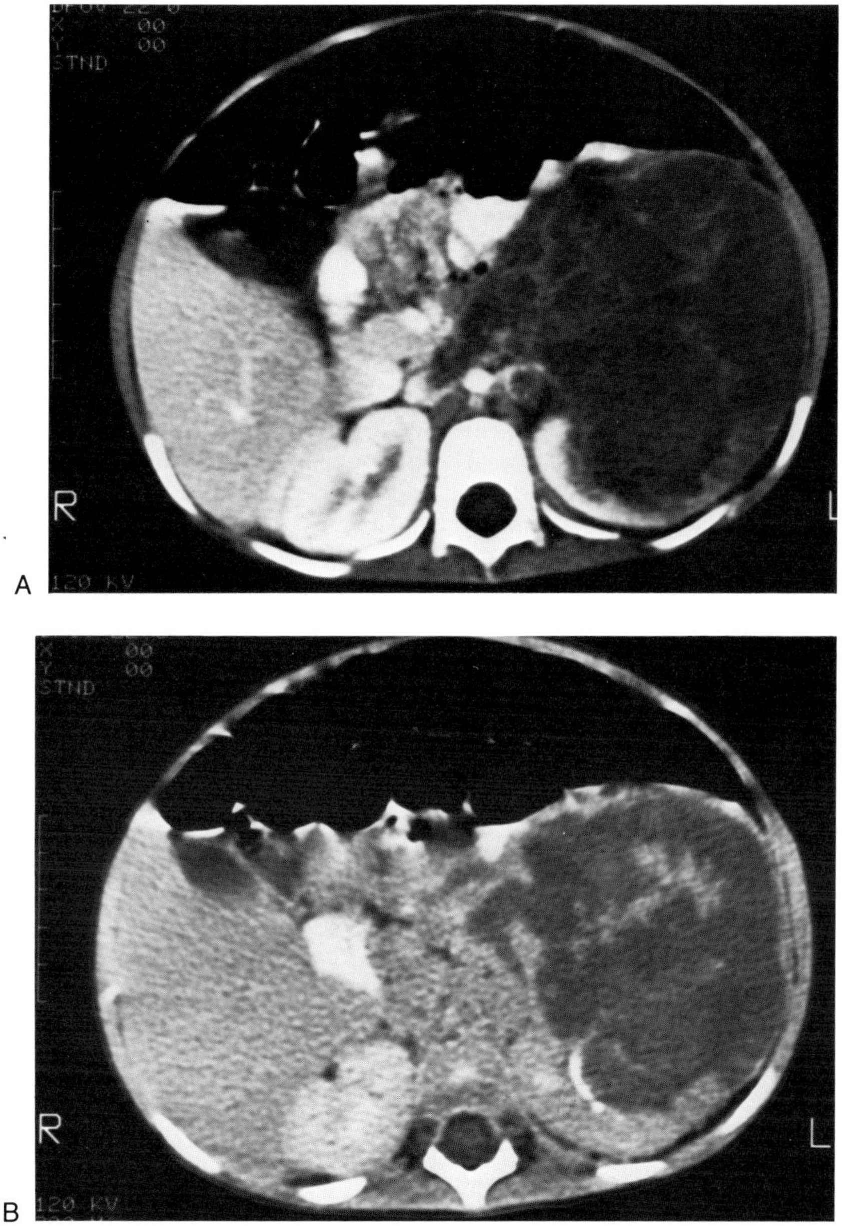

Fig. 6–26 Wilms' tumor. **(A)** Axial CT scan obtained shortly after IV administration of contrast material demonstrates a nephrogram on the right. On the left, a thin, enhancing rim of renal parenchyma is seen posteriorly. The remainder of the kidney is destroyed by a low density mass, which is well circumscribed. **(B)** A delayed image demonstrates distortion of the collecting structures of the left kidney by the large Wilms' tumor.

26). The ability of MRI to obtain coronal images is extremely helpful in identifying the extent of the lesion, liver metastases, and invasion of the inferior vena cava. The goal of surgery is complete resection. Approximately 90 percent of Wilms' tumors are unilateral. They are more likely to occur on the left side. Five percent are multifocal. Staging is usually based on the National Wilms' Tumor Study Group method, which suggests the surgeon stage the patient in the operating room. Pathologic confirmation should occur in less than 48 hours. The histopathology of Wilms' tumor may vary and is either favorable (90 percent, 2-year survival rate) or unfavorable (54 percent, 2-year survival rate). Either synchronous or metachronous bilateral Wilms' tumors occur in approximately 5 percent of affected children. The metachronous lesions have been uniformly fatal, while synchronous lesions have a long-term survival rate of 63 percent. CT continues to be the "gold standard" of follow-up evaluation for recurrence. Bone metastases occur in less than 5 percent of cases.

The other malignant tumor arising from the metanephric ridge is the rhabdomyosarcoma, representing only 3 percent of renal tumors. Bone metastases have been reported with rhabdomyosarcoma.

Cystic nephroma is a multicystic mass easily confused with multicystic dysplastic kidney. This lesion usually presents in children between the ages of 4 months and 2 years. Associated hypertension has been reported. Ultrasound examination is useful in identifying the noncommunicating cysts with sharp walls and echogenic parenchymal tissue between them. Nodules are often noted along the cyst walls. Treatment is surgical excision. The majority of cystic nephromas are benign. Occasionally, a partially differentiated Wilms' tumor is detected within one of the mural nodules during pathologic examination.

Mesoblastic nephroma (fetal renal hamartoma) is the most common renal tumor in the neonate, but it rarely occurs outside of infancy. One-half of the cases are noted during the first week of life as asymptomatic abdominal masses. Occasionally patients may present with congestive heart failure or hypertension. Twenty percent of mesoblastic nephromas arise in multilocular cysts. All cases are unilateral and the right kidney is more commonly affected. Ultrasound examination reveals a mixed echogenicity solid tumor (Fig. 6–27). This appearance is also seen on CT scans, which may reveal contrast material within the mass after IV administration. The treatment of choice is nephrectomy.

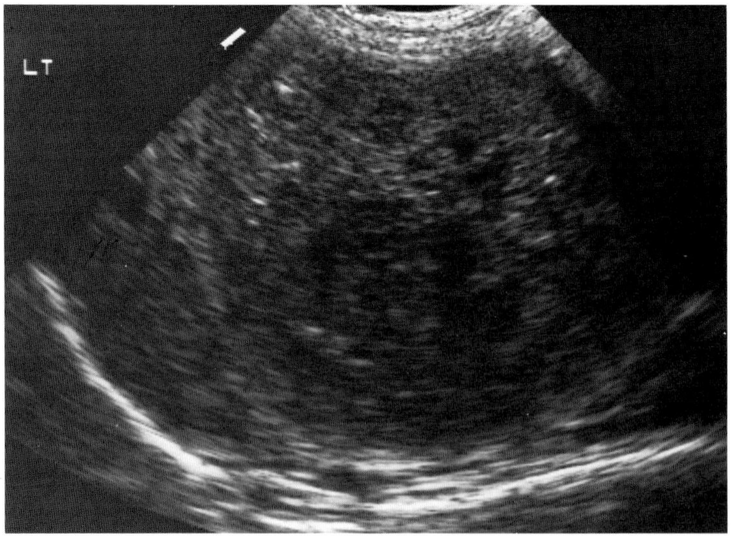

Fig. 6–27 Mesoblastic nephroma. Longitudinal ultrasound of the left renal fossa demonstrates replacement of the kidney by a hyperechoic mass in this newborn infant. Foci of calcification demonstrate posterior shadowing. Small cystic spaces are also noted.

The nodular renal blastema–nephroblastomatosis complex is a condition in which microscopic subcapsular nodules are seen in the cortex of the kidney. These consist of immature metanephric tissue (the blastema). Nodular renal blastema has been associated with trisomies 13 and 18, and with other genitourinary tract abnormalities. Obviously, these lesions are difficult to detect preoperatively. Wilms' tumor has been associated with multifocal nephroblastomatosis. Affected children present with hypertension and are usually less than 2 years old. Both kidneys are enlarged and multifocal parenchymal masses of abnormal echogenicity may be detected. No matter which imaging modality is used it is difficult to differentiate this condition from infantile polycystic kidney disease unless discrete masses are identified. Patients who receive prophylactic chemotherapy have an excellent long-term survival.

Less than 1 percent of all renal cell carcinomas occur in individuals under 20 years of age. Most children are diagnosed in the preadolescent years when they present with either flank pain, fever, or gross hematuria. Renal cell carcinoma has been reported after the treatment of adrenal cortical carcinoma and Wilms' tumor. Unilateral involvement is the rule. Von Hippel-Lindau syndrome has been associated with bilateral renal cell carcinomas arising in multiple cysts. Ultrasonography detects a solid mass of mixed echogenicity. Presurgical imaging includes either CT or MRI to exclude extension of tumor into the inferior vena cava (Fig. 6–28). Treatment is radical nephrectomy.

Neuroblastoma should also be considered in the differential diagnosis of what appears to be a tumor of renal origin. While intrarenal neuroblastoma is extremely rare, the tumor may arise adjacent to the renal hilum or in the perirenal soft tissues and cause massive replacement of the kidney. Calcifications are much more common in neuroblastoma than in any neoplasm of renal origin. Unfortunately, the ultrasound appearance is of a mixed echogenicity solid tumor and may be difficult to differentiate from Wilms' tumor.

The two most common neoplasms to invade the kidney secondarily during childhood are neuroblastoma and lymphoma. Seventy-five percent of children with lymphoma will have kidney involvement during the

A

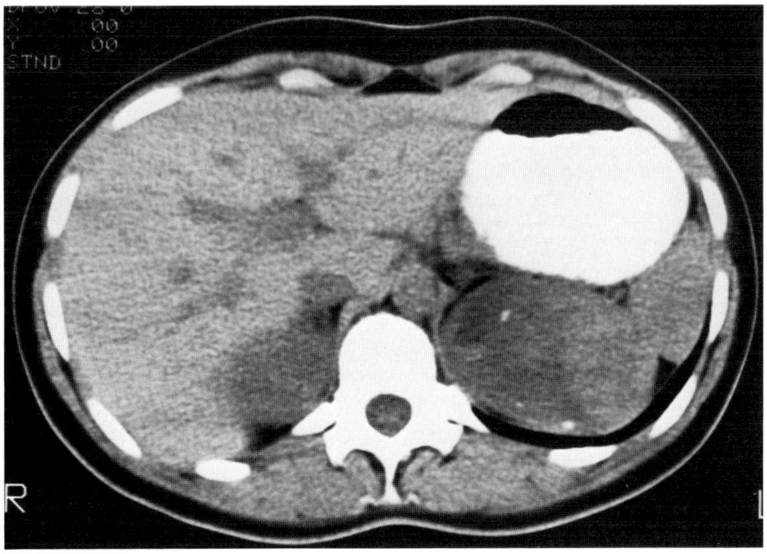

Fig. 6–28 Renal cell carcinoma. **(A)** Noncontrasted CT scan demonstrates an enlarged left kidney with scattered small calcifications. (*Figure continues.*)

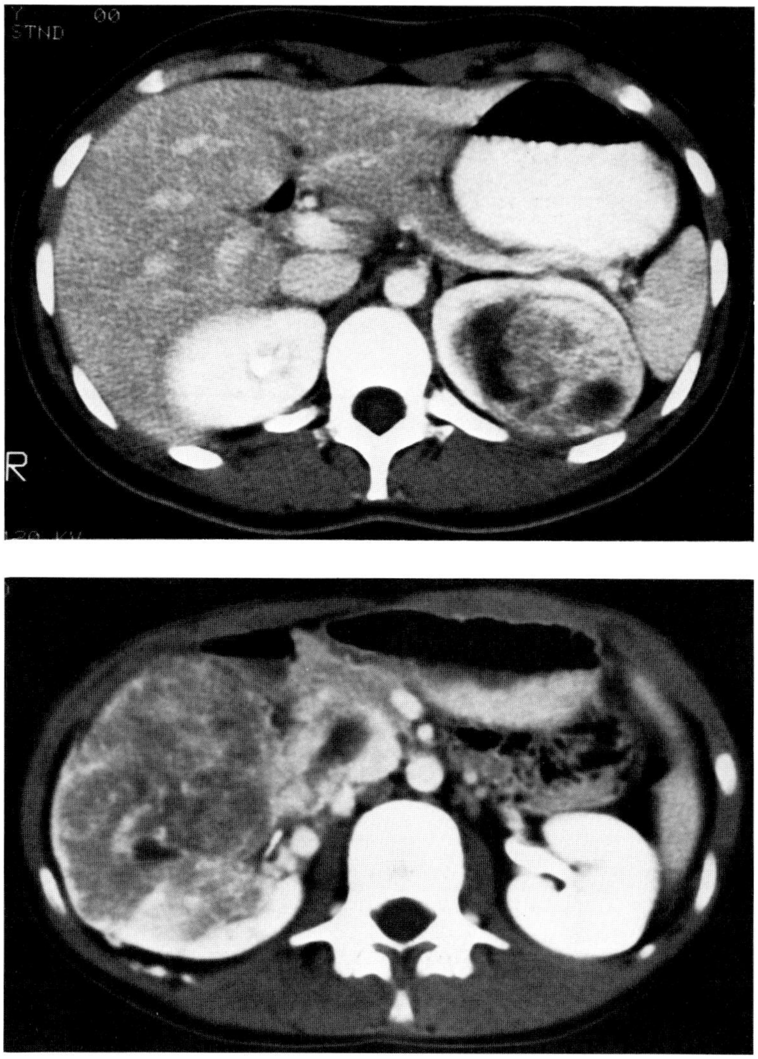

B

C

Fig. 6–28 (*Continued*). **(B)** After injection of intravenous contrast material there is inhomogeneous contrast enhancement of the mass. No extension was identified into the inferior vena cava. **(C)** Enhanced axial CT scan of another patient demonstrates a large inhomogeneous mass distorting the right kidney with extension into the inferior vena cava as evidenced by the hypodense mass within the right side of the lumen.

course of their illness. The disease may be diffuse and infiltrative or present with discrete nodules (Fig. 6–29). Most patients are asymptomatic and infiltrates are detected at autopsy. Rarely, patients may present with acute nephritic syndrome. Leukemia may cause similar renal infiltration.

Generalized/Systemic

The pathologic detection of calcium deposition in the renal parenchyma is common. The term *nephrocalcinosis* is reserved for conditions leading to deposition of calcium in the renal parenchyma that are detectable by imaging. In children, ultrasonography has demonstrated that nephrocalcinosis occurs much more frequently that previously suspected. It resolves spontaneously in a number of cases. Predisposing factors are different in children than in adults. Hypercalcemia may be secondary to steroid therapy or Cushing's disease. Metabolic disturbances (Bartter's syndrome,

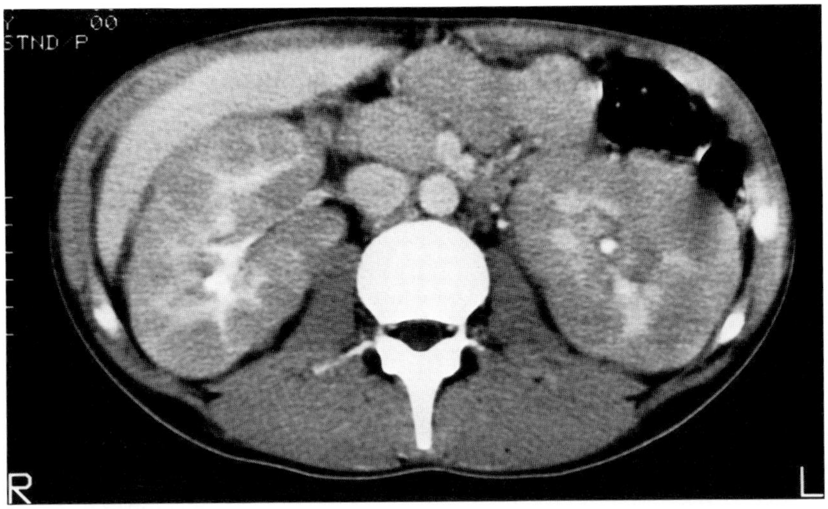

Fig. 6–29 Infiltrative lymphoma. Enhanced axial CT scan through the midabdomen demonstrates bilateral enlargement of the kidneys with replacement of the majority of the renal parenchyma by lymphoma cells. The patient had a newly diagnosed T-cell lymphoma.

cystinosis, fructose intolerance, galactosemia, glycogenosis, hyperparathyroidism, idiopathic hypercalcemia, Lowe's syndrome, tyrosinemia, Wilson's disease) may lead to renal tubular acidosis. Diuretic therapy (furosemide) for bronchopulmonary dysplasia in premature infants may also cause renal tubular acidosis. The conditions lead to the formation of stones with a calcium matrix. Uric acid stones may form in congenital heart diseases. Amorphous calcifications may develop secondary to previous trauma or necrosis, or in tumors. Ultrasound examination may reveal diffuse calcifications throughout the renal parenchyma or increased echogenicity of the medullary pyramids (more common in distal renal tubular acidosis) (Fig. 6–30). Ultrasonography is much more sensitive in the detection of nephrocalcinosis than is

A B

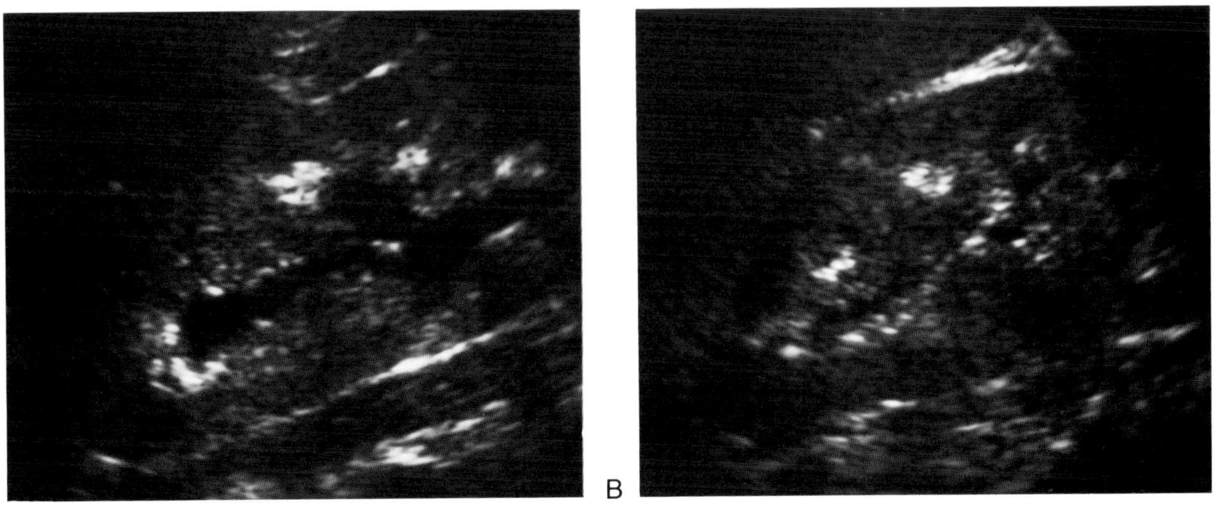

Fig. 6–30 Nephrocalcinosis. **(A)** Note the bright areas of increased echogenicity in the distribution of the medullary pyramids on the longitudinal scan of the right kidney. **(B)** The left kidney shows similar changes consistent with primary hyperparathyroidism.

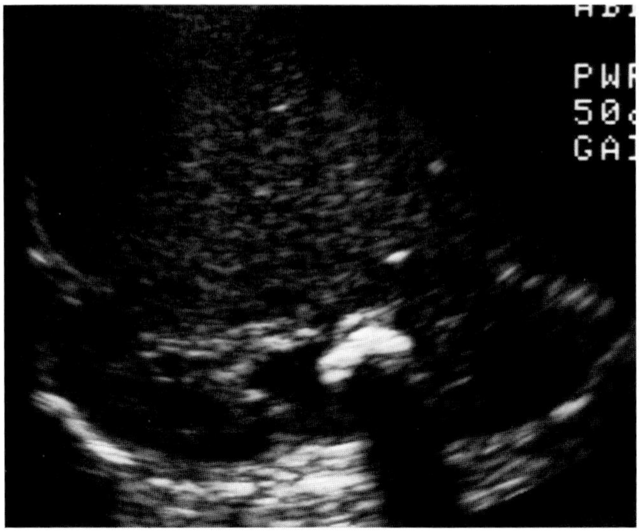

Fig. 6–31 Urolithiasis. Longitudinal ultrasound of the left kidney demonstrates a large echogenic focus with posterior shadowing, which proved after surgery to be a renal stone.

radiography and thus is the modality of choice for suspected cases.

Urolithiasis is the occurrence of stones within the collecting structures of the urinary tract (Fig. 6–31). Predisposing factors include hypercalciuria, urinary stasis, and recurrent urinary tract infection. Urolithiasis is related to urinary tract infection in almost 50 percent of patients. Approximately 40 percent have no etiology apparent and 10 percent have associated metabolic disorders. Urolithiasis may be associated with nephrocalcinosis. The patient usually presents with intermittent flank pain associated with hematuria or with urinary tract infection. Plain radiographs of the abdomen are the most sensitive modality for identifying stones within the collecting structures. Excretory urography is excellent in demonstrating obstruction secondary to urolithiasis. If the preliminary radiograph is obtained using low kilovoltage technique and careful collimation, most stones will be detected. Classic staghorn calculi are unlikely to form in children, but dense calcium compound stones are often detected. Cystine stones have a "ground glass" appearance and are associated with cystinuria, hyperoxaluria, and uricosuria. Uric acid stones, xanthene stones, and mixed composition stones are radiolucent. Uric acid stones are associated with Lesch-Nyhan syndrome and treated malignancies. Mixed composition stones may be associated with chronic gastrointestinal disorders and urinary stasis. Xanthine stones are associated with allopurinol therapy. If obstruction of the collecting structures due to a stone is suspected from the preliminary radiograph or from the patient's history, abdominal compression should not be used during the excretory urogram.

Trauma/Iatrogenic

In the face of blunt or penetrating abdominal trauma, CT stands alone as the imaging modality of choice for delineation of severity and extent of intra-abdominal injury. However, not every patient who experiences abdominal trauma is a candidate for CT. The patient must be hemodynamically stable for the examination. Stable patients with chronic or acute mental status changes leading to a nondiagnostic physical examination and those with an abnormal physical examination or laboratory evidence of intra-abdominal trauma should proceed to CT. If associated injury is suspected, both neurosurgical emergencies and evidence of aortic injury supercede intra-abdominal injury. In these cases, diagnostic peritoneal lavage is the method of choice for determining intra-abdominal trauma. Aortic injury is best evaluated with aortography prior to abdominal CT.

If illness or age prevents patient cooperation, sedation should be administered with the approval of the surgeon. Prior to sedation, the gastrointestinal tract may be opacified with 4 to 12 oz of a 1.5 percent oral contrast solution. After the patient is on the scanner, a digital scout film is followed by several preliminary cuts through the upper abdomen. Intravenous contrast material (in a dosage of 2 mg/kg for most low osmolality agents) is administered. Immediately after administration, axial 10-mm computed tomograms are obtained at 10-mm increments from the diaphragm through the lower poles of the kidneys. If lower abdominal injury is suspected, the study is continued through the pelvis. Dynamic scanning techniques should be utilized to minimize streak artifact if the patient is breathing rapidly.

The most common organs injured in childhood blunt abdominal trauma are the liver and spleen. Renal injuries follow closely. The least common are catastrophic injuries including vascular pedicle disruptions and multiple parenchymal fractures (Fig. 6–32). Although uncommon, major injuries include isolated renal fractures and cortical lacerations involving the

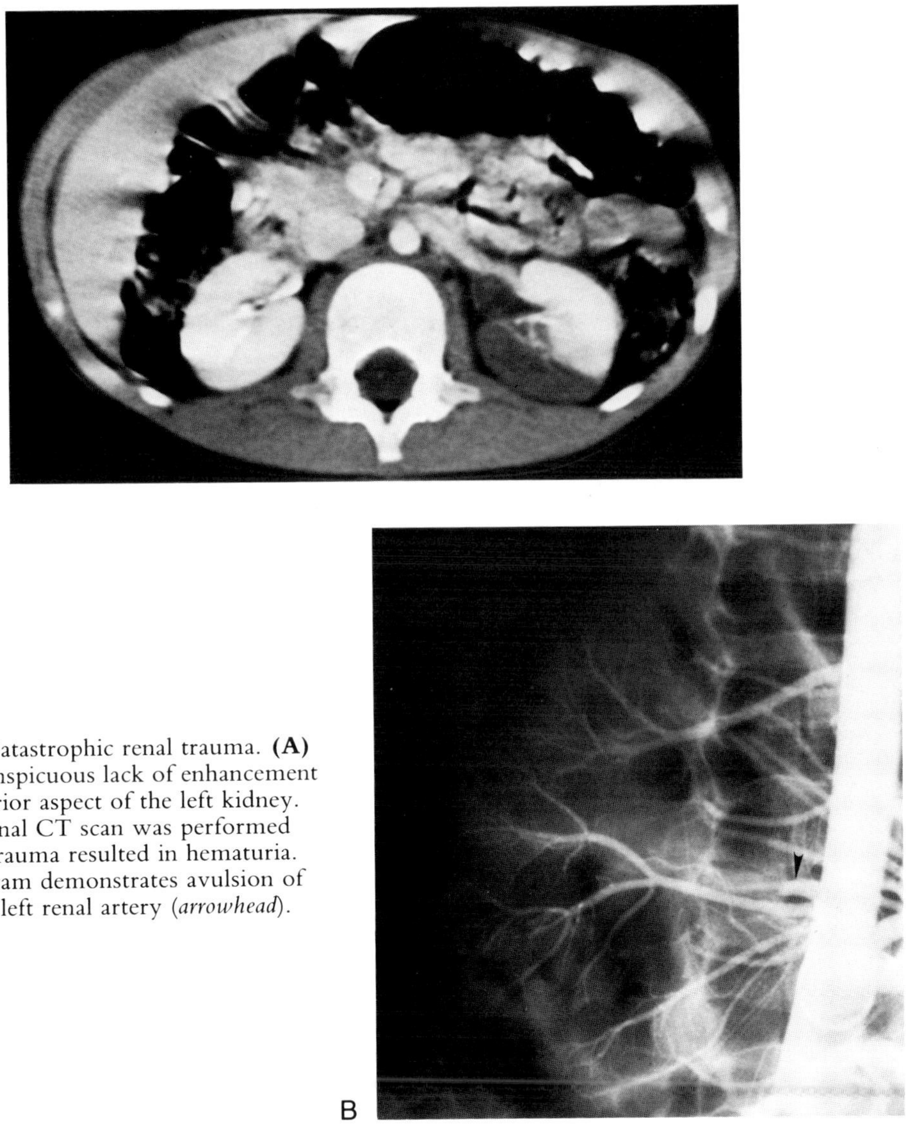

A

B

Fig. 6–32 Catastrophic renal trauma. **(A)** Note the conspicuous lack of enhancement of the posterior aspect of the left kidney. The abdominal CT scan was performed after blunt trauma resulted in hematuria. **(B)** Aortogram demonstrates avulsion of a segmental left renal artery (*arrowhead*).

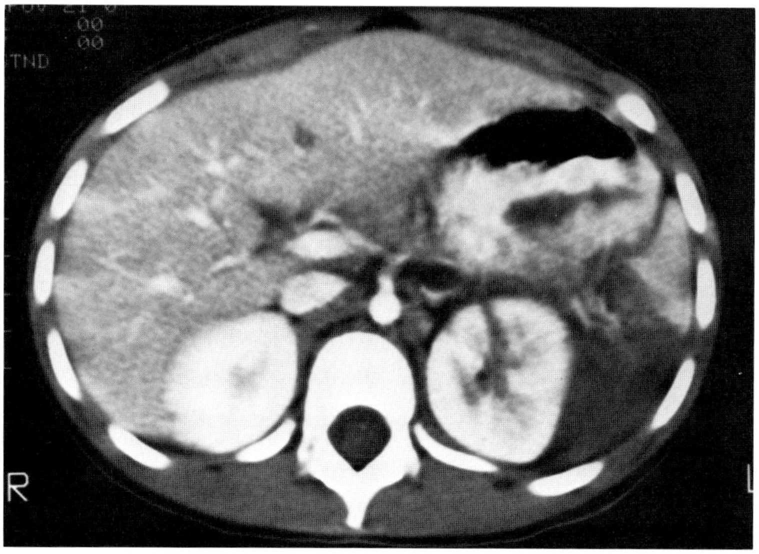

Fig. 6–33 Renal laceration. Enhanced axial CT scan following blunt abdominal trauma reveals a linear lucency through the midportion of the left kidney extending anteriorly. The laceration subsequently resolved with conservative therapy.

collecting structures. Eighty-five percent of renal injuries are minor and include isolated cortical lacerations, contusions, and hematomas. The majority of renal lesions heal without surgical intervention. Excretory urography is nondiagnostic in approximately 20 percent of cases and tends to underestimate severe renal injury. Ultrasound examination is useful for follow-up of injuries once the extent is fully defined by CT.

In fractures, the kidney will be separated into various parts. Lacerations and infarcts appear as geographic regions of decreased attenuation on CT examination (Fig. 6–33). Lacerations extending into the collecting structures are associated with extravasation of contrast material. When hemorrhage leaks into the subcapsular or perirenal space, increased attenuation values is seen prior to contrast administration. The enhancement of extrarenal hematomas lags behind that of the adjacent renal parenchyma. Delayed images of the kidneys may aid in detection. Approximately 10 percent of patients with renal trauma are noted to have pre-existing lesions such as congenital anomalies, cysts, hydronephrosis, or caliceal diverticula. Congenital absence of the kidney must be differentiated from the nonfunctioning kidney associated with renal vascular pedicle disruption.

Subcapsular hematoma causes compression of the adjacent renal parenchyma, which may lead to long-term renal ischemia and shrinkage of the involved kidney. Termed the *Page kidney,* it may be demonstrated by either ultrasonography or CT (Fig. 6–34). Both modalities demonstrate overall enlargement of the involved renal capsule in which a subcapsular mass is identified, with adjacent compression of the kidney. Early evacuation of the subcapsular collection may lead to resolution of ischemia and return of normal renal function. A Page kidney may cause hypertension. In chronic cases with no chance of return of normal renal function, nephrectomy is recommended for treatment.

Chronic renal failure may be the end result of numerous conditions previously discussed. Acceptable forms of therapy for renal failure include peritoneal dialysis, hemodialysis, and renal transplantation. The transplant organ may be from either a cadavaric or living-related donor. Immediately after transplantation, there is a mild increase in the size of both the transplant kidney and the pelvocaliceal collecting structures. Within 48 hours of transplantation both an ultrasound examination and a ^{99m}Tc-DTPA examination are recommended to establish a baseline for follow-up.

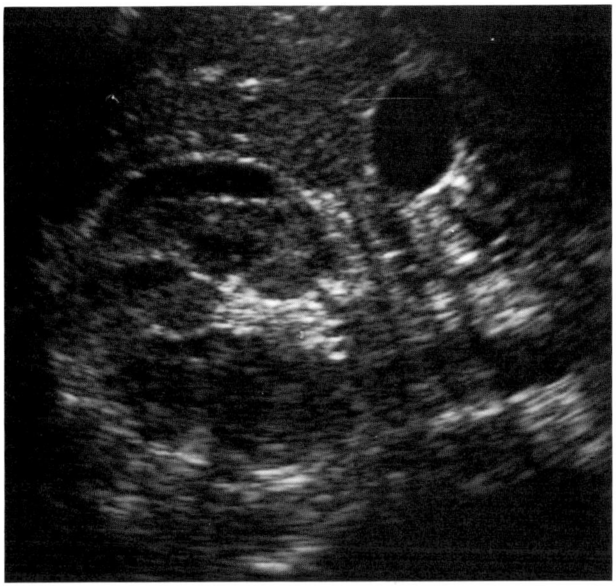

Fig. 6–34 Subcapsular hematoma. Transverse scan of the right kidney demonstrates a superficial, small, hypoechoic fluid collection within the renal capsule. The patient's transient hypertension subsequently resolved as did the hematoma.

Complications that are most common in the first week after transplantation include hyperacute and acute rejection, acute tubular necrosis, vascular obstruction, and urine extravasation. Both seromas and urinomas may be seen in the immediate postoperative period with ultrasound examination and usually spontaneously resolve over time.

The most common complication of renal transplantation is graft rejection. Hyperacute rejection is usually noted before the end of surgery as the transplanted kidney becomes swollen and cyanotic. Acute rejection is the most common form and usually occurs within 12 days after transplantation. Symptoms include increasing serum creatine and blood urea nitrogen levels and oliguria. Unfortunately, neither sonography nor radionuclide imaging is specific for the diagnosis of rejection. It is important to differentiate acute rejection from acute tubular necrosis since acute tubular necrosis is self-limited. Ultrasonographic findings that have been implicated as diagnostic of rejection include a greater than 30 percent increase in the renal volume, enlargement and squaring off of the medullary pyramids, a decrease in the central sinus echoes,

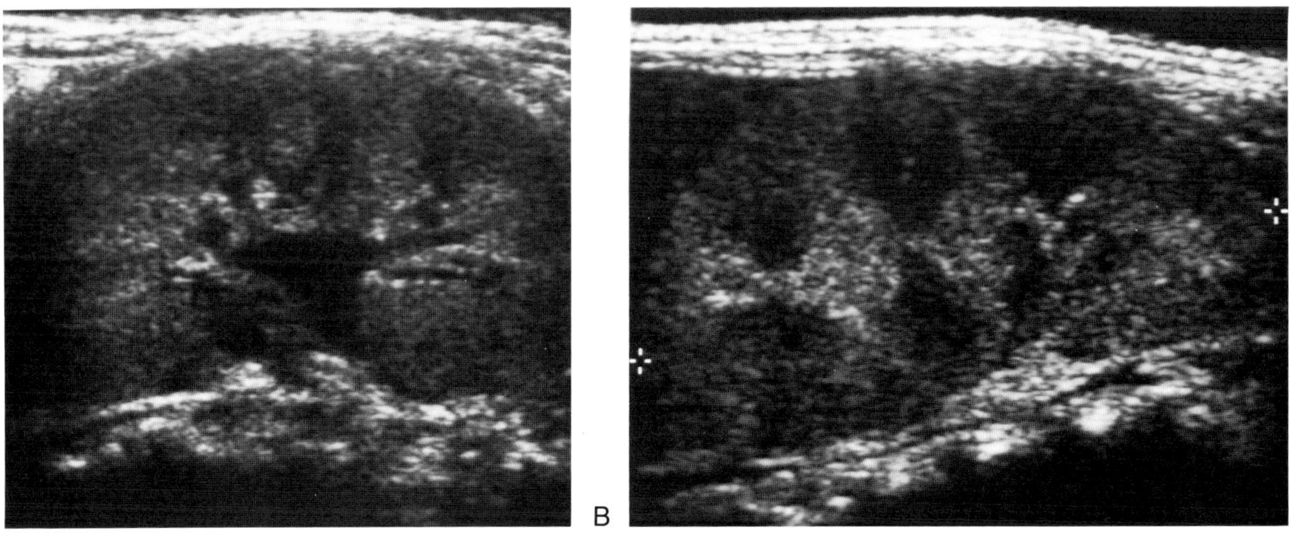

A B

Fig. 6–35 Transplant rejection. **(A)** Note the lack of a distinct corticomedullary junction and squaring off of the renal pyramids in the longitudinal scan of the transplant kidney. **(B)** Note the plump appearance of the transplant kidney in another patient with suspected rejection. The echotexture is increased and homogeneous. *(Figure continues.)*

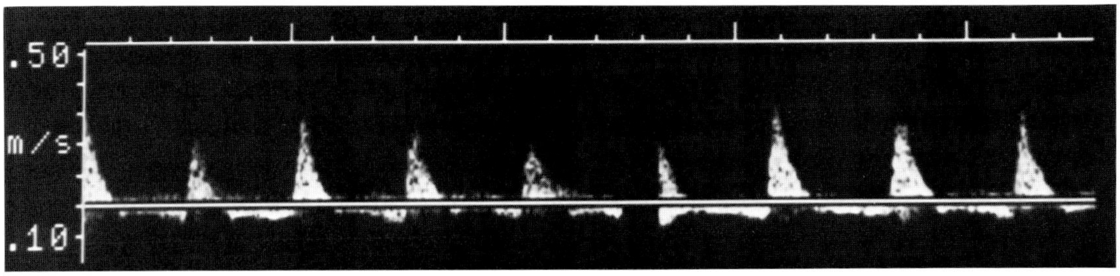

C

Fig. 6–35 (*Continued*). **(C)** Duplex scanning revealed a reversal of arcuate artery diastolic flow consistent with a resistive index of greater than 100 percent. Biopsy revealed rejection resulting in retransplantation.

and abnormal echogenicity of the renal parenchyma (Fig. 6–35). A combination of these findings along with suggestive changes on the Doppler analysis are more useful in diagnosing rejection than any single finding alone. Radionuclide imaging shows decreased perfusion and function with acute rejection. In contrast, acute tubular necrosis shows mild enlargement of the kidney on ultrasound examination with no change in the echogenicity. Radionuclide scanning shows good perfusion but decreased function. Follow-up examinations at frequent intervals are often necessary to differentiate the two conditions.

Duplex scanning has become useful in evaluating the vascular supply of the transplant. It is the modality of choice for the diagnosis of anastomotic arterial stenosis and venous thrombosis. An increase in the resistive index to greater than 90 percent is suggestive of rejection although high resistive indices have been reported in healthy transplants and with acute tubular necrosis on occasion.

Arteriovenous fistula describes an acquired condition in which either accidental or iatrogenic trauma to the kidney results in direct communication between the arteries and veins bypassing the glomeruli. Common conditions leading to the formation of arteriovenous fistula include blunt and penetrating abdominal trauma, renal biopsy, and percutaneous nephrostomy tube placement. The clinical clue to the diagnosis is persistent microscopic hematuria. The injury may be suspected when ultrasound examination reveals a focal abnormality, such as an increase in echogenicity or an increase in blood flow with color Doppler. Spectral analysis reveals rapid change from arterial flow to venous flow. However, selective arteriography is the most sensitive method of diagnosing arteriovenous fistulas and also provides access for embolization therapy.

COLLECTING SYSTEM ABNORMALITIES

Normal

The number or calyces present varies between patients and between kidneys. Incomplete division of the calyces results in dysmorphysm and megacalyces. These variations are more common at the poles than in the midportion of the kidney.

The renal pelvis may extend beyond the medial edge of the renal parenchyma (extrarenal pelvis). This should not be mistaken for pelvic dilatation on ultrasound examination (Fig. 6–36). A small amount of fluid may be seen within the renal pelvis during ultrasound examination. As long as the calyces appear normal, fluid within either an intrarenal or extrarenal pelvis should not be mistaken for mild hydronephrosis. Vascular indentations may appear as linear filling defects about the renal pelvis on excretory urograms. Another cause of filling defects in the region of the ureteropelvic junction are contractions. Kinking may cause filling defects that are relieved by changing the patient's position.

The ureters of children are much more mobile than those of adults. Deviation due to adjacent stool-filled bowel should not be mistaken for a mass unless the deviation is fixed while the patient changes positions.

COLLECTING SYSTEM ABNORMALITIES

Normal
- Calyceal dysmorphism
- Extrarenal pelvis
- Redundant mucosal folds/contractions
- Ureteral deviation

Congenital
- Hydronephrosis
- Ureteral ectopia
- Ureterocele
- Megaureter

Infection/inflammation
- Pylelitis/ureteritis
- Fungus
- Ureteral stenosis

Neoplasm
- Intrinsic
- Extrinsic

Trauma/iatrogenic
- Hematoma
- Perforation
- Air

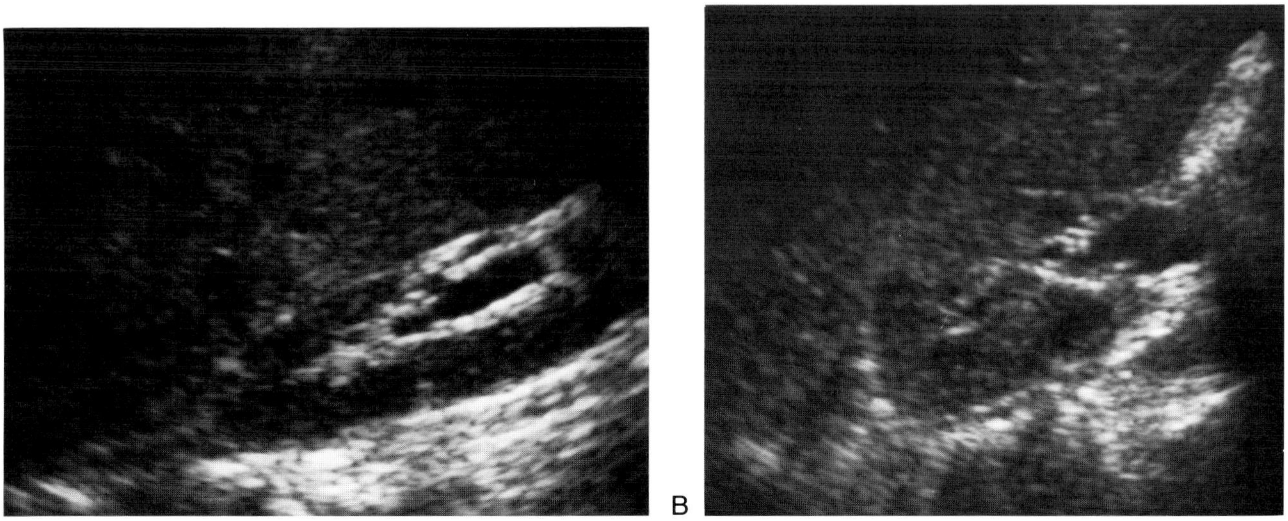

A B

Fig. 6–36 Extrarenal pelvis. **(A)** The longitudinal view of the right kidney demonstrates fullness of the renal pelvis but no corresponding dilatation of the calyces. **(B)** Transverse view demonstrates the extension of the renal pelvis outside the confines of the kidney, which is a normal variant.

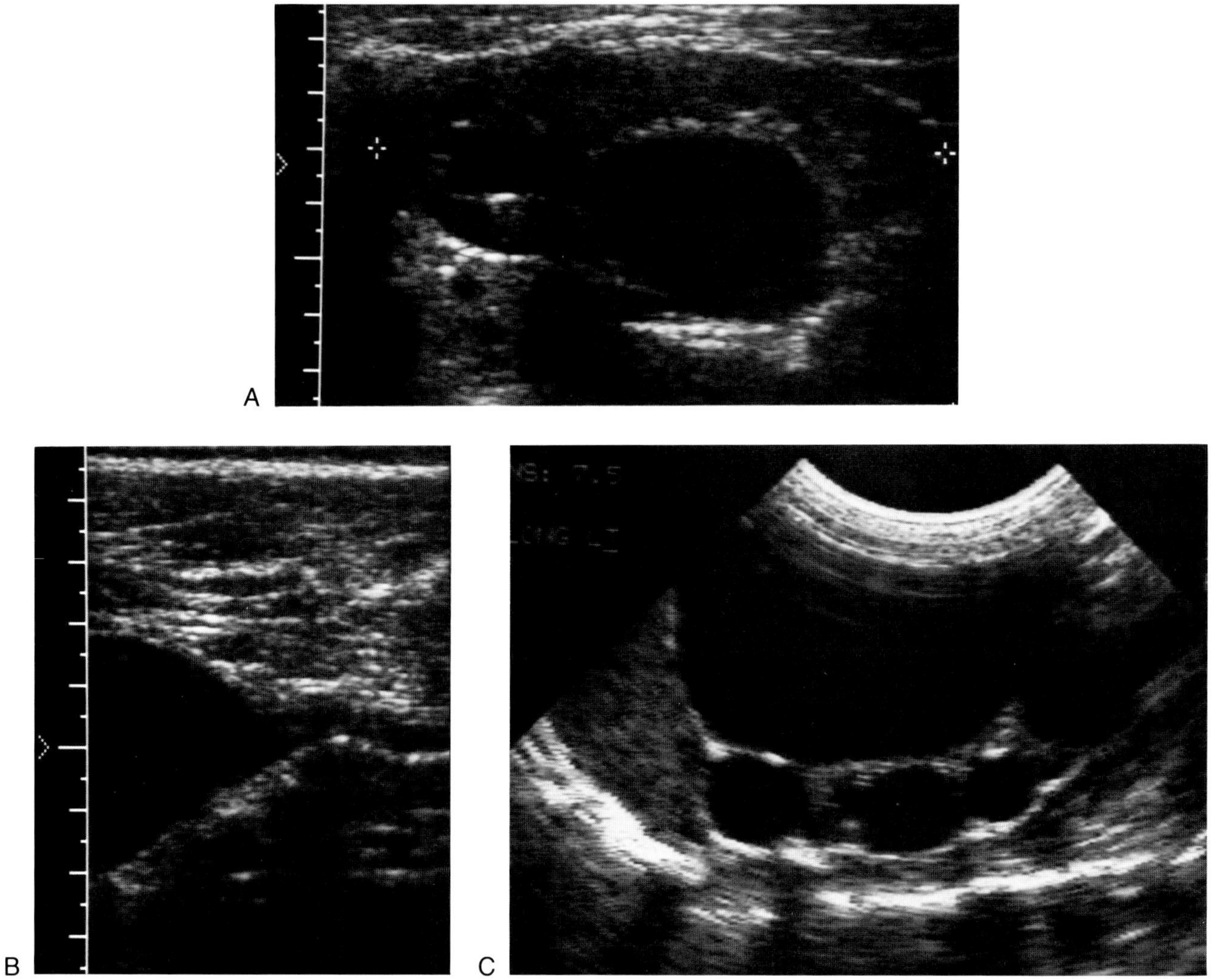

Fig. 6–37 Ureteropelvic junction obstruction. **(A)** Longitudinal ultrasound of the left kidney demonstrates moderate hydronephrosis. **(B)** In this case, the abrupt change in caliber between the distal left renal pelvis and the proximal left ureter was diagnostic upon longitudinal scanning of the left flank. **(C)** By contrast, the longitudinal scan of a multicystic cysplastic kidney demonstrates multiple cysts of varying sizes that do not communicate with each other. Very little renal parenchyma is identified.

Congenital

In childhood the most common causes of hydronephrosis include congenital ureteropelvic junction obstruction, ureterovesicular junction obstruction, bladder outlet obstruction, and vesicoureteral reflux. While obstruction of the pelvis or ureter is easy to recognize with ultrasonography, the cause is difficult to determine without the use of contrast material to opacify the system (Fig. 6–37). Technetium 99m-DTPA is useful in the evaluation of obstructive hydronephrosis since the renal function may be quantitated by this method. Scintigraphy is especially useful in the differentiation of a questionable ureteropelvic junction obstruction versus a multicystic dysplastic kidney.

Ureteropelvic junction obstruction is the most com-

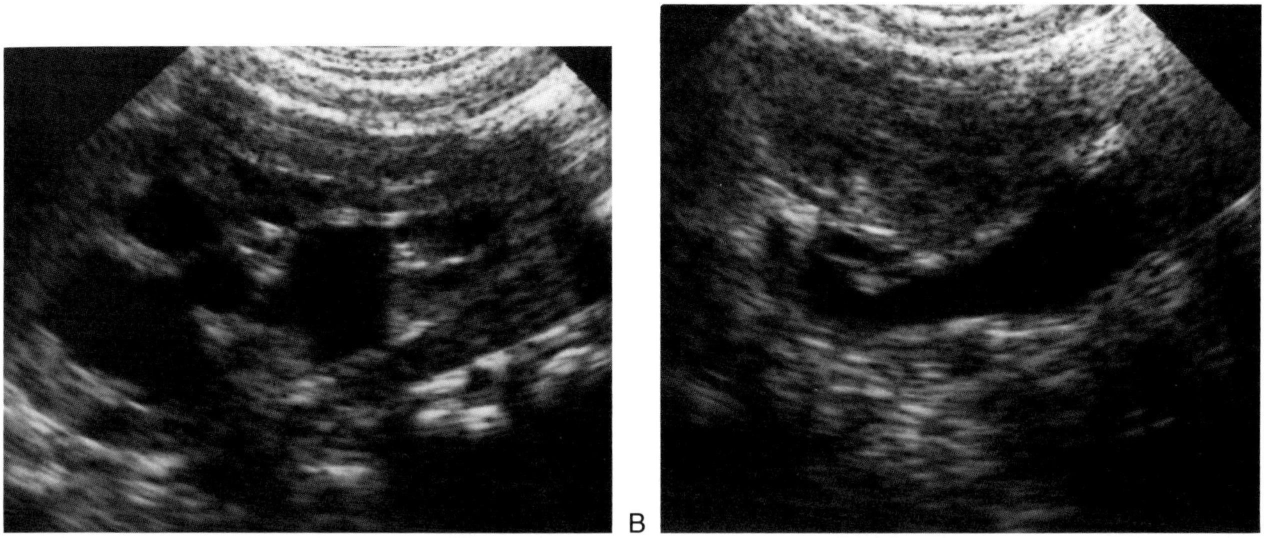

A B

Fig. 6–38 Hydronephrosis. **(A)** Longitudinal scan of the left kidney demonstrates moderate hydronephrosis. The hypoechoic psoas muscle is seen deep to the lower pole of the kidney. **(B)** Slight angulation of the transducer permits visualization of the dilated left ureter, which extended to the pelvis. Vesiculoureteral reflux was confirmed with cystography. Compare this patient with the previous figure (Fig. 6–37B) of ureteropelvic junction obstruction.

mon cause of mechanical obstruction of the urinary tract in children. It is more common on the left than the right side and is bilateral in 10 percent of cases. In utero, a primary stenosis may develop and lead to obstruction that is detectable on prenatal ultrasound examination. Immediately after birth, the neonate becomes dehydrated and mild ureteropelvic junction obstruction may be missed if ultrasonography is performed at this time. Other less common causes of ureteropelvic junction obstruction include localized muscular deficiency resulting in functional obstruction, extrinsic compression, or no obvious cause. A palpable mass in the infant may lead to ultrasound examination, which reveals the typical appearance of the fingerlike dilated calices communicating with the palmlike renal pelvis reminiscent of a "chubby hand." Once upper system dilatation is noted, a diligent search must be performed to rule out hydroureter (Fig. 6–38).

After confirmation of ureteropelvic junction obstruction is made by scintigraphy, invasive intervention follows. If there is a question regarding the significance of a mild ureteropelvic junction obstruction, a Whitaker test may be performed to evaluate urodynamics. This test requires antegrade puncture of the kidney as well as catheterization of the bladder. If renal function is impaired but not absent and dilatation is great, percutaneous nephrostomy tube placement may be performed. Complications include infection, perforation of the collecting system, and vascular injury leading to arteriovenous fistula formation. Advantages include access for antegrade stent placement and acute relief of obstruction leading to improved renal function before surgery. In cases of nonfunction of the involved kidney, nephrectomy is generally performed to decrease the risk of subsequent infection.

Congenital obstruction of the ureter between the ureteropelvic and uretovesicular junctions is rare. In childhood, the most common cause of obstruction at this level is extrinsic compression due to an abnormal course of the ureter or due to mass effect from an intra-abdominal process. Other causes include valves and strictures. The retrocaval ureter is an abnormal course of the right ureter so that it passes posterior to the inferior vena cava and extends anteriorly between the aorta and inferior vena cava before continuing downward anterior to the inferior vena cava. Abnormal development of the inferior vena cava is the cause of the deviated course of the ureter. Often, the entity is clinically unsuspected during childhood and may be incidentally noted when urologic evaluation is performed for another cause. Either ureter may pass behind the iliac arteries and demonstrate obstruction at this level. The hypogastric artery and other vessels may also cause ureteral obstruction with concommitant stricture formation as the patient ages. Treatment is resection of the ureter at the symptomatic level.

Obstruction at the ureterovesicular junction is quite common. Ultrasound examination may easily recognize the characteristic hydronephrosis and hydroureter but may fail to differentiate obstruction, reflux, and megaureter. Diligent scanning in the lower pelvis may reveal ureteral stones or other causes of obstruction such as ectopic insertion. Technetium 99m-DPTA scintigraphy with lasix washout provides additional information since the radiotracer will not clear the obstructed system on delayed images. Retrograde pyelography is the most sensitive method of differentiating ureteral abnormalities. It readily demonstrates intraluminal stones, neoplasms, strictures and atresia. Excretory urography with delayed films is commonly used since complications are rare.

The incidence of vesicoureteral reflux in healthy infants and children is estimated to be approximately 2 percent. A familial relationship has been established in some series, although most cases are sporadic. Infants and children with urinary tract infections have a higher incidence of vesicoureteral reflux (up to 52 percent). In children under 1 year of age, the length of the intravesical section of the ureter is less than 1 cm but increases in length to 1.45 cm in early adulthood. It is generally accepted that the length of the intravesical section is important in the pathogenesis of reflux since this section forms a passive valve. While most nonrefluxing ureters demonstrate an intramural portion six times longer than the ureter diameter, refluxing ureters usually have an intramural segment shorter than the diameter of the ureter. The aim of surgical correction is to lengthen the intravesical portion of the ureter, thus creating a passive valve. The angle of ureteric insertion has been implicated as a causative factor in reflux. If the distal ureter becomes more horizontally oriented, reflux occurs. A horizontal orientation of the ureter is normally seen in infancy (when the intramural portion of the ureter is short), during cystitis, and with periureteral diverticula. In 16 to 57 percent of children with reflux, renal scarring occurs (reflux nephropathy). The voiding cystourethrogram is the most efficient method of demonstrating vesicoureteral reflux. The severity of reflux is directly related to parenchymal damage, thus grading is important in treatment planning.[14] Reflux nephropathy occurs in less than 20 percent of patients with grade I and II reflux, but increases to 79 percent with grades III through V. The lower grades of reflux are associated with spontaneous cessation as the patient ages in up to 80 percent of cases. During the voiding cystourethrogram it is important to notice whether low pressure reflux occurs with early bladder filling or if reflux is only associated with high pressures from complete bladder distention or during micturation. Low pressure reflux is associated with the higher grades of reflux needing surgical correction. After a contrast voiding cystourethrogram has been performed for the diagnosis of reflux, follow-up studies may be obtained using ^{99m}Tc-pertechtenate.

An ectopic ureter is usually associated with a duplex kidney. Ectopic ureters may have an intravesicular or extravesicular insertion site. If the ureteral bud does not separate from the Wolfian duct, then the ectopic ureter inserts in a lower site than normal.

Simple ureteral ectopia is more common in females than males and is associated with continual dribbling of urine when the insertion site is extravesicular. Common locations for the ectopic site include the periurethral region, bladder neck, and vagina. Reflux is more commonly associated with a high insertion site, while incontinence is associated with a lower insertion site. Affected males usually present with symptoms of infection. Incontinence is not a symptom in boys because the ectopic ureter opens proximal to the internal urethral sphincter. The most common insertion site in males is the prostatic urethra (up to 60 percent of cases). Other sites of insertion include the seminal vesicles, vas deferens, and ejaculatory ducts. Occasionally ectopic ureters may enter the rectum. The radiographic demonstration of the presence of a simple ectopia may be difficult. Ultrasound examination of the pelvis with the bladder filled may demonstrate a dilated distal ureter below the level of the bladder trigone. Direct visualization of the ureteral

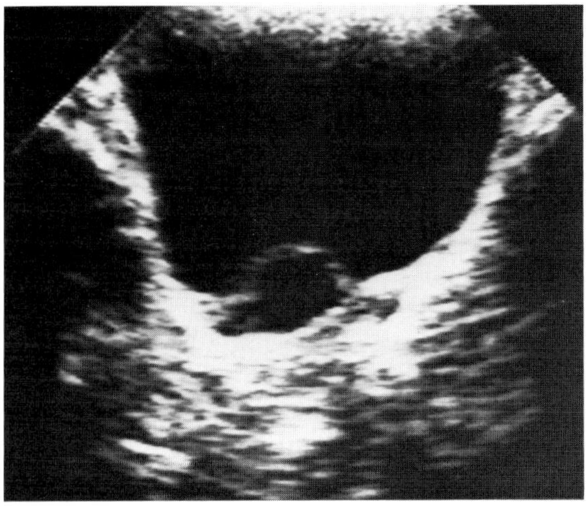

A

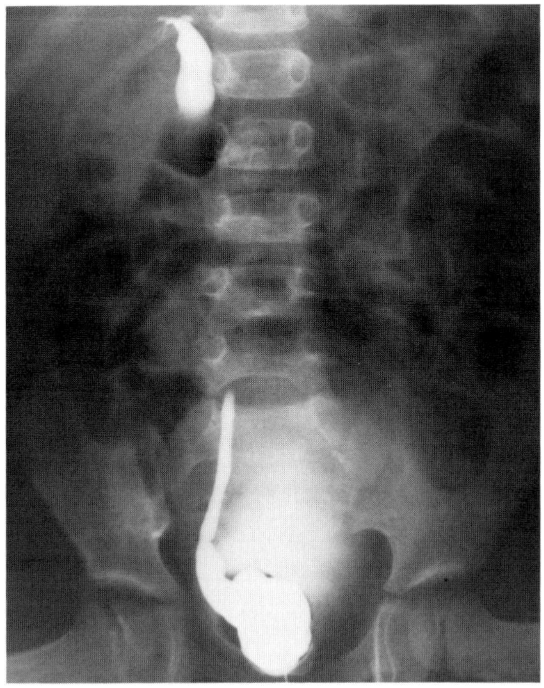

B

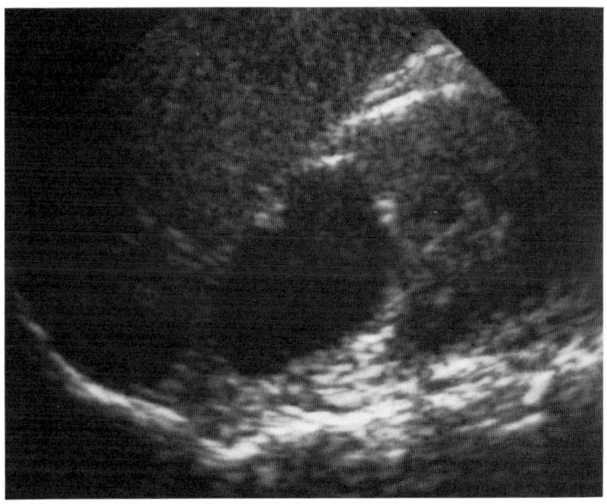

C

Fig. 6–39 Ectopic ureterocele. **(A)** Transverse ultrasound image of the full bladder demonstrates a fluid-filled defect at the level of the trigone. **(B)** Intraoperative catheterization permits retrograde filling of the ectopic ureterocele and the nonfunctional upper pole moiety. **(C)** Longitudinal ultrasound of another patient demonstrates gross dilatation of the upper pole moiety with no identifiable upper pole renal parenchyma of the right duplex kidney. An associated ectopic ureterocele was present.

orifice with cannulation and retrograde opacification is usually necessary for definitive diagnosis.

A ureterocele is a dilatation of the distal ureter. Seventy-five percent of ureteroceles are ectopic, while only 30 percent of ectopic ureters demonstrate a ureterocele. Fifty percent of children with ectopic ureteroceles demonstrate a duplex kidney. Generally the upper pole moeity is associated with the ectopic ureter and ureterocele, which inserts below the trigone. The presence of a ureterocele is readily recognized by ultrasonography. A fluid-filled mass extends into the bladder lumen either at the level of the trigone or along the posterior bladder wall (Fig. 6–39). Differentiation from a Hutch diverticulum (paraureteral diverticulum) is necessary. Ureteroceles are bilateral in 10 percent of the patients. Ectopic ureteroceles occur more frequently in females. Complications include reflux and obstruction. When an ectopic ureter is associated with duplication, treatment is heminephrectomy and ureterectomy.

Simple ureteroceles may be incidentally noted on ultrasound examination or excretory urography. Symptoms rarely occur in childhood and if no evidence of obstruction of the ipsilateral ureter is seen, then no treatment is necessary. If obstruction is evident, the ureterocele is excised and the ureter reimplanted.

Functional obstruction of the vesicoureteral junction, termed *primary megaureter,* may occur as an isolated finding or associated with gross dilatation of the bladder (megacystis). Primary megaureter may or may not be associated with vesicoureteral reflux. Sixty percent of patients present with an abdominal mass, males are affected more than females, and the left side is involved more than the right. Only 20 percent of the patients demonstrate bilateral involvement. Ultrasonography will demonstrate the distal aperistaltic segment, which is narrowed in comparison to the dilated upper ureter (Fig. 6–40). Voiding cystourethrography is useful in demonstrating reflux.

Infection/Inflammation

Pyelitis describes chronic inflammation of the mucosa and submucosa of the renal pelvis and infundibula. Chronic inflammation of the ureter is termed *ureteritis.* Ultrasound examination accurately demonstrates inflammation of the wall of the renal pelvis or ureter as wall thickening (Fig. 6–41). Pyelitis is most commonly associated with chronic pyelonephritis, however, the finding is nonspecific. Ureteritis is associated with congenital anomalies leading to stasis or infection, accidental or iatrogenic trauma, urinary tract infection, and extrinsic inflammation. The terms *pyelitis cystica* and *ureteritis cystica* are reserved for identification of inflammatory cysts lining the mucosa of either the pelvis or ureter that may reach up to 2 mm in size. Both conditions are associated with chronic urinary tract infection. One excretory urography, multiple small, smooth intraluminal filling defects are scattered along the mucosal surface. Ultrasound examination demonstrates fluid within the cysts.

Invasive candidiasis is likely to occur in infants of very low birth weight (less than 1,500 g). Other predisposing factors are parenteral hyperalimentation, antibiotic therapy, long-term IV catheterization, and malnutrition. Nonspecific thickening of the mucosa of the renal pelvis or ureter may be seen. Renal involvement may be the solitary focus or may be part

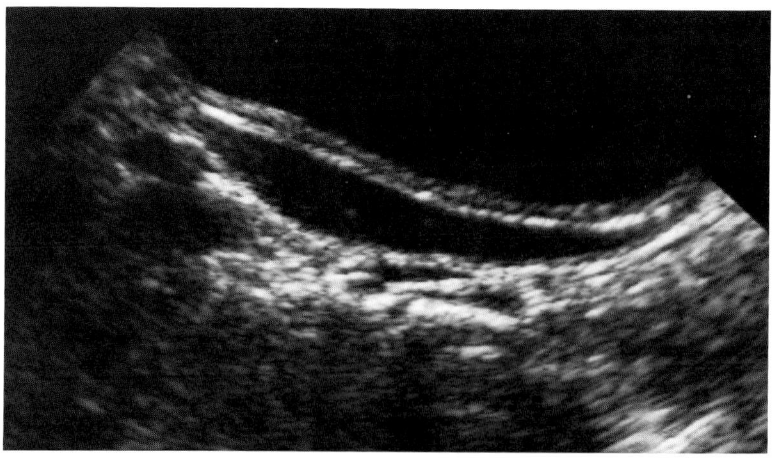

Fig. 6–40 Primary megaureter. Longitudinal scan of the right ureter demonstrates abrupt tapering just before insertion into the bladder. The narrowed segment was aperistaltic.

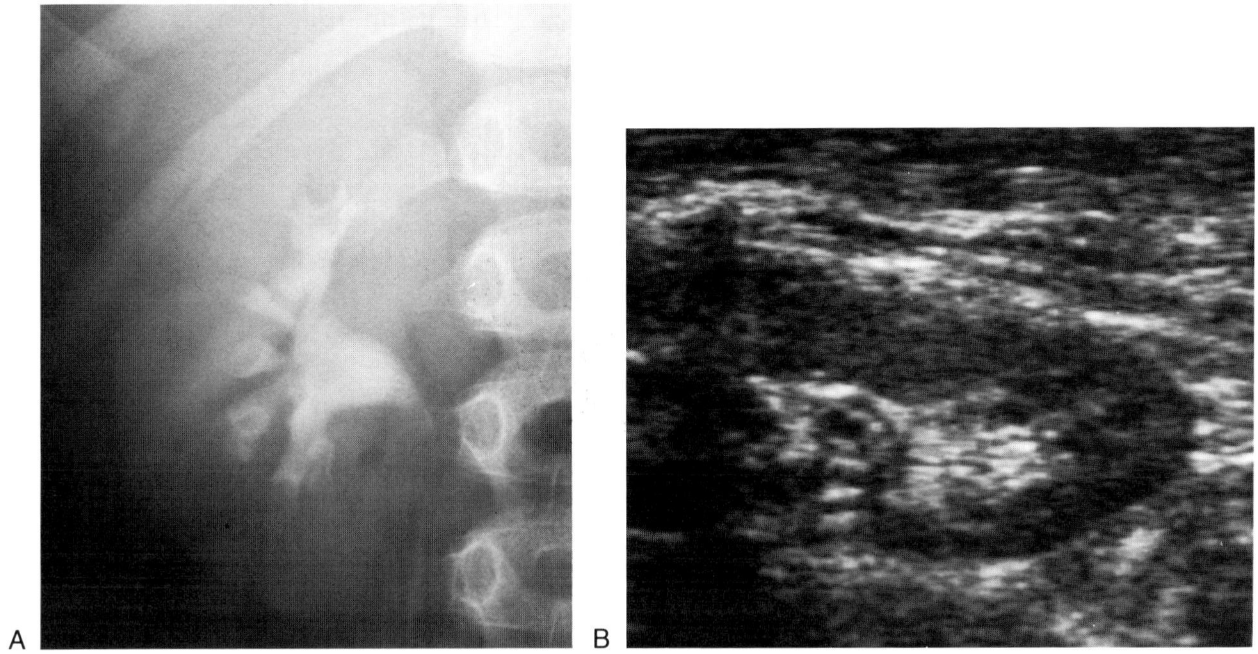

Fig. 6–41 Pyelitis striata. **(A)** The 15-minute radiograph from an excretory urogram demonstrates striation of the right renal pelvis consistent with inflammation of the wall. **(B)** Corresponding longitudinal ultrasound demonstrates the wall thickening as a hypoechoic rim of submucosal edema underlying the hyperechoic mucosa.

of a spectrum of multiorgan infection. Fungus balls within the renal pelvis may cause obstructive uropathy resulting in damage to the renal parenchyma. Rarely, fungus balls may cause bladder outlet obstruction resulting in obstructive uropathy. Diagnosis is usually made on ultrasound examination when an echogenic mass is seen within either the renal pelvis or the bladder (Fig. 6–42). Treatment involves irrigation with amphotericin B and occasionally percutaneous removal of the fungus balls.

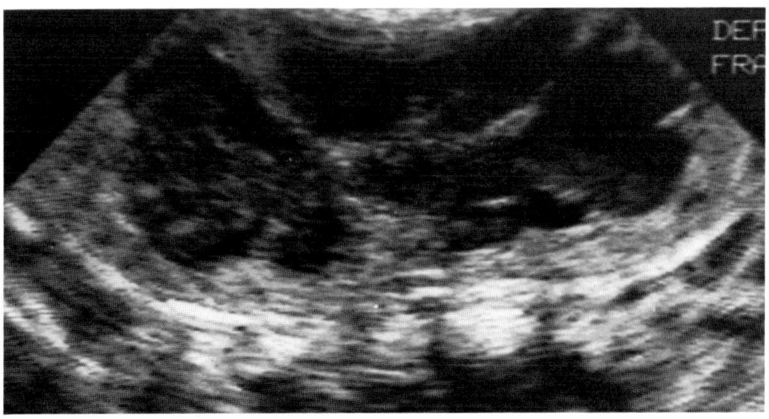

Fig. 6–42 Fungus balls. Note the severe hydronephrosis of a premature infant's right kidney on the longitudinal ultrasound. The echogenic renal parenchyma is compressed by the dilatation. Echogenic filling defects within the collecting structures represent fungus balls.

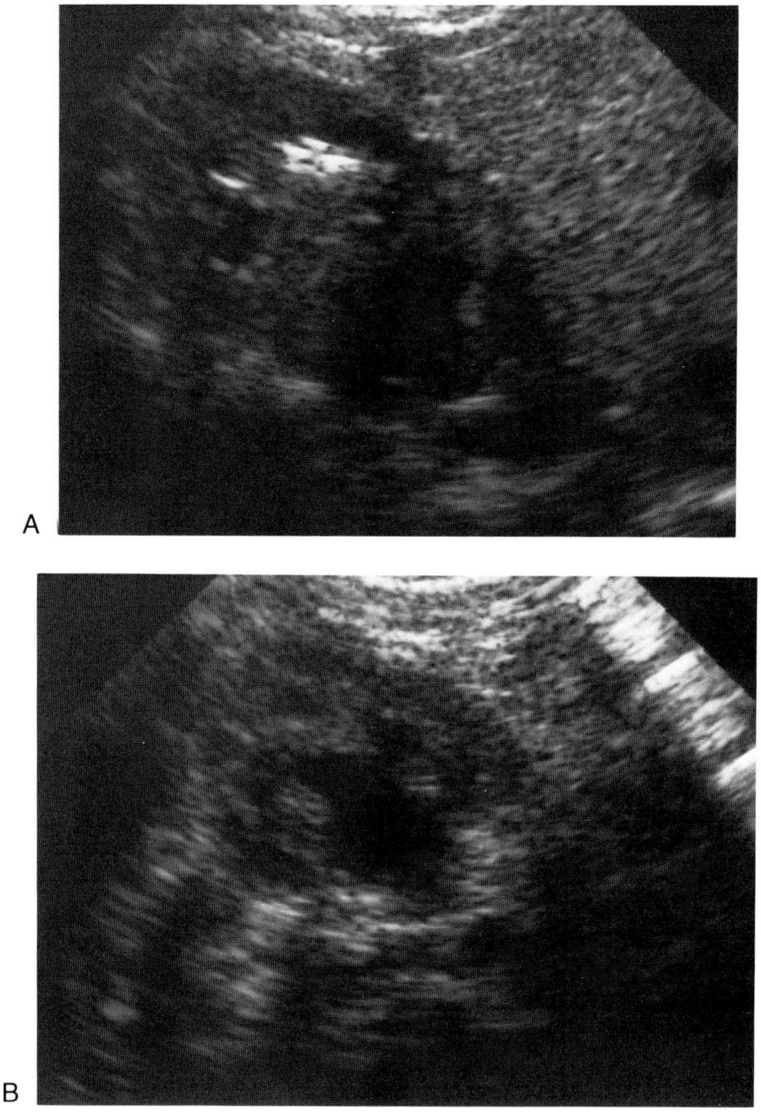

Fig. 6–43 Iatrogenic air. **(A)** Transverse scan of the right kidney following catheterization demonstrates echogenic foci with posterior shadowing in the calyces draining the midportion of the right kidney. **(B)** Repeat examination demonstrates resolution of the air bubbles. Air was confirmed on a concomitant cystogram.

Ureteral stenosis may occur as a result of adjacent ureteral inflammation from many causes of small vessel vasculitis and ischemia. Causes include Henoch-Schönlein purpura, radiation therapy, actinomycosis, retroperitoneal fibrosis, Crohn's disease, and dermatomyositis.

Neoplasm

Intrinsic neoplasms of the renal pelvis and ureter are rare and usually arise from the transitional epithelium. Aside from benign and malignant tumors of the transitional cell line, benign fibrous polyps have also been reported in the upper ureter.

Secondary invasion of the collecting structures by Wilms' tumor is not uncommon. Extrinsic retroperitoneal masses such as neuroblastoma, ganglioneuroma, and teratoma may cause displacement or obstruction of the ipsilateral ureter. Retroperitoneal lymphadenopathy associated with leukemia and lymphoma may also cause extrinsic compression or displacement of the ureter.

Trauma/Iatrogenic

Blunt abdominal trauma may result in hematuria regardless of whether the collecting system is actually damaged. Hematoma formation within the collecting structures is seen as single or multiple filling defects on contrast examination. Occasionally, ureteral obstruction will result from a hematoma lodged at the ureterovesicular junction.

Retrograde procedures may lead to iatrogenic injuries of the ureter and renal pelvis including perforation with urine and contrast extravasation into the periureteral tissue. Occasionally, post-traumatic fibrosis leads to a ureteral stricture, best documented with contrast opacification of the involved ureter.

Accumulation of air within the collecting structures may occur after retrograde procedures such as cystoscopy. If ultrasound is performed following a procedure, echogenic foci may be seen and may be confused with renal calculi (Fig. 6–43). Careful scrutiny of the retrograde pylogram may reveal air bubbles within the collecting structures. Otherwise, a repeat ultrasound examination more than 24 hours after the invasive procedure was performed will demonstrate resorption of the air.

LOWER URINARY TRACT ABNORMALITIES

Normal

When distended with contrast material administered through a retrograde catheter, the normal bladder should appear smooth with no external indentations. The infant bladder is higher in position with the bladder floor above the symphysis pubis. As the child ages, the bladder floor lies at the level of the symphysis pubis. The full bladder should not extend higher than the level of the lumbosacral junction. Bladder capacity varies with age. At birth, a 40-cc capacity is average. Between 1 to 7 years of age, the average bladder

BLADDER ABNORMALITIES

- Normal
  - Position
  - Capacity
  - Configuration
- Congenital
  - Abnormal urachus
  - Diverticula
  - Exstrophy
  - Megacystis
  - Neonatal urine retention
- Infection/inflammation
  - Cystitis
  - Pneumaturia
  - Bladder stones
  - Calcification
- Neoplasm
  - Hemangioma
  - Neurofibroma
  - Rhabdomyosarcoma
  - Transitional cell carcinoma
  - Metastases
- Trauma
  - Rupture
  - Avulsion
- Iatrogenic/miscellaneous
  - Perforation
  - Neurogenic dysfunction

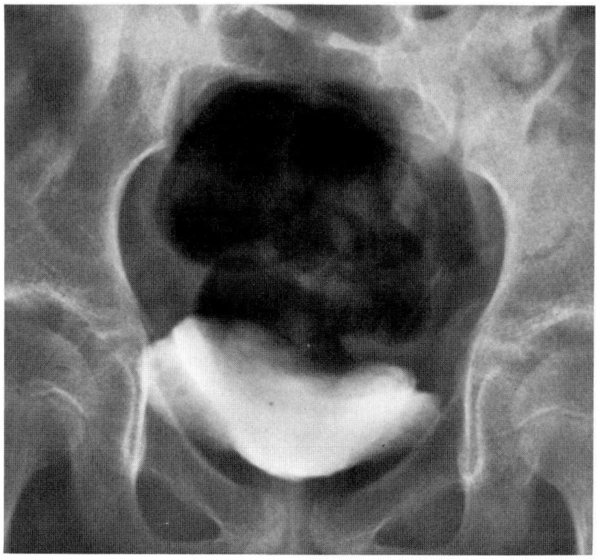

Fig. 6–44 Bladder ears. During the course of an excretory urogram, the partially filled bladder extends inferolaterally into the inguinal regions. As the bladder continued to fill, the bladder ears disappeared.

A
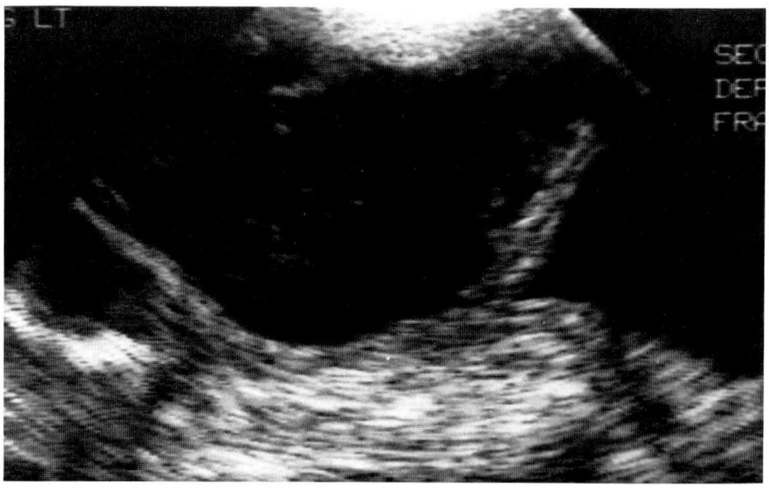

Fig. 6–45 Urachal cyst. **(A)** Longitudinal scan of the abdomen demonstrates a hypoechoic cystic mass with internal debris arising superior to the bladder. (*Figure continues.*)

capacity is 75 to 150 cc. Older children may have a capacity of up to 300 cc. When the bladder is incompletely filled, the inferolateral wall may extend into the femoral or inquinal canals forming "bladder ears." With full distension, the bladder recesses disappear (Fig. 6–44). Extrinsic compression from adjacent bowel and the uterus are most apparent with incomplete filling. The normal bladder may assume various configuration ranging from round to square.

On ultrasound examination, the bladder walls should not exceed 3 mm in thickness when fully distended. The trigone is easily identified and ureteral jets are often demonstrated. Caudal angulation reveals the bladder neck, which frequently contains a small amount of fluid.

Congenital

In embryonic life, the bladder extends up to the umbilical region. With fetal growth it subsequently descends along the anterior abdominal wall. The upper portion (urachus) usually is a fibrous remnant by birth. However, if the tract does not obliterate, the urinary bladder will drain through the umbilicus (patent urachus). The presence of a patent urachus is suspected when the umbilicus continues to be moist outside of the neonatal period. If only a segment of the tract remains, a urachal cyst forms. This may present as swelling of the umbilicus. Umbilical abnormalities are often investigated by ultrasound examination (Fig. 6–45). It is important to identify whether a cyst arises from the gastrointestinal tract (persistent vitelline duct) or whether it communicates with the superoanterior portion of the bladder (urachal remnant). While a patent urachus may be demonstrated with ultrasonography, the anomaly is best evaluated during cystography (Fig. 6–46). Incomplete filling of the bladder during ultrasound examination may cause a patent urachus to be missed. The lateral view during cystography will show reflux of contrast material into the umbilicus. Occasionally the urachus will be closed at the bladder but will continue to communicate through the umbilicus (urachal sinus). Direct catheterization with instillation of contrast material may be necessary for diagnosis. Since the risk of infection with both persistent communications is increased, surgery is recommended for treatment.

B

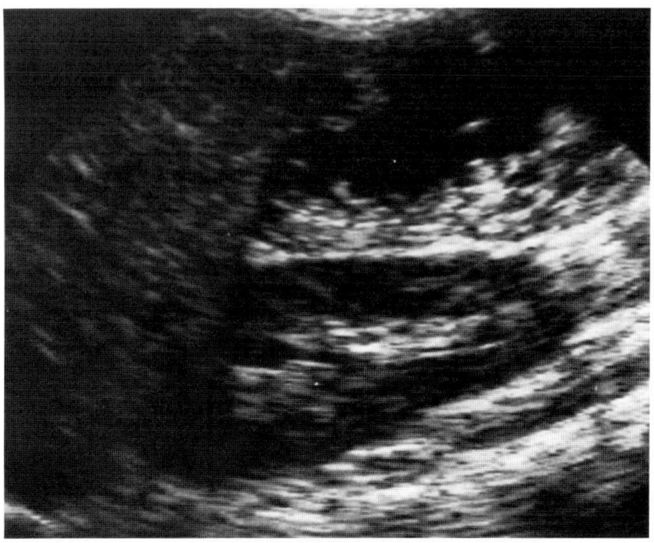

Fig. 6–45 (*Continued*). **(B)** A scan obtained higher in the abdomen demonstrates extension of the mass to the inferior margin of the liver. On physical examination, the patient's umbilicus was inflamed. At surgery, an infected urachal cyst was found.

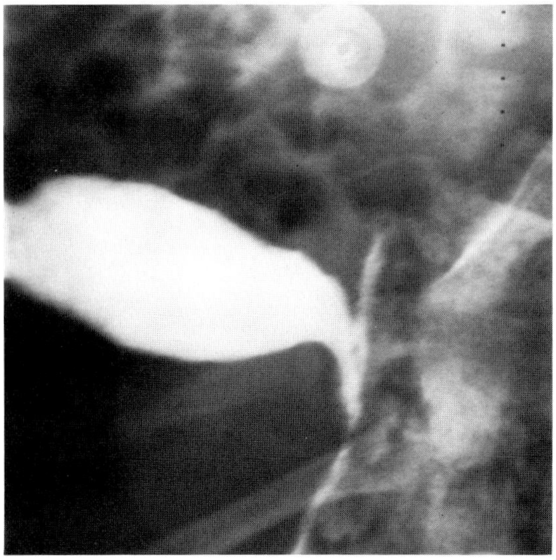

Fig. 6–46 Patent urachus. Lateral view from a voiding cystourethrogram in a girl with meningomyelocele and a single dysmorphic left kidney demonstrates wide patency of the anterior, superior aspect of the bladder, which communicated with the umbilicus.

Primary diverticula of the bladder are responsible for less than 5 percent of all bladder diverticula. Most congenital diverticula are Hutch diverticula arising at the ureterovesicular junction with herniation of the bladder mucosa through a muscular defect. Hutch diverticula are usually asymptomatic but predispose the patient to infection if statis is present. After the diverticulum enlarges, both reflux and obstruction of the ipsilateral ureter are likely to occur. While Hutch diverticula may be detected on ultrasound examination, voiding cystourethrography provides dynamic evaluation (Fig. 6–47). When the diverticulum is small, herniation only occurs during micturation. If the bladder pressure is high, as with neurogenic dysfunction, the diverticulum may be present at all times. This may lead to reflux of the ipsilateral ureter because the detrusor muscle no longer can contract efficiently. If evidence of renal damage is seen, resection of the diverticulum may be necessary. While most diverticula are isolated anomalies, a small percentage are associated with cutis laxa, Ehlers-Danlos syndrome, Menkes' kinky hair syndrome, prune-belly syndrome, and William's syndrome.

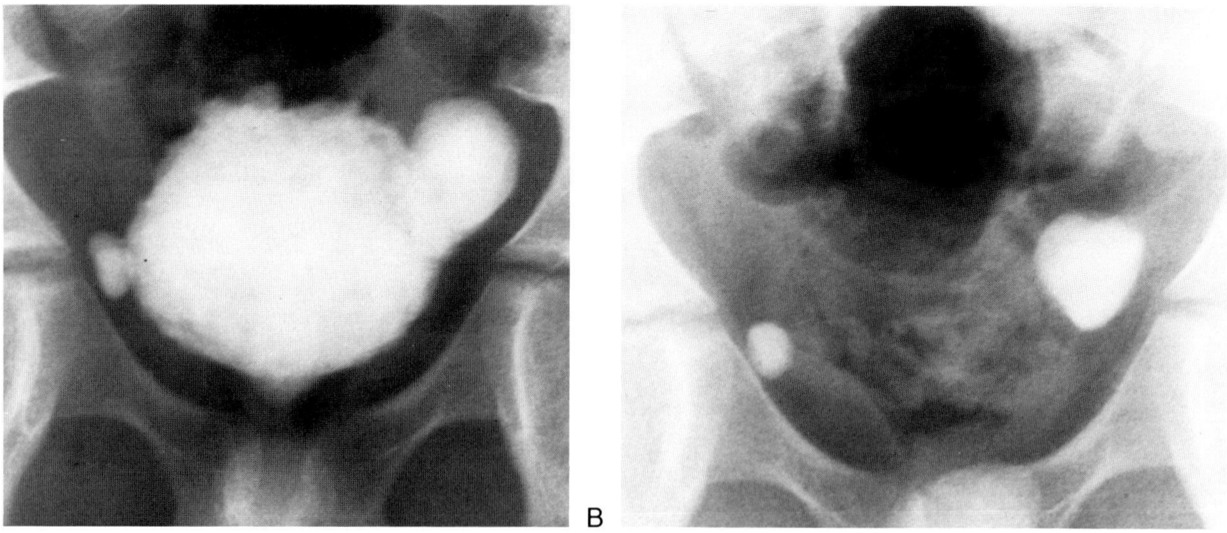

A B

Fig. 6–47 Paraureteral diverticula. **(A)** Radiograph obtained during a voiding cystourethrogram demonstrates opacification of bilateral Hutch diverticula. The paraureteral location was confirmed on oblique views. **(B)** After complete voiding, the diverticula retain contrast material.

Bladder exstrophy represents 4 percent of all lower urinary tract anomalies. Abnormal embryogenesis of the cloacal membrane results in persistent diastasis of the symphysis pubis and failure of midline fusion of the skeletal muscles and fascia of the lower anterior abdominal wall. The spectrum of anomalies encompassed in exstrophy ranges from simple epispadias to a persistent cloaca. Classic bladder exstrophy accounts for 50 percent of anomalies in the extrophy spectrum (Fig. 6–48). Cloacal extrophy is the most severe anomaly in the group and presents with two or more openings in the skin or mucosal surface of the lower anterior abdominal wall. Catheterization of the openings and instillation of contrast material reveals an exstrophied bladder that forms the lateral two pouches of the cloacal anomaly, exstrophied bowel interposed between the two bladders, and large intestine ending in an imperforate anus. The reproductive organs are usually duplicated. Often the sex is anomalous. Exstrophy is associated with other congenital malformations including (in order of decreasing frequency) intestinal anomalies, dysraphism, and other genitourinary anomalies. Primary surgery is directed at urinary and bowel diversion with skin closure over any midline mucosal surface.

Megacystis describes a normal appearing bladder with an abnormally large capacity. While this may represent a normal variant, it is also identified in functional abnormalities such as high-urine-volume states (diabetes insipidus) and in infrequent voiders.

Gross dilatation of the bladder is the major feature in the megacystis-microcolon intestinal hypoperistalsis syndrome. The entity occurs more commonly in females than males and is rare. The neonate presents with abdominal distension, which, revealed by ultrasound examination, is due to a dilated bladder. Barium enema reveals a nonfilled microcolon and generalized abdominal hypoperistalsis. The etiology of the syndrome is uncertain, although a visceral myopathy is suspected.

Neonatal bladder retention is not uncommon in the first weeks of life and usually resolves spontaneously. Bladder retention occurs most often in asphyxiated infants.

Infection/Inflammation

Cystitis describes both acute and chronic inflammation of the bladder. Twenty percent of all patients

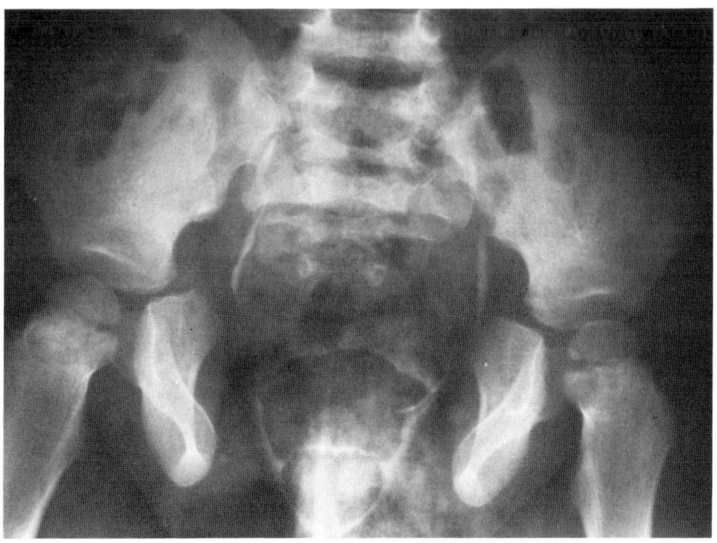

Fig. 6–48 Bladder exstrophy. Anteroposterior view of the pelvis during an excretory urogram demonstrates diastasis of the pubic symphysis with caudal herniation of the bladder consistent with exstrophy.

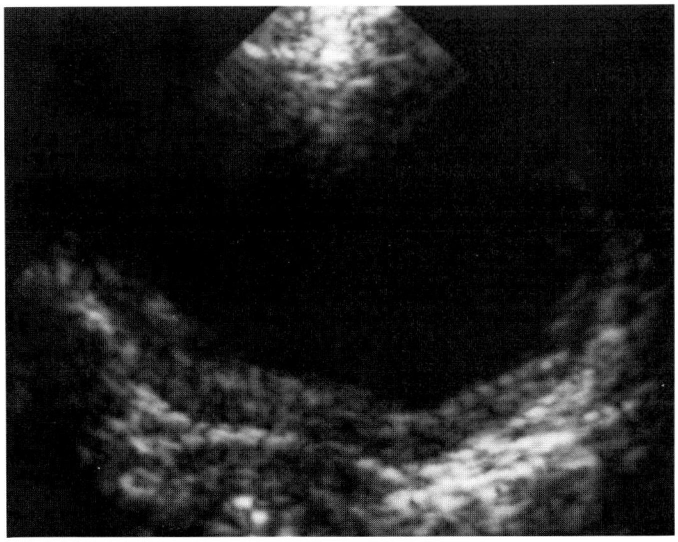

Fig. 6–49 Cystitis. Transverse ultrasound of the bladder demonstrates marked thickening of the wall with a dependent layer of echogenic debris. Tapping the transducer or decubitus positioning mobilized the debris within the infected urine. The echoes in the near field are artifacts.

with nontraumatic hematuria are subsequently diagnosed with hemorrhagic cystitis. Implicated organisms include adenovirus type II, type XI and type XXI, *E. coli,* and *C. albicans.* Up to 35 percent of patients receiving cyclophosphamide chemotherapy develop sterile hemorrhagic cystitis. Ultrasound examination reveals thickening of the bladder wall and debris within the urine (Fig. 6–49). Large, echogenic masses may represent blood clot, exudative inflammatory masses, or fungus balls. The question of whether to perform voiding cystourethrograms in the acutely infected child continues to be debated. It is logical that if the child is experiencing vesicoureteral reflux, then organisms are ascending into the upper collecting systems prior to the instillation of contrast material. No clear-cut evidence exists that performing a voiding cystourethrogram during the acute infection increases the incidence of parenchymal damage.

Chronic cystitis is usually the result of urine stasis. This leads to proliferation of the transitional epithelium of the bladder (cystitis cystica/glandularis) (Fig. 6–50). This may be diagnosed either ultrasonographically or during cystography as a focal irregular thickening of the bladder wall in the region of the trigone. Cysts of varying sizes may be detected in the bladder wall. Occasionally, a villous mass may also be seen. Proliferative cystitis is a predisposing factor for neoplastic transformation of the urethelium. Often, the radiologist cannot distinguish proliferative cystitis from bladder neoplasm (rhabdomyosarcoma). Cystoscopy with bladder biopsy is required for diagnosis.

Pneumaturia describes free air within the bladder lumen, which may be seen on either ultrasonography or contrast cystography. One cause is fermentation by organisms such as *E. coli, Aerobacter aerogenes,* and *C. albicans.* Gas production is more likely to occur with conditions predisposing the patient to glycosuria (poorly controlled diabetes mellitus). Other causes include fistulas between the gastrointestinal and genitourinary tracts secondary to either Crohn's disease or perforated appendicitis and iatrogenic introduction of air into the urinary system.

Calcifications in the region of the bladder are uncommon in childhood. Bladder stones present as smooth, large calcifications within a setting of urinary stasis (large bladder diverticulum or neurogenic bladder). The stones are usually calcium oxalate and have developed de novo within the bladder.

Bladder wall calcification is uncommon in childhood

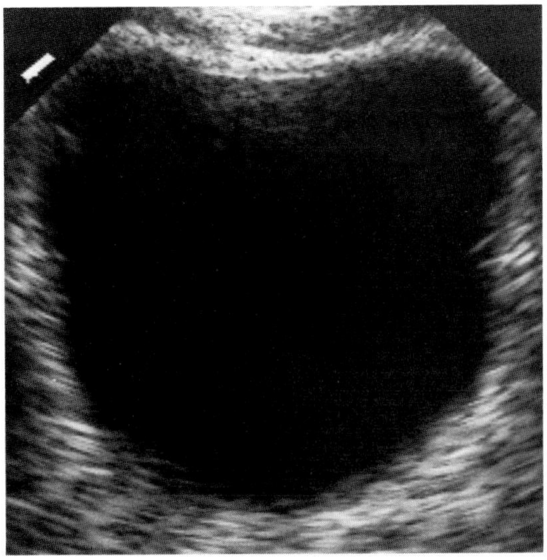

Fig. 6–50 Cystitis cystica. Note the multiple, small cysts arising from the lateral bladder walls on the transverse ultrasound of a lymphoma patient undergoing chemotherapy.

but has been associated with urine stasis in prune-belly syndrome, after cytoxan therapy, and for no apparent reason (idiopathic).

Neoplasm

Both benign and malignant neoplasms of the child's bladder are uncommon. Of the benign lesions, hemangioma is probably the most common. Patients present with hematuria and up to 30 percent of individuals have additional hemangiomas of either the skin or soft tissues. The most common site is at the bladder dome or trigone and the hemangiomas are usually no greater than 1 cm in size. A hemangioma may be detected as a bladder mass in a partially filled bladder on ultrasound examination. Irregular filling defects along the upper half of the bladder wall have been reported during cystographic examination. However, complete filling of the bladder during retrograde studies may compress the hemangioma. Cystoscopy allows direct visualization of the hemangioma, which is often characteristic. Since there is a significant risk of severe hemorrhage with biopsy, open exploration is necessary for tissue diagnosis.

Solitary or multiple filling defects within the bladder and prostate in a child with neurofibromatosis most likely represent multiple neurofibromas. The detection of a neurofibroma within the bladder is virtually pathognomonic of neurofibromatosis. It is unusual for the bladder to be the only involved organ.

The most common bladder neoplasm of childhood is the rhabdomyosarcoma (Fig. 6–51). The lower genitourinary tract is the site for approximately 20 percent of all rhabdomyosarcomas. The two major sites in the pelvis are the bladder and prostate. Patients present with hematuria and the mean age at diagnosis is 5 years. Males are affected more than females. Bladder neck obstruction may be a presenting symptom because of a propensity for development at the trigone. Ultrasound examination reveals focal bladder wall thickening and nodularity of the mucosa. While sarcoma botryoides is the most common form of rhabdomyosarcoma, an infiltrative pattern without polypoid projections also occurs. Since the occurrence of all other bladder neoplasms is rare in comparison to rhabdomyosarcoma, any focal area of wall thickening should be suspicious until cystoscopy has proven otherwise. The lower genitourinary tract is a favorable site for rhabdomyosarcoma with an overall survival rate of 70 to 80 percent. Metastases are most common in the lungs and liver. Both CT and MRI may be helpful in the metastatic workup. However,

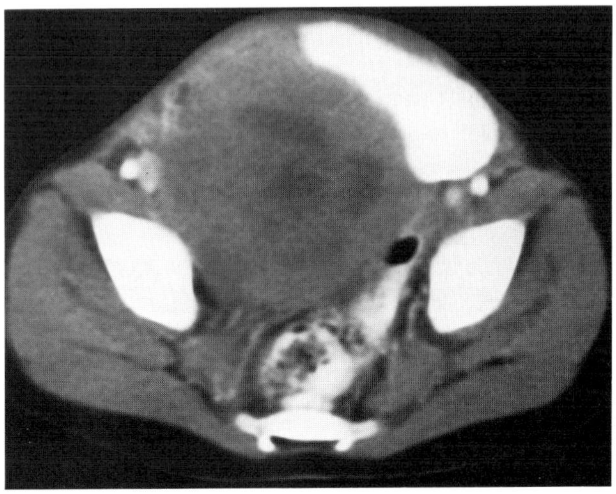

Fig. 6–51 Pelvic rhabdomyosarcoma. Enhanced axial CT scan demonstrates an inhomogeneous, nonenhancing low-density mass arising from the region of the prostate gland. The bladder is displaced anteriorly and to the left. The rectum is displaced posteriorly and to the left. At surgery, the mass was unresectable.

local invasion at the base of the bladder is difficult to evaluate with either modality. MRI appears to be slightly more helpful in local staging due to the ease of obtaining coronal and sagittal images.

Metastases to the bladder are uncommon but are usually due to leukemia or lymphoma. Occasionally, a Wilms' tumor will metastasize to the ureter or bladder.

Trauma

Since catheterization and cystoscopy have become more commonplace in children, mild iatrogenic trauma is not unusual. Complications of invasive procedures include mucosal irritation, infection, and perforation. Stricture formation of the distal ureter procedure may present late as hydronephrosis. Small perforations of the bladder or ureterovesicular junction may present as retroperitoneal pseudocysts.

Nonpenetrating injury of the bladder usually occurs in association with pelvic fracture. Only about 10 percent of pelvic fractures have associated bladder ruptures; a full bladder is more likely to rupture than an empty one. Intraperitoneal, extraperitoneal, and combined ruptures have been described. The intraperitoneal rupture may occur without associated fracture and is diagnosed by performing a retrograde cystourethrogram. After the urethra has been evaluated, the catheter is advanced and the bladder filled using fluoroscopy. Full distension or voiding may be necessary to obviate the tear. Occasionally the tear may not be apparent. In intraperitoneal rupture, the bladder maintains its rounded shape when filled, while extravasated contrast material opacifies the peritoneal cavity. In extraperitoneal rupture, extravasated urine causes extrinsic compression of the bladder. Extraperitoneal extravasated contrast material spreads over the lower half of the bladder in a streaky pattern as it extends upward and outward through the fascial planes. When both injuries are combined, signs of both types of rupture will be detectable.

Avulsions of the ureter or of the bladder neck are unusual and are unlikely to occur as isolated injuries. Patients with frank bladder avulsion present with anuria. Ureteropelvic junction avulsions may be more difficult to diagnose and may present late with pseudocyst formation.

Iatrogenic/Miscellaneous

One of the more common pediatric urologic problems encountered is the neurogenic bladder. Congenital spinal cord anomalies account for the majority of cases and include myelomeningocele, tethered cord, lipomeningocele, dysraphism, and sacral agenesis. Acquired causes include trauma to the spinal cord or nerve roots, pelvic neoplasms, and previous surgery. Any cause may result in dysfunction of the detrusor muscle and the external urethral sphincter. Symptoms may include frequency, enuresis, urine retention, and incontinence. A neurogenic bladder may be suspected when an abnormally small- or large-volume bladder is encountered on ultrasound examination (Fig. 6–52). Trabeculation and thickening of the wall may be apparent. Re-evaluation after the

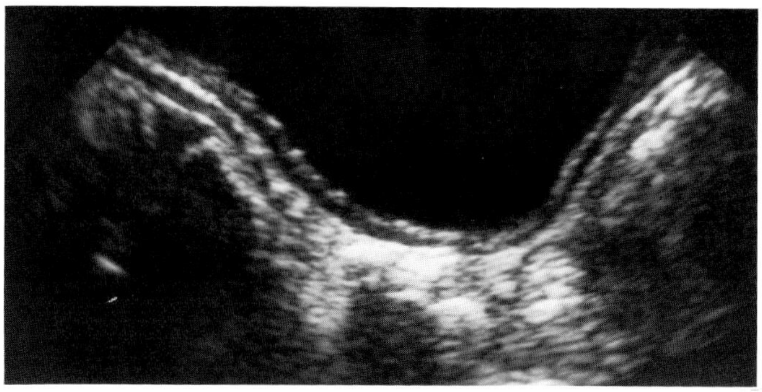

Fig. 6–52 Neurogenic bladder. The midline longitudinal scan of the pelvis demonstrates a large volume bladder with a thick irregular wall after voiding in this patient with neurogenic dysfunction.

patient voids may reveal a residual volume of urine. The voiding cystourethrogram remains the standard screening test for bladder capacity and function. Early in neurogenic dysfunction the bladder may appear normal. Various sizes and shapes of the bladder have been described including the "Christmas tree" configuration, sacculations, pseudodiverticula, and hypertonicity. Atonic bladders with large volumes and smooth walls are uncommon in childhood.

PROSTATIC AND URETHRAL ABNORMALITIES

The female urethra is best evaluated in the lateral position during voiding. While some normal urethras are tubular, others assume a gradual tapering configuration and yet others assume the shape of a spinning top. The female urethra is equivalent to the posterior urethra in the male. However, no verumontanum is present in the female and thus the urethra is radiographically featureless. On voiding studies, reflux into the vagina is a frequent occurrence and is of no clinical significance in the recumbent position.

> **PROSTATIC AND URETHRAL ABNORMALITIES**
>
> Congenital
> - Posterior urethral valves
> - Hypospadias
> - Diverticulum
> - Anterior urethral valves
> - Megalourethra
> - Congenital stricture/stenosis
>
> Infection/inflammation
> - Urethritis
>
> Neoplasm
> - Polyp
> - Rhabdomyosarcoma
>
> Trauma/iatrogenic
> - Rupture
> - Foreign body
> - Mucosal injury
> - Stricture

The male urethra also demonstrates variations in the normal configuration, mainly due to spasm or contraction of the bulbocavernosus muscle and the external urethral sphincter. Normal indentations along the posterior urethra include the verumontanum, inferior urethral crest, and the incisura. The suspensory ligament of the penis divides the anterior urethra into the proximal and distal portions. Since the proximal urethra courses along the bulbocavernosus muscle, contractions of the muscle may cause transient narrowings in this portion of the urethra. A ventral compression defect may be seen at the level of the suspensory ligament. The anterior urethra is featureless except for dilatation distally at the fossa navicularis. The caliber of the posterior urethra may vary markedly during different phases of micturation.

Congenital

The most common cause of obstructive uropathy in infancy is posterior urethral valves. The condition may be suspected on prenatal ultrasound examination, with neonatal abdominal distention, or with weakness of the urinary stream in an older patient. Urinary ascites is most frequently secondary to posterior valves and resultant rupture of the urinary tract. Mortality from posterior urethral valves occurs in up to 40 percent of children presenting before 3 months of age. The most common type of posterior urethral valves is the Young type I, an accentuation of the ridges arising from the verumontanum. The folds originate from the caudal aspect of the verumontanum montanum and extend downward and forward before fusing anteriorly. Young type II are anterior urethral valves that are not thought to cause obstruction if they occur at all. Young type III valves represent a membranous obstruction by a mucosal diaphragm. The type III valve is the most common type found in fatal cases. Thickening of the bladder wall and dilatation of the posterior urethra may be seen during ultrasound examination (Fig. 6–53). Voiding cystourethrography will demonstrate a sharp demarcation between the dilated posterior urethra and the normal anterior urethra. Up to 40 percent of children with posterior urethral valves also demonstrate vesicoureteral reflux. All children demonstrate signs of bladder outlet obstruction including trabeculation and hypertrophy of the bladder. In type I, the verumontanum and the inferior urethral crest are

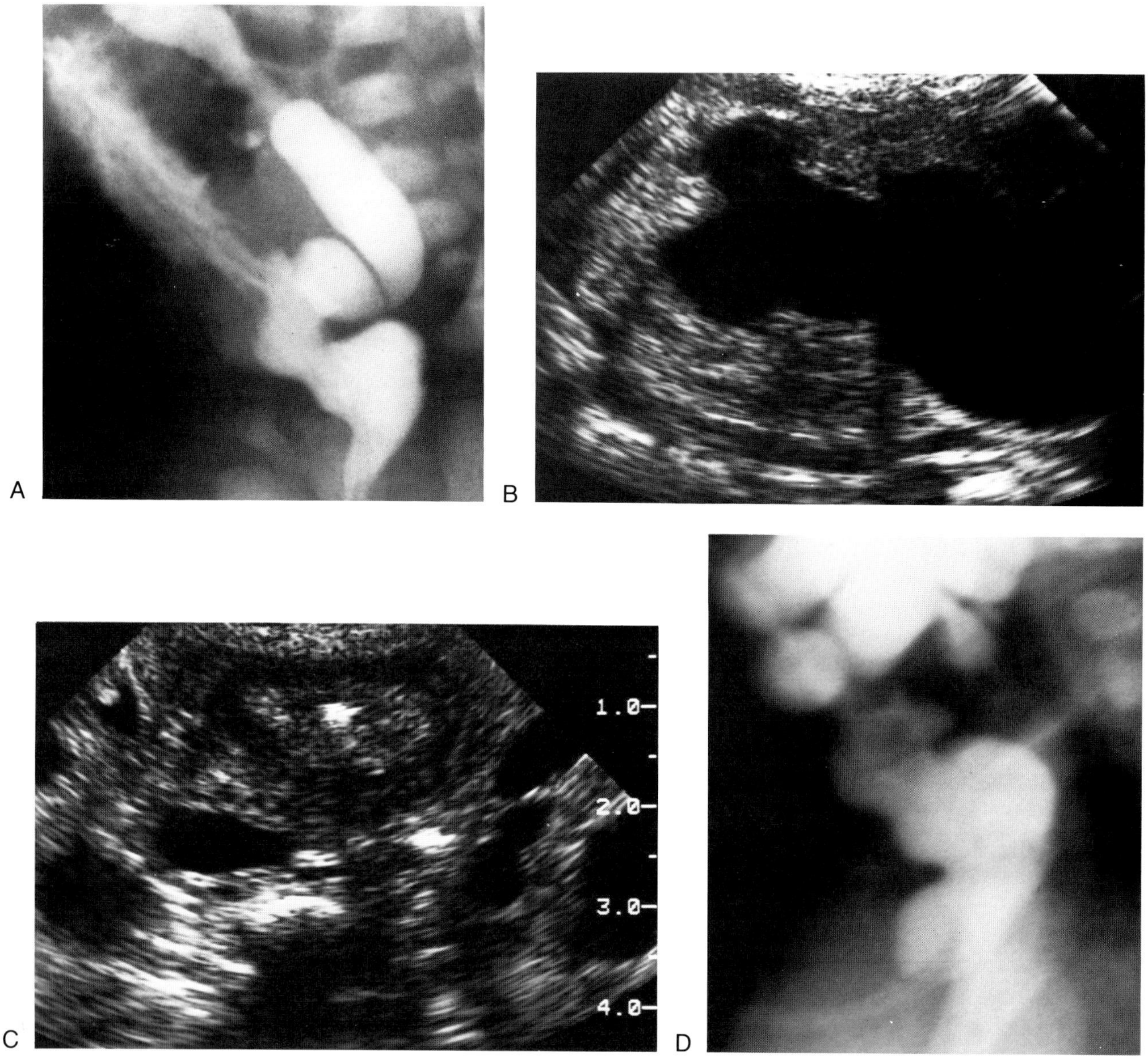

Fig. 6–53 Posterior urethral valves. **(A)** Note the markedly trabeculated bladder, which is elongated and extends up to the level of L4 on the lateral view from a voiding cystourethrogram. Note the marked dilatation of the posterior urethra about the catheter. **(B)** Ultrasound examination of the same patient revealed bilateral hydronephrosis and hydroureter as demonstrated in the longitudinal view of the left kidney. **(C)** Transverse ultrasound of the bladder decompressed by a Foley catheter demonstrates gross thickening of the bladder wall around the catheter. The cystic structures seen bilaterally represent the hydronephrotic ureters. **(D)** As the catheter is removed during lateral urethrography, high pressure injection of the posterior urethra again demonstrates marked dilatation. Definite valves are not seen.

hypertrophic, with the valves appearing as thin radiolucencies. The posterior urethra may also be deformed due to hypertrophy of the bladder neck. The types are differentiated in the lateral position. The appearance of the valves themselves varies during the examination and from patient to patient. Often the diagnosis is inferred by the classic changes in the bladder and posterior urethra rather than actually visualizing the valves. The membrane in the Young type III valve may be located just below the verumontanum or even lower. If it occludes more than one-half of the diameter of the urethra, a windsock deformity develops and may cause herniation into the anterior urethra. If posterior urethral valves occur in females they are Young type III.

One of the more common urethral abnormalities is hypospadias, which results in an abnormal location of the external urethral meatus. In males the meatus is usually located on the underside of the penis, scrotum, or perineum; in females it usually opens into the anterior aspect of the vagina. The urethral meatus may be narrowed in the female resulting in bladder outlet obstruction. Females also experience associated urinary incontinence, affected males do not. The more severe degrees of hypospadias are likely to be associated with intersex anomalies. This is especially true in males also affected by cryptorchidism.

Defects in the corpus spongiosum and corpora cavernosa result in anterior urethral diverticula, valves, and megalourethra. Megalourethra refers to either diffuse or localized ectasia of the penile urethra. The anterior urethral diverticulum is also a localized abnormality of the ventral penile urethra that appears as a wide-mouthed saccular cavity filled with contrast material. With voiding, the diverticulum bulges and causes focal obstruction of the urinary stream. Proximal dilatation is seen above the diverticulum. The anterior lip of the urethral diverticulum is similar in radiographic appearance to the anterior urethral valve. Anterior valves are consistently accompanied by a large diverticulum and sometimes by a partial duplication of the urethra. Posterior urethral valves occur 10 times more frequently than anterior urethral valves.

The presence of stenosis or congenital stricture of the urethra usually occurs close to the meatus and is a frequent lower urinary tract anomaly. Males are affected more commonly than females and present clinically with a poor stream. While voiding cystourethrography will demonstrate a stricture, retrograde urethrography with constriction of the glans penis during voiding gives superior distention of the urethra thus delineating the length of the stricture.

Infection/Inflammation

Infection and inflammation of the prostate and urethra are uncommon in childhood. Early in infancy, hematogenous spread of organisms during sepsis may result in prostatitis. Urethritis is more likely to be secondary to manipulation or foreign body insertion until the age of sexual activity.

Neoplasm

Neoplasms of the urethra are exceedingly uncommon. Fibroepithelial polyps and congenital hypertrophy of the verumontanum are benign causes of tumorlike urethral obstruction. Rhabdomyosarcoma is the most common primary malignant tumor of the prostate in children. Patients present with symptoms of outflow tract obstruction and suprapubic pain. Usually the tumor must bulge into the bladder floor to be detected with conventional voiding cystourethrography. However, ultrasound examination readily demonstrates a pelvic mass and bladder involvement. CT is helpful in identifying pelvic extent and distal metastases.

Trauma

The bulbous and membranous urethra are the most common injured sites due to a straddle injury. Often, rupture results in the inability to void. In this case, retrograde urethrograms become the only method of evaluating injury. Complications of rupture include fistulas, stricture formation, and impotence. Urethral foreign bodies are uncommon in childhood. The most common trauma to the urethra is iatrogenic secondary to catheter placement, cystoscopy, and surgery. The severity of injury ranges from mucosal contusion to perforation. Occasionally, stricture formation may result as a late complication.

REPRODUCTIVE SYSTEM

Anomalies of the reproductive system range from aplasia and ambiguity to duplication and ectopia. Clinical evaluation is combined with extensive radiographic work-up including ultrasound screening, contrast injection of various perineal orifices and, less commonly, CT or MRI. The various facets of reproductive imaging have been discussed at length by other authors.[4, 10]

There are two main reasons why a child is referred for imaging of the pelvis outside of trauma: abdominopelvic pain and a palpable mass (see lists on pages 296 and 307). Two major causes of abdominopelvic pain in children are appendicitis and intussusception. Often, the diagnosis is inferred by characteristic plain radiographic findings such as an appendicolith (appendicitis) or a right lower quadrant mass associated with small bowel obstruction (intussusception). Other differential considerations include gonadal torsion, nephrolithiasis, pyelonephritis, ruptured/hemorrhagic ovarian cyst, pelvic inflammatory disease, pregnancy, and epididymo-orchitis. Ultrasonography is an easy, noninvasive method of evaluating the causes of pain.

ABDOMINOPELVIC PAIN

Infection
- Appendicitis
- Pelvic inflammatory disease
- Epidydimo-orchitis
- Pyelonephritis

Trauma
- Intussusception
- Gonadal torsion
- Incarcerated hernia

Other
- Reproductive organ masses
- Nonreproductive masses

Ultrasound evaluation of the deep pelvis requires a full bladder. If the patient is dehydrated, a Foley catheter may be inserted to fill the bladder, although this is not routinely necessary. With high resolution transducers, the uterus and ovaries are easily discernible in most children. The uterus at birth has a length of approximately 3.5 cm but decreases to less than 3 cm until age 7 at which time hormonal effects begin to cause the uterus and ovaries to mature. The prepubertal ovary rarely has a volume of greater than 1 cc. After puberty, the volume increases to approximately 5.2 cc. Small follicular cysts and a small of amount of free fluid in the cul-de-sac are normal findings throughout childhood.

Comparison of the size of the two ovaries is important in the evaluation of ovarian torsion. Torsion is commonly associated with the acute onset of ipsilateral pain. Most ovarian torsions occur on the right in premenarchal girls. Even small degrees of torsion may lead to venous stasis and edema, which eventually may cause arterial compromise and infarction. The ultrasound appearance of the torsed ovary is variable with the most common pattern being uniformly increased echogenicity (Fig. 6–54). However, septated cysts, solid masses, and simple cysts have been reported. There may be associated fluid in the cul-de-sac. It may be difficult to differentiate a torsed ovary from a large ovarian cyst complicated by either hemorrhage or infection. Acute hemorrhage in a large

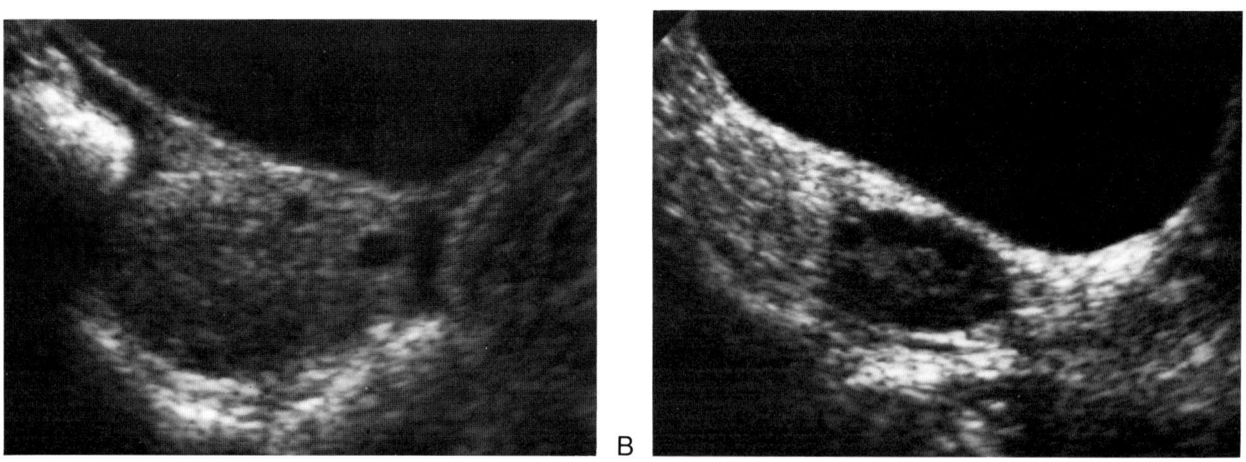

A B

Fig. 6–54 Ovarian torsion. **(A)** This 9-year-old child presented with acute onset of suprapubic pain. Note the increased size and echogenicity of the left ovary in this longitudinal scan. **(B)** Normal right ovary for comparison.

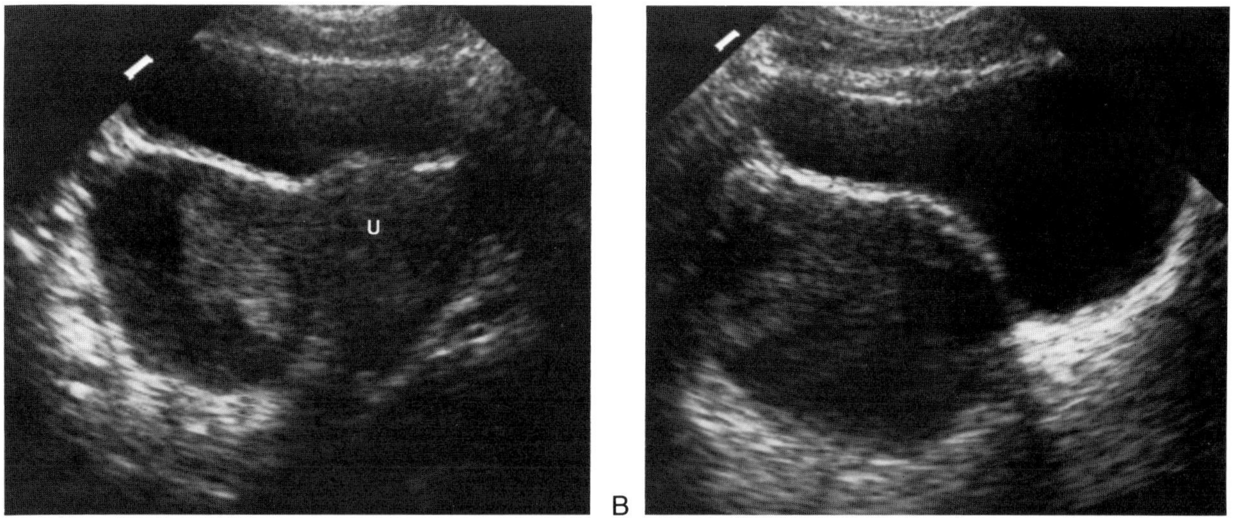

A B

Fig. 6–55 Hemorrhagic ovarian cyst. **(A)** Transverse scan of the pelvic demonstrates enlargement of the right adnexa with a homogeneous area of increased echogenicity located medially. The right adnexa is larger than the adjacent uterus (*U*). **(B)** Longitudinal scan demonstrates the presence of other small cysts in the right ovary caudal to the hemorrhagic cyst.

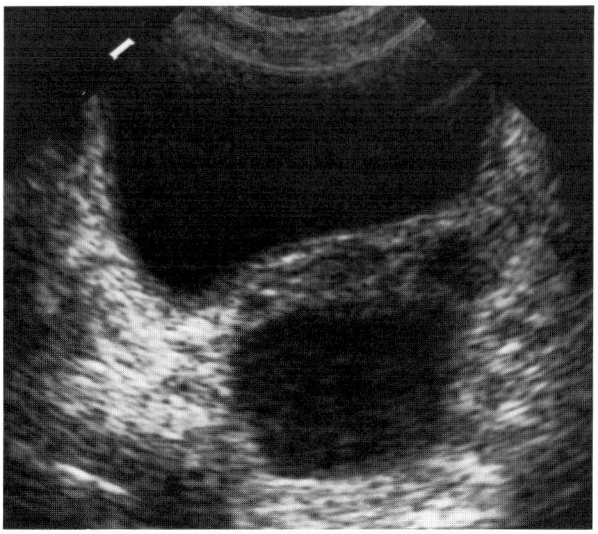

Fig. 6–56 Pelvic inflammatory disease. Transverse ultrasound demonstrates a large, hypoechoic fluid collection containing debris posterior to the uterus and left adnexa. The right adnexa was not identified.

cyst appears as a hyperechoic homogeneous rounded density surrounded by the less echoic ovarian stroma (Fig. 6–55). Subacute hemorrhage within a cyst may appear as a fluid debris level. Other considerations include the corpus luteum cyst associated with pregnancy and ectopic pregnancy. The uterus should also be evaluated for retained fetal parts or a decidual reaction. Pelvic inflammatory disease demonstrates various ultrasonographic appearances (Fig. 6–56). The sonologist may find the margins of the adnexa difficult to separate from the adjacent uterus in some cases. In others, dilated, fluid-filled structures representing tubo-ovarian abscesses may be detected. In any case, if a reproductive cause of pain is not found, the bladder may be emptied and a search for the appendix initiated. A high resolution linear transducer applied to the lower abdomen with graded compression may readily demonstrate an inflammatory mass associated with appendicitis (Fig. 6–57).

The evaluation of scrotal pain may include both ultrasound and radionuclide imaging. Prompt evaluation is in order to rule out testicular torsion since delay in treatment results in a significantly increased morbidity. If surgery is delayed more than 12 hours,

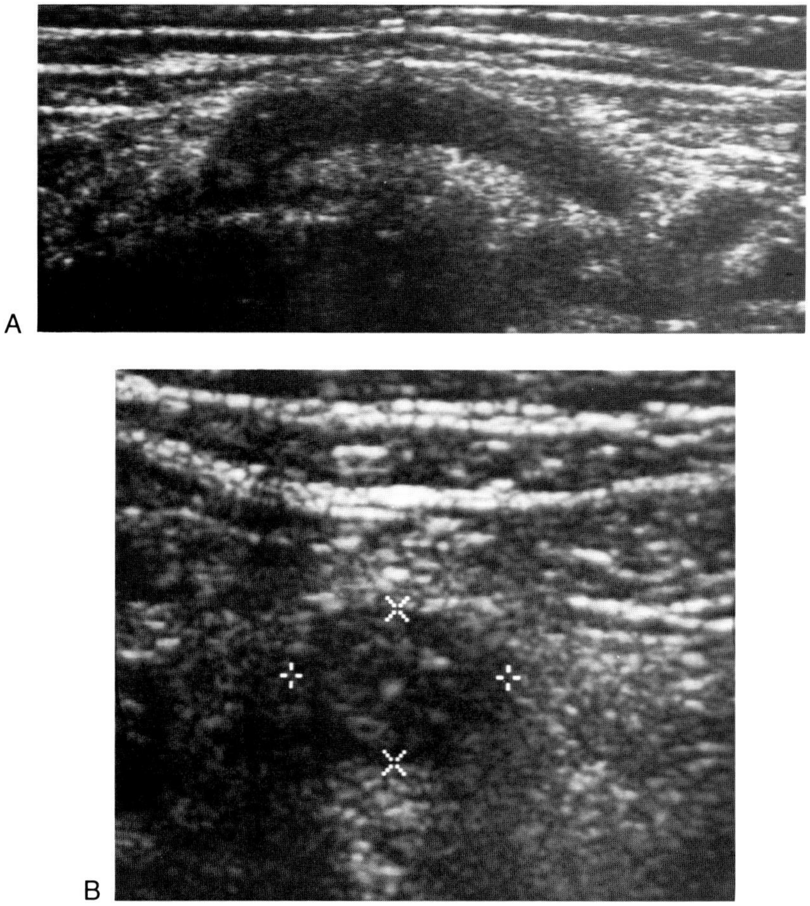

Fig. 6–57 Appendicitis. **(A)** Longitudinal scan of the right lower quadrant demonstrated a sausage-shaped mass measuring 6 cm in length in this patient with acute onset of right lower quadrant pain. **(B)** Transverse scanning demonstrated a noncompressible mass with an echogenic lumen. At surgery, appendicitis was confirmed.

the salvage rate is virtually nil. Two types of testicular torsion are described: torsion of the appendix testis and the more common torsion at the level of the spermatic cord. Approximately 80 percent of cases of testicular torsion are diagnosed between the ages of 12 and 18, although torsion of the appendix testis tends to occur between the ages of 10 and 13. Undescended testicles may also torse. There is a 64 percent incidence of malignant germ cell tumor associated with torsed intra-abdominal testes. The most common ultrasound findings with torsion include slight enlargement and a slight decrease in the testicular echogenicity. The epididymis may also be enlarged. Rarely, the involved testis may demonstrate increased echogenicity in the acute phase (Fig. 6–58). The longer the torsion is missed, the more apparent the decreased echogenicity will become. In chronic cases, testicular atrophy is noted with a homogeneous decrease in the echotexture when compared to the normal testis. Technetium 99m-pertechnetate scintigraphy remains the examination of choice for identification of acute testicular torsion. If torsion has persisted less than 24 hours, decreased perfusion of the testis is demonstrated during the early phases of the imaging. A central photopenic region may be identified representing the testicles surrounded by a rim of normal scrotal activity. Subacute torsion demonstrates normal perfusion in the early phases of imaging and a rim of hyperemia about the photopenic testicle on the delayed scintigram.

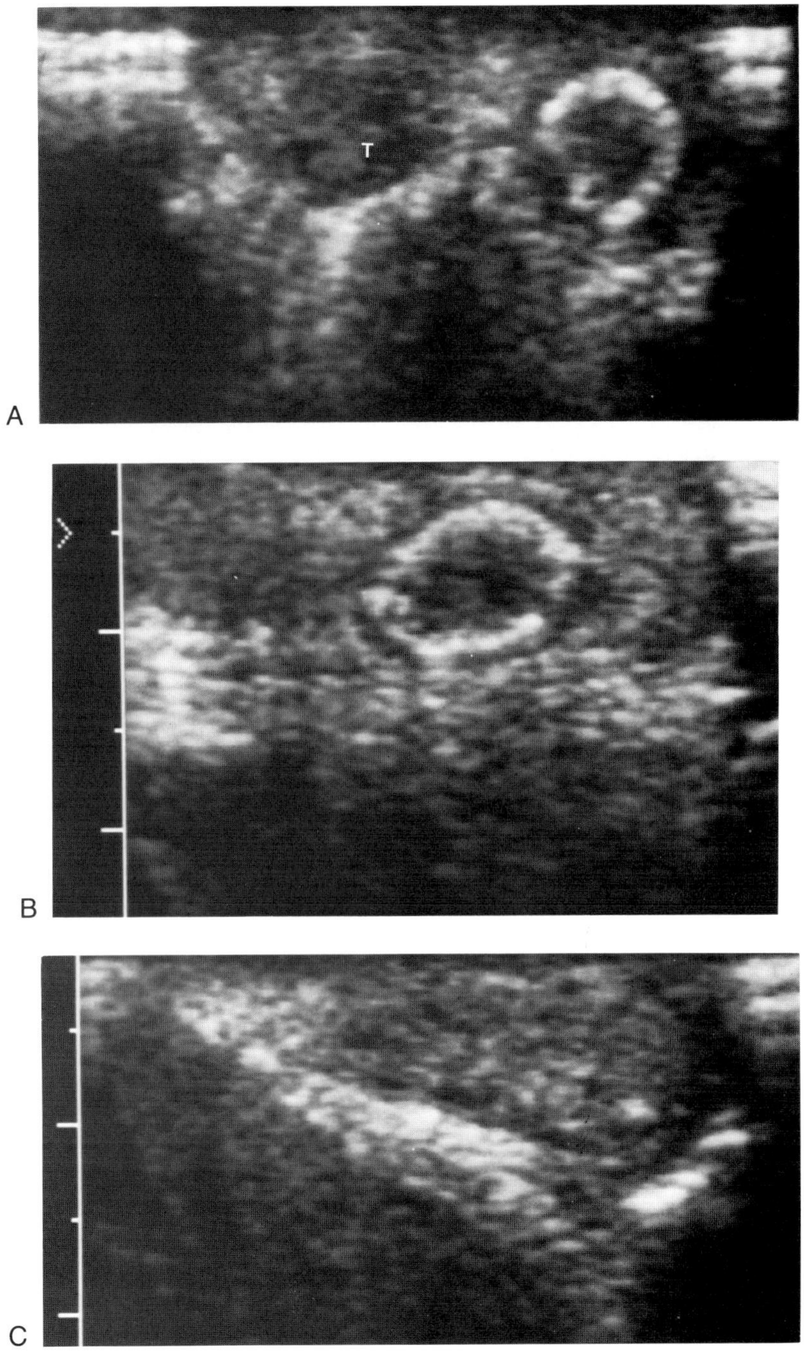

Fig. 6–58 Testicular torsion. **(A)** Transverse view of the scrotum of a newborn demonstrates the normal right testicle (*T*) adjacent to the left testicle, which demonstrates an echogenic rim. **(B)** Longitudinal view of the enlarged left testicle again demonstrates the hyperechoic rim consistent with intrauterine torsion. **(C)** Longitudinal view of the right testicle for comparison.

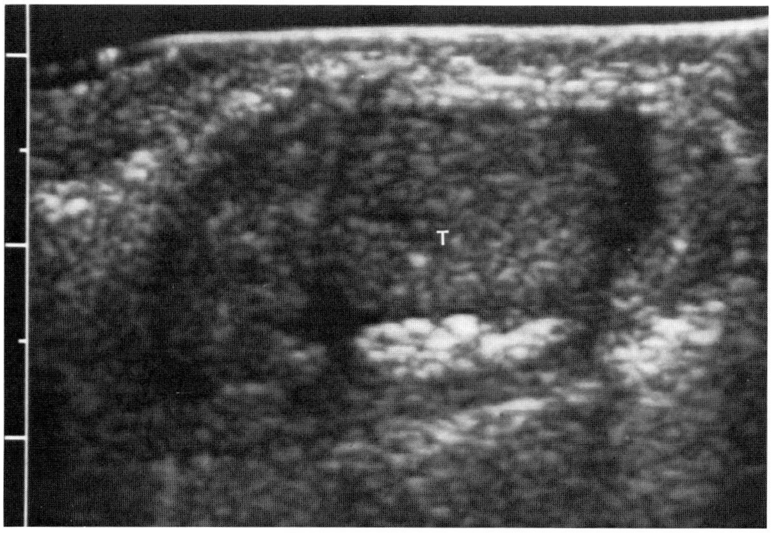

Fig. 6–59 Epididymo-orchitis. Longitudinal ultrasound of a young man's swollen left scrotum demonstrates scrotal wall thickening, a hydrocele, normal appearing testicle (*T*), and an enlarged epididymis superiorly.

Epididymo-orchitis is an uncommon cause of scrotal pain and swelling occurring after puberty. A specific organism is not isolated in most cases. Rarely, gonorrhea, chlamydia, tuberculosis, and the mumps virus are identified. Isolated epididymitis is identified sonographically by a decrease in the echogenicity of the involved epididymis associated with enlargement when compared with the normal side (Fig. 6–59). Testicular inflammation ranges from generalized hypoechoic parenchyma to localized abscess formation. Reactive hydroceles and scrotal thickening may be seen in either epididymo-orchitis or torsion. Radionuclide scanning reveals a diffuse increase in the activity of the involved hemiscrotum. Focal areas of increased activity may be seen in the region of the epididymis or testis. Often the findings of epididymo-orchitis are difficult to differentiate from tumor or trauma. Repeat ultrasound examination at frequent intervals may be helpful in planning an appropriate course of therapy.

The reproductive tract is the most likely site of origin for palpable pelvic masses in the female. Hydrocolpos, hematocolpos, and hydrometrocolpos accounts for 15 percent of pelvoabdominal masses in girls. These conditions describe large accumulations of fluid within either the vagina alone or the vagina and uterus. Sixty-seven percent of cases are due to an imperforate hymen. Other causes include vaginal stenosis/atresia, complete vaginal membrane and, rarely, it is associated with children of mothers exposed to diethylstilbestrol. The imperforate hymen is a thin membrane low in the vagina. Atresia and stenosis result in a thick (greater than 7 mm) septum in the upper third of the vagina, which may be demonstrated by inserting a Foley catheter into the vagina during ultrasound examination. The characteristic ultrasound findings include a large cystic mass arising along the midline, posterior to the bladder and anterior to the rectum (Fig. 6–60). Often, a debris level is seen as well. As with any other large pelvic mass, static scanning may be helpful in fully defining the proportions of the mass. Other masses of uterine origin are uncommon in childhood.

The most common ovarian mass of childhood is an ovarian cyst. Small cysts may be delineated at any age in the ovaries. While a size greater than 6 cm may prompt surgery, most cysts are follicular and will spontaneously resolve. Other ovarian cyst types are simple and lutein. Unfortunately, serous cystadenoma and cystadenocarcinoma may have an identical appearance to benign ovarian cysts. When a cyst is compromised by hemorrhage or infection, a nonspecific ovarian mass is seen with ultrasound. The typical benign ovarian cyst on ultrasound is unilocular with

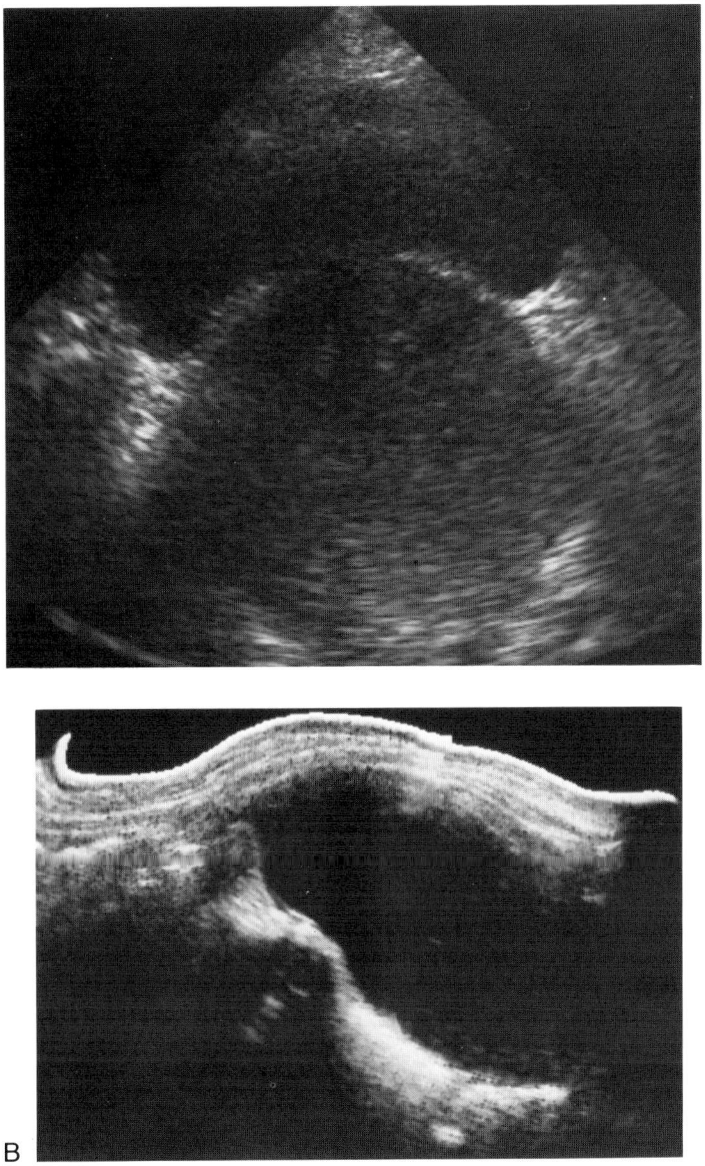

A

B

Fig. 6–60 Hematometracolpos. **(A)** Transverse scan of the pelvis of a young lady with cyclic abdominal pain reveals a hypoechoic midline mass compressing the posterior aspect of the bladder. **(B)** Static scans were performed to delineate the entire length of the mass, which measured 15 cm on this longitudinal scan. Note the debris located posteriorly in the dependent portion of the mass.

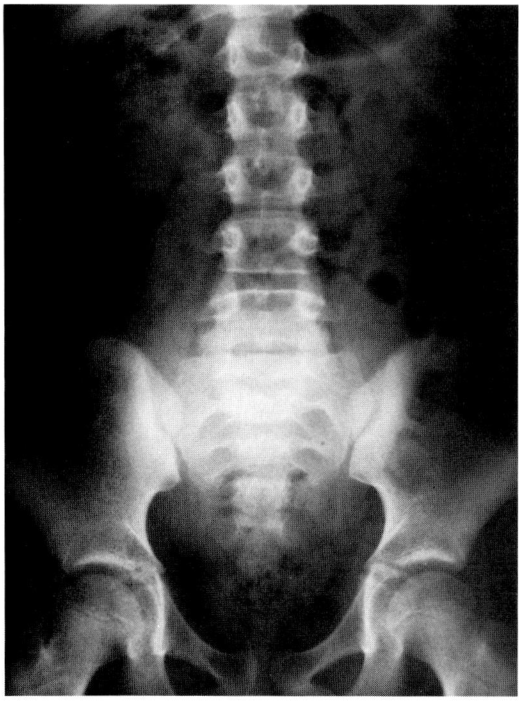

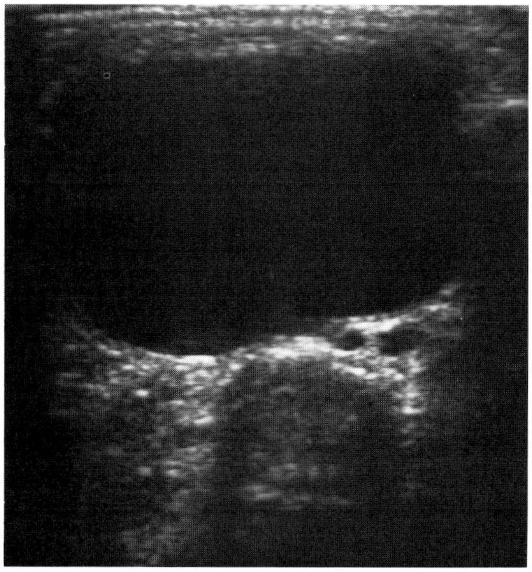

Fig. 6–61 Ovarian cysts. **(A)** This 9-year-old patient presented with abdominal pain and fullness. Note the rounded soft tissue density mass overlying the sacrum. **(B)** Transverse ultrasound image demonstrates a unilocular thin-walled cyst filled with anechoic fluid. The spine is seen posterior to the cyst. On examination of the reproductive organs, the right ovary was not identified. Surgical diagnosis was a benign right ovarian cyst.

a very thin wall and fulfills all the criteria of a cyst (Fig. 6–61). When bilateral simple ovarian cysts are identified, conditions such as untreated hypothyroidism and polycystic ovary disease (including Stein-Leventhal syndrome) should be considered. Simple cysts may also arise from the mesosalpinx and are termed *paraovarian cysts*. These may be indistinguishable from ovarian cysts until the time of surgery but occur much less frequently than ovarian cysts.

Low-grade pelvic inflammatory disease may present as a complex adnexal mass with the inability to identify a normal ovary. As was previously mentioned, ovarian torsion results in adnexal enlargement. Partial torsion of the ovary may result in massive edema due to lymphatic stasis. This condition usually occurs in postpubesent girls and young adults.

Neoplasms of the ovary are uncommon in childhood but are classified in the same manner as adult ovarian neoplasms. Cells of origin include the germ cell, surface epithelium, sex cord, and metastatic cells. The germ cell is the site of origin for 60 percent of all pediatric ovarian neoplasms. Forty percent of the germ cell neoplasms are biologically and histologically malignant. Only the sacrococcygeal region has a higher incidence of germ cell tumors with the ovary being the site of origin for up to 35 percent of all germ cell neoplasms in childhood. Germ cell tumors appear as complex adnexal masses on ultrasound examination (Fig. 6–62). Some, such as the mature teratoma, demonstrate calcifications identifiable on CT or plain radiographics; others demonstrate cystic areas (dermoid cysts, cystic teratoma). Aside from the teratoma, the germinoma is the next most common germ cell tumor arising from the ovary and accounts for 11 percent of all childhood ovarian tumors. This tumor is the equivalent of the testicular seminoma and extragonadal germinoma. Germinoma accounts for 30 percent of childhood malignant ovarian tumors.

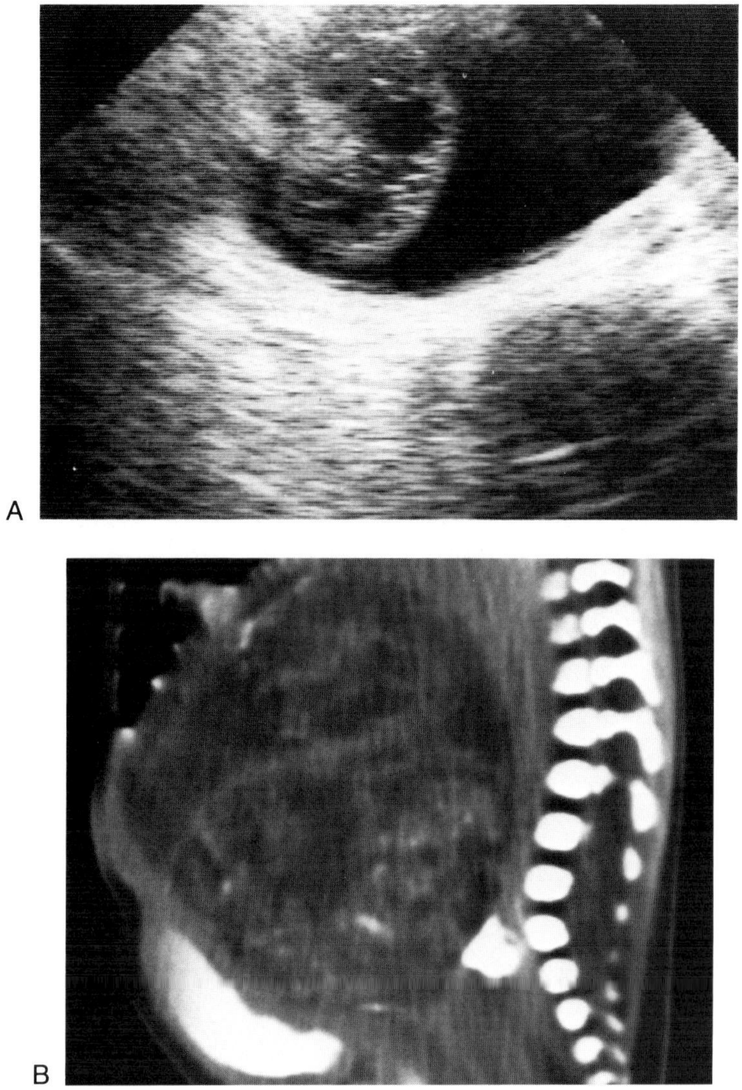

Fig. 6–62 Teratomas. **(A)** Transverse ultrasound of the right pelvis demonstrates a complex adnexal mass that is predominantly cystic. At surgery, a bigerminal teratoma was identified. **(B)** Noncontrasted CT scan of an infant demonstrates a large mixed density mass arising posterior to the bladder that contains calcifications. At surgery, a trigerminal teratoma was identified.

The next most common malignant germ cell tumor is the endodermal sinus tumor, which accounts for 22 percent of all malignant germ cell tumors. This tumor accounts for 5 percent of all germ cell tumors in children and adolescents. The endodermal sinus tumor is more likely to arise in the sacrococcygeal region and testicle but the ovary is the next most common site.

Tumors arising from the surface epithelium are responsible for 20 percent of childhood ovarian tumors and include serous cystadenoma, mucinous cystadenoma, cystadenofibroma, and cystadenocarcinoma. Serous cystadenoma is the most frequently diagnosed of the epithelial tumors in the pediatric population but rarely occur prior to puberty.

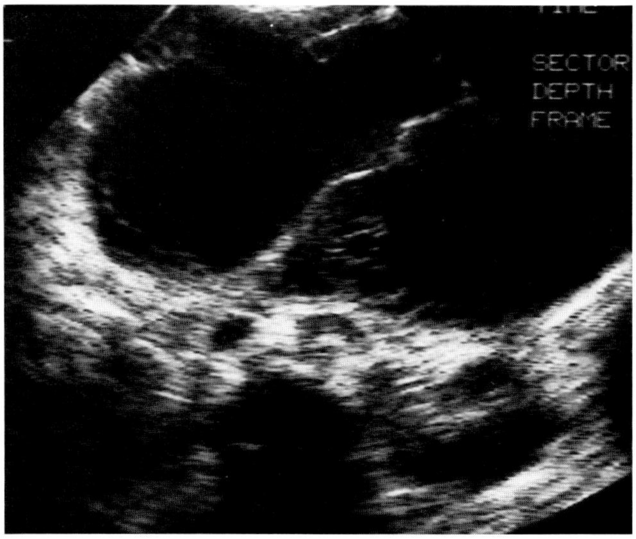

Fig. 6–63 Mesenteric cyst. Transverse ultrasound of the midabdomen of a patient with fever and abdominal pain demonstrates a large multiloculated cystic mass occupying the majority of the abdomen.

Tumors arising from the sex cord account for 12 percent of childhood ovarian neoplasms and include fibromas, juvenile granulosa cell tumors, thecoma, sclerosing stromal tumor, and Sertoli-Leydig cell tumor. The juvenile granulosa cell tumor is the most common of the sex cord tumors in childhood with the fibroma being the second most common. Combined, the two tumors account for 6 percent of pediatric ovarian neoplasms. The unique feature of the sex cord tumors is the ability to synthesize either estrogen or androgens resulting in hormonally related symptoms. Therefore, while most ovarian neoplasms present with either abdominal fullness or pain (which may be due to torsion), these tumors are more likely to present as precocious puberty. Fibromas may be associated with ascites and pleural effusion in Meigs' syndrome. Bilateral fibromas are associated with Gorlin syndrome.

Metastatic tumors of the ovary are exceedingly rare and account for only 1 percent of pediatric ovarian neoplasms. Leukemia and lymphoma are the most common causes of pediatric ovarian metastases. Other primary sites metastasizing to the ovary include breasts, colon, endometrium, and stomach. The Krukenberg tumor is a stomach carcinoma that presents with bilateral ovarian enlargement due to metastases in an adolescent. Metastasis of rhabomyosarcoma and neuroblastoma have also been reported.

Nonreproductive causes of adnexal masses include fluid- and feces-filled bowel loops, pelvic abscesses secondary to inflammatory bowel disease or appendicitis, endometrioma, adenopathy, intestinal duplications, neuroblastoma, rhabdomyosarcoma, sacral meningocele, cerebrospinal fluid pseudocysts associated with a ventriculoperitoneal shunt malfunction, and mesenteric cysts.

Mesenteric/omental cysts (lymphangiomas) are common space-occupying lesions in children. Fifty percent are diagnosed before age 10 and males are affected more commonly than females. The most common location is in the mesentary of the ileum. The lesion is usually a solitary multilocular cyst approximately 10 cm in diameter (Fig. 6–63). The ultrasound findings are characteristic, although multifocal and unilocular cysts have also been described. It may be differentiated from intestinal duplication by the fact that no hypoechoic muscular rim about the periphery of the lesion outside of a mucosal layer is seen.

A pediatric scrotal mass is a neoplasm until proven

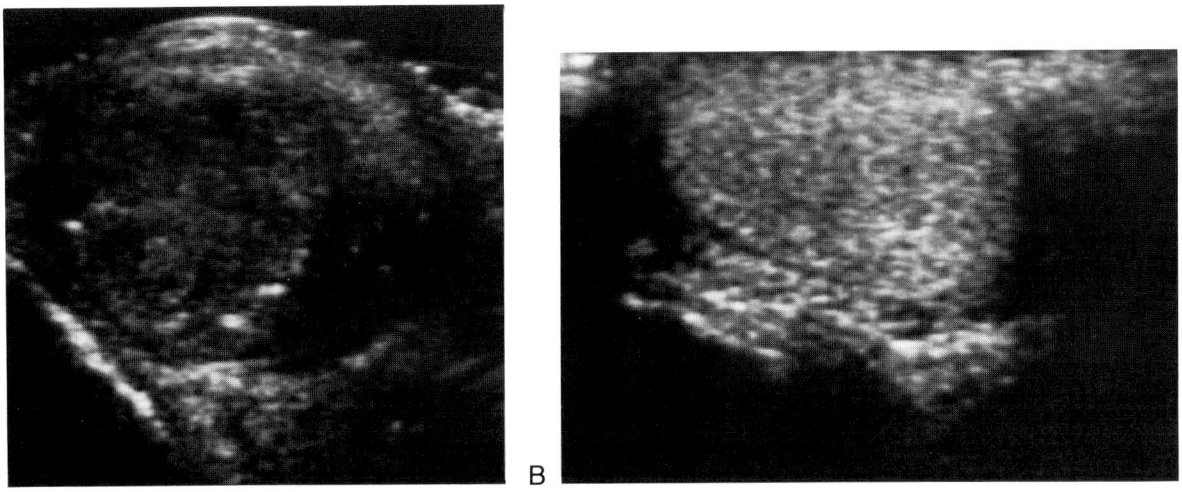

A B

Fig. 6–64 Seminoma. **(A)** This 16-year-old boy had a 4-month history of right testicular fullness. Transverse scrotal ultrasound reveals a mixed echogenicity mass that has replaced the majority of the right testicle. There are hypoechoic, hyperechoic, and calcific areas within the mass. **(B)** Normal left testicle for comparison.

otherwise. Testicular neoplasms account for 5 percent of male pediatric malignant tumors. The tumors may arise from germ cells, the gonadal stroma, paratesticular tissues, or be metastatic. Germ cell tumors account for 70 percent of cases. Two age peaks are noted in the occurrence of scrotal masses, one before age 5 and the other at puberty. Testicular neoplasms are associated with hydroceles and inguinal hernias in up to 25 percent of cases. Cryptorchidism and intersex anomalies are also associated with testicular neoplasms.

Below age 5, pure endodermal sinus tumors and embryonal rhabdomyosarcomas are the most common tumors. Mixed germ cell tumors are more likely to occur at puberty. The stromal tumors are the equivalent of the sex cord tumors in the ovary and are composed of Leydig's cells, Sertoli's cells, or granulosa cells. Paratesticular neoplasms are usually rhabdomyosarcomas, although primitive mesenchymal tumors have also been reported. The most frequent secondary malignancies of the testes in childhood are from leukemia and lymphoma. Less than 1 percent of scrotal masses are due to causes other than neoplasm in the pediatric age group and include inflammatory masses, scrotal meconium, benign mesenchymal tumors, pigmented neuroectodermal tumor, and neuroblastoma. Other causes of scrotal enlargement include incarcerated hernia, benign hydrocele, torsion, hematoma, and epididymo-orchitis. While ultrasonography is sensitive for scrotal pathology, the specificity is low. It is important for the radiologist to convey the possibility of neoplasm to the surgeon prior to surgery, since the risk of spillage of a malignant tumor into the scrotum is greatly decreased by an inguinal rather than a scrotal approach. Children with testicular tumors present with unilateral testicular enlargement, which is documented on ultrasound examination. The testicular mass is usually firm and not painful. Most testicular tumors present as focal hypoechoic areas (Fig. 6–64). However, on occasion, focal areas of increased echogenicity have been reported. Metastatic disease to the testicle may be imaged as focal or diffuse areas of decreased echogenicity. If the testicles appear symmetric in size and echogenicity bilaterally with no distortion of the mediastinum testes, then an extratesticular cause for the scrotal enlargement should be identified. Meconium appears as echogenic foci with shadowing. Inguinal hernias may demonstrate peristalsing bowel within the inguinal canal and may be reducible. However, an incarcerated hernia may cease to peristalse. A hydrocele may be benign (congenital incomplete closure of the processus funicularis or secondary to a benign

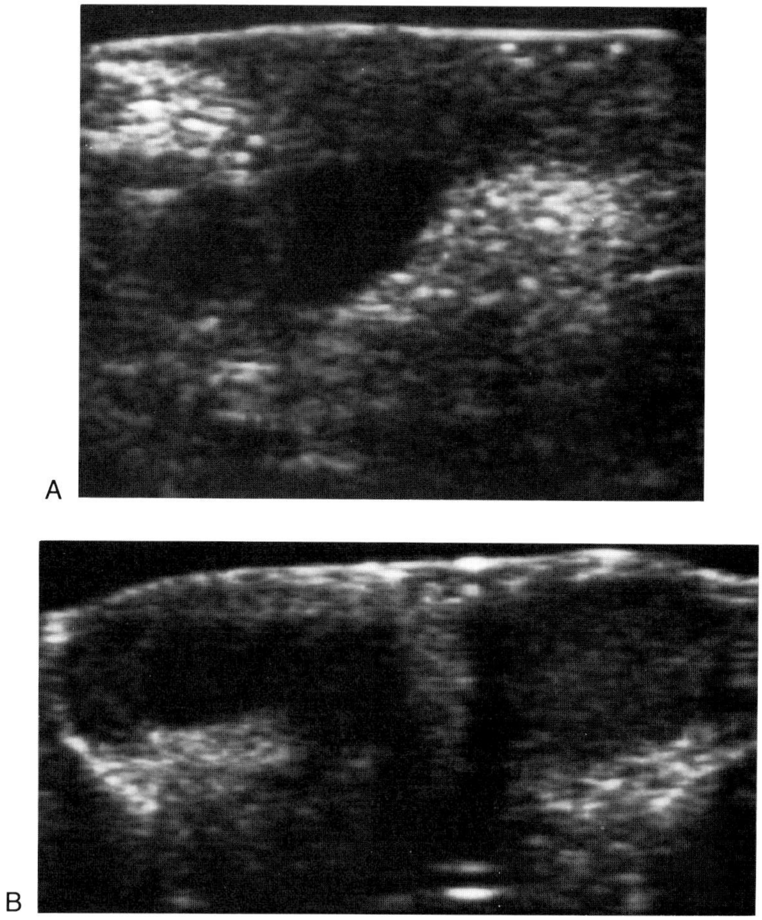

Fig. 6–65 Scrotal fluid. **(A)** Transverse ultrasound demonstrates a fluid collection adjacent to the right testicle. This represented a small hydrocele. Similar findings were seen on the left. **(B)** Transverse ultrasound of a patient with a right scrotal mass demonstrates a cystic collection adjacent to the right epididymis, which represented a spermatocele. The normal left testicle is homogeneous in echotexture.

cause) or associated with neoplasm. While hydroceles are typically fluid collections surrounding the testes, loculated hydroceles do occur and may be difficult to differentiate from large spermatoceles that represent cystic dilatations of the epididymal tubule (Fig. 6–65).

RETROPERITONEAL MASSES

Ultrasonography is a useful screening tool in evaluating the pediatric retroperitoneum. However, it may be necessary to employ either CT or MRI for further evaluation. These modalities may aid in tissue characterization, determine extent of the lesion, and aid in percutaneous biopsy. While the list below is not exhaustive, the more common mass lesions arising from the retroperitoneum are included.

Ultrasound examination of the upper abdomen or genitourinary system may reveal incidental congenital causes of a retroperitoneal mass that are asymptomatic. If accessory spleens are present, they will be identified as rounded masses adjacent to the left kidney demonstrating the same echotexture as the adjacent spleen (Fig. 6–66). If necessary, a ^{99m}Tc-sulphur colloid scan may be performed for correlation. Polysplenia also demonstrates multiple rounded

RETROPERITONEAL MASSES

Congenital
- Polysplenia/accessory spleen
- Meningomyelocele
- Teratoma

Inflammatory
- Abscess
- Pancreatic pseudocyst

Neoplasm
- Neuroblastoma
- Wilms' tumor
- Pheochromocytoma
- Adrenal cortical tumors
- Rhabdomyosarcoma
- Metastases

Generalized/systemic
- Splenomegaly
- Wolman's disease
- Adrenal cortical hyperplasia

Miscellaneous
- Cysts

Trauma
- Adrenal hemorrhage
- Hematoma

homogeneous upper abdominal masses but the normal appearing spleen is absent. Polysplenia is associated with bilateral left-sidedness, dextrocardia, a right aortic arch, and interruption of the inferior vena cava, with azygous continuation. Polysplenia has also been associated with extra hepatic biliary atresia and Kartagener's syndrome. If a rounded homogeneous mass similar in appearance to the spleen is noted in an unusual location the diagnosis of ectopic spleen should be considered. Hypermobility of the spleen is associated with torsion, which may produce a false-negative radioisotope study due to occlusion of the splenic artery. Duplex doppler allows evaluation of the vascular pedicle as well as the splenic parenchyma.

Bony anomalies of the sacrum and coccyx are associated with hereditary presacral teratomas and spinal abnormalities. The scimitar deformity of the sacrum is classically associated with anterior meningoceles (Fig. 6–67). The diagnosis may be made by either contrast myelography or MRI. The sacral region is the most common site for anterior meningoceles and symptoms occur from the mass effect of the meningocele within the pelvis. Occasionally, heterotopic bowel loops or other intra-abdominal organs are found within meningoceles. The split notocord syndrome is the association of persistent anterior vertebral clefts with fistulous communication between the spinal cord and the gastrointestinal tract, neurenteric

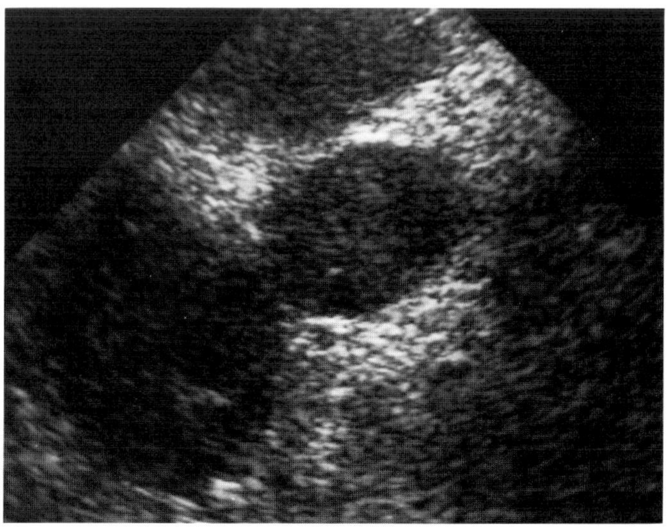

Fig. 6–66 Accessory spleen. Transverse view of the right abdomen in a patient with situs inversus demonstrates a rounded mass just below the splenic tip and medial to the right kidney. The mass is the same echogenicity as the spleen.

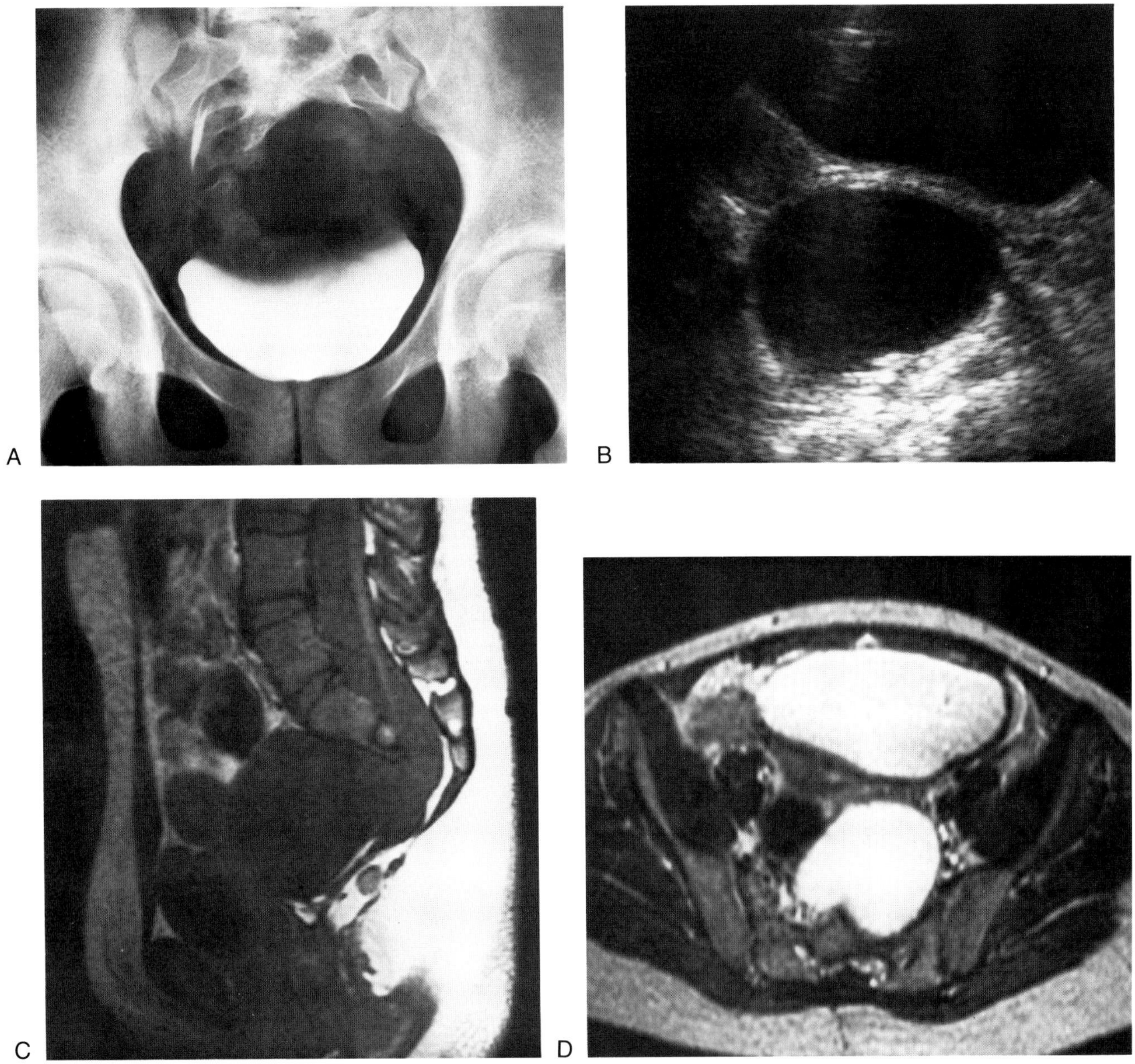

Fig. 6–67 Anterior meningocele. **(A)** Pelvic radiograph from an IV pyelogram demonstrates the scimitar deformity of the sacrum. **(B)** Longitudinal pelvic ultrasound reveals an anechoic mass posterior to the bladder. Along the posterior wall of the meningocele, bony elements cause acoustical shadowing. **(C)** Sagittal T_1-weighted MRI demonstrates widening of the thecal sac and an anterior meningocele. **(D)** Axial T_2-weighted image demonstrates the relationship of the anterior meningocele to the sacral deformity.

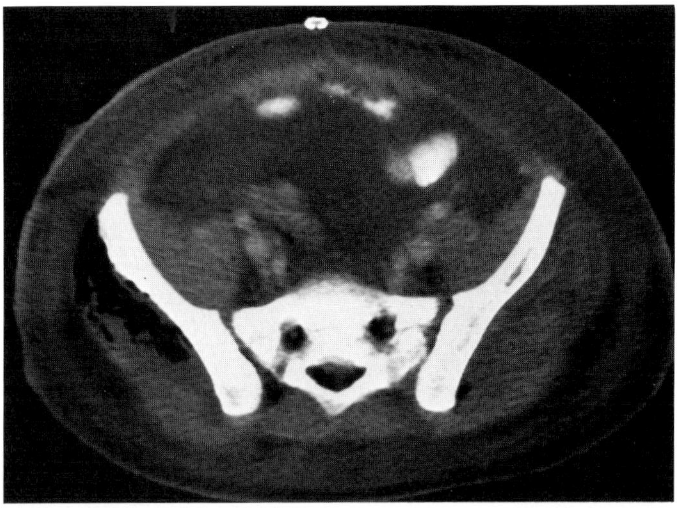

A

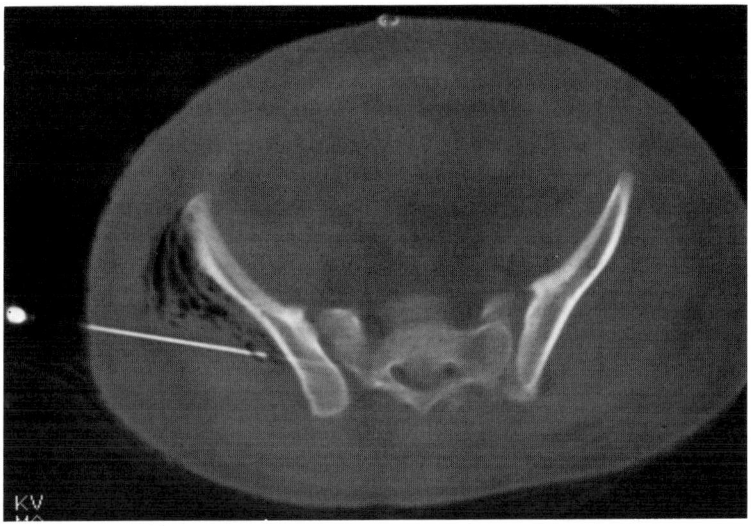

B

Fig. 6–68 Gluteal abscess. **(A)** Axial CT scan demonstrates air and low density fluid distorting the right gluteal muscles. **(B)** Bone window settings during percutaneous biopsy demonstrate adjacent destruction of the cortex of the right iliac crest. The findings are consistent with gas gangrene.

cysts, or dorsal hernias. If a bony protuberance arising from the ilium or ischium is associated with sacral deformity, spinal dysraphism should be highly suspected.

Inflammatory causes of a retroperitoneal mass are not uncommon. Abscess formation may occur in the psoas muscle due to extension of adjacent inflammation of the kidney, appendix, or inflammed bowel. One-half of the cases of primary psoas abscesses occur in children less than 15 years of age. A history of trauma or a previous infection is found in only 20 percent of patients. The exact etiology of primary psoas abscesses remains uncertain. *Staphylococcus aureus* is isolated in 70 percent of reported cases. CT is excellent at delineating the extent of involvement and facilitating percutaneous drainage (Fig. 6–68). Asymmetric enlargement of the involved psoas muscle occurs with a low density fluid collection present. With injection of IV contrast material, an enhancing rim is demonstrated. Abscess formation in the other retroperitoneal organs is much less common. Unilateral enlargement of one of the adrenal glands with a sonolucent appearance and echogenic debris may represent an adrenal abscess that occurs in the neonatal period as a result of sepsis. Bilateral abscesses have also been documented.

Pancreatitis may result in an increase in the echogenicity of the pararenal space. This results from lipolysis of normal retroperitoneal fat by the liberated pancreatic enzymes. If the resultant inflammatory reaction is severe, fluid collections may be seen in the pancreatic and parapancreatic region. If the collections persist, a fibrous capsule develops forming a pseudocyst. Pancreatic fluid collections appear as sonolucent areas of various sizes. Pancreatic pseudocysts may demonstrate scattered internal echoes or a debris level. Pancreatic pseudocysts and abscess formation are rare in childhood, but are usually the result of blunt abdominal trauma. An upper abdominal mass is palpable in 90 percent of children. Surgery is the treatment of choice outside of the acute period when parapancreatic fluid collections are known to resolve spontaneously.

The most common retroperitoneal neoplasm is neuroblastoma, accounting for 10 percent of all neoplasms. The only malignancies more common in pediatric patients are central nervous system and hematopoietic malignancies. The two most common intra-abdominal tumors in childhood are Wilms' tumor and neuroblastoma, which occur with equal frequency outside of infancy. In children less than 1 year, neuroblastoma is four times more common than Wilms' tumor. The peak incidence of neuroblastoma is during the first 3 years of life, with 60 percent occurring in children less than 1 year old. White boys are usually affected. Seventy percent of neuroblastomas arise in the abdomen with 70 percent of abdominal neuroblastomas arising from the adrenal gland. The left side is more commonly involved. Less common retroperitoneal sites include the organ of Zuckerkandl, sympathetic ganglia, and dorsal root ganglia. The typical presentation of neuroblastoma is an asymptomatic abdominal mass. In the neonatal period, hepatomegaly and skin nodules may be detected with stage IV neuroblastoma. Approximately one-half of neuroblastomas demonstrate dystrophic calcifications, which are easiest to detect with CT. If ultrasound is performed it demonstrates an inhomogeneous mass with ill-defined margins that may displace or invade surrounding organs (Fig. 6–69). CT is usually necessary for delineation of tumor extent. The adrenal neuroblastoma will displace the kidney downward in a characteristic pattern. The three most important considerations for prognosis are age at diagnosis, location, and clinical stage. Confirmation of the diagnosis is by abnormal urinary excretion of vanilmandelic acid in 71 percent of patients and homovanillic acid in 75 percent of patients. Staging is based on local extent and the presence of distant metastases; 70 percent of children present with metastatic disease.

Radiographic work-up includes a skeletal survey to rule out bony metastases, which are common. Patients with tumors that do not extend across the midline (stage I, II) are treated with surgery. Radiation and chemotherapy are employed in stage III and stage IV disease prior to resection. Spontaneous regression occurs in 5 percent of all neuroblastomas. The site of origin is important in prognosis as well. An adrenal origin has a worse prognosis than neuroblastoma arising in the neck, chest, and sacrum. Based on clinical staging, the 2-year survival rate for stage I and stage II disease is greater than 90 percent. A subset of stage IV disease (stage IV-S), the occurrence of neuroblastoma limited to the adrenal gland associated with massive hepatomegaly and skin nodules in infancy, has a 2-year survival rate of 65 percent. Intraspinal extension occurs in 15 percent of patients. The other two neural crest tumors that occur in the retroperitoneum (ganglioneuroma and ganglioneuroblastoma) have a much better prognosis, with ganglioneuroma being a well-circumscribed benign lesion. The sharp margins are detectable with ultrasonography, CT and MRI but tissue diagnosis is necessary to rule out neuroblastoma.

Extrarenal Wilms' tumors are uncommon. If Wilms' tumor invades the retroperitoneum, it is usually due to extension outside of the pseudocapsule of the kidney.

The pediatric presentation of pheochromocytoma occurs predominantly in males with symptoms of sustained hypertension and pain. Pheochromocytoma accounts for approximately 5 to 10 percent of childhood neoplasms. Seventy percent of pheochromocytomas arise within the adrenal gland in children and

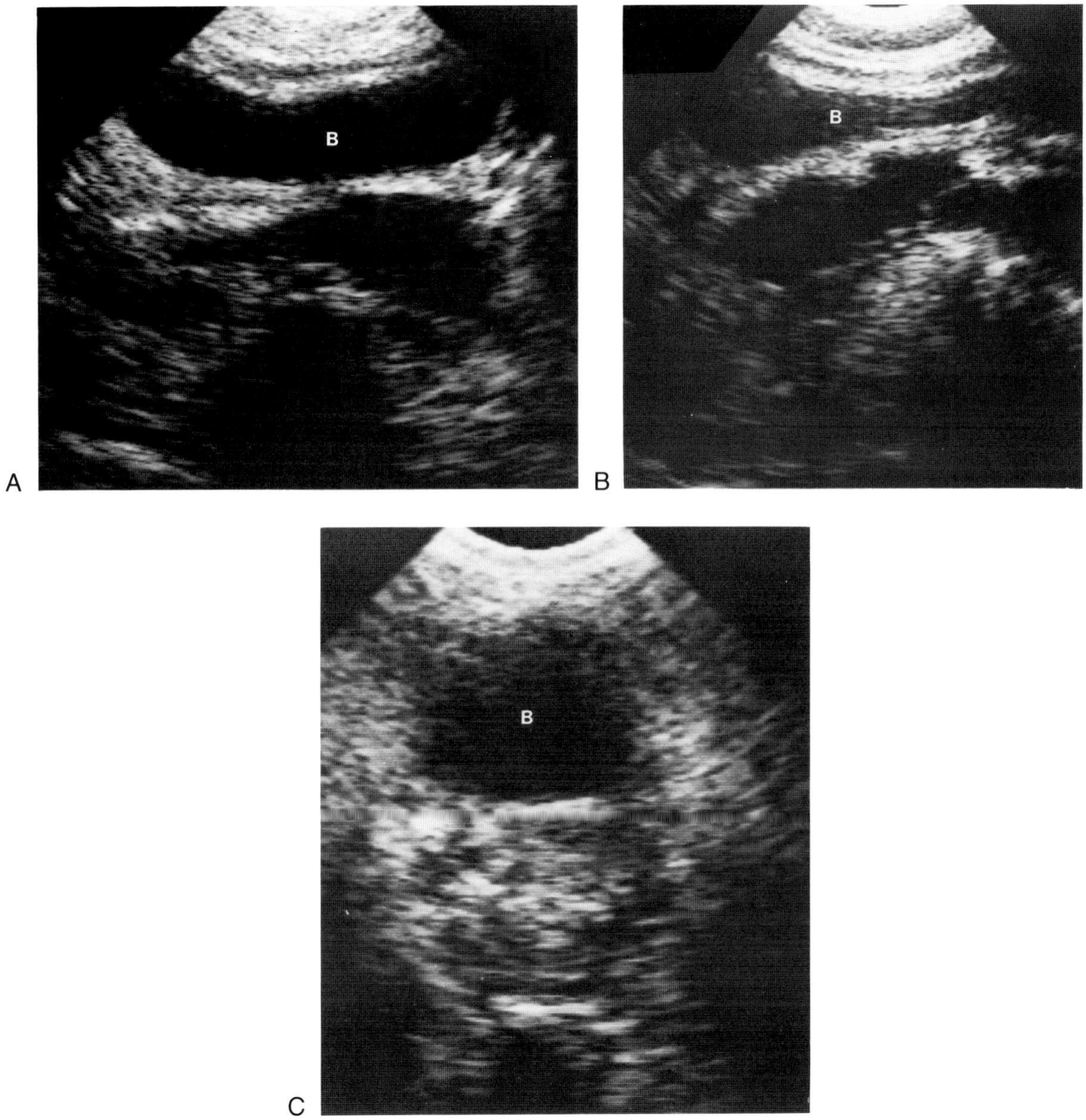

Fig. 6–69 Neuroblastoma. **(A)** Transverse ultrasound image of a boy's pelvis demonstrates a hypoechoic mass deep to the bladder (*B*) and to the left of the midline. **(B)** Longitudinal view of the mass demonstrates echogenic foci with posterior shadowing in the caudal solid portion of the tumor. The bladder (*B*) is compressed anteriorly by the mass. **(C)** After voiding, the solid, inhomogeneous hyperechoic portion of the mass is better appreciated posterior to the bladder (*B*) on this transverse image.

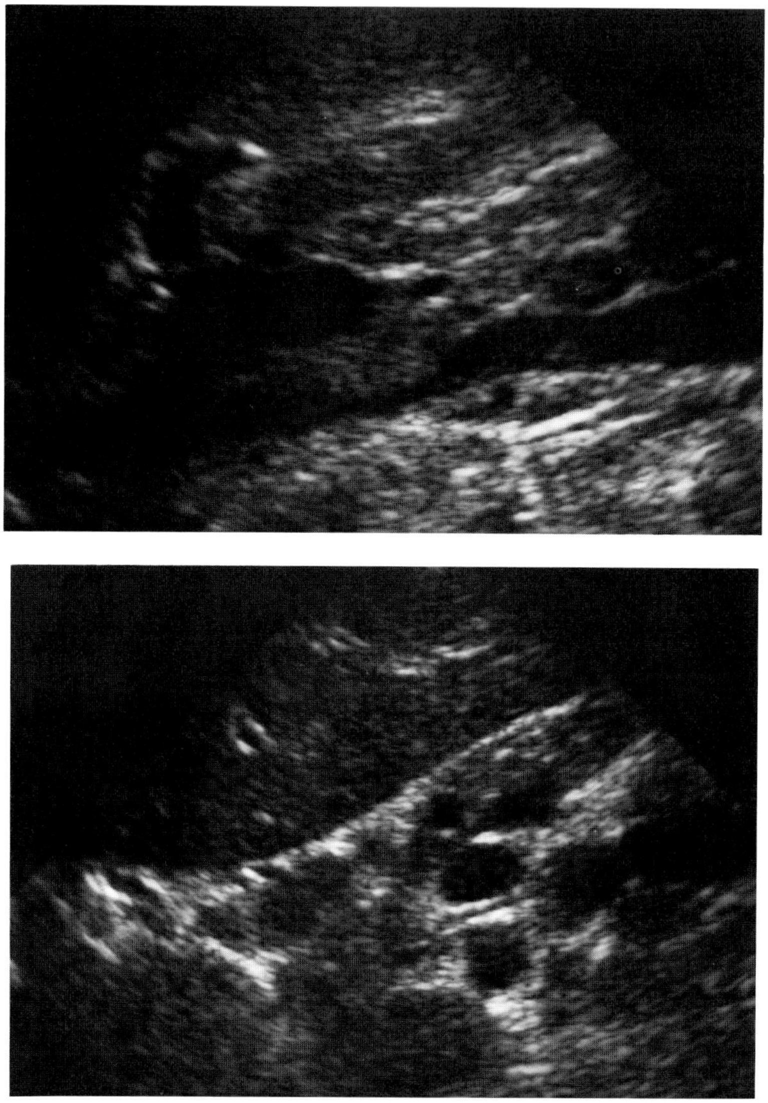

A

B

Fig. 6–70 Retroperitoneal lymphadenopathy. **(A)** Longitudinal scan of the right upper quadrant demonstrates multiple, round, hypoechoic masses compressing the inferior vena cava. **(B)** The spleen is enlarged on the longitudinal scan of the left upper quadrant and multiple, round, hypoechoic masses are identified representing recurrent lymphoma.

are slightly more common on the right than on the left. Adrenal cortical neoplasms such as adenoma or carcinoma are rare in childhood. Most children present with symptoms of Cushing's syndrome with or without virilization. As with other retroperitoneal tumors, ultrasound examination may detect asymmetry of the adrenal glands and a complex appearance to the mass due to hemorrhagic necrosis. CT is equally as effective in identifying primary adrenal tumors and evaluating abdominal metastases. The tumors appear as inhomogenous densities. Pheochromocytomas are usually greater than 2 cm in size and range from solid to cystic. Adrenal carcinomas are usually greater than 4 cm in diameter and are of mixed density. Adenomas range in size from 2 to 5 cm in diameter and because of a high fat content have a lower attenuation.

The third most common tumor in the retroperitoneum is rhabdomyosarcoma, which remains asymptomatic until a large size is attained. Ultrasound examination will demonstrate a predominantly hypoechoic mass lesion with central irregularities consistent with necrosis. While CT and MRI are useful in delineating extent, the tissue characterization is not specific.

Other miscellaneous tumors involving the retroperitoneum include lipomas, hemangiomas, lymphangiomas, fibromas, and neurofibromas. Malignant counterparts may also be encountered.

Metastases to the retroperitoneum are usually due to secondary spread of lymphoma involving the retroperitoneal nodes. CT is the best method for evaluating the retroperitoneal lymph nodes as well as other abdominal organs. When noted incidentally on ultrasound examination, lymphadenopathy may appear as multiple rounded hypoechoic masses in the para-aortic and paracaval region (Fig. 6–70).

Generalized enlargement of the spleen is a common nonspecific finding on both ultrasonography and CT. Causes include hematologic disorders, portal hypertension, infection, and infiltration due to widespread diseases such as leukemia, lymphoma, mucopolysaccharidosis, and histiocytosis X. The echogenicity of the spleen may vary but unless a focal mass is identified, it is not a specific finding. In older children, splenomegaly is most likely secondary to an infiltrative process, while in the neonatal period infection and sepsis account for the overwhelming majority of cases. The incidence of focal splenic masses in children is low. The most common is a simple cyst.

Generalized enlargement of the adrenal glands may be noted on ultrasound examination or CT in several conditions. Wolman's disease is a lysosomal storage disorder resulting in failure to thrive, hepatosplenomegaly, and bilateral enlargement of the adrenal glands with calcification. The disease is almost uniformly fatal by 6 months of age. Bilateral enlarged adrenal glands are also seen in children with adrenogenital syndrome, Cushing's syndrome, and primary aldosteronism (Conn's syndrome). Girls with congenital adrenal hyperplasia are detected at birth due to genital ambiguity. Ultrasound examination will reveal bilateral enlargement of the adrenal glands. Boys, however, will appear normal at birth but develop precocious puberty later in childhood. At this age, the enlarged adrenal glands may be difficult to visualize with ultrasonography. CT will demonstrate thickening of the adrenal limbs with maintenance of a normal pyramidal shape.

Cysts of the retroperitoneum and retroperitoneal organs are rare but do occur. Most are simple cysts with classic ultrasound characteristics (a thin smooth wall, anechoic fluid and back wall enhancement).

A

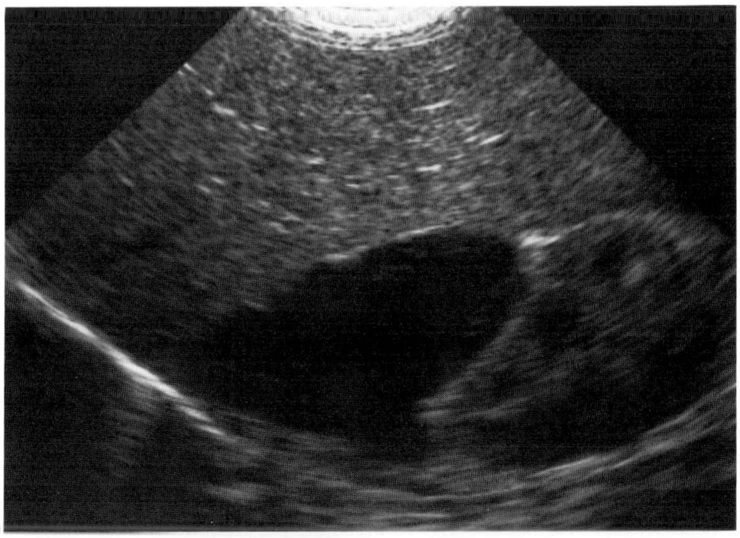

Fig. 6–71 Adrenal hemorrhage. **(A)** Longitudinal ultrasound of a neonate's right upper quadrant demonstrates a hypoechoic mass situated between the liver and kidney consistent with an adrenal hemorrhage. (*Figure continues.*)

B 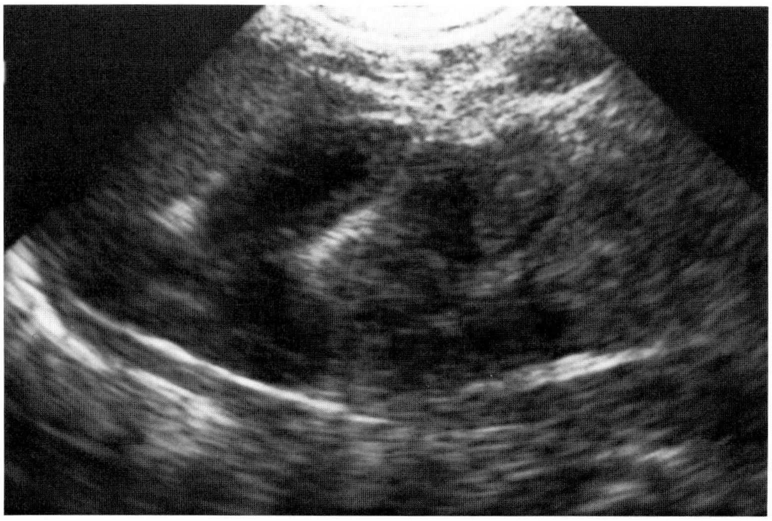

Fig. 6–71 (*Continued*). **(B)** Longitudinal scan of the left adrenal gland demonstrates a smaller hemorrhage with preservation of the pyramidal shape.

Even minor retroperitoneal trauma may result in hemorrhage or hematoma formation. In the newborn period, the prominent adrenal glands are subject to trauma at birth. Small hemorrhages may be noted as incidental findings on ultrasound examination of the kidneys or abdomen. These patients are asymptomatic. When hemorrhage is large, death may rapidly ensue due to exsanquination. Ultrasound is the method of choice to demonstrate adrenal hemorrhage (Fig. 6–71). Adrenal hemorrhage is bilateral in less than 10 percent of cases. Ultrasound usually demonstrates unilateral enlargement of the adrenal gland with the appearance of the hemorrhage varying with its age. Early hemorrhage is echogenic. Evolution of the hematoma results in a decrease in the echogenicity of the mass and eventual decrease in the size. Scarring and dystrophic calcifications are noted in the chronic phase. If the calcifications are of significant

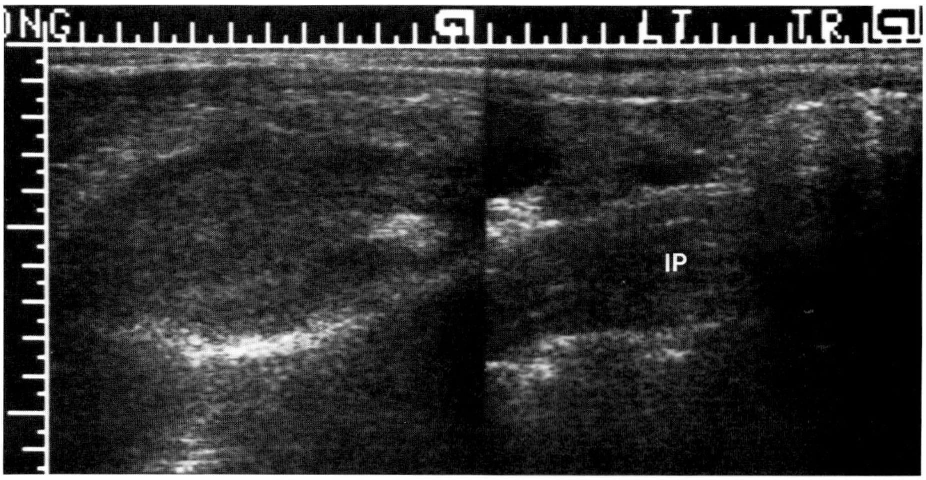

Fig. 6–72 Retroperitoneal hematoma. Longitudinal scans of both iliopsoas muscles are presented on the same screen. The left iliopsoas muscle (*IP*) demonstrates normal striations and a normal wedge-shaped appearance. The right muscle has lost its normal echotexture and bulges secondary to a hematoma in this hemophiliac.

size, they will be noted on plain radiographs of the abdomen.

Blunt trauma to the torso is the usual cause of retroperitoneal hematoma. Children with hemophilia are particularly predisposed to retroperitoneal hematoma formation. While ultrasound examination is useful in identifying a relatively hypoechoic mass with internal debris, CT is superior in delineating the full extent of retroperitoneal hematoma and involvement of the specific muscle groups (Fig. 6–72). An iatrogenic cause of retroperitoneal hemorrhage especially in the psoas muscle is anticoagulation. Acutely, hemorrhage appears echogenic or of high attenuation on CT, while older hematoma demonstrates a low attenuation on CT and decreased echogenicity.

SUGGESTED READINGS

1. Armstrong EA, Harwood-Nash DCF, Ritz CR et al: CT of neuroblastomas and ganglioneuromas in children. AJR 139:571, 1982
2. Babcock DS: Sonography of wall thickening of the renal collecting system: Nonspecific finding. J Ultrasound Med 6:29, 1987
3. Breen JL, Bonamo JF, Maxson WS: Genital tumors in children. Pediatr Clin North Am 28:355, 1981
4. Cremin BJ: Intersex states in young children; the importance of radiology in making a correct diagnosis. Clin Radiol 25:63, 1974
5. Dietrich RB, Kangarloo H: Kidneys in infants and children: Evaluation with MR. Radiology 159:215, 1986
6. Dubovsky EV, Russell CD: Radionuclide evaluation of renal transplants. Semin Nucl Med 18:181, 1988
7. Dun EK, Macchia RJ, Chauhan PS et al: Scintiscan for acute intrascrotal conditions. Clin Nucl Med 11:381, 1986
8. Elkin M, Bernstein J: Cystic diseases of the kidney—radiological and pathological considerations. Clin Radiol 20:65, 1969
9. Graif M, Itzchak Y: Sonographic evaluation of ovarian torsion in childhood and adolescence. AJR 150:647, 1988
10. Haller J, Bass I, Nardi P, Novogroder M: A problem-oriented approach to the imaging of pediatric endocrine disorders. Semin Ultrasound 6:321, 1985
11. Hayden CK Jr, Swischuk LE, Smith TH, Armstrong EA: Renal cystic disease in childhood. Radiographics 6:97, 1986
12. Kuhn JP, Berger PE: Computed tomography of the kidney in infancy and childhood. Radiol Clin North Am 19:445, 1981
13. Lafortune M, Constantine VA, Breton G, Vallee C: Sonography of the hypertrophied column of Bertin. AJR 146:53, 1986
14. Levitt SB, Duckett J, Spitzer A et al: Medical versus surgical treatment of primary vesicoureteral reflux. Report of the International Reflux Study Committee. Pediatrics 67:392, 1981
15. Lebowitz RL, Mandell J: Urinary tract infection in children: Putting radiology in its place. Radiology 165:1, 1987
16. Mahboubi S, Caro PA: Computed tomography in the evaluation of tubo-ovarian abscesses in children. CT 10:67, 1986
17. Mitchell DG, Mintz MC, Spritzer CE et al: Adnexal masses: MR imaging observations at 1.5T, with US and CT correlation. Radiology 162:319, 1987
18. Montgomery P, Kuhn JP, Afshani E: CT evaluation of severe renal inflammatory disease in children. Pediatr Radiol 17:216, 1987
19. Nussbaum A, Sanders R, Jones M: Neonatal urine morphology as seen on real-time ultrasound. Radiology 160:641, 1986
20. Nybonde T, Mortensson W: Ultrasonography of the kidney following renal biopsy in children. Acta Radiol 29:151, 1988
21. Osathanondh V, Potter EL: Pathogenesis of polycystic kidneys Type I due to hyperplasia of interstitial portions of collecting tubules. Arch Pathol 77:466, 1964
22. Osathanondh V, Potter EL: Pathogenesis of polycystic kidneys Type III due to multiple abnormalities of development. Arch Pathol 77:485, 1964
23. Osathanondh V, Potter EL: Pathogenesis of polycystic kidneys Type IV due to urethral obstruction. Arch Pathol 77:502, 1964
24. Sanders RC, Nussbaum AR, Solez K: Renal dysplasia: sonographic findings. Radiology 167:623, 1988
25. Sfakianakis GN, Bourgoignie JJ, Jaffe D et al: Single-dose captopril scintigraphy in the diagnosis of renovascular hypertension. J Nucl Med 28:1383, 1987
26. Sfakianakis GN, Sfakianakis ED: Nuclear medicine in pediatric urology and nephrology. J Nucl Med 29:1287, 1988
27. Warshauer DM, Taylor KJW, Bia MJ et al: Unusual causes of increased vascular impedance in renal transplants: duplex Doppler evaluation. Radiology 169:367, 1988
28. Young HH, Frontz WA, Baldwin JC: Congenital obstruction of the posterior urethra. J Urol 3:289, 1919
29. Zhang G, Day DL, Loken M, Gonzalez R: Grading of reflux by radionuclide cystography. Clin Nuc Med 12:106, 1987

7 Central Nervous System

Lori L. Barr

Pediatric neuroradiology requires the integrated use of all imaging modalities that are appropriate for the patient's age and symptoms. A thorough discussion of each facet of neuroradiology is beyond the scope of this text. The reader is referred to the suggested readings that follow the discussion.

SKULL AND SPINE

Three imaging modalities are commonly used to evaluate the bony covering of the central nervous system: radiography, myelography, and CT. Radiographic evaluation of the pediatric skull requires at least two views that are perpendicular. A systematic approach to interpretation includes evaluation of the size, form, thickness, focal and generalized abnormalities of density, intracranial calcifications, and evaluation of the sella turcica. The following discussion is limited primarily to central nervous system disorders that affect the skull and spine.

Enlarged Head

The most common cause of an enlarged head in the pediatric patient (before suture closure) is hydrocephalus. Hydrocephalus describes any condition causing enlargement of the cerebral ventricles by raising the intracranial pressure. Obstructive hydrocephalus develops when the cerebrospinal fluid (CSF) flow pathway is obstructed from its origin in the lateral ventricular choroid plexus to the fourth ventricular exit foramina. Communicating hydrocephalus implies that the obstruction of flow is beyond the outlet of the fourth ventricle or that cerebrospinal fluid absorption is impaired. Differentiation must be made from cerebral atrophy in which a loss of brain tissue results in subsequent enlargement of both the intracerebral and the extracerebral CSF spaces. Plain radiographic findings of hydrocephalus include spreading sutures, bulging fontanelles, and bony demineralization. After 3 months of age, the coronal suture should not measure more than 3-mm wide (Fig. 7–1).

Once increased intracranial pressure is suspected, ultrasonography is commonly used for screening. Ultrasound imaging is useful in the diagnosis of congenital obstructive hydrocephalus caused by aqueductal stenosis, Foramen of Monroe stenosis, and Chiari malformations. Dandy-Walker cysts and other posterior fossa cysts are easily demonstrated with head ultrasound.

If the fontanelle is closed or the site of obstruction is not discerned, CT and MRI are useful for further evaluation. Hydrocephalus is most often secondary to meningeal adhesions following an episode of meningitis. Trauma may also lead to adhesion formation after subarachnoid bleeding. Intracranial hemorrhage, common in premature infants, may also lead to adhesion formation and subsequent hydrocephalus.

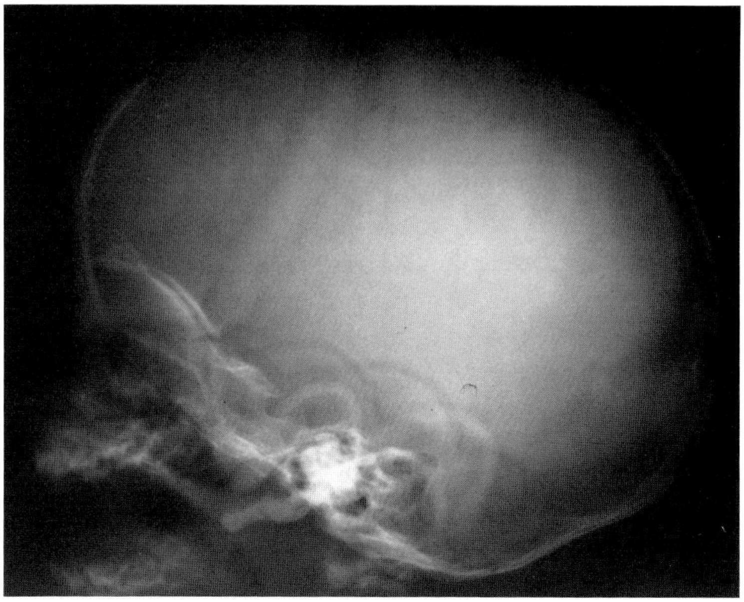

Fig. 7–1 Hydrocephalus. Note the width of the sutures in this 6-month-old patient who has a bulging fontanelle.

Causes of unilateral lateral ventricular obstruction include choroid plexus papilloma, meningioma, intraventricular glioma, and outlet obstruction. Common causes of bilateral foramen of Monro obstruction include adhesions (especially in the premature infant), colloid cysts, and foramen of Monro gliomas. Obstruction at the level of the third ventricle may be secondary to craniopharyngioma, pituitary adenoma, or glioma of the third ventricle.

Aqueductal stenosis results in enlargement of the third and lateral ventricles, while the fourth ventricle remains collapsed. The stenosis is usually congenital due to forking of the aqueduct with multiple channels connecting the third and fourth ventricles.

Obstruction at the level of the fourth ventricle may be due to a posterior fossa tumor or cyst. Tumors may arise the extra-axial region, intra-axially, or within the ventricle. Meningeal adhesions may also obstruct the outlets of the fourth ventricle.

Communicating hydrocephalus describes obstruction of the extracerebral cerebrospinal fluid pathways due to adhesions (secondary to trauma or infection) or Pacchionian granulations (following subarachnoid hemorrhage).

Other less common causes of calvarial enlargement include benign macrocrania, subdural hematoma, the various chondrodystrophies, and syndromes causing enlargement of the brain itself (Beckwith-Wiedemann syndrome, cerebral gigantism, and hemiatrophy).

Small Head

Common causes of a small skull include brain atrophy, craniosynostosis, poor brain growth, or shunt placement. Plain radiographic findings include progressive narrowing of the sutures, a small sella turcica, and overgrowth of the air-filled mastoid air cells and paranasal sinuses. The thickness of the calvaria is increased. When craniosynostosis occurs, the calvaria is small but there is concomitant increased intracranial pressure, which causes increased inner table convolutions, demineralization of the posterior clinoids/dorsum sella, and sometimes, enlargement of the sella.

Intracranial Calcifications

Intracranial calcifications may be physiologic or abnormal. Common sites for physiologic calcifications include the choroid plexus, habenula, pineal gland, and along the falx. Abnormal calcifications may be caused by tumors, infection, vascular disease, the phakomatoses, metabolic disorders, radiotherapy, or chemotherapy.

The highest percentage of tumoral calcifications in the pediatric population occurs in craniopharyngioma (80 to 90 percent). Approximate rates of calcification for other tumors include oligodendroglioma, 50 percent; astrocytoma, 20 percent (the occurrence of low grade astrocytomas is so much more frequent than oligodendrogliomas that they account for most instances of calcified gliomas); ependymoma, 15 percent; meningioma, 10 to 20 percent; pinealoma, 50 percent; chordoma, 25 percent; choriod plexus papilloma, 25 percent; dermoid, 20 percent; and pituitary adenoma, 5 percent.

Prenatal viral infections account for a large number of intracranial calcifications associated with microcephaly and occasionally, with porencephalic cysts. Viruses resulting in varying patterns of calcification include rubella, herpes simplex, chickenpox, measles, and poliomyelitis. Cytomegalic inclusion disease typically results in ventriculomegaly with periventricular calcifications that are either punctate, curvilinear, or stippled (Fig. 7–2). Toxoplasmosis demonstrates tiny calcifications scattered throughout the brain parenchyma. Plaquelike meningeal calcifications and striated basal ganglia calcifications have also been described. Hydrocephalus is seen in 80 percent of patients with toxoplasmosis caused by obstruction of the ventricular system by toxoplasmic granulomas. Congenital human immunodeficiency virus (HIV) classically causes basal ganglia calcification. Trichinosis and cysticercosis cause multiple, small oval calcifications in the encysted larvae. Brain abscesses that heal may result in dense irregular calcifications.

While central nervous system vascular anomalies quite frequently calcify, those identified during childhood most often do not contain calcium. The two major categories of vascular anomalies are aneurysms and arteriovenous malformations. The presentation of intracranial aneurysms in childhood is much less common than in adults. Only 3 percent of all cases occur in children. Aneurysms are multiple in only 5 to 6 percent of children as opposed to 10 to 15 percent of adults. Arterial aneurysms are usually 1 to 3 cm in diameter with the site of rupture occurring in the dilated distal portion rather than the neck. The most common location is at the junction of the internal carotid artery and the posterior communicating branch of the anterior cerebral artery. Rupture during childhood is extremely rare.

Arteriovenous malformations account for 25 percent of spontaneous intracranial hemorrhages in children. Eighty percent of arteriovenous malformations are supratentorial in location with the parietal and frontal regions being the most frequent sites. Infratentorial arteriovenous malformations are likely to occur in the cerebellum or cervical spinal cord. Twenty-five percent of arteriovenous malformations appear calcified on skull radiographs.

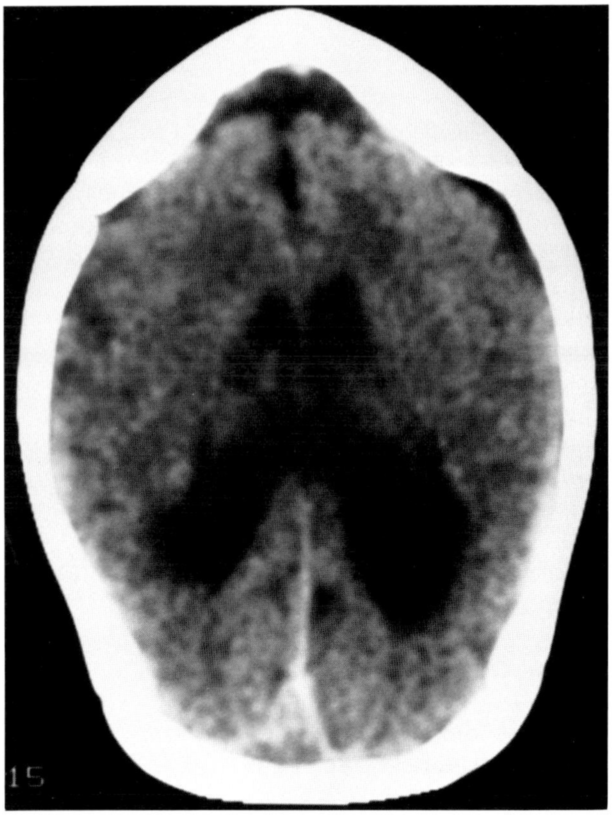

Fig. 7–2 Intrauterine cytomegalovirus infection. Tiny punctate calcifications line the walls of both lateral ventricles. Microcephaly has led to prominent extra-axial fluid spaces and lateral ventricles.

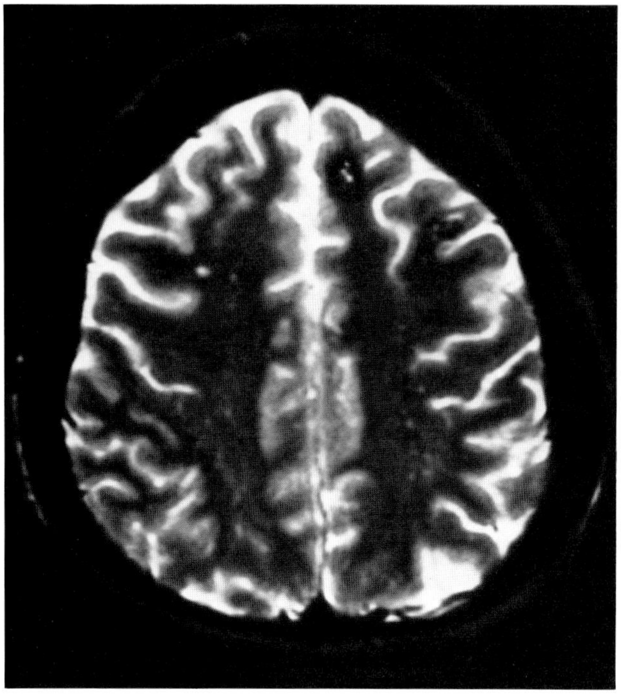

Fig. 7–3 Cavernous angioma. Note the hypointense halo surrounding small foci of increased signal in the left frontal lobe on this T_2-weighted axial image.

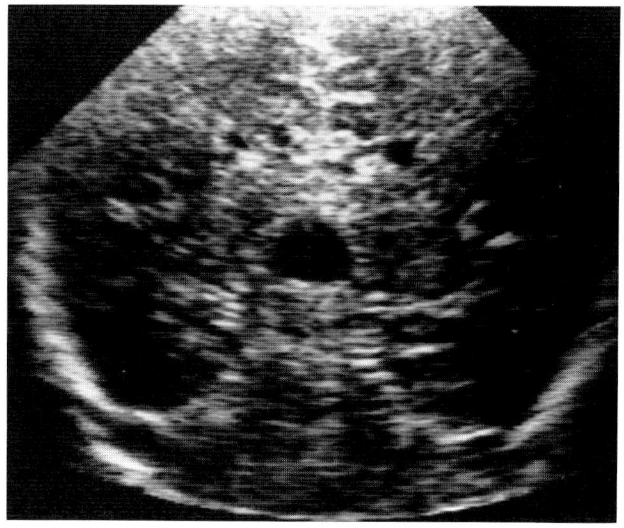

A

Fig. 7–4 Vein of Galen malformation **(A)** Coronal head ultrasound demonstrates a cystic structure posterior to the third ventricle. (*Figure continues.*)

Cerebral cavernous angiomas are vascular hamartomas that before the advent of CT and MRI went undiagnosed until adulthood. On CT a hyperdense round mass without surrounding edema is seen. Very little, if any, enhancement occurs after contrast administration. MRI demonstrates mixed signal intensity in a reticulated pattern with circumferential hypointensity on T_2-weighted images (Fig. 7–3). Surgical resection cures seizures and prevents catastrophic hemorrhage.

The "vein of Galen aneurysm" is actually an arteriovenous fistula. Presenting symptoms range from congestive heart failure because of massive arteriovenous shunting to hydrocephalus (if the malformation is large and obstructs the aqueduct of Sylvius). The most common chest x-ray findings are diffuse cardiomegaly and increased pulmonary venous congestion. The carotid arteries, vertebral arteries, and the jugular veins will be dilated. Thin crescentic calcifications in the pineal region may be noted on skull radiographs. The diagnosis is frequently made by head ultrasound, which shows a large oval sonolucency posterior to the third ventricle (Fig. 7–4). Intracranial Doppler reveals a venous wave form in the region of the malformation and decreased resistive indices in the anterior and posterior cerebral arteries that supply the malformation. Differentiation between the vein of Galen malformation and a thalamic arteriovenous malformation draining into a dilated vein of Galen may require angiography.

The phakomatoses are a group of genetic neurocutaneous disorders commonly diagnosed during childhood. Neurofibromatosis, tuberous sclerosis, von Hippel-Lindau syndrome, Sturge-Weber syndrome, basal cell nevus syndrome, ataxia telangiectasia, occulocutaneous melanosis, and encephalocranial cutaneous lymphomatosis are commonly included in this class of disorders. Tuberous sclerosis, Sturge-Weber syndrome, and von Hippel-Lindau syndrome may demonstrate characteristic calcifications on skull radiographs or CT scans. Moyamoya disease (intracerebral arterial occlusive lesions) has been associated with neurofibromatosis, tuberous sclerosis, and Sturge-Weber syndrome.

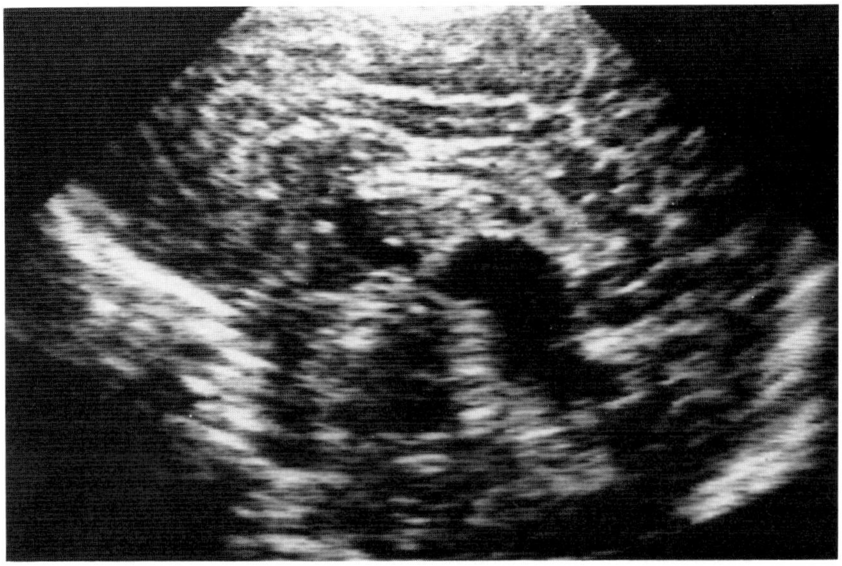

B

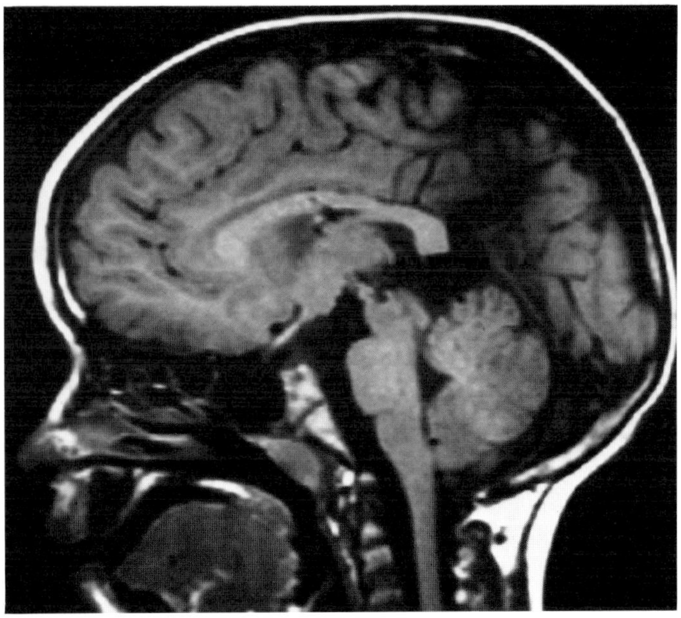

C

Fig. 7–4 (*Continued*). **(B)** Sagittal view demonstrates that the cystic structure corresponds to the vein of Galen. **(C)** T_1-weighted sagittal MRI of another patient demonstrates signal void posterior to the third ventricle consistent with flow in the vein of Galen malformation.

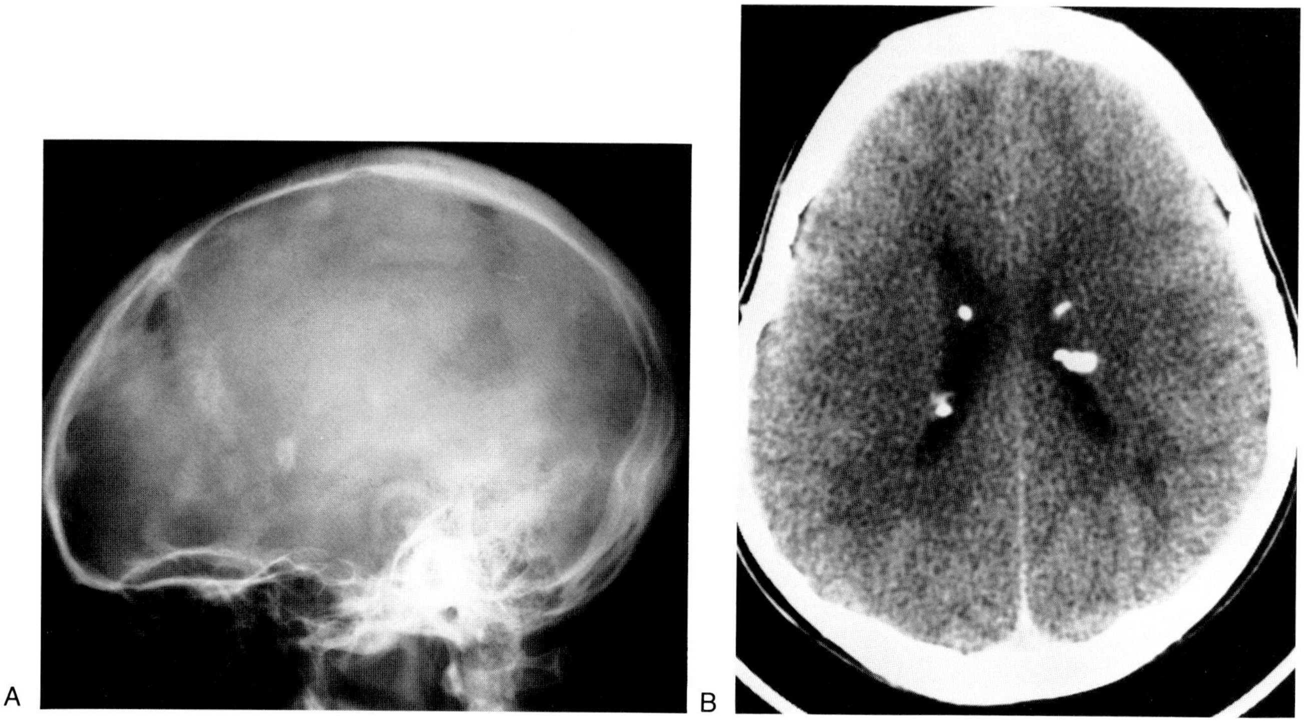

Fig. 7–5 Tuberous sclerosis **(A)** Lateral view of the skull demonstrates vague rounded calcifications overlying both the anterior and posterior portions of the calvaria. **(B)** Head CT scan of another patient demonstrates calcified hamartomas lining the lateral ventricles bilaterally.

In tuberous sclerosis, 75 percent of patients demonstrate calcified hamartomas in the lateral ventricular walls (Fig. 7–5). Other associated abnormalities include renal angiomyolipomas (50 percent of patients), seizures, mental deficiency, and adenoma sebaceum.

Sturge-Weber syndrome demonstrates tram-track calcifications with parallel plaques following the convolutions of the brain cortex (Fig. 7–6). These most commonly occur in the parieto-occipital regions. Associated abnormalities include an ipsilateral facial angioma (port wine nevus), mental retardation, seizures, hemiparesis, and hemiatrophy.

von Hippel-Lindau syndrome results in retinal calcifications and intracranial angiomas. Associated abnormalities include hemangioblastomas of the cerebellum and spinal cord; angiomas of the liver, kidneys and pancreas; pheochromocytomas; and renal tumors.

Calcifications of the basal ganglia usually signify metabolic diseases such as hypoparathyroidism, pseudohypoparathyroidism, and hypervitaminosis D. They may occasionally represent a normal variant and are also seen in congenital acquired immunodeficiency syndrome (AIDS) and in leukemic children after methotrexate therapy (Fig. 7–7). Radiotherapy results in fine amorphous calcifications at sites of parenchymal necrosis.

Sella Turcica

Evaluation of the sella turcica should include assessment of the shape, size, and wall demineralization/erosion. Suspected sellar abnormalities may be investigated by either CT or MRI. CT is especially helpful in identifying calcifications within parasellar masses. Both enhanced and nonenhanced thin cut coronal views are helpful in evaluating the pituitary gland.

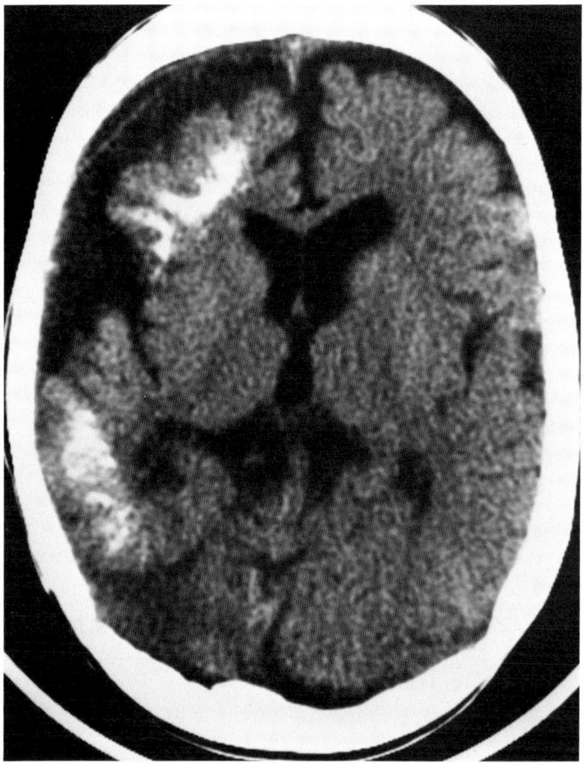

Fig. 7–6 Sturge-Weber syndrome. Axial CT scan demonstrates right cortical hemiatrophy associated with widespread calcifications following the contour of the brain convolutions.

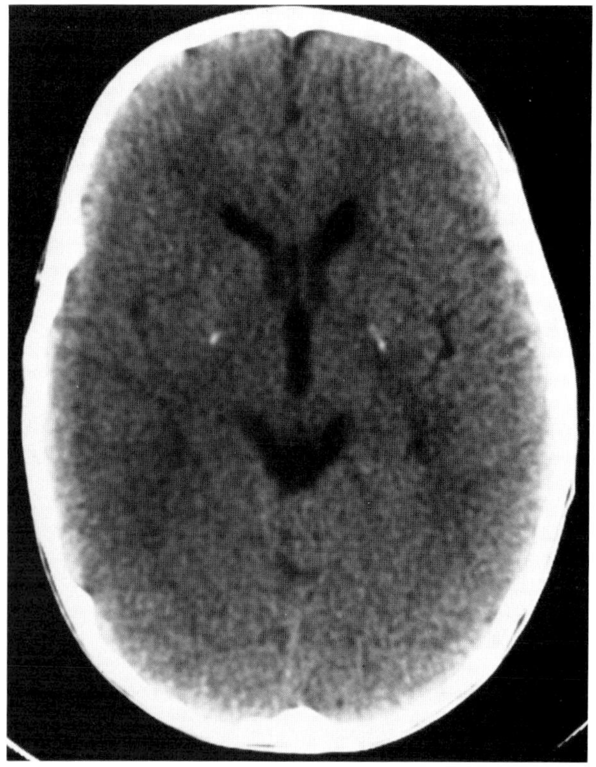

Fig. 7–7 Basal ganglia calcifications. Axial CT scan demonstrates small calcifications in the region of the internal capsule, thought to be a normal variant in this asymptomatic patient.

The most common cause of an enlarged sella turcica in children is an intrasellar tumor arising from the parasellar region. Other causes of an enlarged sella include increased intracranial pressure (an enlarged third ventricle may bulge into the sella turcica), empty sella syndrome, Nelson's syndrome (pituitary gland hyperplasia after adrenalectomy), hypothyroidism, and an intrasellar cyst or neoplasm. Increased intracranial pressure may be diagnosed by demineralization of the posterior floor of the sella and amputation of the dorsum sellae. The differential diagnosis of a parasellar neoplasms is listed below. Perhaps the least common cause of sellar enlargement is an arterial aneurysm. However, it is the most important lesion to differentiate from a neoplasm since resection may prove fatal. Curvilinear calcification, intense contrast enhancement, conspicuous signal void on MRI, and characteristic angiographic findings leave little doubt as to the diagnosis.

Fifty percent of all parasellar masses in the pediatric age group are craniopharyngiomas. This tumor accounts for approximately 10 percent of intracranial neoplasms in children. One-third of all craniopharyngiomas are diagnosed in children with the peak incidence occurring between 5 and 8 years of age. The site of origin is a remnant of Rathke's pouch above the sella turcica. Symptoms may range from headache and loss of visual acuity to the diencephalic syndrome (failure to thrive despite adequate caloric intake, hyperactivity, and unusual happiness). The diencephalic syndrome may occur with any tumor arising anterior to the third ventricle. Craniopharyngiomas com-

CHILDHOOD PARASELLAR NEOPLASMS

Craniopharyngioma
Glioma (optic chiasm/hypothalamus)
Germinoma
Epidermoid cyst
Meningioma
Pituitary adenoma

monly demonstrate coarse calcifications in a matrix of both solid and cystic components. These features are nicely demonstrated on axial CT scans (Fig. 7–8). There is very little enhancement of the solid portion of the tumor after contrast administration. As the tumor enlarges it may depress the optic chiasm, obstruct the lateral ventricles, and compress the pituitary gland. MRI is the most helpful modality for surgical planning, for the sagittal and coronal planes better define the relationship of the lesion to the optic chiasm and to blood vessels. The goal of therapy is complete surgical excision. However, if the tumor is intimately related to surrounding structures, partial resection and radiotherapy may be necessary. Recurrence rates range from 25 to 40 percent.

Gliomas arising from either the optic chiasm or hypothalamus are relatively common in childhood. Most represent slow-growing astrocytomas. Optic chiasm gliomas usually occur in adolescent girls and may be the first indication of neoplasia associated with type I neurofibromatosis. On CT examination, calcifications are usually not noted. The mass may be isodense on the nonenhanced scans (Fig. 7–9). Variable enhancement occurs after IV injection of contrast material. The contour of hypothalamic gliomas is usually irregular but well defined with inhomogeneous contrast enhancement. Low-grade gliomas either do not enhance or demonstrate homogeneous intense enhancement on T_1-weighted MRI

A B

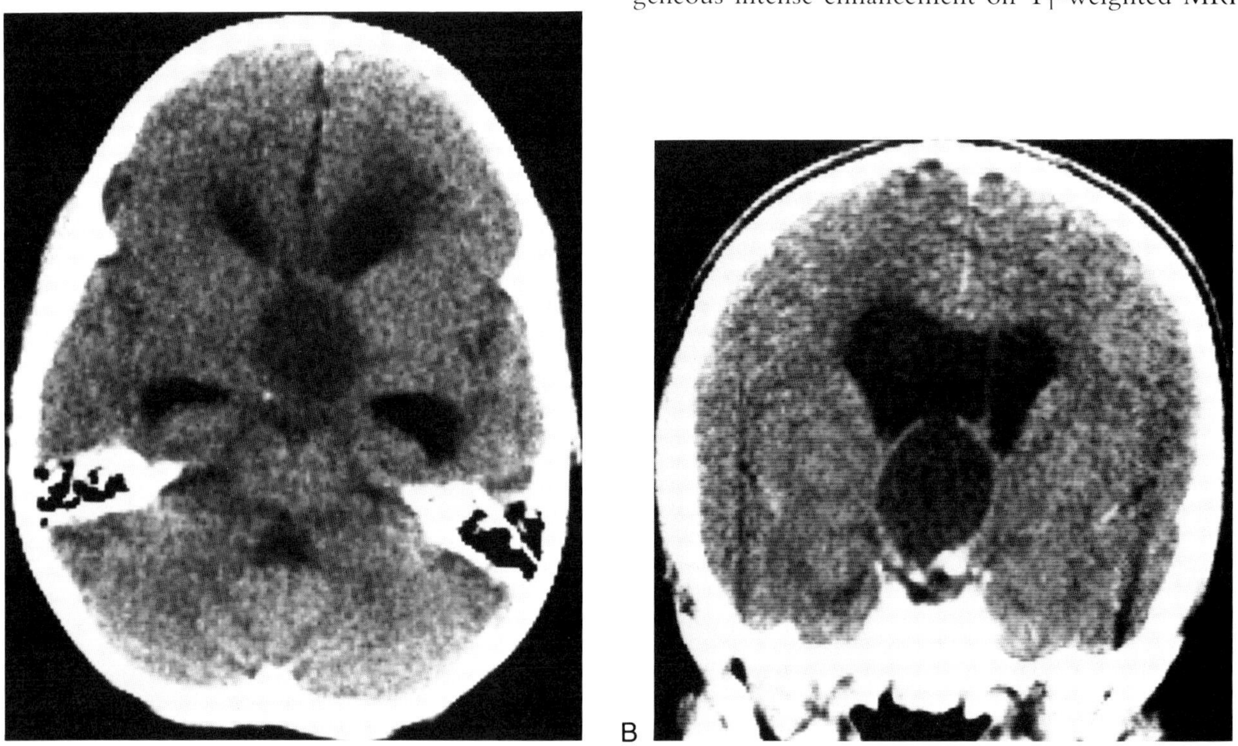

Fig. 7–8 Craniopharyngioma. **(A)** Nonenhanced axial CT scan demonstrates a cystic mass in a region of the third ventricle with a tiny calcification posteriorly on the right. **(B)** Coronal image obtained after administration of contrast material shows a thin rim of enhancement around the cystic portion of the craniopharyngioma.

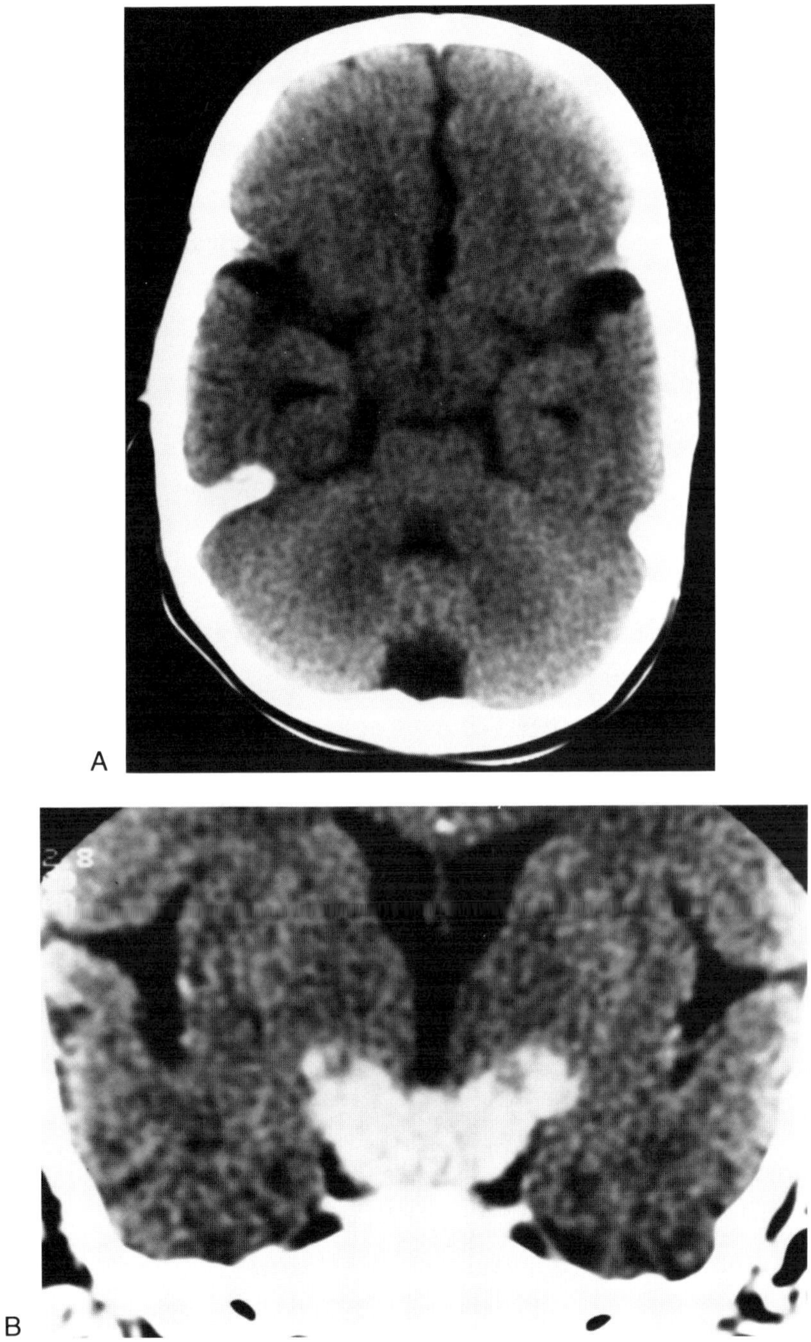

Fig. 7–9 Hypothalamic glioma. **(A)** Axial CT scan demonstrates an isodense suprasellar mass displacing the brain stem posteriorly. **(B)** Coronal enhanced CT scan demonstrates homogeneous contrast enhancement and an irregular margin. Whether the mass arises from the optic chiasm or hypothalamus is difficult to determine.

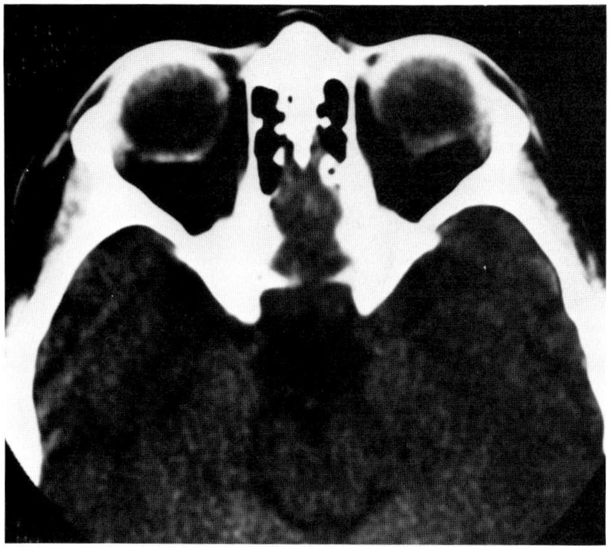

Fig. 7–10 Suprasellar epidermoid. Note the hypodense rounded mass arising in the suprasellar region of this patient being evaluated for sinusitis. This represents an inclusion cyst containing fat.

following gadolinium-diethylenetriaminepentaacetic acid (Gd-DTPA) administration. Patchy enhancement is suspicious for a higher grade of malignancy.

Germ cell tumors, congenital cysts, and meningiomas occur less commonly than the previously described lesions. The germinoma, or ectopic pinealoma, is the most common cell type of germ cell tumor arising in the parasellar region. A variable pattern of CT or MRI contrast enhancement is seen. Radiotherapy is the treatment of choice for this lesion.

It may be difficult to differentiate some craniopharyngiomas from epidermoid cysts because of the mixed density/intensity on both CT and MRI (Fig. 7–10).

Meningiomas account for only 2 to 8 percent of primary central nervous system tumors during the first 2 decades of life. Neurofibromatosis is present in approximately 25 percent of young patients with meningiomas. Meningiomas presenting as supersellar

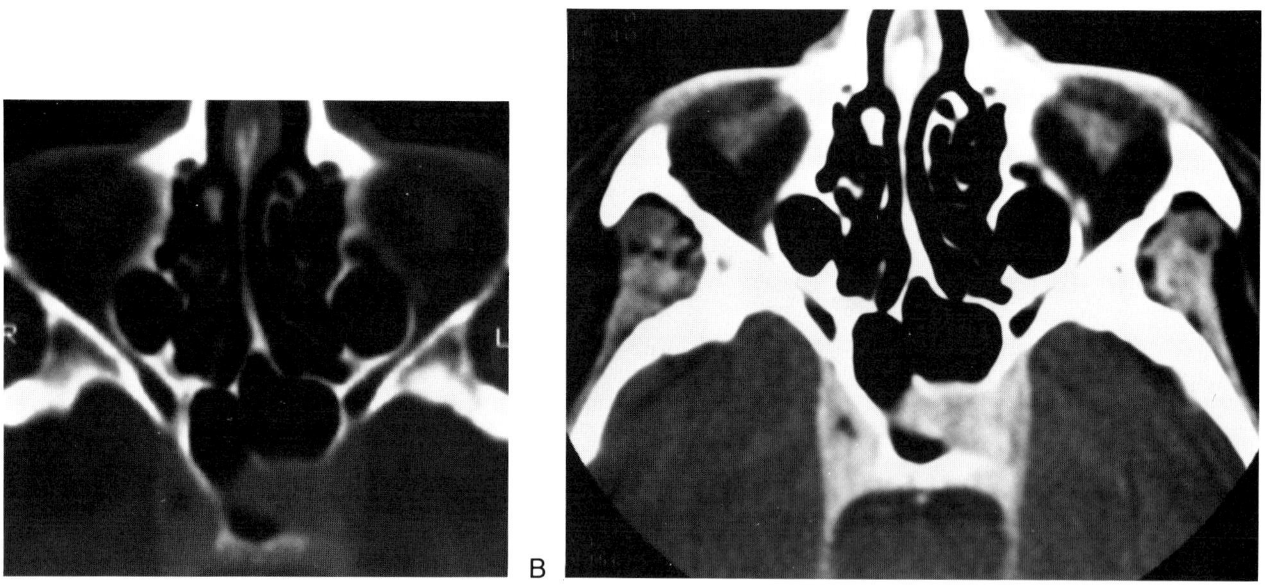

Fig. 7–11 Meningioma. **(A)** Note the slightly hyperdense mass arising from the left planum sphenoidale on a nonenhanced axial CT scan. **(B)** Enhanced axial scan at the same level shows homogeneous hyperdensity. (*Figure continues.*)

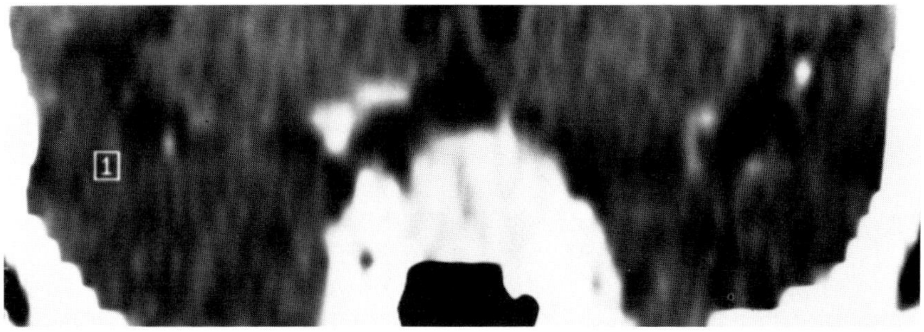

C

Fig. 7–11 (*Continued*). **(C)** Coronal reconstruction demonstrates the full extent of the hyperdense meningioma.

masses may arise from the optic nerve sheath, cerebellopontine angle cistern, sphenoid ridge, tuberculum sellae, and clinoid processes. The mass is isodense or hyperdense on nonenhanced CT and demonstrates homogeneous intense enhancement after contrast material injection (Fig. 7–11). The adjacent bone is usually hyperostotic.

Pituitary adenomas comprise 1 to 2 percent of all intracranial neoplasms in children less than 15 years of age. The incidence increases in the latter half of the second decade of life. Symptoms include delayed puberty and visual disturbances. CT typically demonstrates a sharply circumscribed tumor that is isodense or hyperdense when compared to the surrounding brain. Homogeneous enhancement with contrast material is seen on both CT and MRI (Fig. 7–12). Extrasellar extension is more common in childhood than in adulthood.

In contrast, microadenomas demonstrate a variable pattern of enhancement with injection of contrast material and may be increased, equal, or decreased in intensity when compared with the surrounding pituitary gland on MRI. The presenting symptom is prolactinemia.

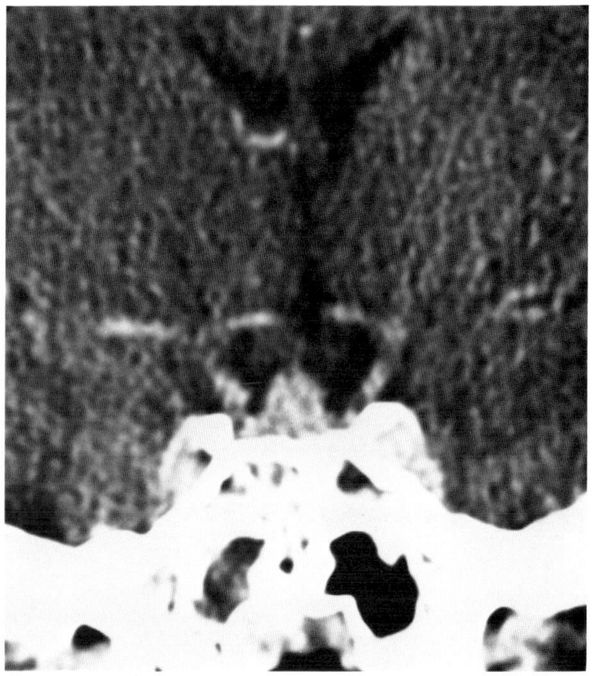

Fig. 7–12 Pituitary adenoma. Note the diffuse homogeneous enhancement of the enlarged pituitary gland on the coronal CT scan of a young woman with delayed puberty.

Causes of a small sella turcica include normal variation, hypopituitarism, brain atrophy, and decreased intracranial pressure.

Spinal Canal

Abnormalities in the size of the spinal canal are reflected by the interpedicular distance. The widest portions of the normal spinal canal on the frontal view are in the cervicothoracic and lumbosacral regions of infants.

The most common cause of a focal increase in the interpedicular distance is meningocele/meningomyelocele. The thecal malformations are associated with failure of fusion of the posterior elements of the spine and may be associated with scoliosis or kyphosis. Other causes include intraspinal space-occupying lesions (cysts, tumor), syringomyelia, diastematomyelia, thinning of the pedicles associated with tumors of neurogenic origin (neuroblastoma, neurofibroma), and arteriovenous malformations.

Abnormal narrowing of the spinal canal is most commonly associated with the chondrodystrophies (achondroplasia, hypochondroplasia). Other causes include arteriohepatic dysplasia, narrow lumbar spinal canal syndrome, and the other dwarfs.

INTRACRANIAL HEMORRHAGE

Intracranial hemorrhage may be detected with either ultrasonography, CT, or MRI. Each imaging modality demonstrates characteristic appearances depending on the age of the hemorrhage. Acute intracranial hemorrhage (less than 7 days) is more echogenic than normal choroid plexus but does not demonstrate acoustic shadowing. The increased echogenicity persists for at least 6 weeks and may last for several months if the bleed is large. As the hematoma ages, the echogenicity gradually decreases and becomes inhomogeneous. The hematoma also decreases in size with the central portion becoming sonolucent first.

INTRACRANIAL HEMORRHAGE

Grade I
: Subependymal hemorrhage

Grade II
: Subependymal hemorrhage or choroid plexus hemorrhage, with intraventricular hemorrhage, but without ventricular dilatation

Grade III
: Subependymal hemorrhage or choroid plexus hemorrhage, with intraventricular hemorrhage and ventricular enlargement

Grade IV
: Intraparenchymal hemorrhage with or without grade III hemorrhage

This sequence of findings is extremely useful in the detection and follow-up of pathology associated with prematurity.

Before the age of 32 weeks gestation, the germinal matrix represents a vascular bed located between the caudate nucleus and caudothalamic notch that is extremely sensitive to changes in intracranial pressure. The trauma of birth may cause germinal matrix hemorrhage that is graded based on extent and prognosis,

A

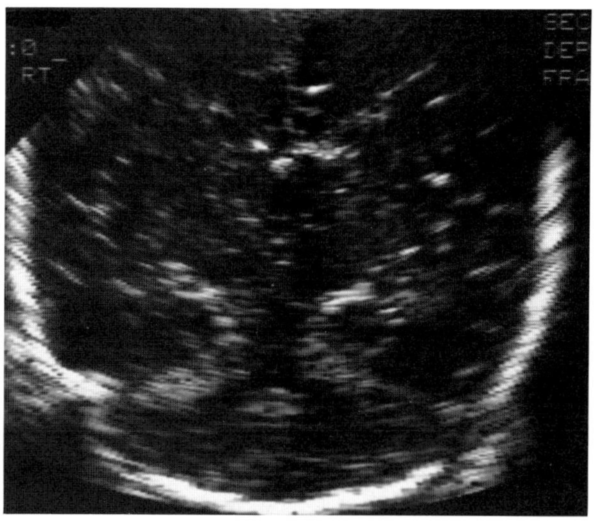

Fig. 7–13 Intracranial hemorrhage. **(A)** Coronal head ultrasound demonstrates indistinctness of the choroid plexus in the floor of the left lateral ventricle. Compare this with the normal choroid plexus in the right lateral ventricle and in the roof of the third ventricle. (*Figure continues.*)

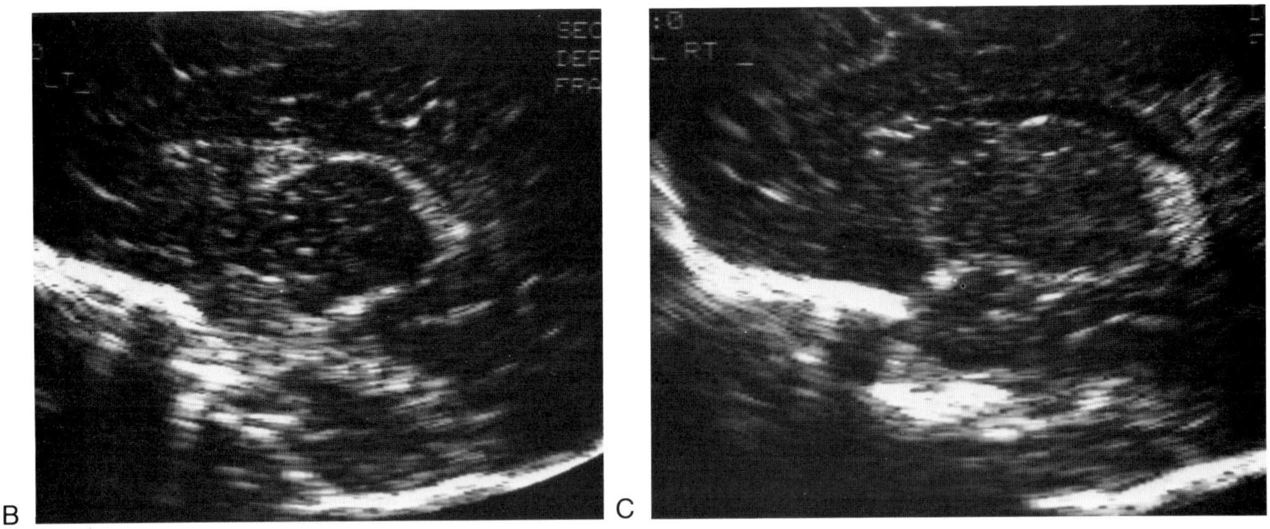

Fig. 7–13 (*Continued*) **(B)** Left parasagittal image demonstrates increased echogenicity in the region of the germinal matrix (caudothalamic groove). **(C)** Right parasagittal ultrasound image demonstrating normal caudothalamic groove for comparison.

(see list). The optimum time for routine detection of intracranial hemorrhage is between 7 and 14 days of age (Fig. 7–13). Detected hemorrhages may be followed-up weekly to assess for posthemorrhage ventriculomegaly and hematoma resolution/extension. The grade of the hemorrhage does not always correspond with the long-term clinical outcome of the patient. In general, premature infants suffering only from intracranial hemorrhage rarely have marked disability. Seventy percent of patients with interventricular hemorrhage develop posthemorrhagic obstructive hydrocephalus.

In contrast, children suffering from periventricular leukomalacia (the result of ischemia in the watershed areas between the anterior, middle, and posterior cerebral arteries) often have a poor prognosis. Periventricular leukomalacia occurs in only 10 to 20 percent of newborns. Acutely, increased echogenicity is seen in the peritrigonal occipital white matter and/or adjacent to the foramen of Monroe (Fig. 7–14). Hemorrhage may occur in up to 20 percent of cases

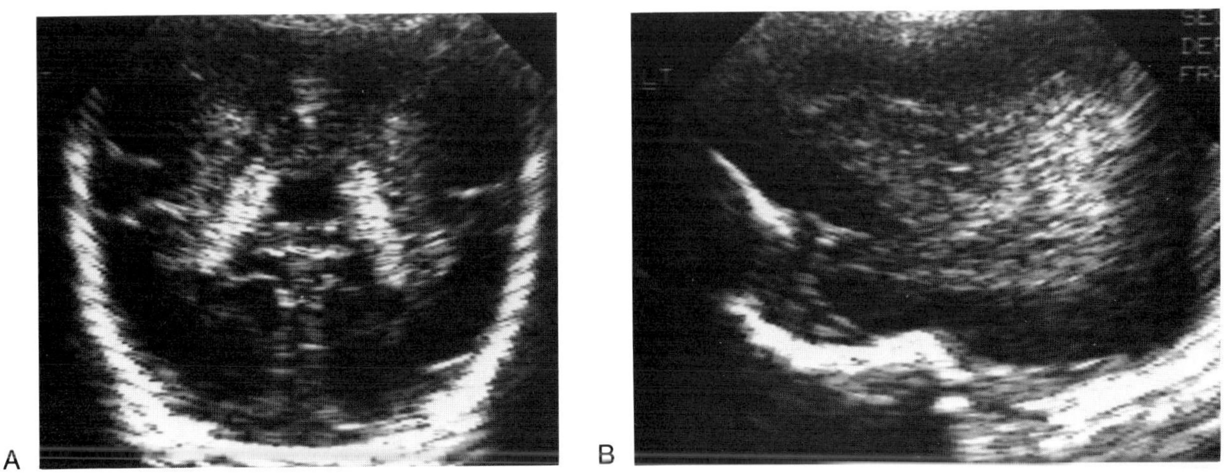

Fig. 7–14 Periventricular leukomalacia. **(A)** Coronal view from a screening head ultrasound demonstrates increased echogenicity lateral to the choroid plexus of the lateral ventricles. **(B)** Ill-defined areas of increased echogenicity are confirmed on parasagittal scans lateral to the lateral ventricles.

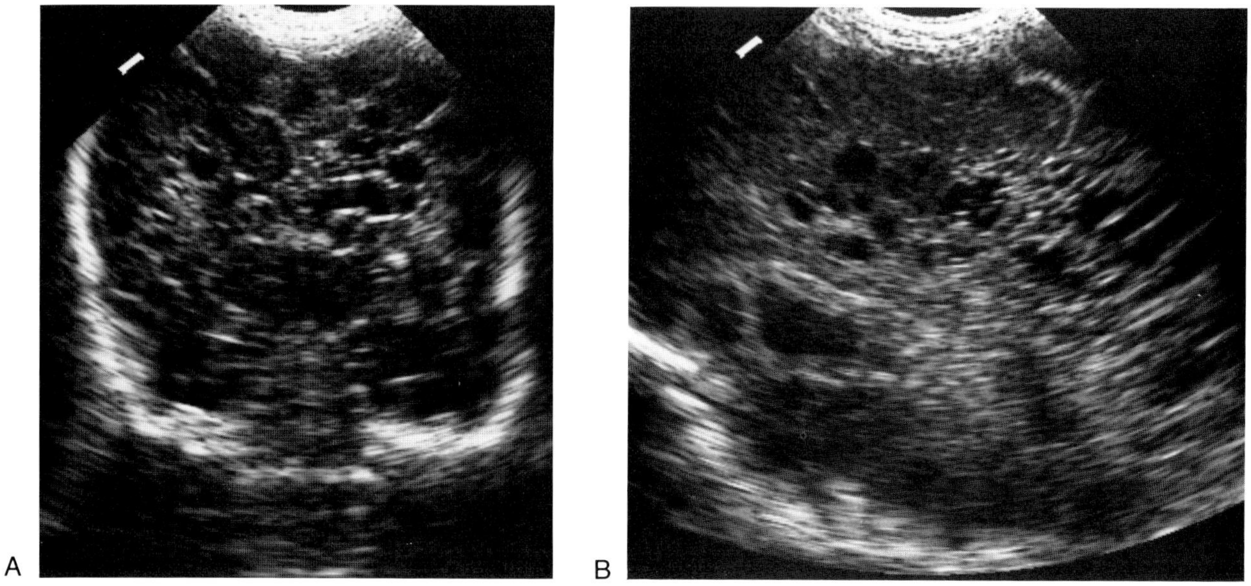

Fig. 7–15 Cystic periventricular leukomalacia. **(A)** Coronal scan on a follow-up ultrasound image of a child with periventricular leukomalacia demonstrates bilateral cysts scattered diffusely throughout the cortex. **(B)** Right parasagittal view lateral to the lateral ventricle confirms the periventricular location of the cysts.

and, when present, indicates significant infarction. The incidence of germinal matrix hemorrhage and periventricular leukomalacia occurring together is low. Two to three weeks after the ischemic event occurs, multiseptated cysts may occur adjacent to the ventricles confirming the diagnosis (Fig. 7–15). While some cysts may resolve, most persist and may communicate with the ventricles.

Cortical hemorrhages secondary to arteriovenous

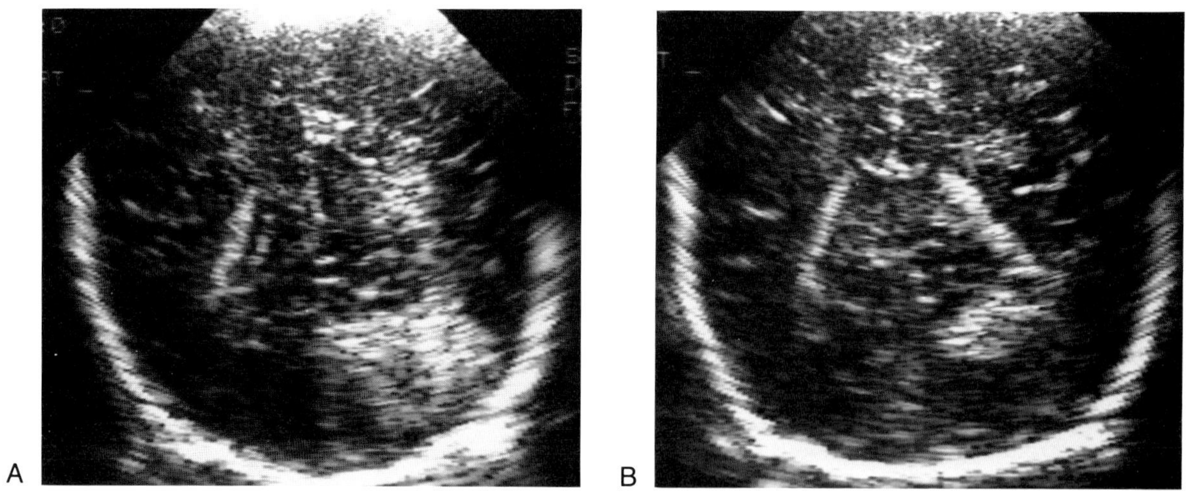

Fig. 7–16 Intraparenchymal hemorrhage. **(A)** This infant was suffering from *E. coli* meningitis. Bulging fontanelles prompted head ultrasound imaging. Coronal view angled posteriorly demonstrates a wedge-shaped area of increased echogenicity in the left occipital lobe. **(B)** Mass effect shifts the choroid plexus of the left lateral ventricle laterally. The hemorrhage is equal in echogenicity to the choroid plexus.

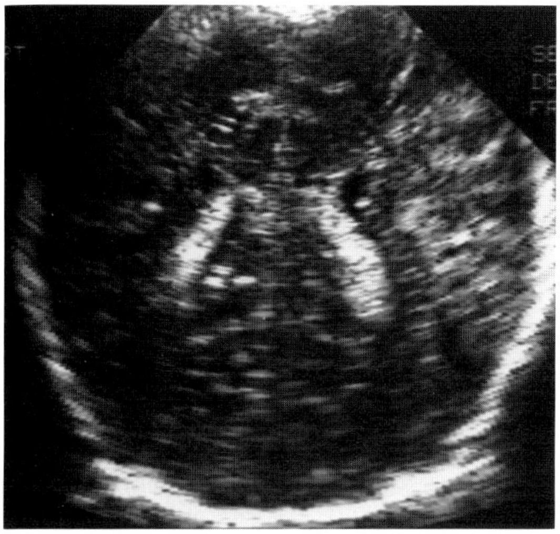

A

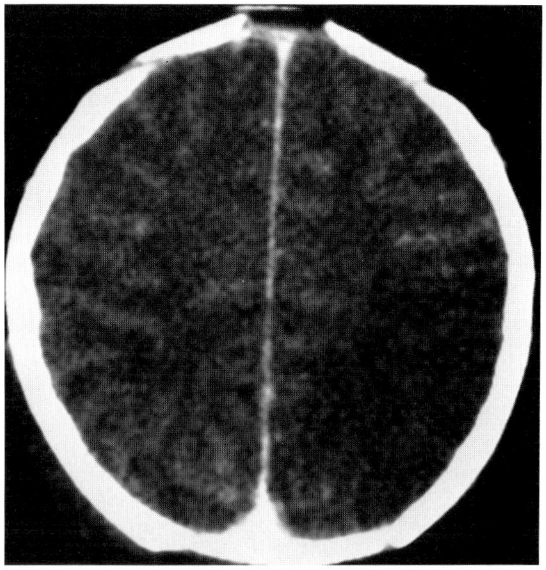

B

Fig. 7–17 Hemorrhagic infarction. **(A)** Coronal head ultrasound demonstrates a wedge-shaped area of increased echogenicity in the distribution of the left middle cerebral artery. Echogenic foci within the lesion approach the echogenicity of the adjacent choroid plexus. **(B)** Enhanced axial head CT image demonstrates the infarction as a wedge-shaped area of decreased attenuation in the left parietal lobe.

malformation, inflammation, trauma, and tumor are easily detectable and demonstrate the same ultrasound characteristics described above (Fig. 7–16). Cerebellar subarachnoid and brain stem hemorrhages may be overlooked if a careful search in these areas is not conducted. Unfortunately, epidural and subdural hematomas must be at least 1-cm thick for accurate sonographic detection. Suspected but unconfirmed hemorrhage should be assessed with CT or MRI (Fig. 7–17). After the anterior fontanelle closes, CT is often the first method used for brain imaging.

The assessment of extracerebral hematomas includes shape, density, and location. Classically, subdural hematomas may cover the convexity of a hemisphere with variable extension into the infratemporal fossa or along the tentorium. The inner margin of the subdural hematoma is usually concave (Fig. 7–18). The acute collection usually is hyperdense as compared with the adjacent brain (80 HU). A gradual decrease in density occurs until about the third week after injury at which time the lesion is isodense with the adjacent brain. Even at this time, midline shift and adjacent ventricular compression are clues that a subacute subdural hematoma is present. After about 6 weeks of age, the collection becomes hypodense as compared with the adjacent brain. Administration of IV contrast material may reveal slight opacification of the compressed cortical sulci or the membrane surrounding the hematoma.

High-field strength MRI may reveal acute subdural hematomas as isointense lesions on T_1-weighted images and hypointense on T_2-weighted images as compared with the adjacent brain. It may be easier to detect interhemispheric blood and tentorial subdural hematomas on the coronal images. Subacute and chronic subdural hematomas appear as hyperintense collections on both T_1-weighted and T_2-weighted images (Fig. 7–19).

In contrast, acute epidural hematomas are more localized and have a lentiform shape. Epidural hematoma has a high association with skull fracture. Injury to the venous sinuses or the middle meningeal artery may result in epidural hematoma. Underlying hemorrhagic brain contusion is common. Often in the acute phase, there may be mixed swirls of high density and lucency within the clot. Once the clot stabilizes,

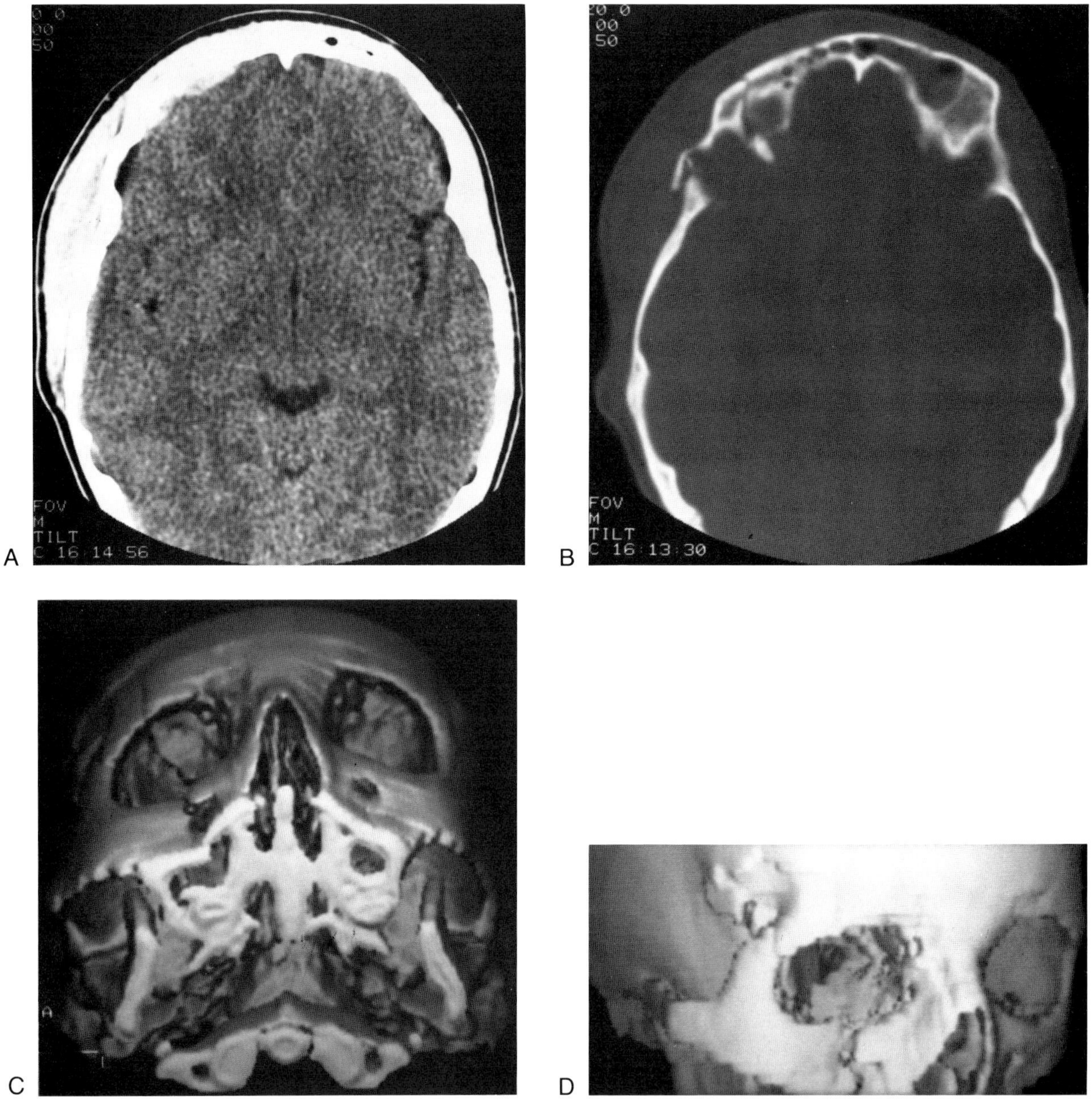

Fig. 7–18 Subdural hematoma. **(A)** Note the small hyperdense collection adjacent to the right frontal lobe indicating acute subdural hematoma. The blood in the adjacent scalp is hyperdense as well. **(B)** Bone window settings demonstrate comminution of the adjacent frontal bone. **(C)** Three-dimensional reconstruction better demonstrates the extent of the right tripod fracture. Note the interruption of the superior orbital rim. **(D)** The depressed skull fracture is best seen in an oblique 3-dimensional reconstruction image. (*Figure continues.*)

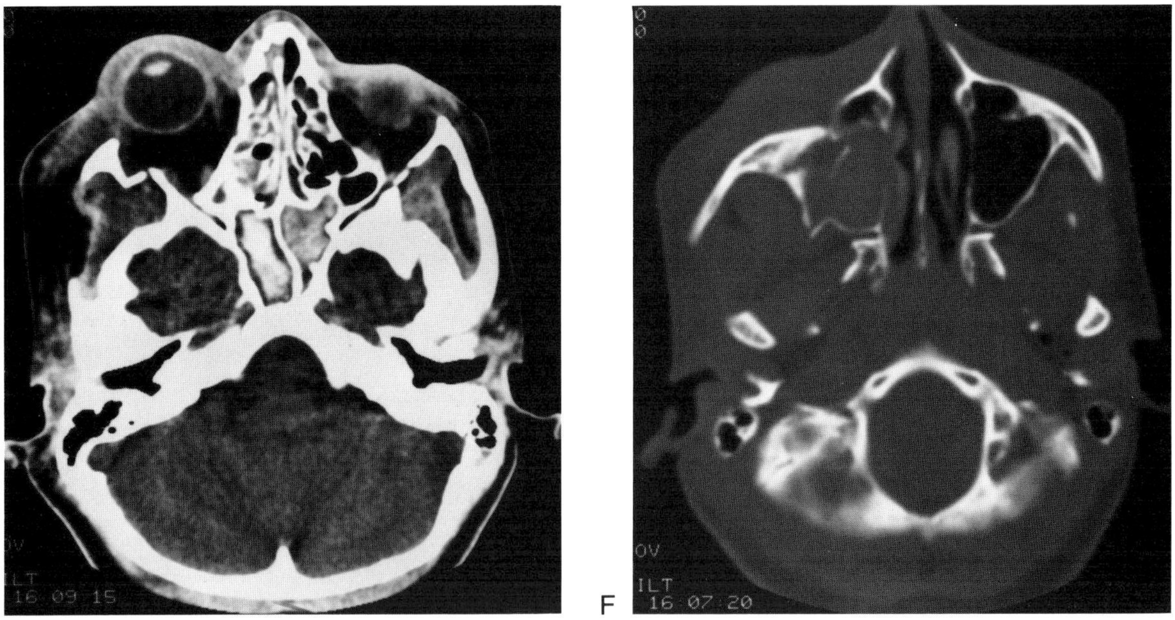

E F

Fig. 7–18 (*Continued.*) **(E)** Preseptal edema overlies the right orbit on an axial scan. Note the hyperdense blood filling the sphenoid sinus and right ethmoid air cells. The lateral orbital rim is comminuted. **(F)** Bone window settings demonstrate comminution of the right maxillary sinus walls.

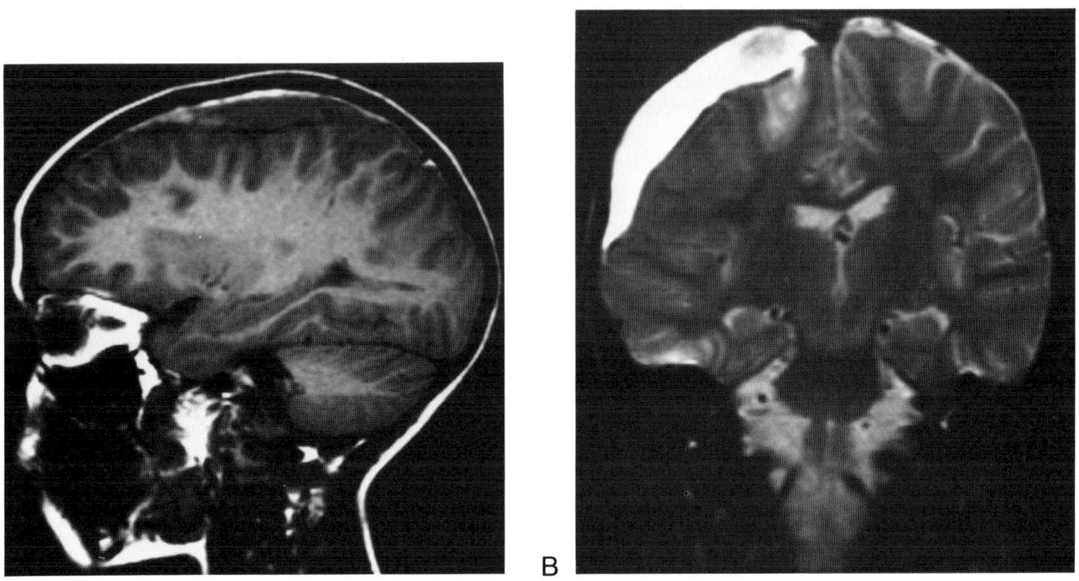

A B

Fig. 7–19 Subdural hematoma. **(A)** T_1-weighted right parasagittal MRI demonstrates a right subdural hematoma that is both isointense and hyperintense in signal intensity. **(B)** Coronal T_2-weighted image demonstrates mixed hyperintensity and isointensity consistent with evolution from the acute to subacute phase. Note the increased intensity of the underlying right frontal cortex due to cerebral contusion.

it becomes homogeneously increased in density as compared with the adjacent brain. In the subacute phase, the clot becomes isodense as compared with the adjacent brain and hypodense in the chronic phase. Contrast enhancement will demonstrate the displaced dura.

On MRI, epidural hematoma can be differentiated from subdural hematoma by the low-intensity fibrous dura seen between the collection and adjacent brain. Acutely, the hematoma will be isointense on T_1-weighted images and hypointense on T_2-weighted images. In the subacute phase, the collection is increased in intensity on both T_1- and T_2-weighted images. After about 3 weeks of age, the collection becomes relatively decreased in intensity on T_1-weighted images as compared with the acute phase. There is also a relative decrease in the T_2-weighted intensity, although it still may be hyperintense when compared with the adjacent brain. Epidural hematomas usually resolve completely without chronic residual change.

Subarachnoid hemorrhage in and of itself is of little consequence but signifies the presence of a previously unsuspected vascular anomaly, tumor, or trauma. Tiny foci of parenchymal hemorrhage may be noted as vague areas of increased density that result in a small amount of surrounding edema. Occasionally, contusion may be nonhemorrhagic and result in a localized area of low attenuation with a variable amount of mass effect.

While traumatic parenchymal hemorrhagic brain lesions are less common in children than in adults, the incidence of mortality and morbidity is higher in pediatric patients who have a combination of cerebral edema and focal parenchymal hemorrhages. The findings are suggestive of shearing injury, which is responsible for 4 percent of pediatric head injuries. The mechanism of injury is abrupt deceleration leading to abrupt cranial acceleration. On impact, one cerebral hemisphere moves in relationship to the other resulting in axonal shearing through the junction of the cortex and the white matter. Small hemorrhages may be seen in the corpus callosum, internal capsule, deep nuclear gray matter, upper brain stem, and at the corticomedullary junction (Fig. 7–20). If the patient survives the acute phase, atrophy of the cortex results in enlargement of the sulci and ventricles.

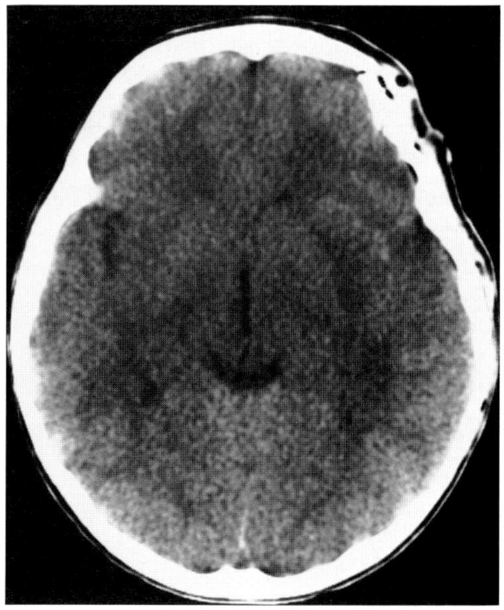

Fig. 7–20 Shearing injury. Axial head CT scan from a patient who fell from a third-story window demonstrates small areas of increased density in the left parietal lobe consistent with shearing injury.

Seventy-three percent of pediatric patients with shearing injuries die.

Brain contusions may be the result of coup or contracoup injuries. Coup contusions occur when the calvarial surface strikes the underlying soft cerebral tissue. A contracoup contusion results at a site remote from the point of cranial impact and may be exactly opposite from the point of impact. Contusions result from the brain's motion within the calvaria and are most likely to occur in the frontal lobes and temporal tips following occipital impact. Hemorrhage into contusion is less common in the infant and young child than in the adolescent. The overall incidence of brain contusions in childhood is approximately 23 percent following depressed skull fracture.

CONGENITAL CENTRAL NERVOUS SYSTEM MALFORMATIONS

Classification of congenital central nervous system malformations may be based on the gestational age at which morphologic derangement occurs. The classification listed in Table 7–1 is modified from that devised by van der Knaap and Valk.[30] An understand-

Table 7–1 Congenital Central Nervous System Malformations

Embryologic Event	Disorder
Dorsal induction	
Primary neurulation (3–4 weeks GA)	Anencephaly Chiari malformation Craniorachischisis totalis Encephalocele Hydromyelia Myelomeningocele Myeloschisis
Secondary neurulation (4–40 weeks GA)	Anterior dysraphic disturbances Caudal regression syndrome Dermal sinus with or without dermoid or epidermoid cyst Diastematomyelia/diplomelia Lipoma Meningocele/lipomeningocele Myelocystocele Tethered cord/tight filum terminale syndrome
Ventral induction (5–10 weeks GA)	Atelencephaly Cerebellar hemisphere hypoplasia/aplasia Cerebellar vermis hypoplasia/aplasia Cerebral hemisphere hypoplasia/aplasia Craniosynostosis Dandy-Walker syndrome/Dandy-Walker variant Diencephalic cyst Holoprosencephaly Lobar hypoplasia/aplasia Septo-optic dysplasia Septum pellucidum agenesis
Migration (2–5 weeks GA)	Corpus callosum hypoplasia/aplasia Lissencephaly Neuronal heteropias Pachygyria Polymicrogyria Schizencephaly
Neuronal proliferation/differentiation (8–20 weeks GA)	Aqueduct stenosis Colpocephaly Congenital central nervous system tumors Congenital vascular malformations Hydranencephaly Megalencephaly Micrencephaly Multicystic encephalopathy Neurocutaneous syndromes Porencephaly Unilateral megalencephaly
Myelination	Hypomyelination Retarded myelination
Unclassified	Arachnoid cyst

Abbreviation: GA, gestational age.
(Modified from van der Knaap and Valk,[30] with permission.)

ing of fetal neural development is the key to logical classification of the disorders.

Dorsal Induction

At approximately 3 weeks gestational age, the notochordal process causes thickening of the embryonic ectoderm to form the neural plate. Primary neurulation describes the formation of the neural tube from the neural plate that begins caudally and extends upward. Secondary neurulation describes canalization and differentiation of the neural tube below the distal notocord resulting in the segments below L1 to L2. While canalization occurs during weeks 4 to 7 of gestation, the process of retrogressive differentiation that follows continues even after birth.

Disorders of dorsal induction usually result from incomplete separation of the embryologic ectoderm from the endoderm resulting in a spectrum of dysraphic or myelodysplastic states. Anomalies of neural tube closure are associated with an elevated maternal serum alpha-fetoprotein level. Fetal ultrasound is quite sensitive to dorsal induction disorders, especially the more severe varieties such as anencephaly, encephaloceles, and large myelomeningoceles.

Anencephaly describes absence of the cerebral hemispheres (telencephalon) with sparing of the midbrain and brain stem (mesencephalon). The cranial vault is absent but the skull base is normally formed. Anencephaly is the most common central nervous system anomaly with an incidence of 1 in 1,000 births. Associated defects include vertebral dysraphism (50 percent of patients), club foot, cleft palate, and umbilical hernias. Polyhydramnios is associated in 50 percent of cases past 26 weeks gestational age. Occasionally, oligohydramnios develops.

Encephaloceles develop from smaller calvarial defects and are characterized by location and contents (Fig. 7–21). Seventy percent of cases occur in the occiput.

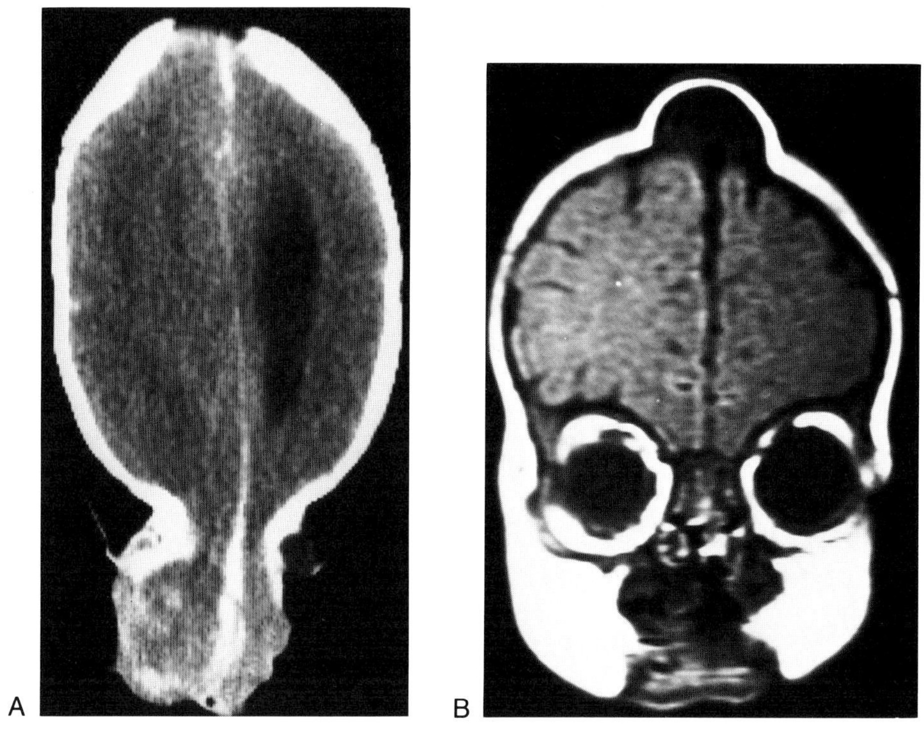

Fig. 7–21 Cephaloceles. **(A)** Note the extension of the falx and cortex from both hemispheres through the bony occipital defect demonstrated on an axial CT image (occipital encephalocele). **(B)** T_1-weighted coronal MRI of another patient demonstrates a frontal cephalocele containing cerebrospinal fluid but no brain parenchyma.

The frontal, parietal, and basal portions of the skull account for 10 percent of cases each. The incidence of cephaloceles is 1 in 2,000 live births. Fetal ultrasound imaging is useful in diagnosis, delivery planning, and prognosis. A large cephalocele may prompt cesarian section. Absence of brain tissue within the sac is a favorable prognostic sign. After birth and prior to repair, MRI may be useful in identifying the contents of the sac. In cases in which the cephalocele size approaches the resolution limits of MRI, contrast material may be injected into the thecal sac. If contrast accumulates in the cephalocele (as indicated by CT), then the diagnosis of communication is assured. Associated anomalies include corpus callosum dysgenesis, hydrocephalus, Dandy-Walker syndrome, and Meckel's syndrome.

The Chiari malformations are anomaly complexes involving multiple central nervous system sites. The Chiari II malformation describes dysgenesis of the hindbrain, which is almost always associated with meningomyelocele and obstructive hydrocephalus. Caudal elongation of the dysplastic cerebellum occurs, resulting in classic findings demonstrable with ultrasonography, CT, or MRI (Fig. 7–22). The foramen magnum is large. Herniated into it are the buckled medulla, compressed portion of the fourth ventricle, and a portion of the cerebellum. Anterolateral growth of the cerebellum causes bulging superiorly through the incisura and extension anterior and lateral to the brain stem. The fused colliculi form the tectal beak. The tentorium is hypoplastic with a low insertion, large incisura, and shortened straight sinus. The upper fourth ventricle may dilate and form a diverticulum. The falx is hypoplastic and commonly interdigitated. The frontal horns of the lateral ventricles are squared laterally and pointed inferiorly. There is prominence of the pineal recess and a large massa intermedia. Ninety percent of patients demonstrate hydrocephalus with a typical pattern of colpocephaly (asymmetric enlargement of the lateral ventricles). Occasionally, the hydrocephalus will not become apparent until after the meningomyelocele has been repaired. Other associated central nervous system anomalies include dysgenesis of the corpus callosum, an increased number of cortical gyrations, and syringohydromyelia.

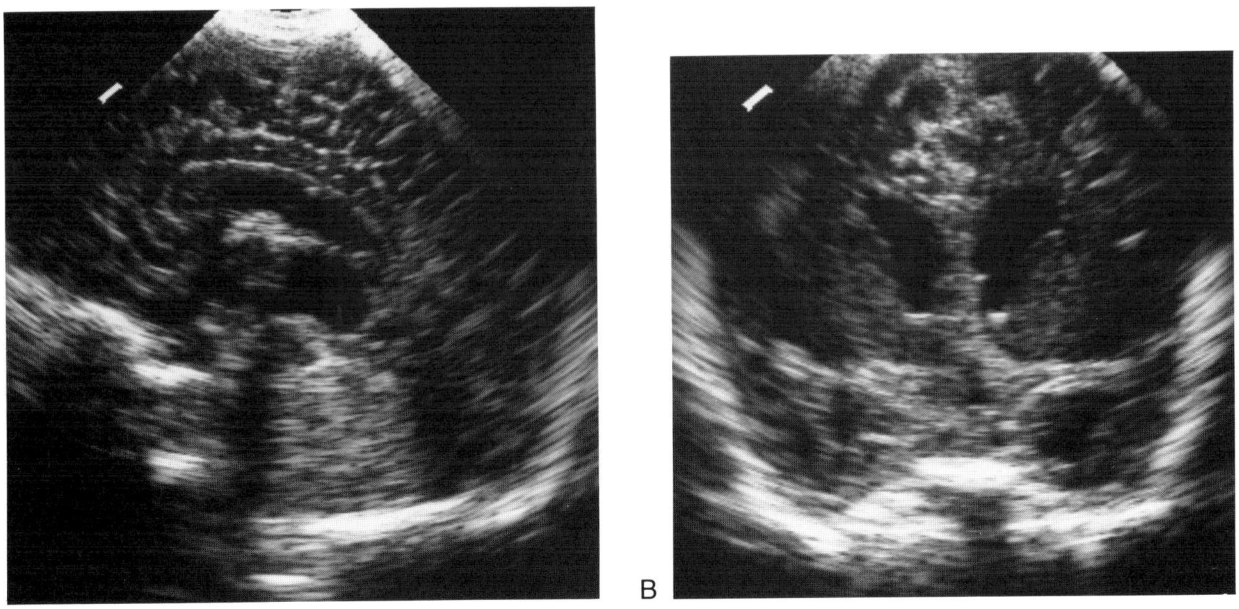

A B

Fig. 7–22 Chiari II malformation. **(A)** Midline sagittal ultrasound image demonstrates prominence of the massa intermedia and an absence of the cerebrospinal fluid usually seen in the cisterna magna. Instead, the cerebellum rests on the occipital bone. **(B)** Coronal image demonstrates inferior pointing of the lateral ventricles and squaring-off of the anterior horns. Note the interdigitation of the frontal lobes due to hypoplasia of the falx. (*Figure continues.*)

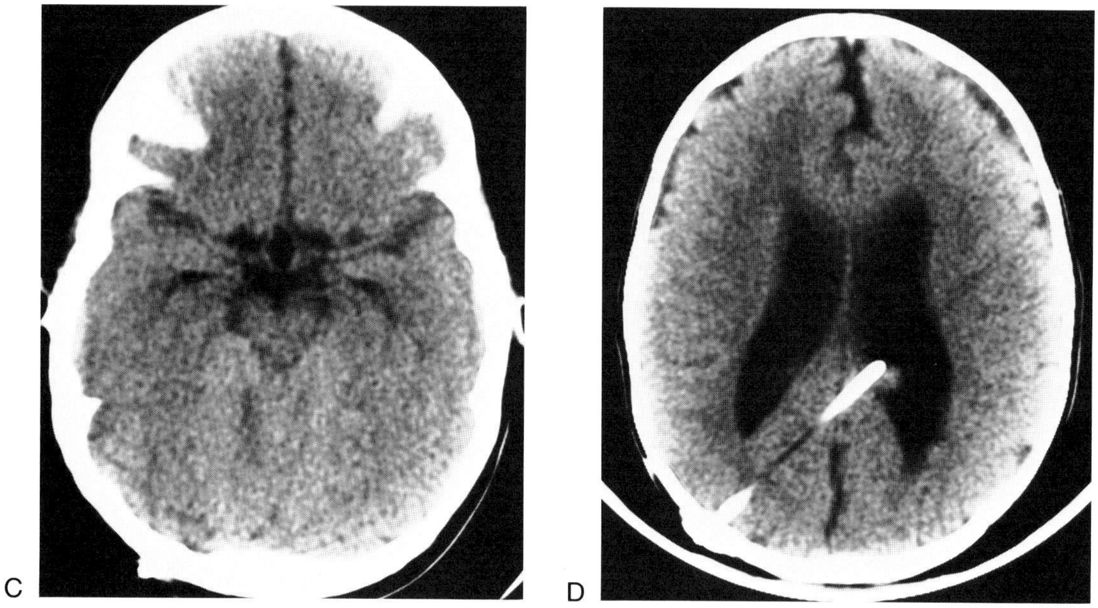

Fig. 7–22 (*Continued*). **(C)** CT scan of the same patient demonstrates tectal beaking due to the fused colliculi. **(D)** Higher axial image demonstrates shunted hydrocephalus.

The Chiari III malformation is more severe and describes herniation of the cerebellum through a cervicooccipital bony defect (Fig. 7–23).

Spina bifida cystica is the spectrum of spinal dysraphic states, which are similar to the cephaloceles. The average incidence is 1.2 per 1,000 live births. Seventy percent of cases occur below the second lumbar vertebral body with more than one-half at the lumbosacral junction. Fetal ultrasound imaging may disclose a

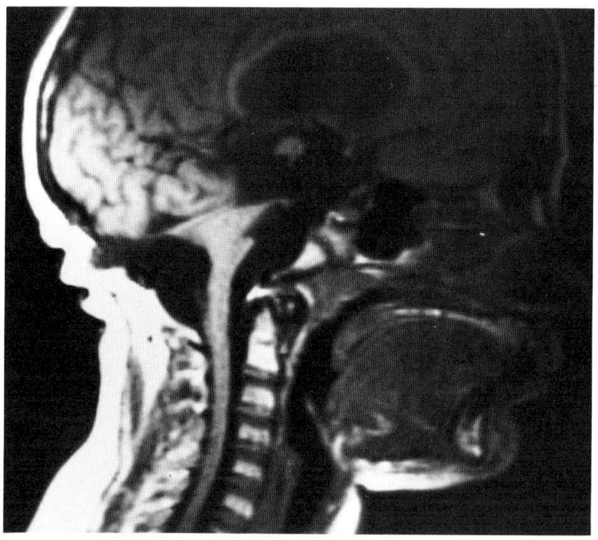

Fig. 7 23 Chiari III malformation. Note the herniation of the fourth ventricle through the small cervicooccipital meningocele on this T_1-weighted sagittal MRI. The cerebellar vermis is completely absent. The cerebellar hemispheres were also hypoplastic. The supratentorial findings were similar to those seen with Chiari II malformation.

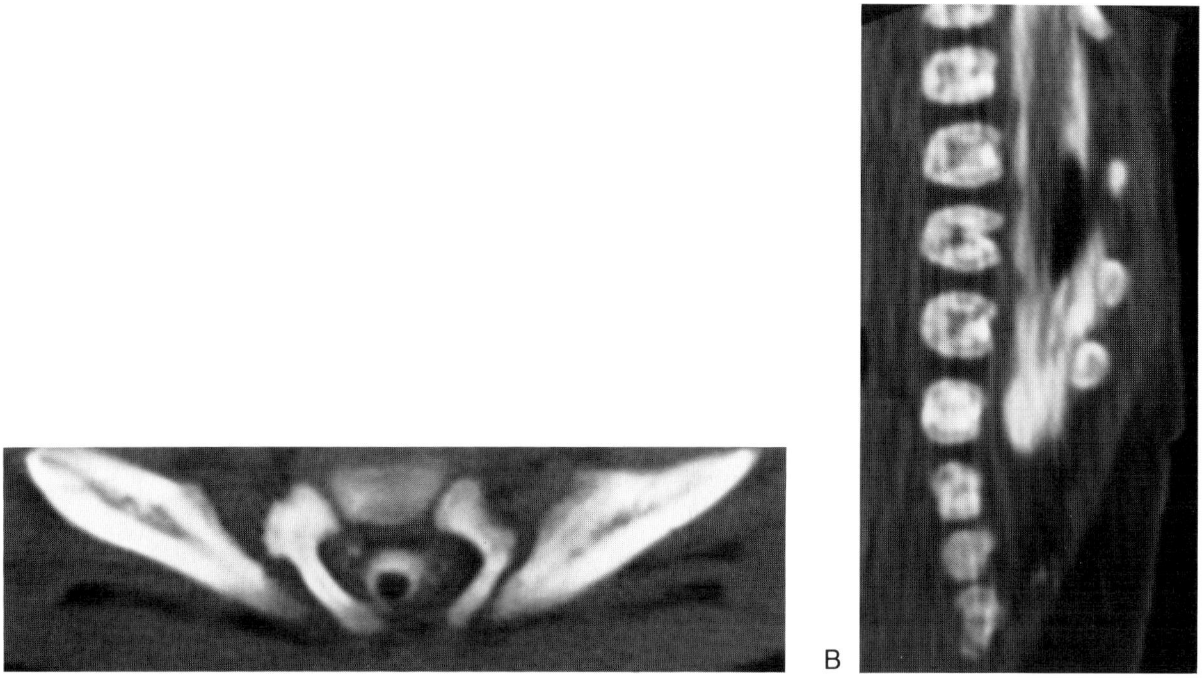

A B

Fig. 7–24 Spina bifida cystica. **(A)** Axial CT image demonstrates vertebral dysraphism at the lumbosacral junction. **(B)** Direct sagittal CT scan demonstrates thickening of the filum terminale associated with a low density lipoma. The cord is tethered posteriorly. Note the absence of the posterior elements at multiple levels in the lumbosacral region.

cystic structure at the caudal end of the spinal cord associated with vertebral body anomalies. After birth, ultrasonography is useful in screening for associated abnormalities including hydrocephalus, Chiari malformations, dislocated hips, club foot anomalies, gastrointestinal anomalies, and genitourinary anomalies. If the sac is rather firm, direct scanning may reveal the location of the neural placode and its relationship to the nerve roots. If this is not sufficient, CT or MRI is useful in identifying these structures (Fig. 7–24). Sixty to ninety percent of meningoceles and myelomeningoceles are associated with hydrocephalus. The association is greatest with lumbar myelomeningoceles. Aqueductal stenosis is the cause of associated hydrocephalus in the majority of cases. Spina bifida cystica is most likely to be posterior in location although occasionally meningoceles form anteriorly, presenting as pelvic masses.

The other neurulation disorders may not be as easy to recognize antenatally. Instead, tell-tale skin changes may be noted after birth including a hairy patch, subcutaneous lipoma, sinus tract, and abnormal skin pigmentation on the back. Since the vertebral bodies in the neonatal period are not completely ossified, ultrasound imaging is useful for screening patients with skin changes or radiographic diagnoses of vertebral anomalies. The cord is readily identified within the spinal canal and the level of the conus is apparent. At birth, the conus medullaris lies at L2 to L3, migrating to L1 to L2 by 3 months of age. Pulsations of the cord and location are useful in determining tethering. Lipomas are identified as hyperechoic space occupying lesions, which may extend beyond the confines of the spinal canal.

The identification of a hypoechoic longitudinal protuberance posteriorly may signify external diastematomyelia. This term describes splitting of the spinal cord by a fibrous, cartilaginous, or bony spur arising posteriorly. The cord is tethered to the spinal canal at the level of the spur. Associated vertebral anomalies include widening of the interpediculate distance, hemivertebrae, butterfly vertebra, block vertebra, spina

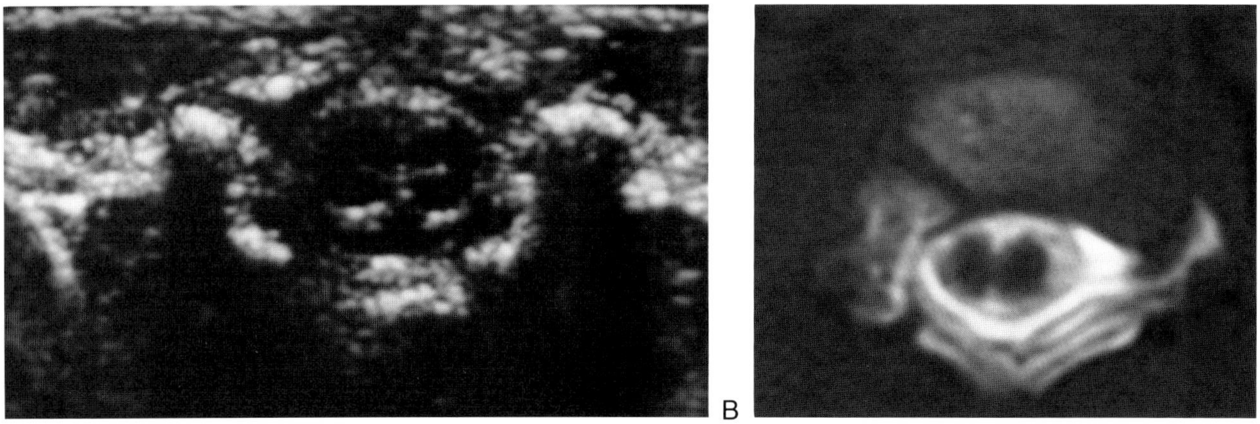

Fig. 7–25 Diastematomyelia. **(A)** Transverse ultrasound of a newborn demonstrates two cords within the thoracolumbar region. No bony spur was identified. **(B)** CT-myelography scans at bone window settings confirm the diagnosis of internal diastematomyelia.

bifida, and segmentation/fusion anomalies. Diastematomyelia is most common in the thoracolumbar region but it may occur at any level. Internal diastematomyelia describes focal splitting of the cord into two portions, each covered by its own dura (Fig. 7–25). Tethering does not occur at the level of the split but may occur at the filum terminale. A posterior spur is not associated.

Most patients who demonstrate ultrasound abnormalities will benefit from MRI. The multiplanar imaging capabilities provide more complete visualization of the cord, nerve roots, and surrounding structures, allowing for surgical planning.

Ventral Induction

Between 5 and 10 weeks gestational age, the rostral end of the primitive brain develops. This development also induces formation of the face. Induction leads to formation of the forebrain, midbrain, and hindbrain. The forebrain forms the two cerebral hemispheres and lateral ventricles. Other structures influenced by ventral induction include the third ventricle, thalamus, hypothalamus, and cranial nerves I and II.

Most of the cerebellar anomalies result from abnormal ventral induction. The cerebellar hemispheres arise from lateral primordia. If either does not develop, varying degrees of cerebellar agenesis will result. If the lateral primordia do not fuse at the midline, vermian hypoplasia or aplasia will result. The cystic posterior fossa malformations account for 30 percent of all congenital brain malformations.

The Dandy-Walker malformation accounts for 14 percent of malformations. In this anomaly, cystic dilatation of the fourth ventricle is associated with absence of the foramen of Magendie and malformation of the foramen of Luschka. The posterior fossa is enlarged and the relationship between the torcula and the lambda is reversed. The cerebellar hemispheres and vermis are hypoplastic. In true Dandy-Walker malformation, the enlarged fourth ventricle does not communicate with the perimedullary cistern. Involved infants present with dolicocephaly. MRI demonstrates the enlarged posterior fossa with a huge fourth ventricle displacing the small hypoplastic cerebellar hemispheres anterolaterally (Fig. 7–26). Only the superior vermis is present and it is displaced anterosuperiorly into the incisura. The tentorium will insert above the lambda with a more vertical orientation of the incisura. The petrous pyramids may also be scalloped. A careful search should be made for septa behind the cerebellum. Absence of any septa is consistent with the true Dandy-Walker malformation. Twenty-five percent of cases demonstrate one or more of the following associated cerebral anomalies: corpus callosal dysgenesis, holoprosencephaly, and cortical dysplasia. Hydrocephalus develops in most patients if given time.

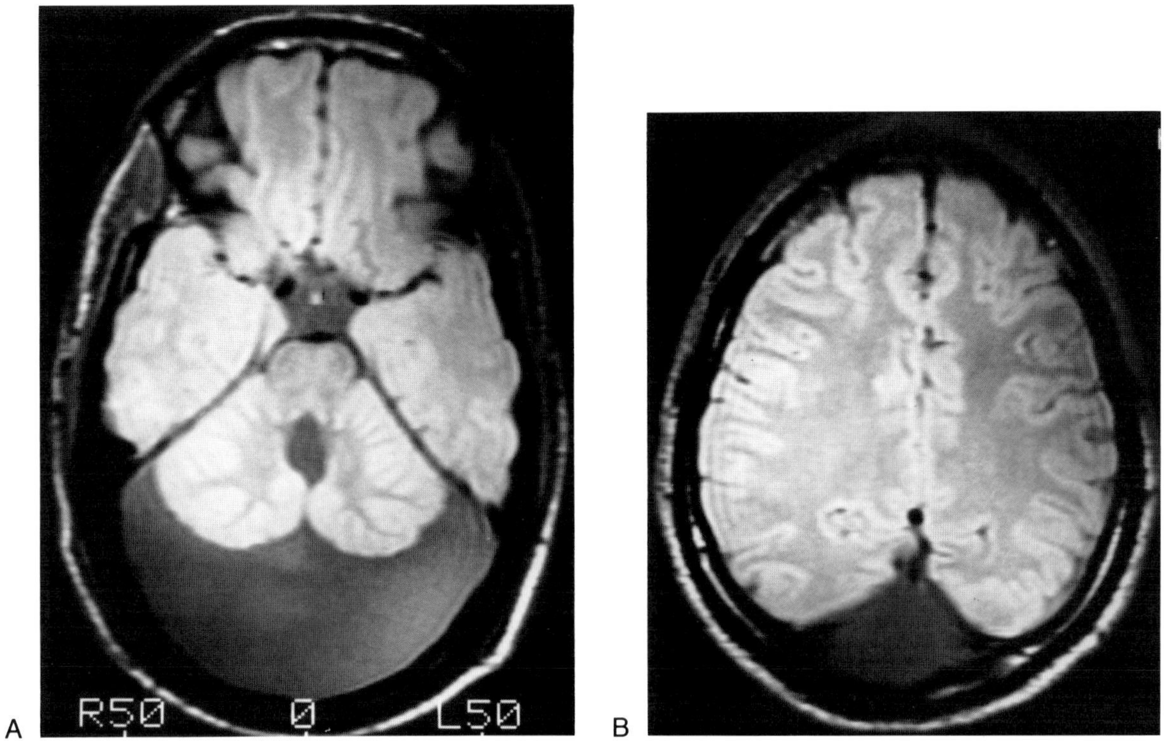

Fig. 7–26 Dandy-Walker malformation. **(A)** First echo from an axial T_2-weighted MRI sequence demonstrates anterior displacement of the hypoplastic cerebellar hemispheres by the dilated fourth ventricle. **(B)** A higher axial image demonstrates the insertion of the tentorium well above the lambda.

A more common posterior fossa cystic anomaly is the Dandy-Walker variant. In the variant, the fourth ventricle is not quite as dilated as in the true malformation and communicates freely with the basal cistern through the patent foramen of Magendie. Thirty-three percent of cystic posterior fossa malformations are Dandy-Walker variants. The posterior fossa is usually not enlarged. The cerebellar vermis is hypoplastic. The tentorium may be high or dehiscent.

The telencephalon forms the cerebral hemisphere by dividing into two parts. The hemispheres then roll over to form the temporal lobes and lateral fissures before joining together via the corpus callosum. Cerebral disorders resulting from incomplete ventral induction include holoprosencephaly, agenesis of the septum pellucidum, and lobar hypoplasia.

Holoprosencephaly results from failure of lateral and transverse cleavage. Three categories are described: alobar, semilobar, and lobar. Since induction of the forebrain does not occur, the face is also affected. Facial changes associated with holoprosencephaly include a spectrum of abnormalities ranging from cyclopia to hypotelorism associated with cleft lip.

Alobar holoprosencephaly is the most severe form and results in a single ventricle bordered anteriorly by a mantle of undifferentiated brain parenchyma and posteriorly by a large dorsal cyst (Fig. 7–27). The third ventricle is not present since the thalami are fused. The brain does not function and seizures are always present. The life span is short and many infants are stillborn. Both the septum pellucidum and corpus callosum are absent. Associated syndromes include trisomy 13 and 18.

The semilobar form describes partial formation of the posterior aspect of the interhemispheric fissure,

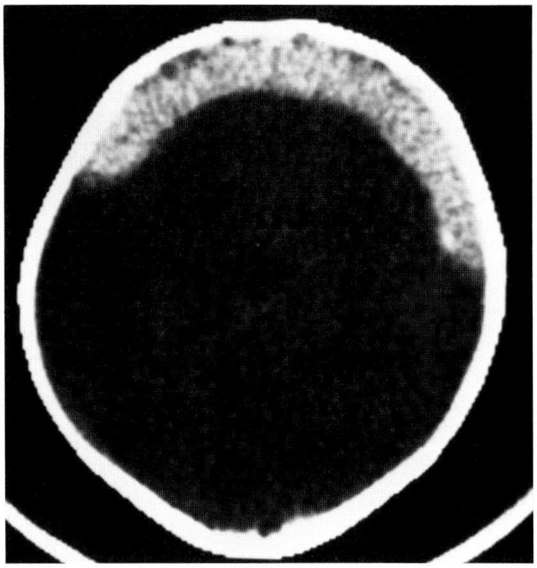

Fig. 7–27 Alobar holoprosencephaly. Note the mantle of brain parenchyma anterior to the large dorsal cyst.

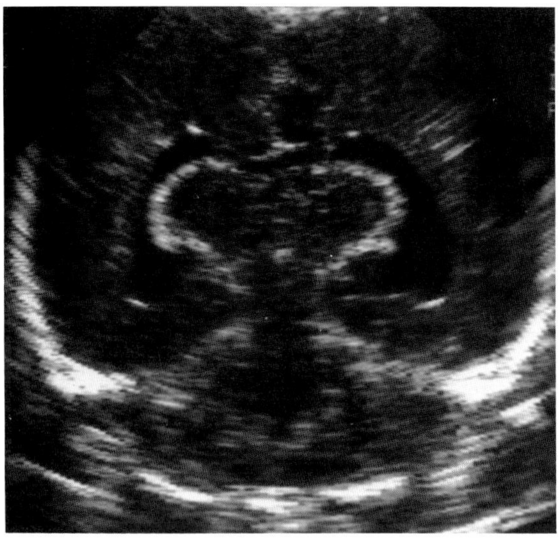

Fig. 7–28 Semilobar holoprosencephaly. Coronal ultrasound image demonstrates partial fusion of the thalami. the lateral ventricles were fused anteriorly.

falx cerebri, and incomplete separation of the thalami (Fig. 7–28). A small third ventricle is present but the corpus callosum and septum pellucidum are absent.

Lobar holoprosencephaly results in further anterior extension of the formed interhemispheric fissure and falx cerebri. Absence of the septum pellucidum and dysplasia of the anterior falx cerebri are present. The frontal lobes may be hypoplastic and partially fused or dysmorphic.

Absence of normal diencephalic development may result in a spectrum of abnormalities, including septum pellucidum agenesis. This abnormality may occur alone or with holoprosencephaly, septo-optic dysplasia, corpus callosal agenesis, schizencephaly, and some of the embryologic destructive lesions.

Septo-optic dysplasia describes the association of septum pellucidum agenesis and optic nerve hypoplasia (Fig. 7–29). Sixty-six percent of patients have associated hypothalamic or pituitary dysfunction. Visual symptoms most commonly bring the patients to medical attention including diminished acuity or nystagmus. Opthalmalogic exam reveals hypoplastic optic discs. Both CT and MRI demonstrate the squared-off appearance of the frontal horns with rapid tapering of the inferior margins of the lateral ventricles. Sagittal MRI is useful in demonstrating hypoplasia of the pituitary stalk and absence of the neurohypophysis. Hypoplasia of the optic nerves, canals, and chiasm may be noted on either CT or MRI.

Migration

After the nerve cells are formed in the periventricular layers of the brain parenchyma, migration to the superficial cortex and deep nuclei follows. This process is seen in both the cerebrum and cerebellum. If migration is abnormal or incomplete it will alter the gyral pattern. Cerebral migration is intimately linked with migration of the corpus callosum.

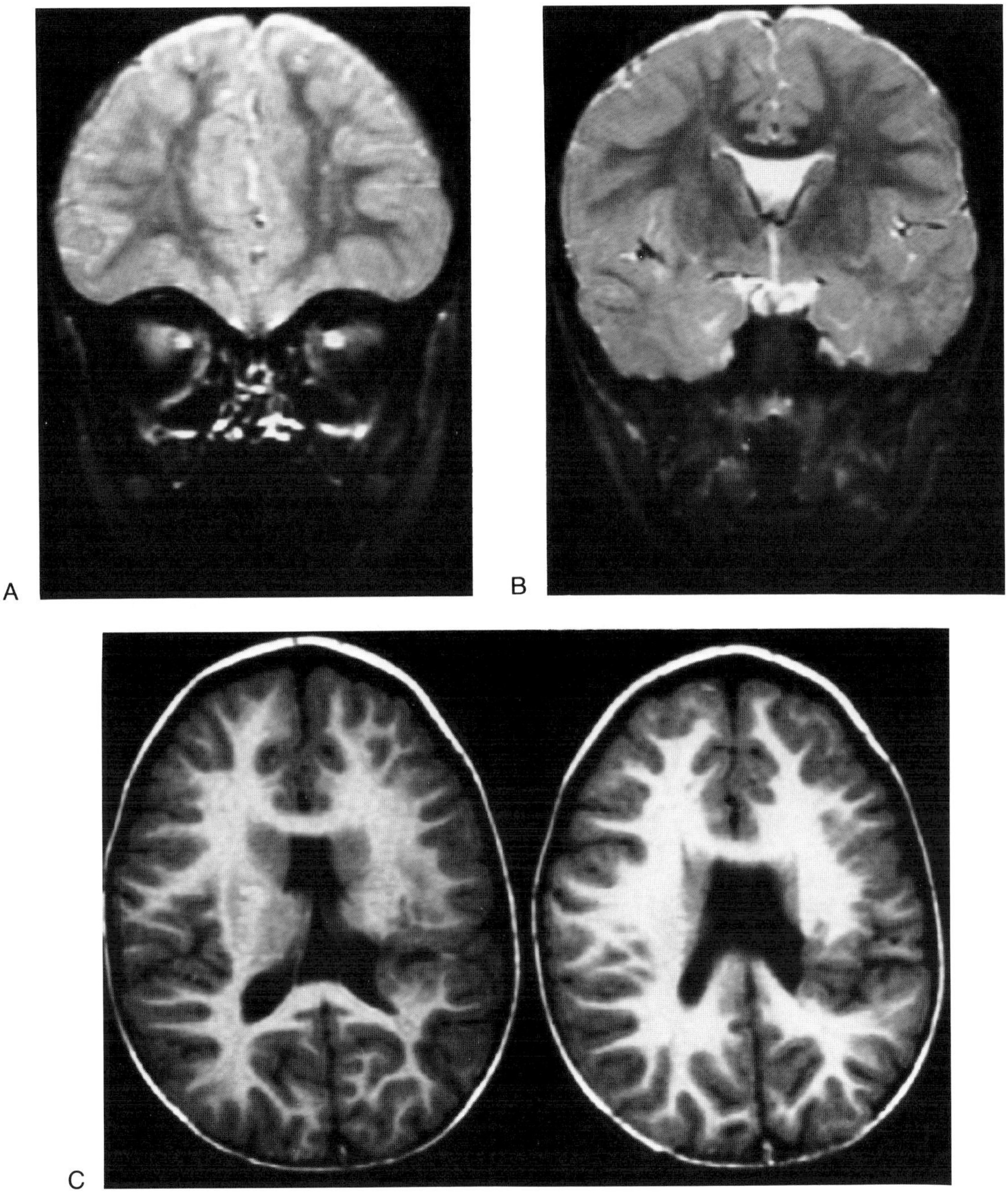

Fig. 7–29 Septo-optic dysplasia. **(A)** Coronal T_2-weighted MRI demonstrates hypoplasia of the optic nerves (right smaller than left). **(B)** At a more posterior location absence of the septum pellucidum is noted. **(C)** An axial T_1-weighted image demonstrates "closed-lip" schizencephaly in the left parietal lobe. Note the gray matter lining the lips of the cleft.

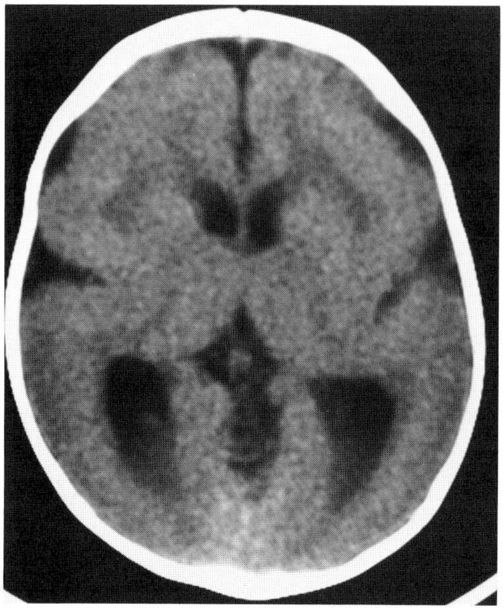

Fig. 7–30 Lissencephaly. Note the absence of sulci and the wide Sylvian fissures on axial head CT scan of a patient with lissencephaly.

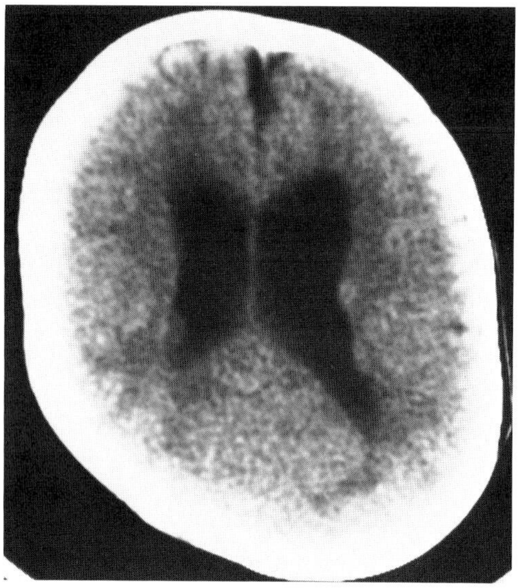

Fig. 7–31 Heterotopic gray matter. Axial CT scan of a patient presenting with seizures demonstrates multiple rounded densities within the ventricles demonstrating the same attenuation values as the cortical gray matter.

Lissencephaly describes the most severe migrational disorder with complete absence of gyri and a smooth cortical surface (Fig. 7–30). Pachygyria results in broad, shallow gyri that are reduced in number. The number of enfoldings is decreased as well. Polymicrogyria describes multiple, tiny gyri, which are increased in number. The small gyri may have fused surfaces and thus may be confused with pachygryia on imaging studies. Heterotopic gray matter may occur at any level from the germinal matrix to the brain surface and the patient usually presents with seizures (Fig. 7–31).

Schizencephaly describes a diverticulum extending from the inner table of the skull inward to the lateral ventricle. The closed lip variety results in a cleft with fusion of the lips of gray matter lining the cleft walls. The open lip variety results in a larger CSF space. The key imaging finding in schizencephaly is gray matter lining the length of the cleft (see Fig. 7–29). Up to 90 percent of patients with schizencephaly also demonstrate absence of the septum pellucidum.

Neuronal Proliferation and Differentiation

An increase in the number of neural cells occurs concomitantly with migration and differentiation into various cell types. Both genetic and teratogenic effects occurring during the second through the fifth gestational months may result in malformation.

Congenital tumors may result from residual embryonic neural cells (chordoma, craniopharyngioma, hamartoma, and medulloblastoma). Residual embryonic cells within the cranial vault that are not neural precursors result in the formation of dermoids, epidermoids, germinomas, and teratomas.

Congenital vascular malformations, neurocutaneous disorders, and cystic disorders appear to have their onset at the same time as neuronal proliferation and differentiation. While the origin of these lesions remains controversial, it is convenient to discuss them within this time frame.

The neurocutaneous disorders (phakomatoses) are thought to arise from dyshistiogenesis resulting in abnormal cell proliferation. Both the skin and central nervous system are involved.

Neurofibromatosis is the most common neurocutaneous syndrome with an incidence estimated at 1 in 2,500 live births. Most cases occur as spontaneous mutations in normal families. The condition is inherited as an autosomal dominant trait. Two types of neurofibromatoses are described. Neurofibromatosis I is von Recklinghausen disease, which accounts for greater than 90 percent of cases. Diagnosis requires two or more of the following: at least six café au lait spots greater than 5 mm in diameter; one plexiform neurofibroma or two or more nonplexiform neurofibromas; axillary or inguinal freckling; optic glioma; Lisch nodules; bone abnormalities; and a parent, sibling, or offspring with the same disease. The skin changes are the first to develop. Neurofibromatosis II is associated with bilateral acoustic schwannomas and is usually diagnosed in adulthood. Both CT and MRI may be used to demonstrate the masses arising from the eighth cranial nerves. Schwannomas of other cranial nerves and meningiomas may also be present. The imaging procedure of choice is contrast enhanced MRI, which shows intense homogeneous enhancement after contrast administration on the T_1-weighted images of both meningiomas and schwannomas. On nonenhanced T_1-weighted images schwannomas are equal or less than the intensity of gray matter. On T_2-weighted images the intensity of the schwannoma increases so that it is greater than that of gray matter. Focal areas of abnormal increased signal intensity on T_2-weighted images are identified in the brain stem, centrum semiovale, cerebellum, globus pallidus, internal capsule, and thalamus (Fig. 7–32). These lesions do not cause mass effect and their exact etiology is unclear. They may represent dysmyelination, gliomatosis, or dysplastic hamartomas. The spine may also be affected by paraspinal neurofibromas, ependymomas, or meningiomas. Again, contrast-enhanced MRI is superior in demonstrating enhancement of the ependymomas and meningomas.

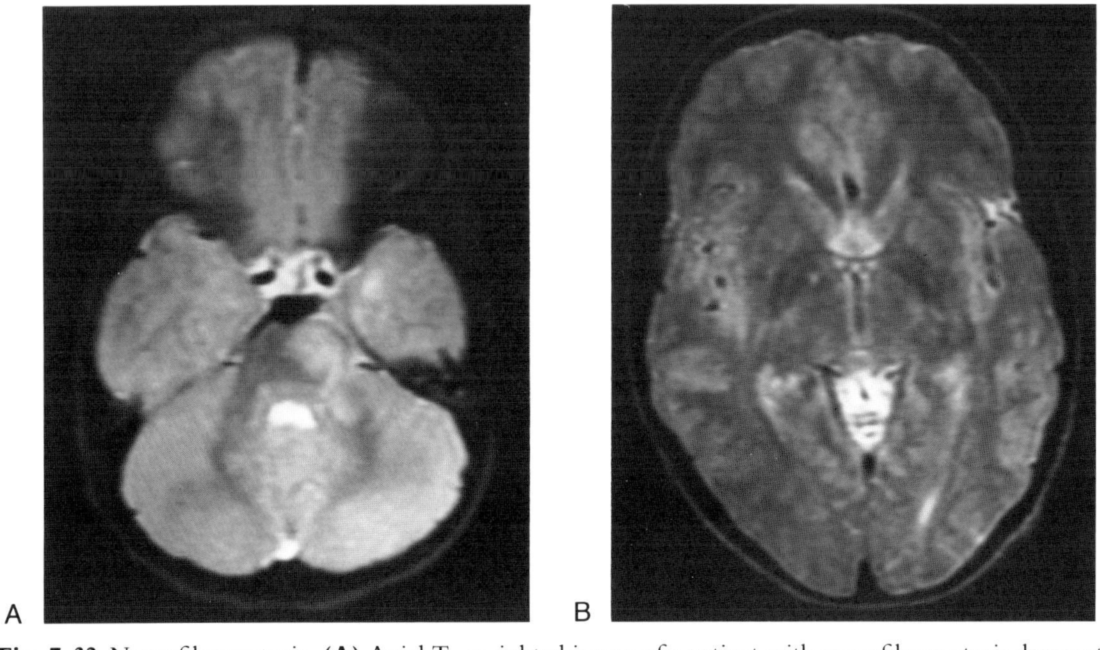

Fig. 7–32 Neurofibromatosis. **(A)** Axial T_2-weighted image of a patient with neurofibromatosis demonstrates abnormal increased signal intensity in the left brain stem and left cerebellar peduncle consistent with a glioma. **(B)** Another patient demonstrating a focus of increased signal intensity in the right internal capsule on the T_2-weighted image characteristic of neurofibromatosis.

Myelination

Myelination of the brain begins during the third trimester and continues into adulthood. Myelin first appears in the brainstem and central cerebellum. At birth, the thalamus, posterior limb of the internal capsule, cerebellar hemisphere, optic radiations, and centrum semiovale are myelinated. Myelin continues to spread outward into the subcortical white matter into early adulthood. Factors that may induce dismyelination include congenital infection, hydrocephalus, inborn errors of metabolism, and malnutrition. Congenital dismyelination must be differentiated from external causes of demyelination. MRI is highly sensitive to myelin disorders and is the mainstay of imaging in these conditions. At birth, the appearance of the neonatal brain on MRI is almost exactly opposite that of the adult brain. By 18 to 24 months of age myelination should be grossly normal and an adult appearance is usually achieved. T_2-weighted images are useful in identifying white matter disease.

The primary dismyelinating diseases seen in childhood are the result of familial biochemical disorders leading to a progressive degeneration of neurologic function. While some white matter disorders are difficult to classify, characteristic findings are seen in certain cases.

One of the more common leukodystrophies is X-linked adrenoleukodystrophy, which occurs almost exclusively in preadolescent boys. Increased signal intensity will be seen in the occipital white matter and splenium of the corpus callosum associated with adrenal insufficiency (Fig. 7–33).

Another common neurodegenerative disease of childhood is metachromatic leukodystrophy. Up to 70 percent of cases are diagnosed in patients between 6 months and 2 years of age with death occurring around 6 years. Unfortunately, the white matter involvement is diffuse and nonspecific. On CT, diffuse low attenuation is seen in the cerebral white matter associated with generalized atrophy. Hypointensity is seen on the T_1-weighted images in the subcortical white matter and extensive hyperintensity is seen on the T_2-weighted images indicating abnormal myelin and accumulated sulphate esters.

A

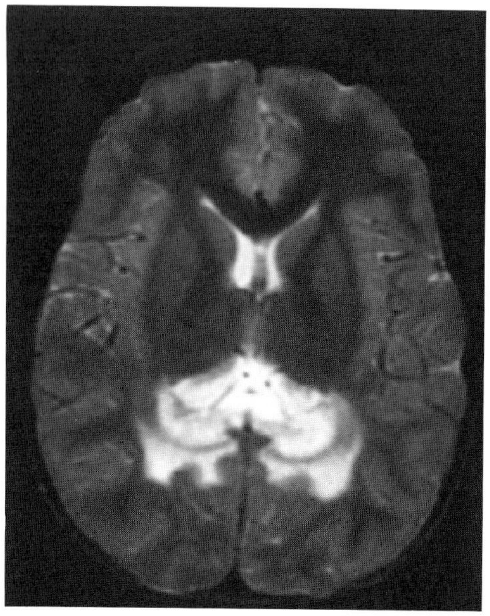

B

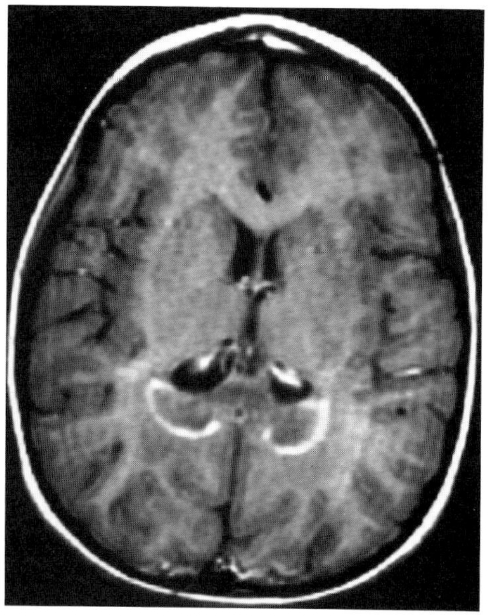

Fig. 7–33 Adrenal leukodystrophy. **(A)** T_2-weighted axial image demonstrates increased signal intensity in the splenium of the corpus collosum and in the occipital white matter. **(B)** After administration of Gd-DTPA, an enhancing rim of disruption of the blood-brain barrier is identified on the T_1-weighted image.

Macrocephalic children with suspected white matter disease either have Canavan's spongy sclerosis or Alexander's disease (fibrinoid leukodystrophy). Canavan's disease presents with diffusely affected white matter whereas Alexander's disease shows a predilection for the frontal regions. In both conditions, the brain is diffusely enlarged.

Krabbe's disease is another leukodystrophy that results in an excess of galactocerebroside in early childhood. CT demonstrates increased density in the caudate nuclei, corona radiata, and thalami. MRI findings include confluent periventricular, high signal intensity on T_2-weighted images. The MRI findings appear prior to the classic CT abnormalities.

Unclassified Disorders

The arachnoid cyst may result purely from abnormal CSF flow in the early stages of embryologic development, leading to a blind pocket in the arachnoid membrane. However, minor inflammation or a traumatic injury could cause an adhesion of the arachnoid membrane and a resultant arachnoid cyst. Arachnoid cysts expand since the cells lining the walls secrete CSF. The most common location is in the Sylvian fissure (50 percent occurance). In the spine, arachnoid cysts are most likely to occur in the thoracic region. As they expand, some degree of obstruction results. On both CT and MRI, a sharply circumscribed rounded lesion that behaves exactly like CSF will be identified. Differentiation from porencephaly may be made by identification of the cyst wall (Fig. 7–34). Intrathecal injection of contrast material results in identification of a sharp smooth border between the cyst and surrounding CSF. In the spine, the cyst may demonstrate a higher signal intensity than the adjacent CSF due to a relative lack of CSF pulsations. Intraoperative ultrasound imaging is useful in assuring cyst puncture since a swirling motion of the fluid will be seen when wall perforation occurs. Twenty-five percent of arachnoid cysts occur in the posterior fossa and must be differentiated from Dandy-Walker malformation/variant. The arachnoid cyst will always be separate from the fourth ventricle.

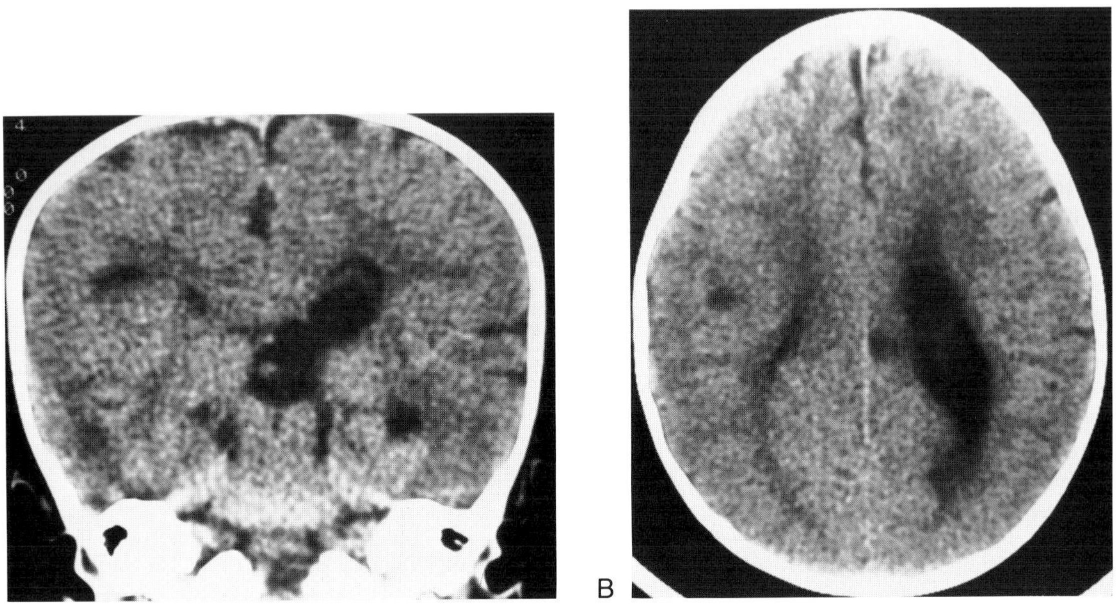

A B

Fig. 7–34 Arachnoid cyst. **(A)** Note the bilobed hypodense area extending superiorly from the level of the quadrigeminal plate cistern into the body of the left lateral ventricle on this coronal CT image. **(B)** Axial CT scan better demonstrates the cyst walls. The cyst obstructs the occipital horn of the left lateral ventricle.

CENTRAL NERVOUS SYSTEM NEOPLASMS

In childhood, central nervous system tumors are second in occurence only to leukemia. Twenty-two children out of every million will be affected by a tumor of the brain or spinal cord. Three age peaks are seen in childhood. In the neonatal period, a supratentorial location is favored with a predominance of astrocytomas and teratomatous tumors. Five percent of all intracranial neoplasms in childhood occur in the neonate. Between the ages of 3 and 5 years infratentorial tumors occur most often. The brain stem glioma and cerebellar astrocystoma are most common. The third age peak occurs between the ages of 10 and 12 years and supratentorial lesions predominate.

The imaging method most commonly used to screen for suspected neoplasms is CT. Even if 5-mm contiguous sections are obtained through the posterior fossa, MRI remains superior for visualization of abnormalities in this region. For the remainder of the brain, 1-cm thick contiguous slices before and after administration of IV contrast material are usually sufficient. Coronal images may be helpful for evaluation of the parasellar region.

The multiple imaging planes provided by MRI are extremely helpful in the preoperative planning of brain tumor resections. T_1-weighted sagittal images may be followed by axial T_2-weighted images. Axial T_1-weighted images should be obtained before and after administration of Gd-DTPA. T_1-weighted images may also be obtained in the coronal or sagittal planes (depending on tumor location) following contrast administration.

In the immediate postoperative period, CT scans are obtained to evaluate ventricular size, bleeding at the operative site, and obvious residual tumor. Long-term follow-up is best accomplished with unenhanced and enhanced MRI. The timing of the follow-up studies may correspond to oncologic protocol or to the acute onset of new symptoms, which may be due to recurrent tumor or metastasis. Contrast-enhanced MRI has detected residual tumor in patients following surgery that was not suspected on precontrast images.

In contrast, only 5 to 7 percent of all spinal cord tumors occur in the first two decades of life. The highest incidence of primary spinal cord neoplasms occurs in children less than 5 years of age. Intramedullary tumors tend to occur in the cervical and cervicothoracic regions. Approximately one-half of childhood spinal cord tumors are gliomas. Congenital tumors are also common.

Of particular interest is the association of the neurocutaneous syndromes with central nervous system tumors. Neurofibromatosis is associated with optic nerve gliomas, acoustic nerve schwannomas, and meningiomas. Tuberous sclerosis is associated with subependymal giant cell astrocytomas and giant Drusen. von Hippel-Lindau syndrome is associated with hemangioblastoma of the cerebellum and/or spinal cord. Turcot's syndrome and Gorlin's syndrome are associated with medulloblastoma and glioblastoma multiforme.

Glial Tumors

The most common glial tumor in childhood is the astrocytoma. Characteristic childhood locations are different from those in adults. Favored childhood sites are the brain stem, cerebellar hemispheres, hypothalamus and the optic chiasm/nerve. The low-grade astrocytoma is also the most common primary intramedullary spinal cord tumor. Other less common tumors arising from glial cells include choroid plexus tumors, ependymal tumors, glioblastoma multiforme, gliomatosis cerebri, mixed gliomas, and oligodendrogliomas.

The most common infratentorial neoplasm in childhood and adolescence is the brain stem glioma. Cerebellar astrocytoma is the second most common tumor followed by an equal occurrence of medulloblastoma and ependymoma. Common presenting symptoms include ataxia, headache, and secondary evidence of increased intracranial pressure.

Unfortunately, the critical location of brain stem gliomas is much more of a prognostic indicator than the cell type. The most common cell type is the astrocytoma. Even with a favorable histology, tumor-related mortality is 85 to 90 percent.

It is difficult to evaluate the brain stem with CT due to beam hardening artifact from the petrous ridges. Nevertheless, a hypodense or isodense focal expansion of the brain stem may be seen. Anterior displacement of the basilar artery and posterior displacement of the fourth ventricle are present. If 50 percent or more of the basilar artery is covered by brain stem tissue, it is highly suggestive of a brain stem neoplasm. Calcification is rare and contrast enhancement is variable. The intra-axial portion of the tumor usually remains the same density as on the unenhanced images. Exophytic tumor tends to enhance somewhat.

MRI is far superior to CT in evaluation of brain stem neoplasms (Fig. 7–35). Sagittal and coronal T_1-weighted images are best for evaluation of the superior and inferior extent of the lesion. Axial images are useful in evaluating lateral extent. A sharply demarcated, homogeneously hypointense mass is identified on T_1-weighted images. Foci of high signal indicate hemorrhage into the tumor, foci of low signal may indicate cysts. Homogeneous hyperintensity is demonstrated on the T_2-weighted images. Exophytic components tend to be lower in intensity on T_1-weighted images and higher in intensity on the T_2-weighted images and may be difficult to separate from surrounding cerebrospinal fluid. Low-grade gliomas tend to demonstrate two patterns of enhancement after Gd-DTPA administration on T_1-weighted images; either they do not enhance at all or intense homogeneous enhancement occurs. Patchy enhancement is suspicious for a higher grade of malignancy. Following radiation therapy, a reduction in the size and normalization of signal intensity are usually seen. Calcification may occur.

The peak frequency of cerebellar astrocytomas occurs between the ages of 3 and 8 years. Symptoms include ataxia, incoordination, and secondary signs of increased intracranial pressure. On CT, cerebellar astrocytomas usually appear as single or multiloculated well-defined cysts associated with a mural nodule or a mass. The fourth ventricle is displaced anteriorly and away from the eccentric mass within one of the hemispheres (Fig. 7–36). After administration of contrast material, the solid tumor or nodule usually enhances intensely. Enhancement of the cyst wall is variable. Twenty percent of cerebellar astrocytomas demonstrate calcification. It is not uncommon for cerebellar astrocytomas to arise as solid tumors in the midline from either the medial cerebellar hemisphere or the vermis. Tiny cysts are sometimes identified within the midline tumors. The solid tumor may be of any density on the noncontrasted CT and homogeneous moderate enhancement is seen after contrast administration.

T_1-weighted MRI demonstrates an inhomogeneous lesion of low signal intensity. Occasionally the mural nodule or solid portion of the mass may be isointense. On T_2-weighted images both the cystic and solid components are hyperintense. Local meningeal extension and spread of recurrent tumor through the ventricular system are common occurrences.

Thirty percent of all childhood supratentorial brain tumors are hemispheric astrocytomas. Ten to fifteen percent of pediatric supratentorial tumors are astrocytomas arising from optic chiasm or hypothalamus. The favored location is in the temporal or parietal lobe. Other common supratentorial sites include the hypothalamus, thalamus, and third ventricle. Approximately one-half of cases demonstrate a cystic component with imaging characteristics similar to cerebellar astrocytomas. Most astrocytomas arise from either the white matter or a subcortical location. Unfortunately, no characteristic imaging features have been described to differentiate hemispheric astrocytomas from other supratentorial gliomas. On MRI, the mass appears dark on T_1-weighted images and bright on T_2-weighted images. Injection of Gd-DTPA demonstrates the same pattern of enhancement previously described for astrocytomas.

The second most common glial tumor of childhood is the ependymoma, accounting for 8 to 10 percent of all primary childhood brain neoplasms. The four most common sites of involvement are the lateral ventricle, fourth ventricle, spinal cord, and cauda equina. Up to 95 percent of childhood ependymomas arise intracranially and 70 percent of these occur below the tentorium cerebri. The average age at diagnosis for ependymomas varies with the primary site. Those arising in the fourth ventricle have a mean age of approximately 2 years, lateral ventricle 6 years, and

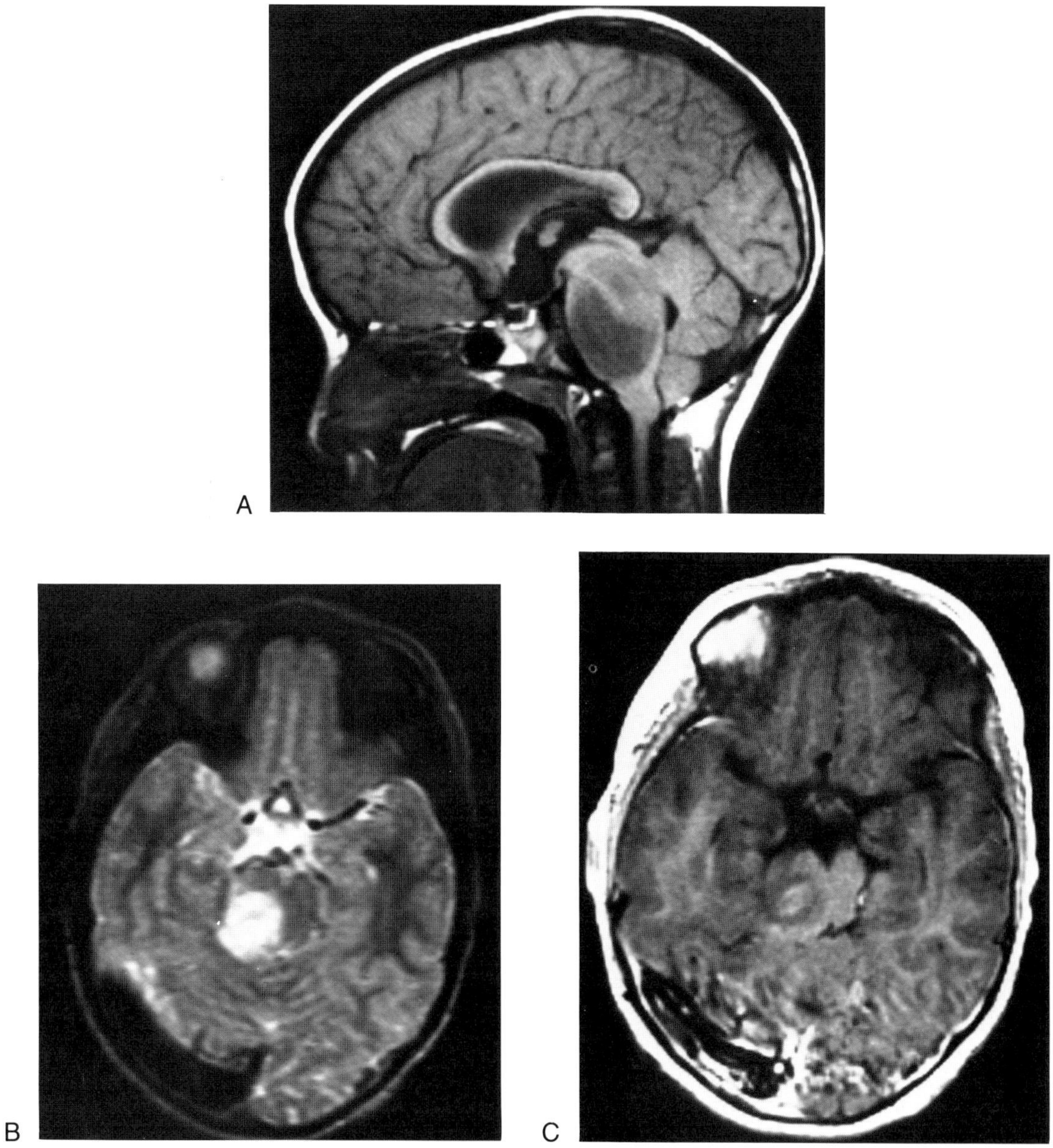

Fig. 7–35 Brainstem glioma. **(A)** T_1-weighted sagittal image demonstrates enlargement of the brainstem by a mixed intensity mass involving both the midbrain and the pons. **(B)** T_2-weighted axial image demonstrates increased signal intensity to the right of the midline representing tumor and edema. **(C)** After injection of contrast material, the edema appears hypointense on the T_1-weighted image, while the tumor enhances moderately.

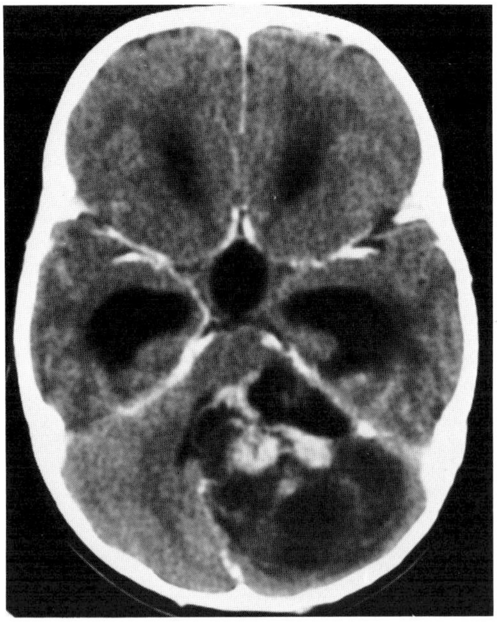
A

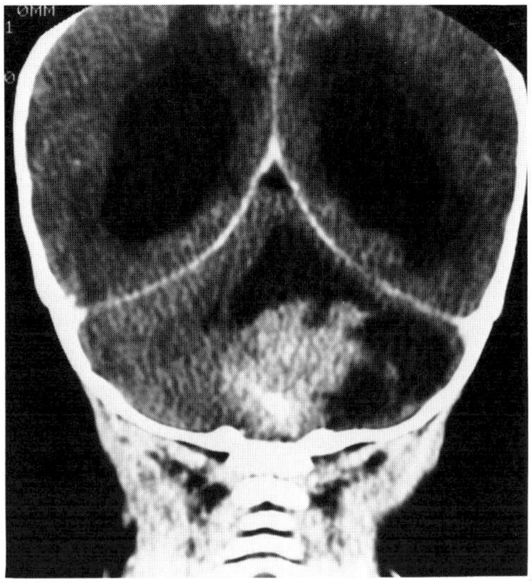
B

Fig. 7–36 Cerebellar astrocytoma. **(A)** Enhanced axial CT image demonstrates an eccentric mass displacing the brain stem and the fourth ventricle anteriorly and to the right. Note the homogeneous intense contrast enhancement of the solid portion of the multicystic tumor. **(B)** Direct coronal image demonstrates displacement of the fourth ventricle to the right. Note the combined solid and cystic components typical of an astrocytoma.

cauda equina 14 years. Spinal cord ependymomas are more likely to occur in adults. The most common presenting symptoms are secondary to increased intracranial pressure. Ependymomas demonstrate an infiltrative pattern of growth and tend to extend into the adjacent brain parenchyma rather than into the ventricle. Most of the tumors are solid but pliable and do not contain calcium. Prognosis is partially determined by the site of origin. Tumors arising in the region of the fourth ventricle have the worst prognosis. Spinal cord tumors demonstrate local recurrence but have a better long-term survival rate. Surgery and radiation are the primary treatment modalities. Subarachnoid seeding rarely occurs with benign ependymomas. Noncontrast CT images classically demonstrate an isodense or hypodense fourth ventricular mass (Fig. 7–37). Calcifications occur in one-half of cases. Cysts may be identified. Rarely, the mass may be hyperdense. Injection of contrast material results in imhomogeneous moderate contrast enhancement. A surrounding halo of low attenuation (CSF) is seen but occurs in any tumor located within the fourth ventricle. T_1-weighted MRI demonstrate an inhomogeneous hypointense mass with areas of both high and low signal intensity. Inhomogeneous hyperintensity is seen with T_2-weighted images. The tissue characteristics on both CT and MRI are nonspecific for supratentorial ependymomas and the exact same findings may occur with primitive neurocutaneous tumors. Posterior fossa ependymomas have a predilection for extension through either the foramen of Magendie or the foramen of Luschka. When extension is seen on either CT or MRI, the diagnosis of ependymoma is more likely. Infrequently, medulloblastomas may have a similar appearance extending through the foramen of Luschka.

The remainder of the tumors of glial origin are uncommon in childhood. Of interest is the choroid plexus papilloma/carcinoma, which accounts for 2 to 3 percent of childhood intracranial neoplasms. The papilloma is by far more common than the carcinoma. Hydrocephalus is the most common presenting symptom with 20 percent of cases being diagnosed in the first year of life and 50 percent recognized by age 10. Almost 90 percent of lesions are located in

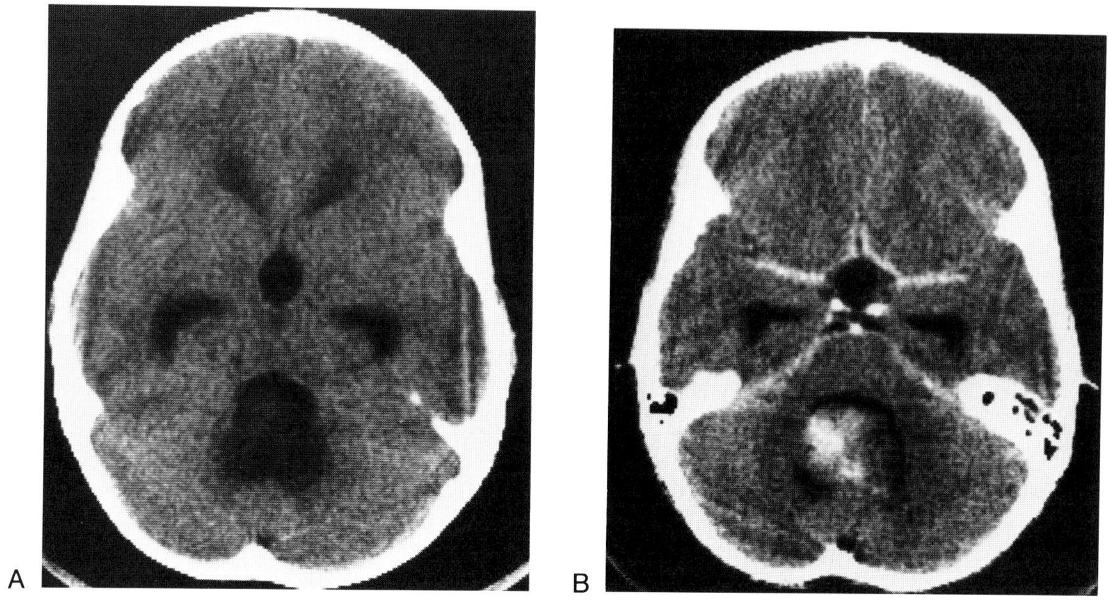

Fig. 7–37 Ependymoma. **(A)** Axial CT demonstrates a hypodense mass in the region of the fourth ventricle with evidence of obstructive hydrocephalus. **(B)** Inhomogeneous enhancement occurs. The hypodense halo represents surrounding cerebrospinal fluid in the fourth ventricle from which the tumor arises.

the lateral ventricles with an increased incidence on the left. The cerebellopontine angle and fourth ventricle are more common sites in older children and adults. On CT, an isodense or slightly hyperdense mass with tiny calcifications is identified in close proximity to the lateral ventricle. The ipsilateral ventricle is asymmetrically enlarged. The mass will enhance homogeneously after injection of contrast material. Intraventricular extent is much more common than intraparenchymal extent of tumor. The malignant variety demonstrates a more irregular border and is less homogeneous both before and after injection of contrast material. These findings are also demonstrated on MRI. Differentiation of choroid plexus carcinomas from primitive neurocutaneous tumors may be very difficult in the region of the fourth ventricle.

Primitive Neuroectodermal Tumors

Primitive neurocutaneous tumors are a spectrum of neoplasms thought to derive from a progenitor neural stem cell. The most common member of the group is the medulloblastoma, which accounts for 12 to 25 percent of childhood central nervous system neoplasms. The mean age at diagnosis is between six and eight years. In younger children, medulloblastoma most commonly presents as a midline posterior fossa mass. In older patients, it is more commonly lateralized to one of the cerebellar hemispheres. On both CT and MRI a vermian mass is seen separating the cerebellar tonsils (Fig. 7–38). In contrast to the glial tumors, the medulloblastoma is usually homogeneous and hyperdense as compared with normal brain parenchyma on noncontrast CT images. There will be anterior displacement of the fourth ventricle with impingement superiorly obstructing CSF flow. Hydrocephalus is present in the majority of cases due to obstruction of the roof of the fourth ventricle. The tumor may extend laterally through the foramina of Luschka or downward through the foramen magnum. Injection of IV contrast material causes marked homogeneous tumor enhancement in almost all cases. Sagittal MRI best demonstrates the origin from the inferior medullary velum along the roof of the fourth ventricle. The key to diagnosis is the compressed fourth ventricle anteriorly and superiorly but not posteriorly. Medulloblastomas are usually hypointense on T_1-weighted images and of variable hyperintensity

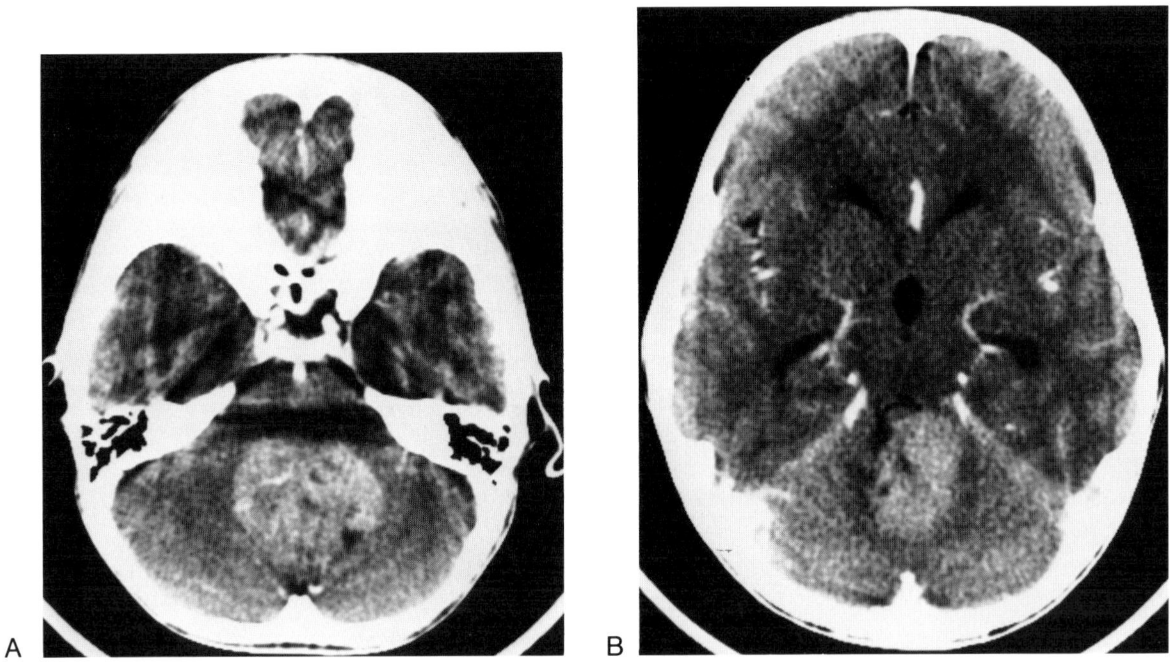

Fig. 7–38 Medulloblastoma. **(A)** Enhanced axial head CT scan demonstrates an enhancing lesion in the posterior fossa surrounded by a halo of low density. **(B)** On a higher cut, the fourth ventricle is compressed anteriorly by the enhacing mass.

on T_2-weighted images (Fig. 7–39). Some degree of enhancement is noted after IV Gd-DTPA administration. T_1-weighted MRI following contrast material is the best way to demonstrate metastases within the central nervous system. Drop metastases to the spinal cord are common as is leptomeningeal involvement. Extraaxial spread is seen as brightly enhancing foci both intracranially and in the intradural, extramedullary portion of the spinal canal. Most metastases or recurrences are detected within 2 years of the initial diagnosis with late recurrences being uncommon. The 3-year-survival rate ranges from 40 to 80 percent. Placement of a ventriculoperitoneal shunt may lead to systemic metastases, which occur in 5 percent of cases.

Aside from medulloblastoma, the remaining primitive neurocutaneous tumors comprise less than 5 percent of childhood supratentorial neoplasms. The tumors have nonspecific imaging characteristics and dismal prognoses. The CT appearance is usually an inhomogeneous hyperdense, deep, white-matter lesion that shows variable contrast enhancement. MRI demonstrates a well-marginated rim separating the tumor from surrounding edema. Inhomogeneity is seen on both pre- and postcontrast MRI.

Pineal Masses

Most of the tumors occurring around the pineal gland and in the vicinity of the third ventricle arise from either the pineal cells or are germ cell neoplasms. The pineoblastoma is a primitive neurocutaneous tumor that has been associated with rapid dissemination of tumor through the CSF and death within 1 year. The incidence is higher in young females and it has been associated with bilateral familial retinoblastoma. Pineocytomas occur more commonly in adults and are less aggressive tumors. The two tumors are indistinguishable from each other on imaging studies. A lobulated isodense or hyperdense mass containing small calcifications will be seen in the midline posterior to the third ventricle. Homogeneous contrast enhancement is demonstrated. On T_1-weighted MRI the lesions are hypointense to isointense. On T_2-weighted images the lesions become hyperintense.

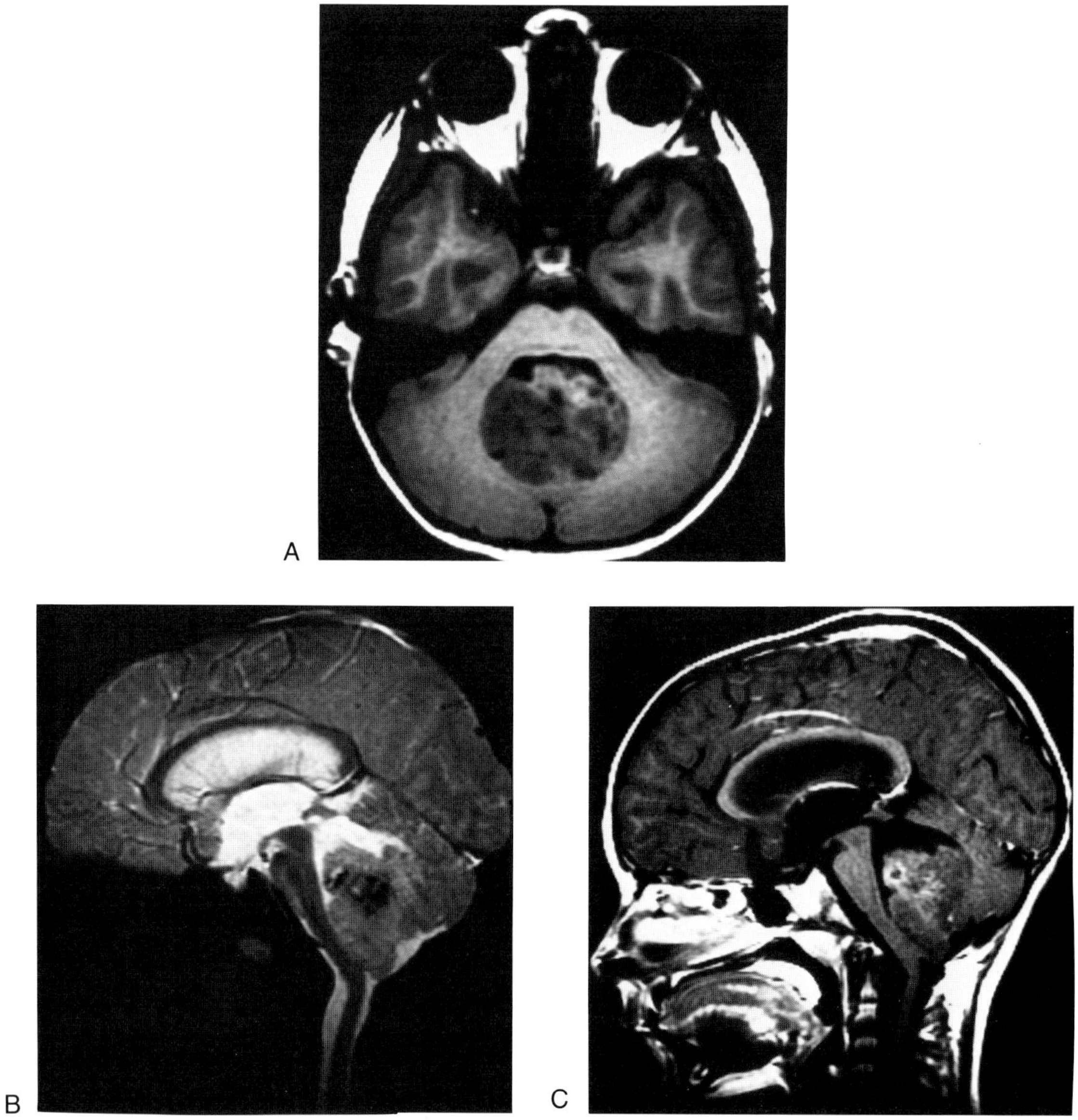

Fig. 7–39 Primitive neuroectodermal tumor. **(A)** Axial T_1-weighted image demonstrates a mixed hypointense and isointense mass arising in the region of the fourth ventricle. The fourth ventricle is displaced anteriorly. **(B)** The sagittal T_2-weighted image demonstrates anterosuperior displacement of the fourth ventricle by the mass. Note the indistinctness of the cerebellar interface suspicious for medulloblastoma. **(C)** Sagittal T_1-weighted image after admininstration of Gd-DTPA demonstrates a small amount of enhancement that is irregular and inhomogeneous.

Pineoblastomas tend to be larger than pineocytomas. Germ cell tumors are usually hyperdense solid masses on noncontrast CT and enhance markedly. An inhomogeneous hypointense mass is seen on T_1-weighted MRI with an isointense appearance on T_2-weighted images (Fig. 7–40). Injection of MRI contrast material will help define subarachnoid metastases. Other mass lesions of the pineal region include arachnoid cysts, hamartomas, gliomas, and metastases.

Malformative Tumors

Included in this classification are all types of embryologic inclusion cysts, hamartomas, and the most com-

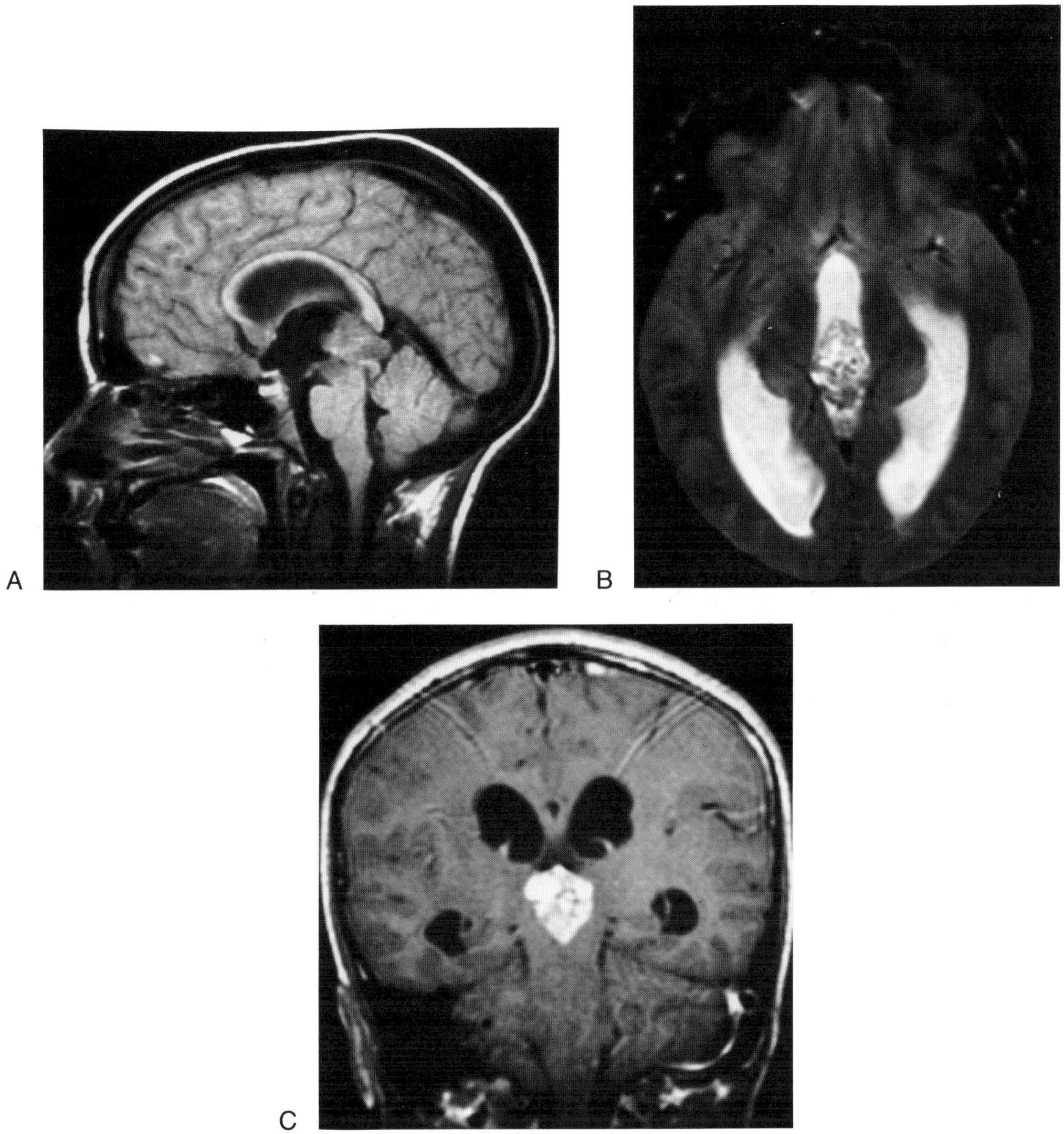

Fig. 7–40 Mixed malignant germ cell tumor. **(A)** T_1-weighted sagittal image demonstrates an inhomogeneous isointense mass arising from the pineal region. **(B)** The lesion is of mixed intensity (predominantly hypointense) on the T_2-weighted axial image. **(C)** After injection of Gd-DTPA, homogeneous enhancement of the tumor is seen on the coronal T_1-weighted image.

mon of the malformative tumors, the craniopharyngioma. Craniopharyngiomas account for 10 percent of intracranial neoplasms in children. Fifty percent of all parasellar masses in the pediatric age group are craniopharyngiomas. Eighty-five percent of craniopharyngiomas are partially cystic. This feature is apparent on both CT and MRI. On CT images, calcification will be identified in more than 90 percent of cases. Mixed areas of isodense tissue and low density cysts will also be identified. The solid portions of the tumor almost always enhance with contrast administration. T_1-weighted MRI demonstrate inhomogeneous signal intensity consistent with both cystic and solid components. The solid portion is usually isointense or hyperintense. On T_2-weighted images the cystic component ranges from isointense to hyperintense. Classification in relationship to the optic chiasm (prechiasmatic, postchiasmatic, or involving both areas) is critical to surgical planning. The intensity of the cyst varies directly with the amounts of cholesterol, hemorrhage, and keratin debris (hypointense, isointense, or hyperintense).

Differentiation from epidermoid tumors is possible with CT since epidermoid tumors will not enhance after contrast. The epidermoid cyst may arise anywhere along the dura at the base of the brain or at the cerebellopontine angle. Dermoid cysts are more likely to be located in the midline of the posterior fossa.

Meningeal Tumors

Meningiomas account for 2 to 8 percent of all primary central nervous system tumors during the first 2 decades of life. Twenty to twenty-five percent of patients diagnosed in this age group with meningiomas will also have neurofibromatosis or tuberous sclerosis. Up to 80 percent of cases occur intracranially with the remainder in the spinal cord or orbit. They present as large irregular isodense or hyperdense masses on noncontrast CT studies. Homogeneous contrast enhancement is seen frequently after injection of IV contrast material on CT. Cystic and necrotic components do not regularly enhance. On MRI the ill-defined mass will appear isointense with gray matter on both the T_1- and the T_2-weighted sequences. Intense enhancement is seen on postcontrast T_1-weighted images. A unique feature of the meningioma is the fact that at least part of the blood supply is derived from dural vessels arising from either the external carotid artery, internal carotid artery, or vertebral artery. The arteries with increased flow become tortuous and dilated dividing into multiple vessels at the tumor edge. There is a homogeneous tumor

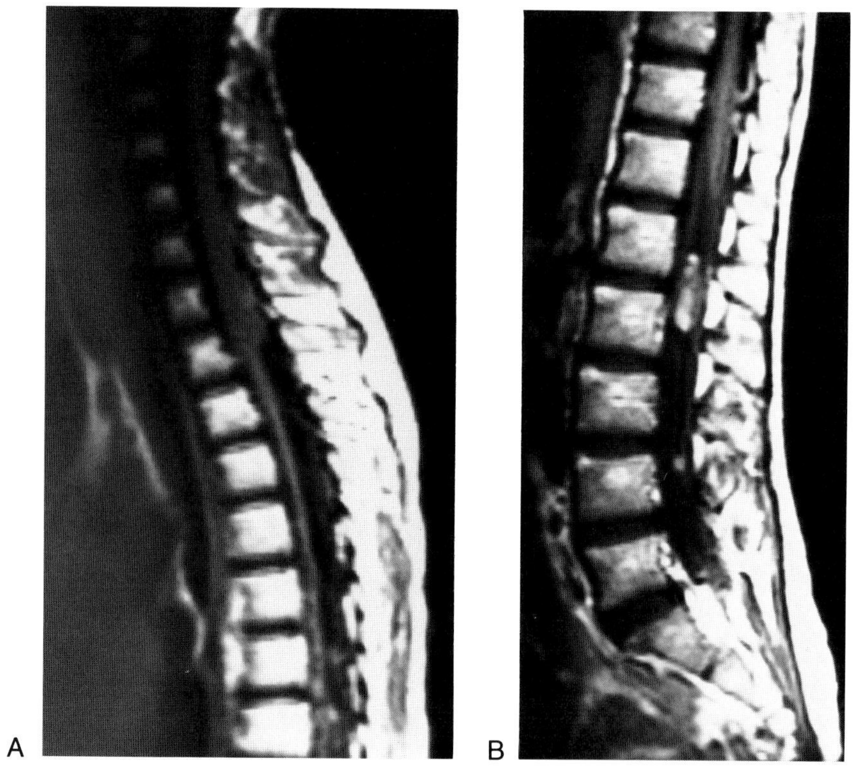

Fig. 7–41 Spinal metastases. **(A)** Enhanced T_1-weighted sagittal MRI demonstrates multiple foci of increased intensity in the thoracic region. **(B)** Enhanced T_1-weighted sagittal MRI of the lumbosacral spine demonstrates other hyperintense drop metastases from the patient's fourth ventricular ependymoma.

stain in the late arterial phase that persists into the late venous phase due to the numerous small vessels in meningiomas studied by arteriography.

Metastatic Tumors

The incidence of intracranial metastases in children with disseminated malignant tumor is only 6 percent. The primary lesions are usually round cell tumors such as neuroblastoma, soft tissue sarcoma, and embryonal cell malignancies.

In the spine, 30 to 35 percent of metastatic tumors are neuroblastomas. Other metastases to the spine include embryonal rhabdomyosarcoma, Ewing sarcoma, lymphoma, medulloblastoma, and ependymoma (Fig. 7–41). Only the medulloblastoma has a predilection for the intramedullary location.

CENTRAL NERVOUS SYSTEM INFECTION/INFLAMMATION

The sites of infection in a child's central nervous system vary according to the route of infection. Middle ear or paranasal sinus infections may lead to contiguous spread of organisms into the adjacent epidural space. The brain may be directly contaminated due to an open fracture or during surgical intervention. Brain abscesses, epidural empyemas, and subdural empyemas may result. Hematogenous spread of organisms accounts for 15 percent of brain abscesses and for most cases of spinal epidural abscesses in children.

The overall incidence of brain abscesses during the first 2 decades of life is 20 to 40 percent. The peak incidence occurs between the ages of 5 and 7. Prior to age 2, brain abscesses are uncommon. However, infants with major intestinal insult such as necrotizing enterocolitis have an increased incidence of *Candida* brain abscesses. The other common pathogens during infancy are gram-negative organisms. The most commonly isolated organisms in older children are group B *Streptococcus* and *Staphylococcus aureus*. Predisposing factors in older children include paranasal sinus infections, tetralogy of Fallot, transposition of the great vessels, other cyanotic heart lesions, and conditions predisposing patients to chronic pulmonary infections. Immunocompromised children are at risk for fungal infections from *Aspergillus, Candida,* and mucormycosis. While the frontal or temporal lobes are involved in 60 percent of patients, children are at greater risk for posterior fossa abscesses due to the high incidence of ear infections as compared with adults.

Both CT and MRI have distinct advantages in central nervous system infection imaging. MRI is extremely effective in demonstrating subdural and epidural fluid collections along the spinal canal (Fig. 7–42). T_1-weighted sagittal images will not only demonstrate an inflammatory collection that is slightly brighter than CSF but isointense with the cord. On T_2-weighted images, the collection will be hyperintense as compared with the adjacent spinal cord but less intense than the cerebrospinal fluid.

In contrast, if contiguous spread from a paranasal sinus infection into the epidural space of the calvaria is suspected, CT is superior for demonstrating bone destruction (Fig. 7–43). The noncontrast CT appearance of empyemas varies with age and may be isodense or hypodense as compared with the underlying brain. After contrast administration, enhancement of the capsule will be seen.

Commonly, the child with suspected brain abscesses is clinically unstable and may be difficult to image with MRI. A combination of unenhanced and enhanced axial CT scans rapidly defines intraparenchymal inflammation. The precursor of the brain abscess is a focus of cerebritis usually located at or near the corticomedullary junction. The rapidity with which CT can detect cerebritis depends somewhat on the virulence of the organism. The CT appearance of the brain may be normal for up to 7 days after the onset of symptoms. The first CT finding is a poorly defined area of low attenuation and inhomogeneity of contrast enhancement. As the blood-brain barrier deteriorates, gray matter enhancement progresses. Encapsulation is detected as ring enhancement on the images obtained after contrast administration. Edema usually surrounds the abscess capsule.

There is no doubt that MRI is more sensitive to changes in the water density of the brain seen in early cerebritis. The inflamed parenchyma will appear

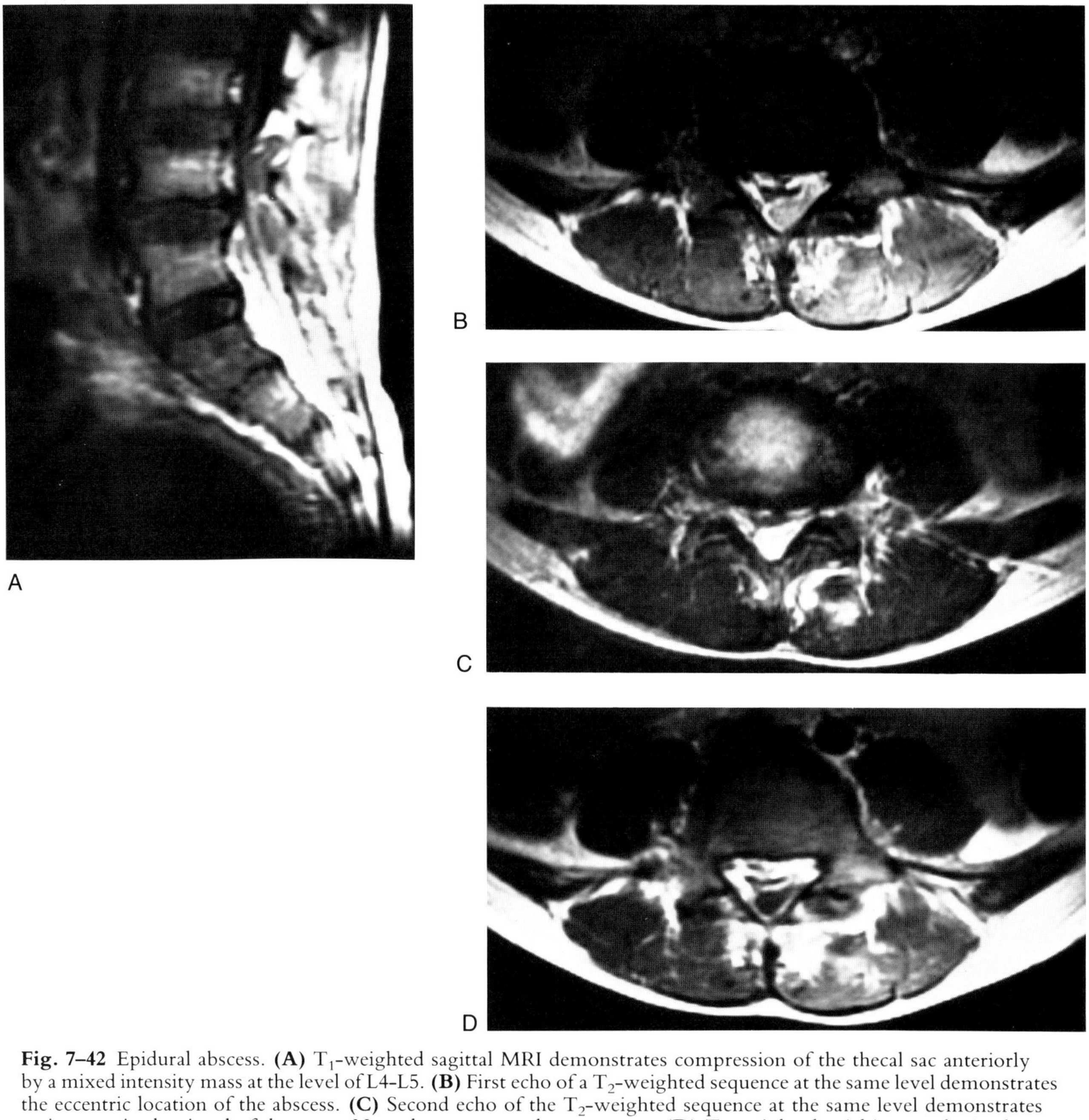

Fig. 7–42 Epidural abscess. **(A)** T_1-weighted sagittal MRI demonstrates compression of the thecal sac anteriorly by a mixed intensity mass at the level of L4-L5. **(B)** First echo of a T_2-weighted sequence at the same level demonstrates the eccentric location of the abscess. **(C)** Second echo of the T_2-weighted sequence at the same level demonstrates an increase in the signal of the mass. Note the compressed nerve roots. **(D)** T_1-weighted axial image obtained after administration of Gd-DTPA demonstrates an enhancing rim.

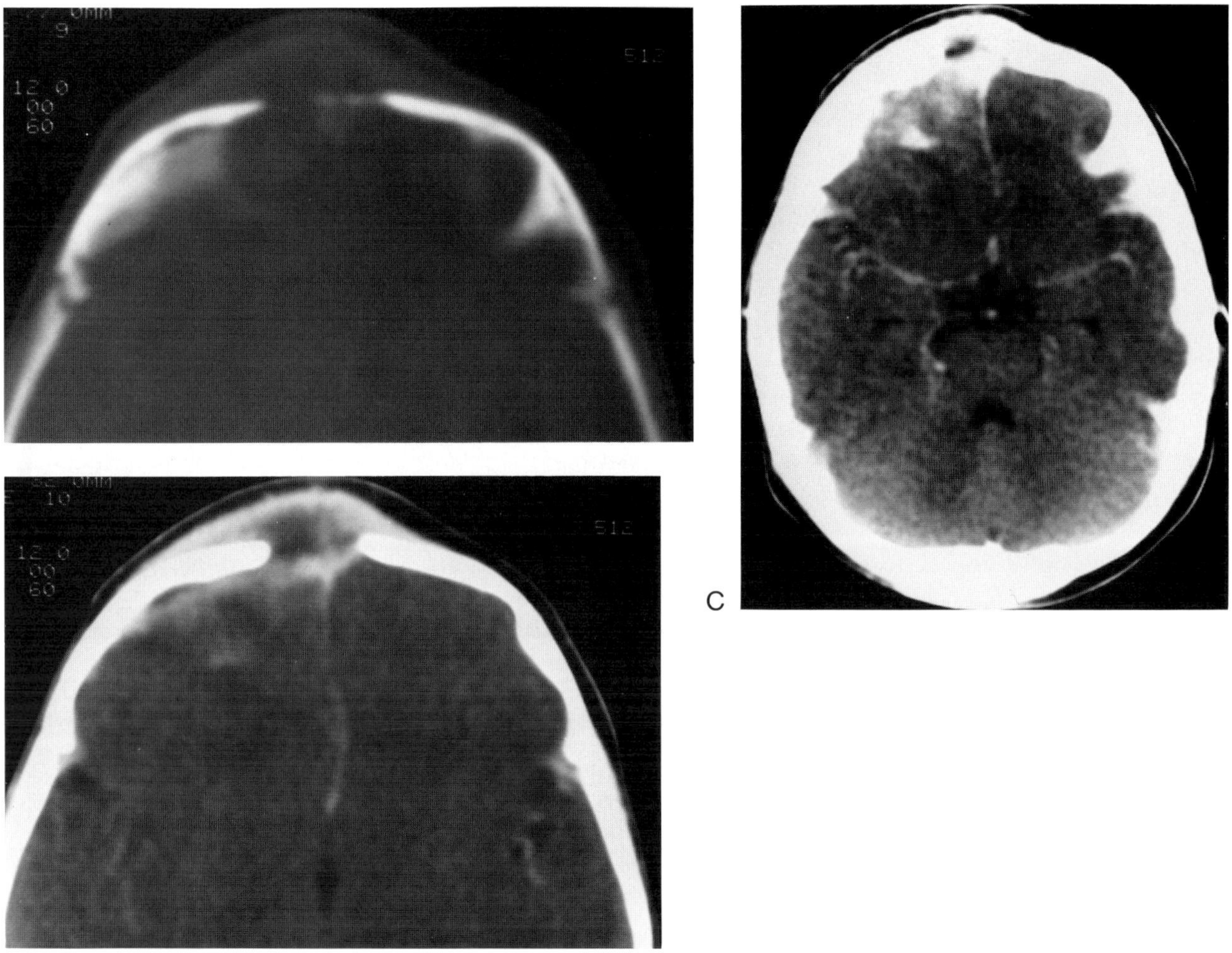

A

B

C

Fig. 7–43 Frontal osteomyelitis. **(A)** Transaxial CT scan at bone window settings demonstrates destruction of the frontal bone associated with a low density mass extending into the superficial soft tissues and the epidural space. **(B)** Administration of contrast material and soft tissue window settings better define the abscess cavity. **(C)** Evaluation of the remainder of the brain demonstrates focal cerebritis of the right frontal lobe on a lower axial image.

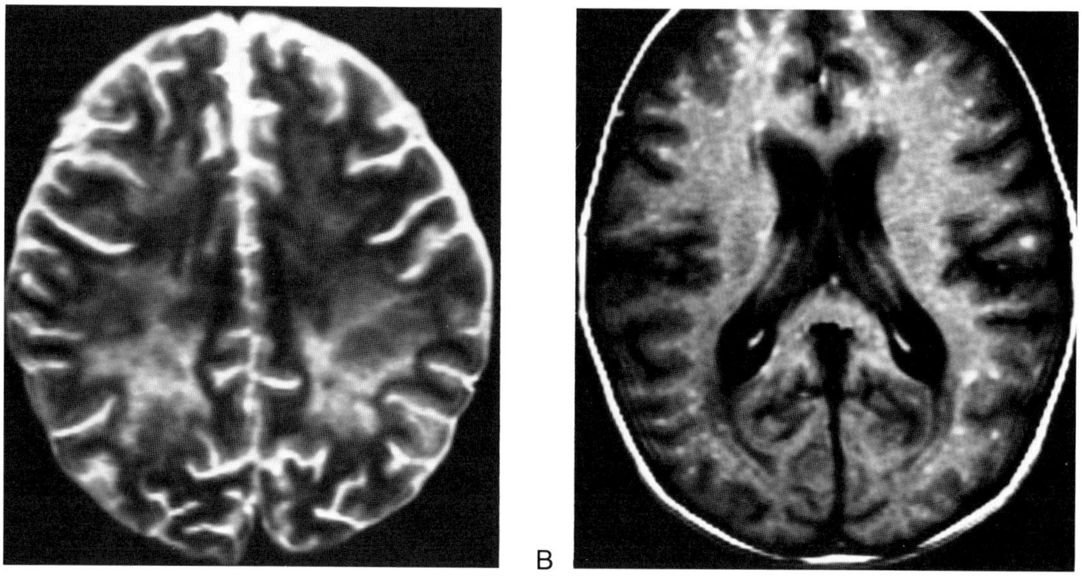

A B

Fig. 7–44 Rickettsial encephalitis. **(A)** T_2-weighted image demonstrates patchy increased signal in the white matter of both parietal lobes. **(B)** Enhanced T_1-weighted image demonstrates multiple tiny enhancing foci at the gray/white matter interface. These findings are consistent with acute widespread inflammation.

as a poorly defined area of hyperintensity on both T_1- and T_2-weighted images (Fig. 7–44). As the abscess capsule forms, the wall appears hyperintense on the T_1-weighted images but hypointense on the T_2-weighted images. As the capsule matures, the signal intensity decreases somewhat so that it becomes isointense on T_1-weighted images and hypointense on T_2-weighted images (Fig. 7–45). Contrast administration will result in ring enhancement at all stages of abscess formation.

While brain abscesses are rare in infants, they are usually larger since infection is poorly controlled at this age. Any infant with an enlarging head should be screened with ultrasound for signs of meningitis, ventriculitis, or abscess formation. Bacterial intracranial infections are the most common type in infancy. Group B streptococci and *Escherichia coli* are common in the neonate. *Haemophilus influenzae* is the most common cause of infection of the central nervous system outside the neonatal period.

While meningitis is the most common form of infection involving the central nervous system, during the first year of life it may be intimately associated with underlying encephalitis. Early on, the head ultrasound may appear normal. Mild cerebral edema may be evidenced by alterations in the appearance of the cortical parenchyma and compression of the ventricles. Increased echogenicity of the meninges may be present. Subdural effusions and/or echogenic purulent exudates may be visualized. Many infants will proceed to ventriculitis and will demonstrate an echogenic lining of the ventricular system. Septations may be noted within the ventricles as exudate accumulates. Late sequelae include hydrocephalus, subdural effusions, and cystic encephalomalacia, all of which may be followed using repeat ultrasound examinations. If inflammatory cells invade the lining, venous thrombosis may develop. This may lead to widespread ischemia and infarction of the underlying brain. The ultrasound image may reveal sharply marginated zones of increased echogenicity in the region of infarction.

The corresponding CT findings include a mild decrease in attenuation due to cerebral edema, contrast enhancement of the meninges and/or ventricular lining, and the "delta sign" of sinus thrombosis (when

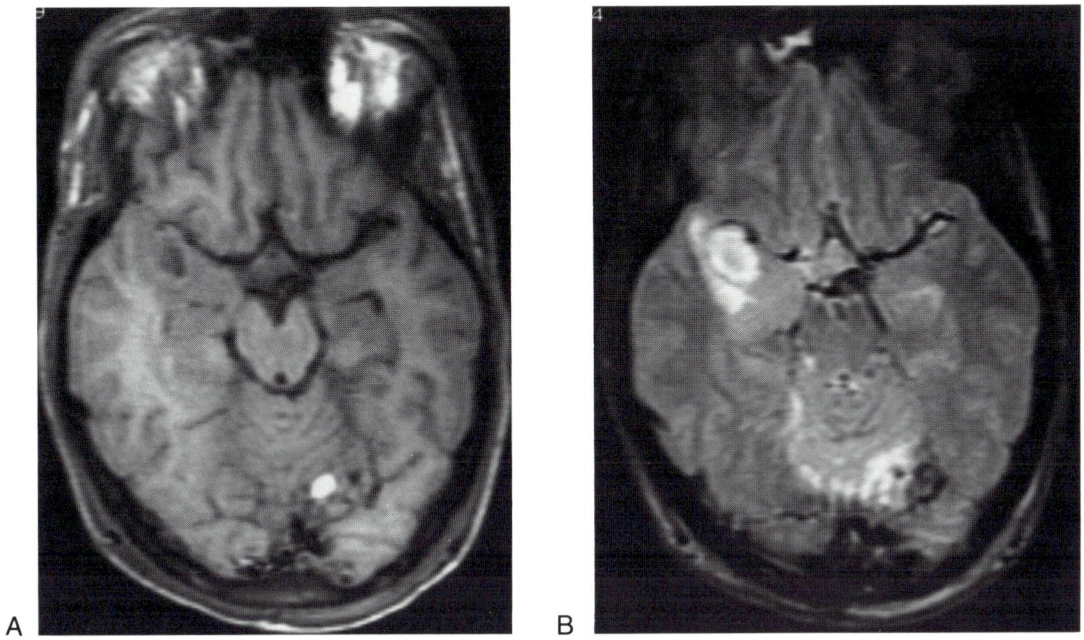

Fig. 7–45 Right temporal lobe abscess. **(A)** Note the ring-shaped area of isointensity with inner hypointensity in the right temporal lobe on the T_1-weighted image. **(B)** With T_2-weighting, the abscess becomes hyperintense as does the surrounding edema.

present). The delta sign is decreased density in the posterior portion of the superior sagittal sinus after contrast administration indicating no flow of contrast through the venous sinus. If the clot is fresh, increased attenuation will be seen in the superior sagittal sinus on the noncontrast images. Focal gyral enhancement after contrast administration may indicate venous infarction and may correspond to a vague area of low attenuation on the noncontrasted scan. If arachnoid necrosis occurs, subdural empyemas will develop. On enhanced CT images, a subdural membrane borders the exudate, which will appear hyperdense as compared with the cerebrospinal fluid.

Most cases of encephalitis are due to viral infections and for the most part are self-limited. Enteroviruses and mumps are most commonly implicated in aseptic meningitis. Of special note is herpes simplex encephalitis, which may be caused by either type I or type II herpes simplex. Roughly one-third of all cases of herpes simplex encephalitis occur in the first two decades of life. After an innocuous prodrome, neurologic symptoms develop, which are often localized to either the temporal or frontal lobes. While the most severe hemorrhagic and necrotic changes occur in the temporal lobes, the entire central nervous system is involved. The first imaging method in a patient with suspected herpes encephalitis should be MRI. Focal areas of increased signal intensity will be seen in the inferior portions of the frontal and temporal lobes on T_2-weighted images. The coronal planes are especially helpful in evaluating these regions. The putamen is spared. Unilateral involvement is more common than bilateral involvement. CT scans are usually not sensitive to herpes encephalitis until almost 1 week after neurologic symptoms have developed. Findings include low attenuation in the anteromedial temporal lobes with extension into the insular cortex. Again, sparing of the putamen is noted. Hemorrhage may be visualized as tiny foci of increased attenuation scattered throughout the regions of low density. After administration of contrast material, gyral enhancement will be seen in the involved areas.

Children infected by HIV are prone to specific neurologic syndromes including nonfocal HIV dementia, subacute encephalopathies, peripheral neuropathies, opportunistic infections, and neoplasms. Widespread central nervous system infection by HIV is responsible for the majority of childhood neurologic complications. An antigen on the virus precipitates an inflammatory reaction. CT findings include basal ganglia and white matter calcifications, cortical atrophy and enlargement of the CSF spaces.

MRI is more sensitive in identifying both the meningeal and parenchymal changes in early opportunistic infections. Unfortunately, it is not specific in differentiating underlying neoplasms from foci of infection. Cytomegalovirus encephalitis is common. Localized infectious lesions and neoplasms are uncommon. *Cryptococcus neoformanus* is a common cause of meningitis. Other reported organisms responsible for parenchymal involvement are *C. albicans* and *Toxoplasma gondi*. The major role of CT and MRI in focal parenchymal disease is to localize an ideal lesion for biopsy. Intraoperative ultrasound may be utilized after opening the calvaria to assure a successful biopsy.

Differentiation of infection from primary brain and spinal cord lymphoma may be difficult prior to biopsy. The incidence of primary CNS lymphoma is exceedingly uncommon outside of the children with either primary or secondary immunodeficiency disorders. Primary malignant lymphoma occurring in AIDS patients may be either a solitary mass or diffusely infiltrative. Most tumors are of the large cell variety and involve the deep brain parenchyma rather than the periphery. Nonenhanced CT scans demonstrate single or multiple hyperdense masses, which demonstrate one of two enhancement patterns after injection of contrast material. The most common pattern in AIDS patients is a rim enhancement difficult to differentiate from brain abscesses since both lymphoma and abscesses have accompanying edema and mass effect. The second pattern is one of homogeneous contrast enhancement. On T_1-weighted MRI, hypointense areas may be identified, which are usually ill-defined. These become hyperintense on T_2-weighted images. The enhancement pattern after injection of Gd-DTPA is similar to that of inflammatory lesions and varies from inhomogeneous to a ring-pattern.

ORBIT

The spectrum of orbital diseases of childhood is different than that found in adults. In the pediatric population, benign masses, congenital malformations, and suppurative inflammation are much more common than primary and secondary malignancies.

The orbit may be divided in reference to the septum (the continuation of the periosteum lining the bony orbit onto the tarsal plates of the eyelids). The space anterior to the septum is considered preseptal while the space posterior to the septum is considered postseptal. The postseptal space is then divided into the intraconal compartment (cone formed by the extraocular muscles posterior to the globe) and the extraconal compartment (space external to the cone).

The most accurate and sensitive means of evaluating the entire orbit at the present time is CT, which provides excellent resolution of both the bony and soft tissue anatomy. Ultrasonography is useful in evaluating intraocular processes. MRI provides separation of the various soft tissue densities without the need for ionizing radiation and is superior in the diagnosis of certain orbital lesions such as lymphangioma.

Contiguous 3-mm or 5-mm CT scans in the plane parallel to a line extending from the external auditory meatus to the floor of the orbit should be obtained from the upper maxillary antrum through the orbital roof. The scan time should be minimized so that eye motion artifact is decreased. One and one-half-mm thick contiguous CT scans may be obtained to further visualize the optic nerves and canal. When necessary, direct coronal sections may be obtained with hyperextension of the neck. Care should be taken to avoid amalgam fillings in the teeth, which degrade the images. A combination of both enhanced and nonenhanced images provide the most complete study but may be unnecessary in cases of infection.

Intraocular Lesions

Common clinical presentations of childhood intraocular lesions include leukocoria, periorbital inflammation, and strabismus. While the most common cause of leukocoria is retinoblastoma, it may also be seen in other intraocular masses of congenital, inflammatory, or traumatic origin. Retinoblastoma accounts for 1 percent of all childhood malignancies and is the most common intraocular neoplasm during the first 15 years of life. Ninety percent of the tumors are recognized before age 5 with the average age at diagnosis being 2 years. Seventy percent of retinoblastomas are unilateral and up to 15 percent of unilateral retinoblastomas are hereditary. Retinoblastomas arise from the retinal layer and are neurocutaneous tumors. Extension may be anterior or posterior. The incidence of calcifications within retinoblastomas ranges between 50 and 100 percent in various series. Seeding of the subarachnoid space may lead to distant metastases in the spinal canal, while hematogeneous spread may lead to long bone metastases.

Ultrasound examination will reveal an echogenic mass arising from the retina extending into the posterior vitreous space. Calcification, if present, will be hyperechoic with posterior shadowing. Areas of tissue necrosis are hypoechoic. The limitation of ultrasound is in the detection of intracranial extension of the tumor.

CT examination reveals a normal orbital size in most cases unless the tumor is quite large (Fig. 7–46). The wall of the eye is thickened and posterior extension occurs into the choroid and sclera. If the tumor penetrates the wall, an exophytic mass may be present and, with continued growth, may fill the bony orbit. CT detection of calcifications occurs in up to 96 percent of cases and is a good indicator of a favorable prognosis. The pattern of calcification is variable. Noncalcified portions of the tumor are usually hyperdense when compared to the surrounding vitreous (25 to 35 HU). Moderate enhancement is usually seen after injection of contrast material although enhancement patterns vary between tumors. Contrast injection is essential for detection of extraocular and intracranial extension of tumor. A careful survey of the opposite eye may reveal subtle contralateral involvement such as plaquelike thickening of the retina. Coronal images are useful in evaluating the superior and inferior aspects of the contralateral eye, which are difficult to visualize with the axial projection. Early local infiltration of the optic nerve sheath may not be detectable with CT. However, with increasing involvement, the sheath enlarges and becomes ir-

A 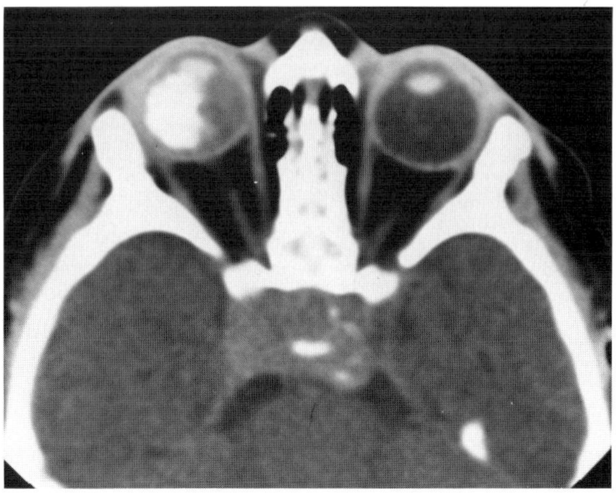 B 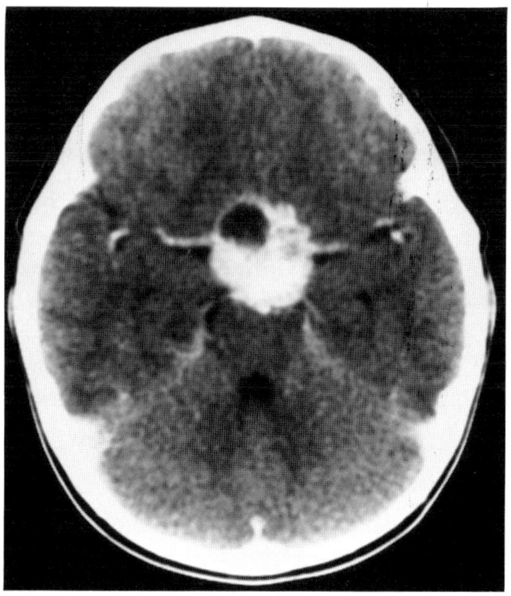

Fig. 7–46 Retinoblastoma. **(A)** A nonenhanced CT scan of the orbits reveals an increase in the density of the contents of the right globe. The intracranial portions of the optic nerve tracts are asymmetric. A calcified mass is seen in the region of the optic chiasm and extends to the left of midline. **(B)** Enhanced CT scans obtained at a higher level demonstrates suprasellar extension of the retinoblastoma with marked homogeneous enhancement of the solid portion of the tumor. Both a calicified and a cystic component are noted.

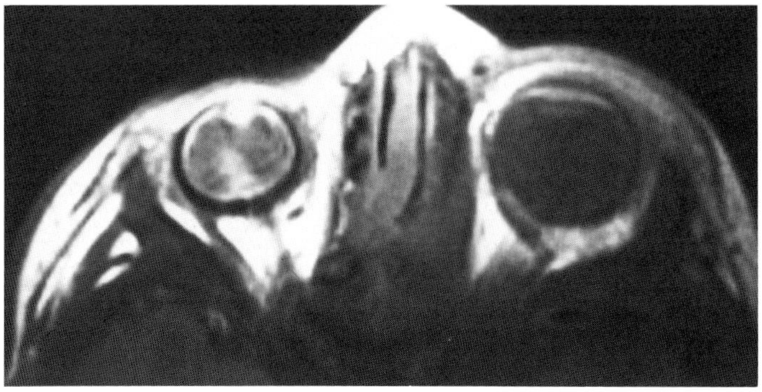

Fig. 7–47 Persistent hyperplastic primary vitreous. T_1-weighted axial MRI demonstrates right microphthalmia associated with a vertical septum. The orbital fluid is increased in signal intensity when compared to the left globe.

regular. MRI reveal a high intensity tumor on T_1-weighted sequences with low intensity on T_2-weighted sequences as compared with the surrounding vitreous.

Trilateral retinoblastoma describes a third site of synchronous tumor involvement in the pineal region associated with bilateral retinoblastomas. Whether this represents metastasis or a second, closely-related tumor remains controversial.

After the diagnosis has been surgically confirmed, CT is the method of choice for follow up. Not only will CT detect local recurrence and distant metastases but complications such as inflammation or those related to the orbital prosthesis may also be detected.

Persistent Hyperplastic Primary Vitreous

Neonates with this congenital malformation are usually recognized shortly after birth because of leukocoria and micro-opthalmia. Unilateral involvement predominates. Deformity occurs because of an arrest in maturation of the primary vitreous and the primary hyaloid artery. After the hyaloid artery supplies the developing optic nerve, posterior bulb, primary vitreous, and posterior lens, it regresses and is usually not apparent at the time of birth.

The characteristic features of persistent hyperplastic primary vitreous include micro-opthalmia, a septum dividing the lobe into two vertically oriented halves, increased attenuation of the posterior vitreous space, and minimal enhancement of the septum after injection of contrast material. The findings are similar on MRI (Fig. 7–47). The septum contains remnants of the hyaloid artery, which cause the enhancement. Reported complications include retinal detachment and chronic retinal hemorrhage. Calcification is not frequently reported in association with persistent hypertrophic primary vitreous. Milder cases with persistent partial hyaloid remnants and a normal secondary vitreous may be overlooked on CT images.

Coats' Disease

Coats' disease is a primary vascular anomaly of the retina with telangiectasias, neovascularization, collateral formation, exudates, and retinal detachment. Ninety-six percent of cases have unilateral involvement alone. Both CT and ultrasonography demonstrate nonspecific findings. A curved echogenic line represents the retinal detachment on ultrasound images. A layer of mixed echogenicity beneath the detached retina represents the exudate. Two patterns of detachment are seen on CT. The most common pattern is a hyperdense V shape with the apex of the V pointing posteriorly at the optic disc. Circumferential detachment results in a ring shaped mass of hyperdensity with a smooth inner margin. A central area of low density represents the remaining vitreous. The exudate does not enhance. Calcification and extraocular extension do not occur in Coats' disease. T_2-weighted MRI demonstrates the proteinaceous subretinal exudate as an area of homogeneous hyperintensity. If any focus of low signal intensity appears within the higher signal proteinaceous exudate, the diagnosis of retinoblastoma should be considered. A Coats-like reaction may be the presenting feature of retinoblastoma. The definitive diagnosis is made by fluorescein angiography, which identifies the abnormal vascularity.

Retrolental Fibroplasia

Prolonged high plasma oxygen concentrations necessary for the treatment of hyaline membrane disease of premature infants leads to toxic retinopathy, termed *retrolental fibroplasia*. Retinal vasoconstriction leads to ischemia and neovascularization of the posterior vitreous and retina. The new vascularity leads to hemorrhage, scarring, retinal retraction, and exudate formation. End-stage retrolental fibroplasia appear similar to the findings seen in Coats' disease since there is exudative retinal detachment. Both orbits are usually involved, although the degree of involvement may vary from side to side. The globes are usually normal in size unless damage is very extensive, in which case they are contracted. Retinal detachment begins in the temporal quadrants of the globe and may appear as either a hyperdense or hypodense nonenhancing subretinal mass. Calcification is rare. Extensive vitreous hemorrhage following retinal detachment may lead to complete replacement of the posterior vitreous space by a high attenuation mass.

Phakomatoses

Ocular disease can be found in each of the neurocutaneous syndromes or phakomatoses. Retinal glial hamartomas are found in both neurofibromatosis and tuberous sclerosis. They may be solitary or multiple and involve the retina or optic nerve disc. Ultrasound examination reveals an echogenic mass involving the retina or optic nerve disc. Calcifications may be present resulting in echogenic foci with posterior shadowing. CT examination reveals nonenhancing retinal plaques.

Choroidal hemangiomas may be found in Sturge-Weber disease. Capillary angiomas may be seen in von Hippel-Lindau syndrome. Both hemangioma and capillary angioma appear as enhancing peripheral masses in the posterior vitreous space and may or may not be accompanied by retinal detachment and subretinal exudate.

Drusen

Focal calcification in the hyaline bodies of an abnormal retinal basement membrane is referred to as an optic nerve drusen. Whether the drusen represents a developmental defect or retinal degeneration remains controversial. Three-fourths of cases are bilateral and 87 percent of patients experience visual field defects. Giant drusen are large unilateral calcified hamartomas near the optic nerve head in tuberous sclerosis. Ultrasound examination reveals increased echogenicity in the region of the calcification without any evidence of an associated soft tissue mass. Unenhanced CT reveals thin, plaquelike, circular calcifications conforming to the optic nerve head (Fig. 7–48). If any soft tissue mass is associated, the diagnosis of retinoblastoma must also be entertained.

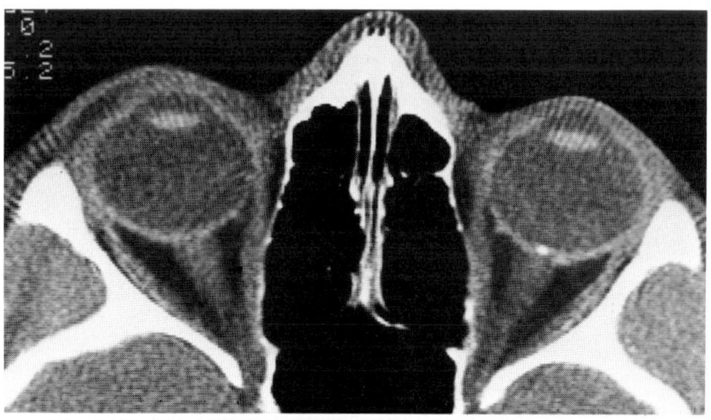

Fig. 7–48 Optic drusen. Note the small calcification in the left optic nerve on this nonenhanced axial CT image.

Pediatric Orbital Masses

The most common masses inside the bony orbit but outside of the globe in childhood are benign, although certain malignant neoplasms also demonstrate a predilection for the orbit. Common benign masses are dermoid, hemangioma, inflammation, lymphangioma, and neurofibroma. Common malignant neoplasms include leukemia, lymphoma, metastatic neuroblastoma, optic nerve glioma, and sarcoma.

The capillary hemangioma is the most common benign mass arising within or adjacent to the orbit in children less than 10 years of age. Ninety percent of hemangiomas are recognized before 6 months of age when the infant is noted to have unilateral proptosis. Hemangiomas may increase rapidly in size and, if symptoms are severe, corticosteroid therapy or operative intervention is indicated. Spontaneous regression is the natural history of the lesion. The most common location for hemangiomas is along the upper lid in the preseptal space. CT examination reveals a crescentric mass within the lid or in the medial or lateral epicanthus that is well-defined. The mass is slightly hyperintense and, following administration of contrast material, homogeneous enhancement is seen. Prominent superficial vessels along the cheek and nasal bridge are common. Calcification is typically absent. The second common location of orbital hemangiomas is in the postseptal region (Fig. 7–49). Involvement of the intraconal and/or extraconal compartments may occur. Concomitant preseptal involvement and intracranial extension are uncommon. Again, CT examination shows a well-defined, slightly hyperintense lesion with homogeneous, hyperintense contrast enhancement and prominent vessels.

The second most common benign tumor of the orbit in children less than 10 years of age is the dermoid. Three types are recognized in the orbit: conjunctival dermoid (located medially), episcleral dermolipoma, and epithelial choristoma. The most common cell type is the epithelial choristoma, which arises laterally. This dermoid may lie outside of the lateral bony orbital wall, within the bone, or within the lacrimal fossa. The conjunctival dermoid is indistinguishable from the epithelial choristoma on both physical examination and imaging studies. On CT scans, a thin, isodense rim surrounds the low attenuation center which ranges from fat to soft tissue density (Fig. 7–50). Bone destruction and erosion are absent. After administration of contrast material, the thin rim enhances moderately. The center of the lesion remains unchanged. Episcleral dermolipomas present as soft, fatty, conjunctival masses located temporally. On CT scans, a crescentric mass with a thin, well-defined rim and a low attenuation center is seen. The attenuation values for the center are fat density. Minimal rim enhancement follows contrast administration.

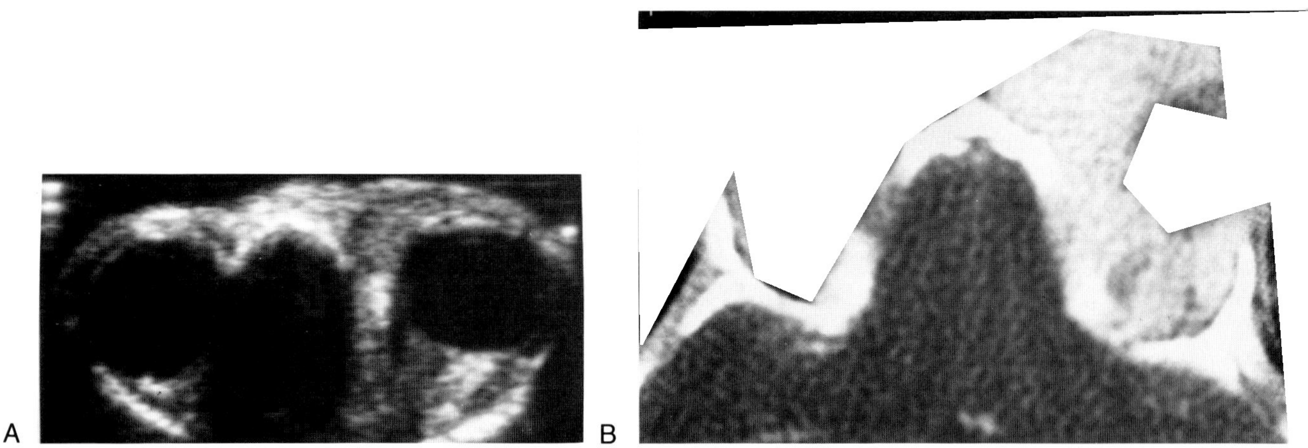

Fig. 7–49 Postseptal hemangioma. **(A)** Ultrasound imaging demonstrates proptosis of the left orbit due to a echogenic mass involving both the intraconal and extraconal compartments. **(B)** Enhanced axial CT scan demonstrates homogeneous enhancement of the capillary hemangioma displacing the left globe.

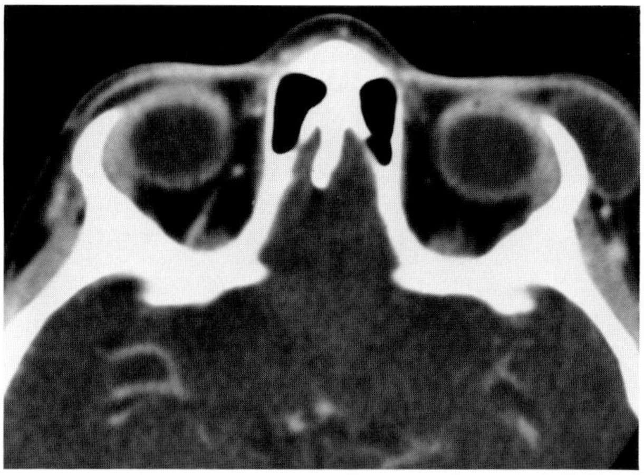

Fig. 7–50 Orbital dermoid. Note the hypodense mass arising just outside the lateral wall of the left orbit. The thin enhancing rim is diagnostic of an orbital dermoid.

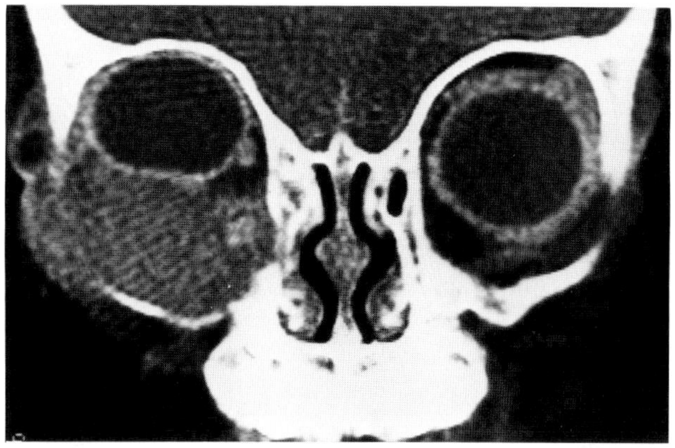

Fig. 7–51 Orbital rhabdomyosarcoma. Coronal head CT scan demonstrates a large, ill-defined mass arising from the inferior aspect of the right orbit. Note the expansion of the orbit, with destruction of the inferolateral orbital rim. The medial orbital rim is also destroyed. The globe is compressed superiorly.

Another cause of infantile proptosis is the presence of an orbital lymphangioma. CT evaluation generally demonstrates a mass arising in the superior aspect of the orbit posterior to the globe without calcification. Occasionally, phleboliths may be detected within the venous spaces. The mass begins in the extraconal compartment but, with enlargement, it may infiltrate and fill the intraconal space. Septal extension is also common. Variable contrast enhancement occurs with the nonenhancing areas of low attenuation representing dilated lymphatics. The mixed attenuation, variable enhancement, and poorly defined margins help to differentiate lymphagiomas from capillary hemangiomas.

MRI is highly sensitive in the detection and follow-up of orbital lymphangiomas. Areas of previous spontaneous hemorrhage demonstrate decreased signal intensity on T_1-weighted images and increased intensity on T_2-weighted images. Since spontaneous hemorrhage is uncommon in other infiltrating mass lesions of the orbit, its presence is highly suggestive of lymphangioma.

Orbital neurofibromas are most commonly associated with neurofibromatosis. Other commonly associated lesions of the orbit include dural ectasia, Schwann cell tumors, meningiomas, and optic nerve gliomas. Sphenoid wing hypoplasia/aplasia may produce pulsating exopthalmos. Neurofibromas may arise from any nerve within the orbit but the supraorbital and infraorbital nerves are most commonly involved. CT evaluation reveals a homogeneous, slightly hyperdense, smoothly marginated lesion that demonstrates moderate enhancement following IV contrast administration.

The most common primary malignant tumor of the orbit in childhood is rhabdomyosarcoma, which accounts for 10 percent of all mass lesions in this site. One-fourth of all head and neck rhabdomyosarcomas arise in the orbit or periorbital region. The average age at diagnosis is 7 to 8 years. The incidence is higher in white males. The presenting symptoms include ptosis, swelling, redness, and unilateral exophthalmos. As opposed to the other described orbital tumors, rhabdomyosarcoma commonly causes bone destruction. CT is the best method of evaluation prior to surgery (Fig. 7–51). The most common location is in the upper eyelid or medial epicanthal area (preseptal). However, the tumor may be postseptal and involve the intraconal and extraconal regions. The malignant, aggressive nature of the lesion is revealed by rapid contiguous bone destruction. Tumor extension into the intracranial vault, paranasal sinuses, and superficial soft tissues of the face may make the site of origin difficult to determine. When small, the lesions demonstrate attenuation values similar to normal muscle. As the tumor size increases, necrosis causes decreased attenuation in some areas. The contour is irregular with infiltration of the surrounding soft tissues. Mild to moderate enhancement occurs after IV contrast administration. The enhancement pattern is not distinguishable from that seen with other less common orbital malignancies.

Inflammation

Paranasal sinusitis may lead to the development of periorbital cellulitis. Contiguous spread is the usual pathway by which organisms reach the septal space. Preseptal cellulitis is confined to the space anterior to the orbital septum and does not require CT evaluation. However, if conjunctivitis, proptosis, limited range of motion, loss of visual acuity, or diplopia are present, postseptal cellulitis should be suspected. Emergent IV antibiotic administration is necessary to insure that no permanent ocular damage occurs.

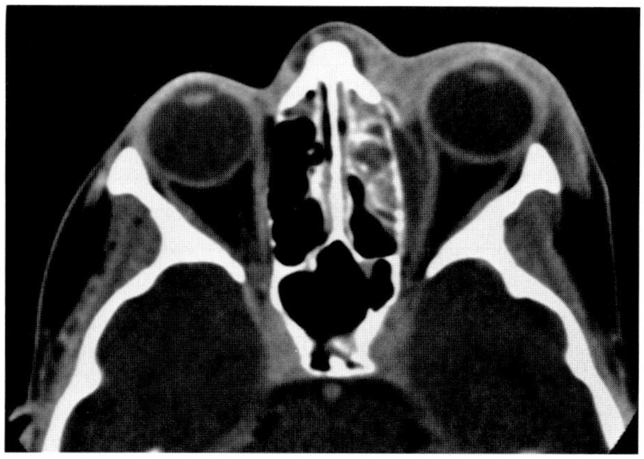

Fig. 7–52 Orbital cellulitis. Note the preseptal edema associated with opacification of the left ethmoid air cells. An inflammatory mass bows the medial rectus muscle laterally. At surgery, this contained pus.

Immediate nonenhanced axial CT scans provide the information necessary for diagnosis and treatment. If only preseptal cellulitis is present, edema expands both the upper and lower eyelids. Inhomogeneous minimal contrast enhancement is seen. The postseptal space and paranasal sinuses are usually normal. In contrast, postseptal cellulitis leads to the presence of an inflammatory mass usually located between the medial rectus muscle and the lamina papyracea (Fig. 7–52). The soft tissue mass may be hypodense or isodense with adjacent muscle. Lateral bowing of the medial rectus muscle is common. Adjacent paranasal sinus disease is present in most cases. Occasionally, the inflammatory mass may arise along the lateral aspect of the orbit. Frank erosion or dehiscence of the lamina papyracea is uncommon. In fact, bony sclerosis, erosion, or remodeling should suggest other diagnoses such as granulomatous inflammation, osteomyelitis, or neoplasm. If an abscess is detected, immediate surgical drainage is indicated. It may be difficult to differentiate postseptal cellulitis from a postseptal abscess. Low attenuation within the extraconal mass may be seen in both cellulitis and in early abscess formation. The most reliable sign of an orbital abscess is the presence of air or an air/fluid level within the mass. Intracranial extension may occur along the superior orbital fissure, optic canal, or by venous propagation. Complications include epidural abscess, subdural empyema, focal cerebritis, brain abscess, and meningitis. Cavernous sinus thrombosis and meningismus also occur. It is prudent to evaluate the brain with contrast CT scans at the same time the orbits are imaged.

A nonspecific inflammatory reaction of uncertain etiology may occur in children resulting in lymphoid hyperplasia within the orbit. This is termed *orbital pseudotumor* and may simulate a neoplasm both clinically and on imaging studies. Symptoms include the rapid onset of unilateral proptosis, orbital pain, and swelling. Up to 20 percent of cases are diagnosed during the first 2 decades of life. The CT appearance of orbital pseudotumor is variable in children and may consist of a well-defined mass in the region of the lacrimal gland, a retrobulbar mass with or without scleral involvement, optic nerve sheath involvement, extraocular muscle myositis, or multiple sites of involvement. Nonenhanced CT scans may reveal either an isodense or slightly hyperdense solid mass as compared with the extraocular muscles. The posterior margin of the sclera may be thickened and irregular. Cylindrical enlargement of the optic nerve sheath may be present. Diffuse enlargement of the extraocular muscle may also be seen. Administration of steroids leads to complete resolution of the problem in many cases. However, in some cases, biopsy may be necessary to separate pseudotumor from infiltrative malignancy.

SUGGESTED READINGS

1. Babcock DS, Han BK: Cranial Ultrasonography of Infants. Williams & Wilkins, Baltimore, 1981
2. Baierl P, Muhlsteffen A, Haustein J, et al: Comparison of plain and Gd-DTPA-enhanced MR-imaging of children. Pediatr Radiol 20:515, 1990
3. Ball WS Jr, Towbin RB: MRI of pediatric central nervous system neoplasms. p. 177. In Thomas S, Pomeranz SJ, Clark R (eds): Craniospinal Magnetic Resonance Imaging. Year Book Publishers, Chicago, 1988
4. Belman AL, Ultmann MH, Horoupian D, et al: Neurological complications in infants and children with acquired immune deficiency syndrome. Ann Neurol 18:560, 1985
5. Brown EW, Riccardi VM, Mawad M, et al: MR imaging of optic pathways in patients with neurofibromatosis. AJNR 8:1031, 1987
6. Buckingham MJ, Crone KR, Ball WS, Berger TS: Management of cerebral cavernous angiomas in children presenting with seizures. Child's Nervous System 5:347, 1989
7. Burstein J, Papile L, Burstein R: Intraventricular hemorrhage and hydrocephalus in premature newborns: a prospective study with CT. AJR 132:631, 1979
8. Cremin BJ, Lamont AC: Neurosonography in full-term cerebral hemorrhage. Br J Radiol 58:111, 1985
9. Cubberley DA, Jaffe RB, Nixon GW: Sonographic demonstration of galenic arteriovenous malformations in the neonate. AJR 3:435, 1982
10. Daniels DL, Herfkins R, Gager WE, et al: Magnetic resonance imaging of the optic nerves and chiasm. Radiology 152:79, 1984
11. Davidson HD, Steiner RE. Magnetic resonance imaging in infections of the central nervous system. AJNR 253:393, 1985
12. Dubowitz LM, Bydder GM, Mushin J: Developmental sequence of periventricular leukomalacia: correlation of ultrasound, clinical and nuclear magnetic resonance functions. Arch Dis Child 60:349, 1985
13. Gomori JM, Grossman RI, Goldberg HI, et al: Intracranial hematomas: imaging by high field MR. Radiology 157:87, 1985
14. Grant EG, Schellinger D, Richardson JD, et al: Echogenic periventricular halo: normal sonographic finding or neonatal cerebral hemorrhage. AJR 140:793, 2983
15. Haimes AB, Zimmerman RD, Morgello S, et al: MR imaging of brain abscesses. AJNR 10:279, 1989
16. Hedges TR, Pozzi-Mucelli R, Char DH, Newton TH: CT demonstration of ocular calcification: correlations with clinical and pathological findings. Neuroradiology 23:15, 1982
17. Hesselink JR, Dowd CF, Healy ME, et al: MR imaging of brain contusions. A comparative study with CT. AJNR 9:269, 1988
18. Johnson MA, Pennuck JM, Bydder GM, et al: Clinical NMR imaging of the brain in children: normal and neurologic disease. AJR 141:1005, 1983
19. Kilgore DP, Strother CM, Starshak RJ, Haughton VM: Pineal germinoma: MR imaging. Radiology 158:435, 1986
20. Kingsley DPE, Brooks GB, Leung AWL, Johnson MA: Acoustic neuromas: evaluation by MR imaging. AJNR 6:1, 1985
21. Nowell JA, Grossman RI, Hackney DB, et al: MR imaging of white matter disease in children. AJNR 9:503, 1988
22. Price DB, Inglese CM, Jacobs J, et al: Pediatric AIDS: neuroradiologic and neurodevelopmental findings. Pediatr Radiol 18:445, 1988
23. Radkowski MA, Naidich TP, Tomita T, et al: Neonatal brain tumors: CT and MR findings. J Comput Assist Tomogr 12:10, 1988
24. Rumack CM, Manco-Johnson ML, Manco-Johnson MJ, et al: Timing and course of neonatal intracranial hemorrhage using real-time ultrasound. Radiology 154:101, 1985
25. Sano K, Wakai S, Ochiai C: Characteristics of meningioma in childhood. Childs Brain 8:98, 1981
26. Siegel MJ, Shackelford GD, Perlman JM, Fulling KH: Hypoxic-ischemic encephalopathy in term infants: diagnosis and prognosis evaluated by ultrasound. Radiology 152:395, 1984
27. Sze G, Abranson A, Krol G, et al: Gd-DTPA in the evaluation of intradural, extramedullary spinal disease. AJNR 9:153, 1988
28. Trounce JQ, Fagan D, Levene MI: Intraventricular hemorrhage and periventricular leukomalacia: ultrasound and autopsy correlation. Arch Dis Child 61:1203, 1986
29. Valk J: Gd-DTPA in MR of spinal lesions. AJNR 9:345, 1988
30. van der Knaap MS, Valk J: Classification of congenital abnormalities of the CNS. AJNR 9:315, 1988
31. Vion-Dury J, Vincentelli F, Jiddane M, et al: MR imaging of epidermoid cysts. Neuroradiology 29:333, 1987
32. Weingarten K, Zimmerman RD, Becker RD, et al: Subdural and epidural empyemas: MR imaging. AJNR 10, 81, 1989
33. Zimmerman RA, Bilaniuk LT, Bruce D, et al: CT of craniocerebral injury in the abused child. Radiology 130:687, 1979

8 Musculoskeletal System

Susan D. Stansberry

JOINTS

Joint Space Widening

The most common cause of joint space widening in children is the presence of fluid within the joint, which most commonly occurs in the hip and shoulder joints. The intra-articular fluid may consist of blood, pus, or serous effusion. Pyogenic arthritis is one of the most common causes of joint fluid and is of the most urgent concern because proteolytic enzymes released by the organisms and inflammatory cells lead to rapid cartilage destruction if early therapy is not instituted. Septic arthritis frequently accompanies osteomyelitis in the neonate and young infant; in the very young it often lacks the characteristic fever and leukocytosis, and therefore, the detection of a widened joint space is critical for early diagnosis.

Joint space widening from hemarthrosis is most commonly caused by trauma (Fig. 8–1). Bleeding disorders such as hemophilia, synovial tumors, and chronic synovial inflammation may also result in blood within the joint.

Serous joint effusions may be caused by a variety of conditions. In children younger than 2 years, transient synovitis is a common cause of a hip effusion. Clinically these patients tend to be much less ill than those with pyogenic arthritis, and the effusion in this condition is much less likely to produce joint space

JOINT SPACE WIDENING

Congenital/developmental
- Congenital dislocating joint
- Winchester syndrome
- Larsen's syndrome

Inflammatory
- Pyogenic arthritis
- Toxic (transient) synovitis
- Rheumatoid arthritis
- Tuberculous arthritis
- Fungal arthritis
- Pigmented villonodular synovitis

Neoplasm
- Synovial tumor

Trauma/surgery
- Post-traumatic effusion or hemarthrosis
- Traumatic dislocation

Systemic/metabolic
- Neuromuscular disease
- Lipogranulomatosis (Farber's)
- Hemophilia (bleeding disorders)

Miscellaneous
- Legg-Perthes disease

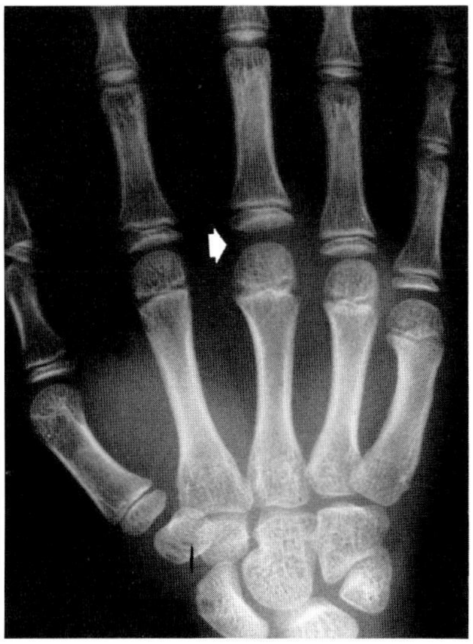

Fig. 8–1 Hemarthrosis. Widening of the third metacarpophalangeal joint (*arrow*) as a result of post-traumatic hemorrhage.

widening. This is a self-limiting condition thought by many investigators to be caused by a viral infection. Serous effusions may also be seen with Legg-Perthes disease, rheumatoid arthritis, and other chronic arthritides.

When joint space widening at the hip is detected on plain radiographs, ultrasonography is useful for identifying and quantifying the presence of intra-articular fluid. Coronal images of the hip clearly demonstrate the hypoechoic fluid within the joint (Fig. 8–2). The character of the fluid, however, usually cannot be determined by ultrasound examination.

Joints other than the hips and shoulders have strong ligaments and joint capsules and are generally not easily displaced by intra-articular fluid. Therefore, one must rely on fat pad displacement and periarticular increased density on plain radiographs to suggest

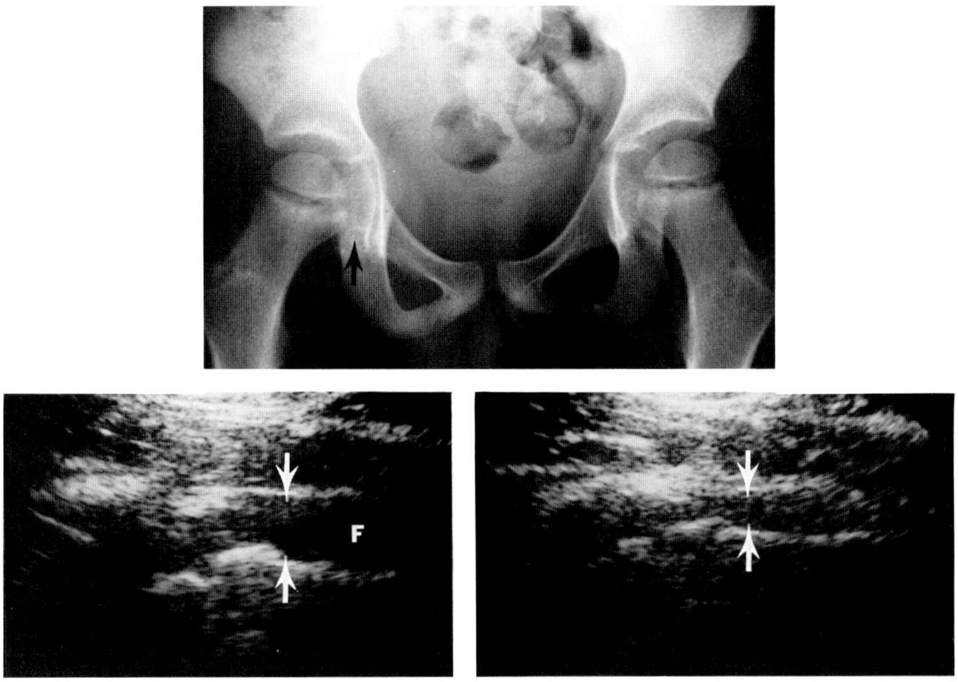

B C

Fig. 8–2 Septic arthritis. **(A)** Plain radiographs show slight widening of the joint space of the right hip (*arrow*). **(B)** Sagittal ultrasound image of the painful hip shows increased fluid (*F*) in the right hip joint (*arrows*) as compared with **(C)** the normal left hip.

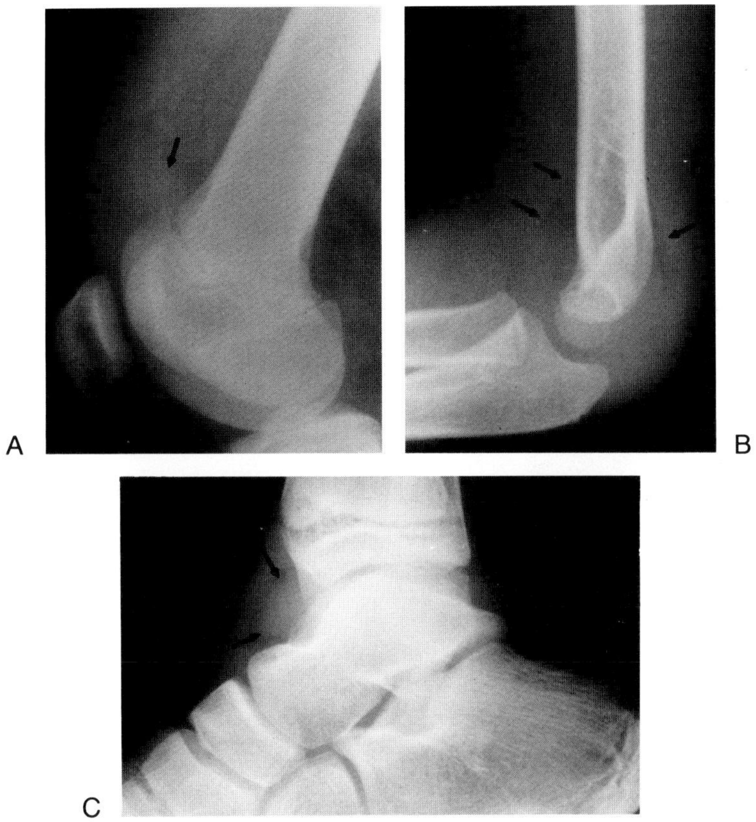

Fig. 8–3 Post-traumatic joint effusions. **(A)** Increased density in the suprapatellar region because of a joint effusion accompanying an epiphyseal-metaphyseal injury (*arrows*). **(B)** Fluid in the elbow joint causing elevation of the anterior fat pad and visualization of the normally hidden posterior fat pad (*arrows*). **(C)** Ankle fluid causing outward displacement of the anterior and posterior fat pads (*arrows*).

the presence of joint fluid. A moderate amount of fluid is usually detectable in the knee, elbow, and ankle on plain radiographs (Fig. 8–3).

Synovial thickening can also lead to widening of the joint space. In children, this is most often caused by rheumatoid arthritis, hemophilic arthropathy, or tuberculous arthritis. Widening of the intercondylar notch of the distal femur from erosion by the hypertrophied synovium is characteristic of the latter two conditions. Winchester syndrome, Farber's lipogranulomatosis, and pigmented villonodular synovitis are rare causes of synovial thickening in childhood. Longstanding synovial thickening eventually leads to cartilage destruction and therefore, joint space narrowing.

Dislocation of a joint may be congenital or post-traumatic. Congenital dislocation of the hip is more common in female infants and in infants who deliver in a breech position. This condition is thought to be part of a generalized instability of the pelvis, most likely secondary to excessive maternal estrogens. Accumulation of these hormones results in ligamentous laxity and joint instability predominantly affecting the hip. Clinically, this condition is suggested by the detection of a click when abducting and internally rotating the leg (Ortolani maneuver).

Radiographically, the findings of a congenitally dislocating hip may be difficult to detect. A vertical line drawn through the lateral edge of the acetabulum

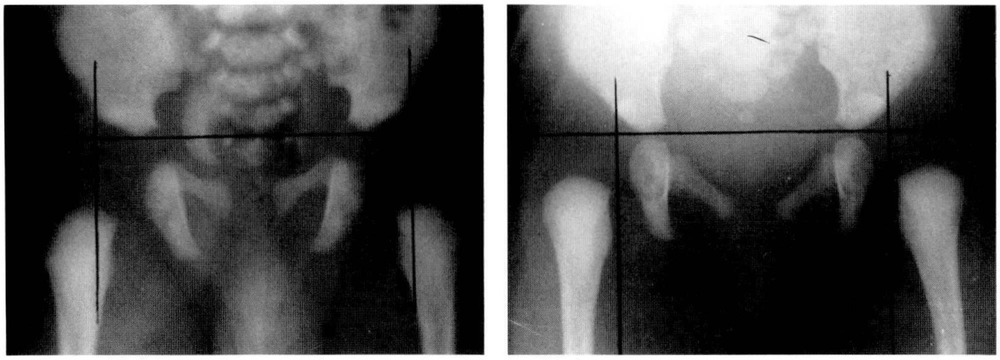

A B

Fig. 8–4 Perkin's line. **(A)** The vertical lines pass through the medial aspect of the proximal femurs in this normal patient. **(B)** Lateral positioning of the femurs with respect to Perkin's line indicates bilateral hip dislocation in this patient with congenitally dislocating hips.

(vertical line of Perkins) should normally pass through the medial aspect of the upper femur (Fig. 8–4). If the femur lies completely lateral to this line, the hip is dislocated. Dynamic imaging is often requested to try to detect dislocatability in hips that otherwise appear normal.

More recently, ultrasonography has been used to diagnose a congenitally dislocating hip. The cartilaginous femoral head in its relationship to the acetabulum is easily identified in both the transverse and coronal planes (Fig. 8–5). Real-time sonography also allows dynamic imaging using a flexion-stress maneuver to attempt to displace the hip posteriorly.

Trauma may lead to joint dislocation in children, although epiphyseal-metaphyseal fractures are the more common result. Rupture of the ligamentum teres in the hip results in lateral displacement of the femur. Occasionally, an unossified fragment of cartilage may remain in the joint and cause persistent joint space widening. These fragments can be identified by CT or MRI. Birth trauma from a traumatic delivery can occasionally result in injury to the bra-

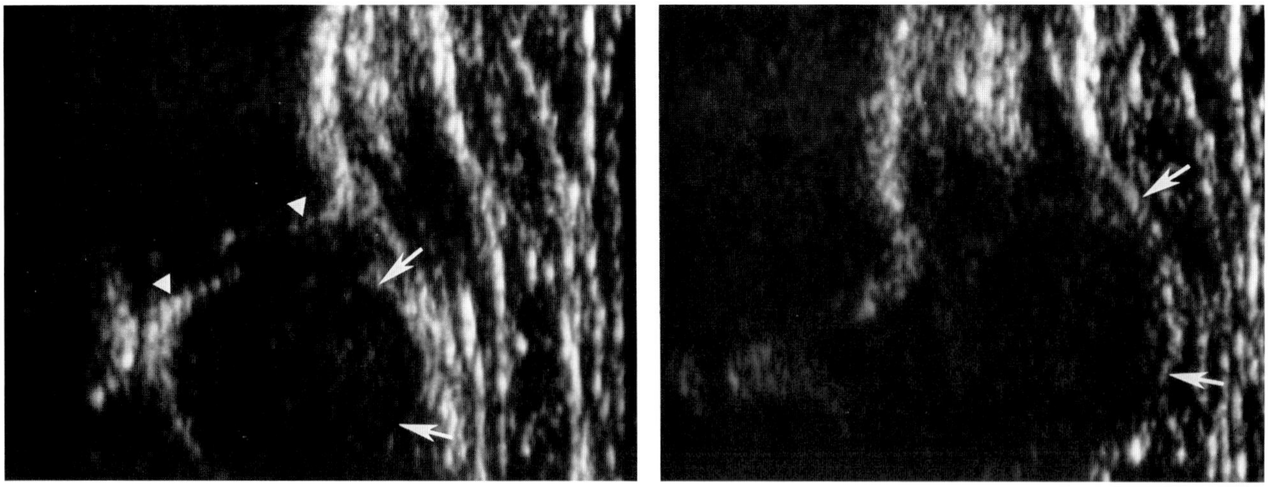

A B

Fig. 8–5 Ultrasonography of congenitally dislocating hip. **(A)** Ultrasonography in the coronal plane with the hips flexed in a normal patient clearly shows the unossified cartilaginous femoral head (*arrows*) in good alignment with the acetabulum (*arrowheads*). **(B)** With hip dislocation, superolateral positioning of the head is seen with displacement of the joint capsule (*arrows*).

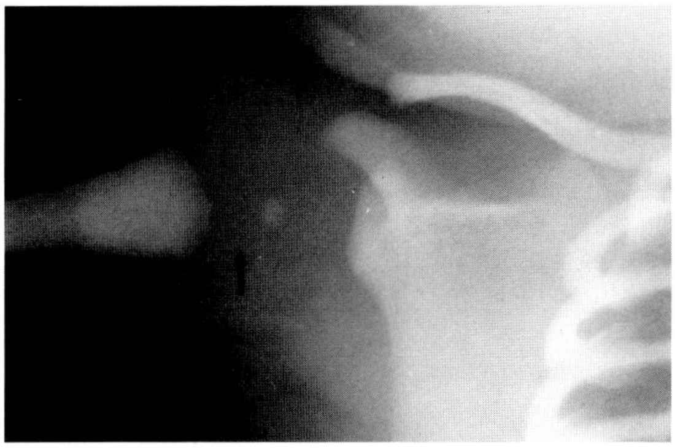

Fig. 8–6 Erb's palsy. Widening of the right shoulder joint caused by brachial plexus injury during delivery. Widening of the epiphyseal-metaphyseal junction of the right proximal humerus indicates a concomitant Salter-Harris I fracture (*arrow*).

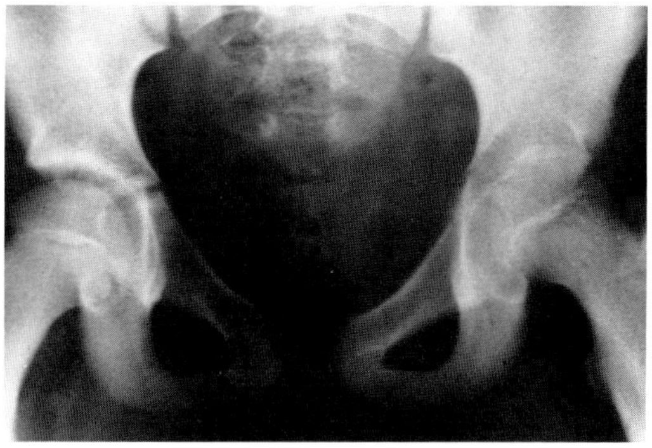

Fig. 8–7 Septic arthritis. Severe joint space narrowing resulting from cartilage destruction caused by pyogenic arthritis of the left hip.

chial plexus (Erb's palsy), which can manifest as a widened shoulder joint (Fig. 8–6). The joint laxity that accompanies various neurologic and neuromuscular diseases can also cause joint space widening.

Joint Space Narrowing

Joint space narrowing is usually the result of cartilage destruction, which may accompany a variety of conditions. Rapid cartilage destruction and joint space narrowing are seen with pyogenic arthritis (Fig. 8–7). The narrowing that occurs with rheumatoid arthritis, hemophilic arthropathy, and tuberculous arthritis progresses more slowly. Fungal arthritis, pigmented villonodular synovitis, slipped capital femoral epiphysis, and certain syndromes are uncommon causes of joint space narrowing in children. The joint space may also be narrowed due to osteoarthritis that results as a long-term complication of aseptic necrosis (e.g., Legg-Perthes disease) and trauma.

In some cases of traumatic joint dislocation, the joint space will appear to be narrowed because of overlap of the bones on a single view. A second view taken at right angles to the first should clearly demonstrate the dislocation.

JOINT CALCIFICATION

Calcifications in or around a joint are quite uncommon in children. The most common intra-articular

---

JOINT CALCIFICATION

Congenital/developmental
- Tumoral calcinosis*

Inflammatory
- Synovial inflammation†

Neoplasm
- Synovial chondromatosis†
- Synovial tumors†

Trauma/surgery
- Avulsion fracture†
- Burns*

Systemic/metabolic
- Ochronosis†
- Oxalosis†
- Dermatomyositis*
- Hypervitaminosis D*
- Hyperparathyroidism*

Miscellaneous
- Osteochonditis dissecans†
- Idiopathic

* Periarticular.
† Intra-articular.

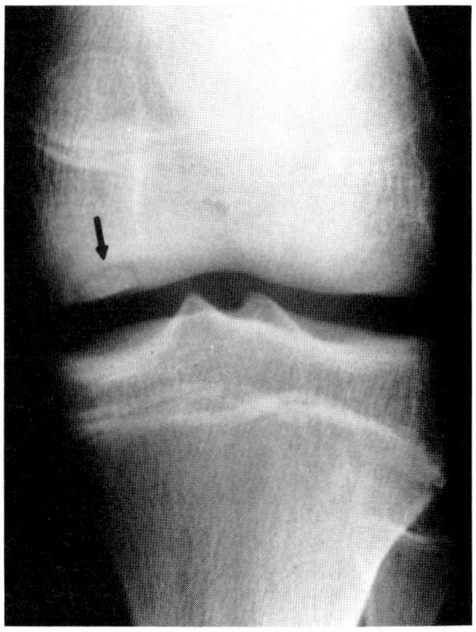

Fig. 8–8 Osteochondritis dissecans of the knee. The defect in the medial femoral condyle (*arrow*) is typical of this condition.

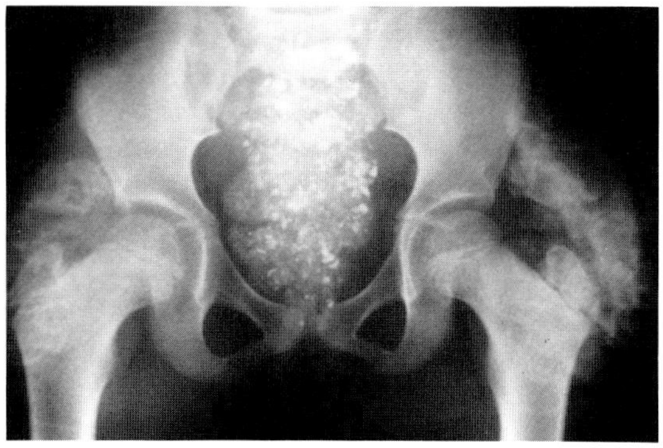

Fig. 8–9 Tumoral calcinosis. Characteristic nodular, masslike periarticular calcification around the hips of a patient with tumoral calcinosis.

calcification is the fragment associated with osteochondritis dissecans, in which avascular necrosis of a fragment of articular cartilage and its underlying subchondral bone occurs. Trauma, ischemia, and constitutional predisposition are all factors that may be involved in the development of osteochondritis dissecans. Often, only the cartilaginous defect in the articular surface of the bone is visible, without evidence of calcification. The lateral surface of the medial femoral condyle in the knee is the most commonly affected site, although other joints can be affected (Fig. 8–8).

Traumatic avulsion fractures may result in calcifications in or near a joint. Other causes of intra-articular calcifications are rare. Idiopathic calcifications have been seen in the hips of infants, but most of these cases are thought to have been caused by inadvertent injection of drugs into the joint from a nearby venous infusion catheter.

Periarticular calcifications are also rare in childhood. These are occasionally seen in patients with burns, rheumatoid arthritis, hyperparathyroidism, hypervitaminosis D, and collagen vascular diseases such as dermatomyositis. Tumoral calcinosis is a rare hereditary condition that may be caused by abnormal phosphorus metabolism and results in masses of multinodular calcifications in the juxta-articular regions (Fig. 8–9).

Genu Varum (Bowed Legs)

Bowed legs are common in childhood, particularly in toddlers younger than 4 years old. In many of these children, the deformity is actually an exaggeration of the physiologic tibial torsion present in infants. The tibia and ankle are tilted medially causing toeing in and compensatory bowing at the knees. This deformity usually occurs in well developed infants who often walk early. The problem is usually self-limiting and spontaneously resolves by the age of 3 to 4. It should be noted, however, that many of these children will develop knock-knees, which also tend to resolve spontaneously by 7 years of age (Fig. 8–10).

Femoral anteversion is a similar "physiologic" cause of bowed legs, in which exaggerated anterior torsion of the femurs leads to toeing in and bowing of the knees; it is less prominent than that accompanying tibial torsion. The degree of anteversion can be determined by measuring the angle between the femoral neck and shaft on the lateral view or by CT. The degree of anteversion tends to decrease as the patient

GENU VARUM (BOWED LEGS)

Congenital/developmental
- Tibial torsion (physiologic)
- Femoral anteversion
- Metaphyseal dysostoses
- Bone dysplasias (e.g., achondroplasia, osteogenesis imperfecta, diastrophic dwarfism)
- Blount's disease

Inflammatory
- Osteomyelitis

Trauma/surgery
- Epiphyseal-metaphyseal injuries

Systemic/metabolic
- Rickets
- Hypophosphatasia
- Hyperparathyroidism
- Hyperphosphatemia

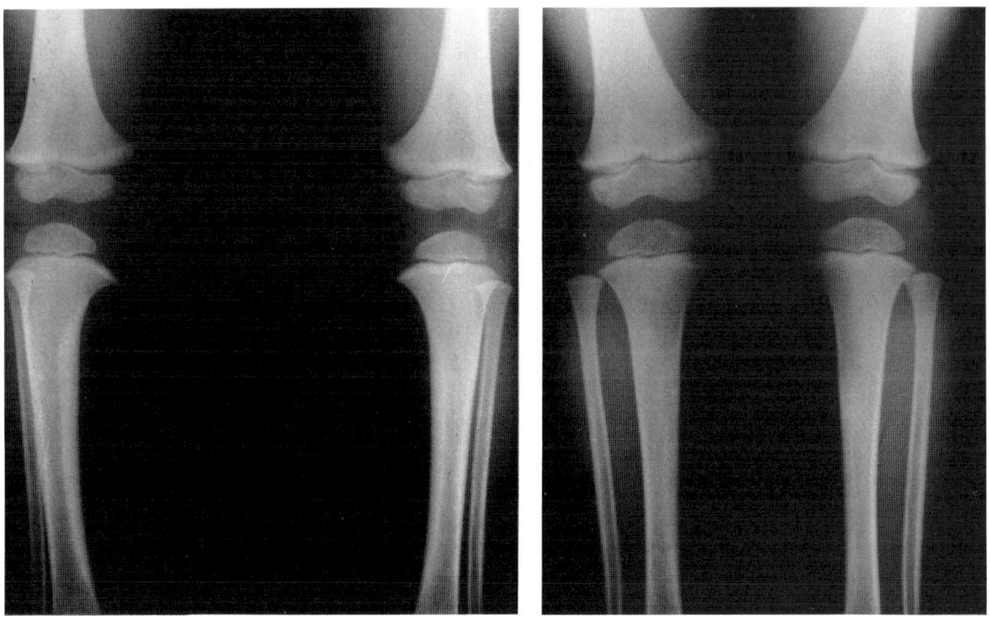

A B

Fig. 8–10 Physiologic bowing of the lower extremities. **(A)** At 2 years of age, genu varum deformity was present with mild beaking of the medial metaphyses about the knees. **(B)** By 3 years of age, the bowing deformity has corrected and mild knock-knee deformity has resulted. This deformity also corrects spontaneously in most cases.

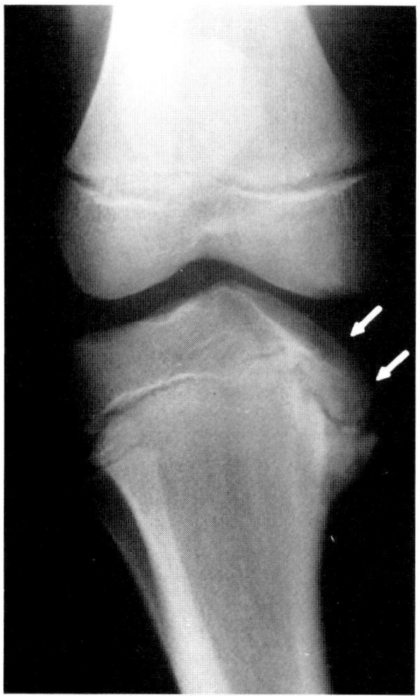

Fig. 8–11 Blount's disease. Growth disturbance of the medial tibia has resulted in marked sloping of the medial tibial epiphysis and metaphysis (*arrows*). This deformity results in a marked bowing deformity at the knee.

ages. If deformity persists, derotational osteotomies are used for correction.

When bowing deformity does not spontaneously resolve, Blount's disease must be considered. Blount's disease (tibia vara) is a developmental abnormality resulting from a growth disturbance of the medial aspect of the proximal tibial epiphysis. In addition to the prominent varus deformity that progresses, this condition is characterized by caudal sloping of the medial tibial metaphysis, terminating in a prominent beak (Fig. 8–11). The medial portion of the epiphysis is small and also slopes caudally. Blount's disease may be unilateral or bilateral, and sometimes requires a wedge osteotomy to correct the deformity.

Abnormal bone mineralization leading to soft bones may also result in bowing deformity. This is most commonly the result of rickets, but can also be seen with hyperparathyroidism, hypophosphatasia, and hyperphosphatemia. Bowed bones leading to bowed extremities are characteristic of a number of bony dysplasias or syndromes. If the bowing is unilateral, some type of injury to the growth plate (e.g., infection, trauma) is often responsible.

LONG BONES

Generalized Increased Bone Density

A generalized increase in the density of the bones is most often the result of either a bone dysplasia or a metabolic abnormality resulting in excessive calcium deposition in the bones. The classic bone dysplasia

GENERALIZED INCREASED BONE DENSITY

Congenital/developmental
- Osteopetrosis
- Pyknodysostosis
- William's syndrome
- Robinow's syndrome
- van Buchem's disease
- Tubular stenosis syndrome
- Melorheostosis
- Pachydermoperiostosis
- Engelmann's disease
- Craniodiaphyseal dysplasia

Inflammatory
- Neonatal intrauterine infection

Neoplasm
- Leukemia (myelofibrosis)

Systemic/metabolic
- Renal osteodystrophy (healing)
- Hypervitaminosis D
- Hypothyroidism
- Heavy metal intoxication
- Mucopolysaccharidosis
- Mucolipidosis
- Fluorosis
- Mastocytosis
- Sarcoidosis

Miscellaneous
- Idiopathic osteosclerosis of newborn

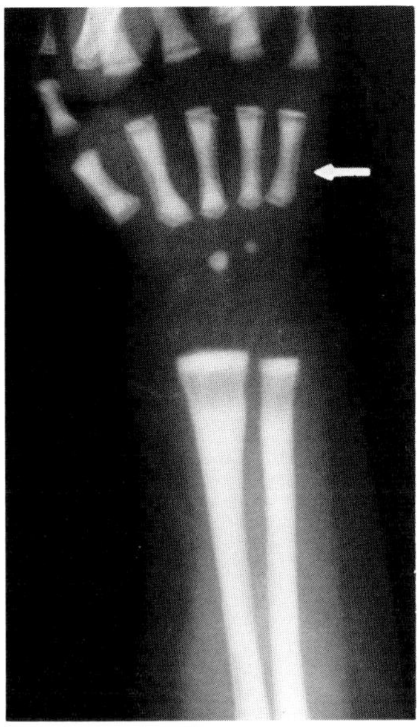
A

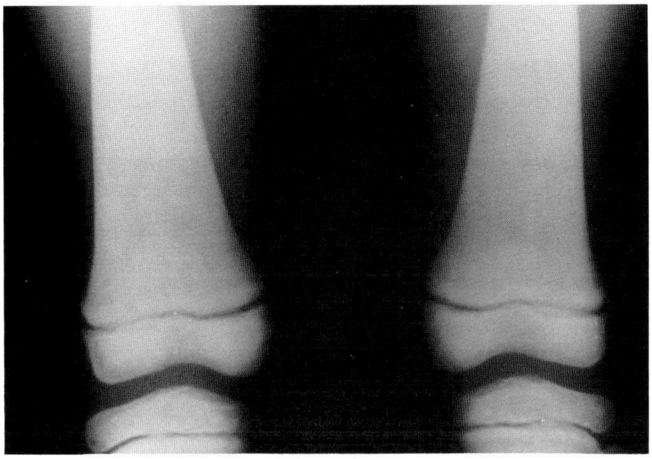
B

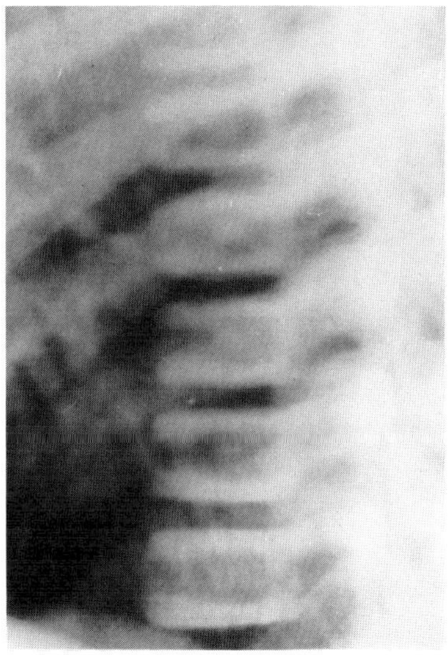
C

Fig. 8–12 Osteopetrosis. **(A)** The hand of this newborn with osteopetrosis shows the characteristic bone within bone appearance (*arrow*). The bones of the forearm are markedly dense, except for transverse bands of radiolucency in the metaphysis. These changes are sometimes mistaken for the trophic bands seen in the long bones of patients with congenital infections such as syphilis. **(B)** An older child with osteopetrosis demonstrates homogeneously dense bones with mild Erlenmeyer flask deformity. The vertebrae may be uniformly dense or **(C)** may demonstrate increased density along the end plates only, as in this patient.

resulting in increased bone density is osteopetrosis (Albers-Schönberg disease). Osteopetrosis is thought to be caused by abnormal osteoclast activity, leading to failure of normal resorption of the primary spongiosa. The bones become extremely dense and eventually the medullary cavity is obliterated. Encroachment on the medullary cavity as well as a hemolytic component lead to profound anemia and hepatosplenomegaly in these patients. Marked calvarial thickening can lead to narrowing of the cranial nerve foramina with nerve compression. A characteristic bone-within-bone appearance has been described (Fig. 8–12). Although the bones appear dense, they are actually quite brittle and tend to fracture easily.

Pyknodysostosis is a bone dysplasia that results in dense bones similar to osteopetrosis. Nevertheless, no hematologic abnormalities occur in this dysplasia. In William's syndrome, idiopathic hypercalcemia can result in generalized osteosclerosis. Supravalvular aortic stenosis and an elfin facies are also a part of this syndrome. Several congenital syndromes result

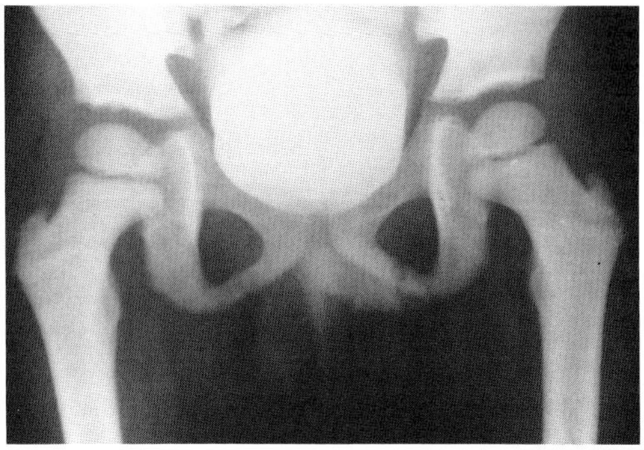

Fig. 8–13 Hematologic disease. Increased density of the long bones in a child with granulocytic leukemia.

in osteosclerosis that predominantly involves the diaphysis. These include tubular stenosis syndrome, melorheostosis, pachydermoperiostosis, hyperphosphatemia, craniodiaphyseal dysplasia, and Englemann's diaphyseal dysplasia.

Most of the other conditions that result in increased bone density involve metabolic abnormalities that affect the deposition of calcium in the bones. Patients on dialysis because of chronic renal disease often develop dense bones. Other metabolic causes include hypervitaminosis D, hypothyroidism, mucopolysaccharidosis, and mucolipidosis. Chronically increased intake of heavy metals or fluoride may also cause dense bones.

In the newborn, a normal transient form of osteosclerosis can occur, probably because of a larger percentage of spongiosa in the bones of these infants. This must be differentiated from the increased bone density that may be seen in neonatal infections, primarily rubella and syphilis.

Hematologic disease is an uncommon cause of osteosclerosis in children. Occasionally, leukemia accompanied by myelofibrosis can cause increased bone density (Fig. 8–13). Multiple bone infarcts in older children who have sickle cell disease can, rarely, lead to patchy areas of sclerosis, which may eventually become confluent.

Generalized Decreased Bone Density

A generalized decrease in the density of the bones because of abnormal calcium content may be due to either osteoporosis or osteomalacia. These two conditions differ in pathogenesis and, in their pure form, have distinct radiographic characteristics. However, it is not uncommon for both processes to be present simultaneously.

Disease processes that result in the abnormal formation or loss of bone matrix result in osteoporosis. In children, osteoporosis is most commonly caused by atrophy that occurs with immobilization. When the normal forces on a bone are removed, osteoblastic activity decreases relative to osteoclastic activity, gradually leading to bone loss and demineralization. Hyperemia can also result in bone atrophy. Such hyperemia in children is usually associated with trauma, infection, or inflammation. Rarely an arteriovenous fistula may lead to hyperemia and focal osteoporosis. Elevated steroids (exogenous or endogenous), certain bone dysplasias, and disease processes that result in marrow hypertrophy or replacement (e.g., chronic anemia, storage diseases) may also lead to osteoporosis.

Radiographically the deficiency of bone matrix results in a decreased number of trabeculae with prominence of the remaining trabeculae. The bone cortex is thinned but appears dense compared to the spongy bone (Fig. 8–14).

Osteomalacia results in a radiographic pattern that is quite different from osteoporosis. The bone cortex is demineralized but not thinned. The cortex and the trabecular pattern are indistinct in children. While enchondral bone growth still occurs, characteristic changes occur in the metaphyses. The growth plate appears widened, the normal zone of provisional calcification is lost, and the metaphysis is splayed, cupped, and irregular (Fig. 8–15).

The various types of rickets are the most common cause of osteomalacia in children. Vitamin D dependent rickets and vitamin D deficiency due to nutritional disturbances most commonly occur in infants.

OSTEOPOROSIS

Congenital/developmental
- Osteogenesis imperfecta
- Turner's syndrome
- Winchester syndrome
- Progeria
- Ehler-Danlos syndrome

Inflammation
- Hyperemia with inflammation or infection

Neoplasm
- Hepatic tumors

Trauma/surgery
- Disuse (immobilization)

Systemic/metabolic
- Poor nutrition (failure to thrive)
- Chronic anemia
- Collagen vascular disease
- Idiopathic hypercalcemia
- Cushing's syndrome
- Mucopolysaccharidoses
- Mucolipidoses
- Hyperthyroidism
- Gaucher's disease
- Scurvy
- Neimann-Pick disease
- Pseudo- or pseudopseudohypoparathyroidism
- Mastocytosis
- Homocystinuria
- Phenylketonuria
- Hyperphosphatemia
- Farber's lipogranolomatosis

Miscellaneous
- Steroid therapy
- Idiopathic juvenile osteoporosis
- Sudek's atrophy

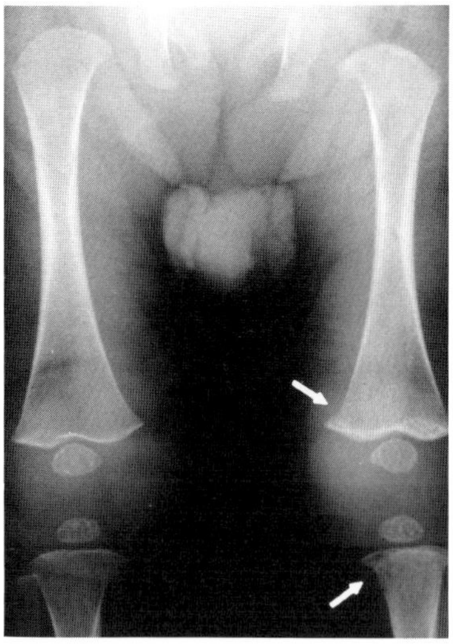

Fig. 8–14 Nutritional osteoporosis in a 2-month-old infant. The long bones demonstrate diffuse demineralization with thin, but dense, cortical bone. Weakening of the bones has resulted in metaphyseal fractures (*arrows*).

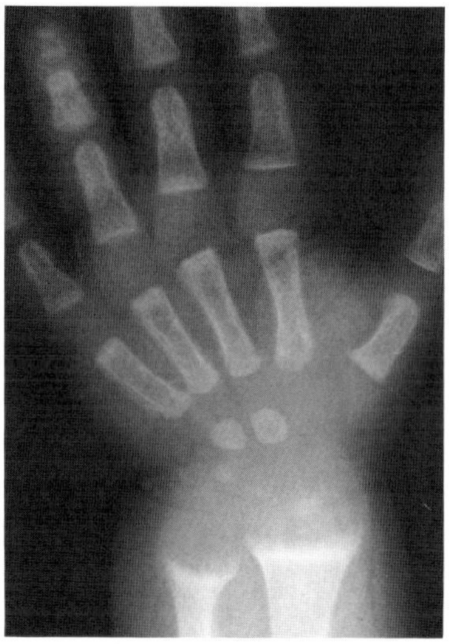

Fig. 8–15 Rickets in a 9-month-old infant. Note the characteristic splayed, cupped, and frayed metaphyses, widened distal radial growth plate, and indistinct bone cortex.

Rickets due to proximal renal tubular acidosis may also present in infancy. Familial hypophosphatemic rickets, renal osteodystrophy, and rickets secondary to cystinosis and anticonvulsive drug therapy generally appear later in childhood.

Hyperparathyroidism, most often secondary to renal osteodystrophy, is another common cause of osteomalacia in children. In these children, the typical changes of rickets are combined with subperiosteal bone resorption, seen best along the middle phalanges

OSTEOMALACIA

Congenital/developmental
- Fibrogenesis imperfecta

Systemic/metabolic
- Rickets
- Hyperparathyroidism
- Hypophosphatasia
- Gangliosidosis
- Mucolipidosis II
- Metaphyseal chondrodysplasia (Jansen)

of the hand, the medial aspect of the proximal tibial metaphysis, the distal radius and ulna, and the femoral neck (Fig. 8–16). Resorption along the lateral ends of the clavicles, the ribs, and the flat bones is not uncommon. Primary hyperparathyroidism is rare in children. Gangliosidosis, mucolipidosis type II, and Jansen's metaphyseal dysplasia are three conditions that produce bony changes typical of hyperparathyroidism in infancy. Nevertheless, hyperparathyroidism is not a part of these conditions and as the patient matures, the bones tend to appear more osteoporotic than osteomalacic.

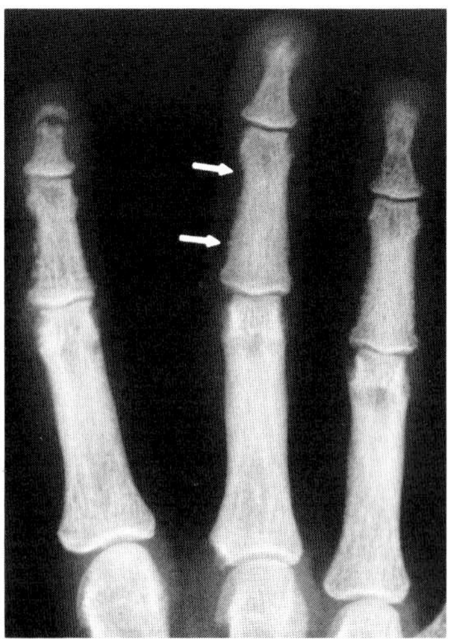

Fig. 8–16 Hyperparathyroidism. Advanced subperiosteal resorption of the phalanges (*arrows*) and fractures of the terminal tufts in a patient with renal osteodystrophy.

SHORT BROAD BONES

Congenital/developmental
- Achondroplasia
- Metaphyseal dysplasia
- Pseudoachondroplasia
- Dyschondrosteosis
- Turner's syndrome
- Cornelia de Lange syndrome
- Hypochondroplasia
- Chondrodysplasia punctata congenita
- Asphyxiating thoracic dystrophy
- Achondrogenesis
- Thanatophoric dwarfism
- Kniest syndrome
- Diastrophic dwarfism
- Campomelic dwarfism
- Larsen's syndrome
- Phocomelia (toxic embryonopathy)

Systemic/metabolic
- Storage diseases
- Hypothyroidism
- Rickets (hypophosphatemic)
- Hyperphosphatemia
- Hypophosphatasia

Short Broad Bones

Shortening of the long bones may be either focal or generalized. When focal, the most likely causes include congenital hypoplasia, trauma, and infection. Generalized long bone shortening encountered in the neonatal period is usually due to one of a number of bone dysplasias or dwarfing syndromes. The most common of these conditions is achondroplasia, an inherited disorder characterized by abnormal enchondral bone growth; the long bones are shortened with flared metaphyses (Fig. 8–17). Other typical findings include rectangular vertebral bodies and a narrowed lumbosacral spinal canal, shortened ribs with flared anterior ends, squared and hypoplastic iliac wings, flattened acetabular angles, and underdevelopment of the base of the skull and foramen magnum.

Many other bone dysplasias and dwarfing syndromes cause long bone changes similar to that of achondroplasia. Generally the appearance of the spine can be

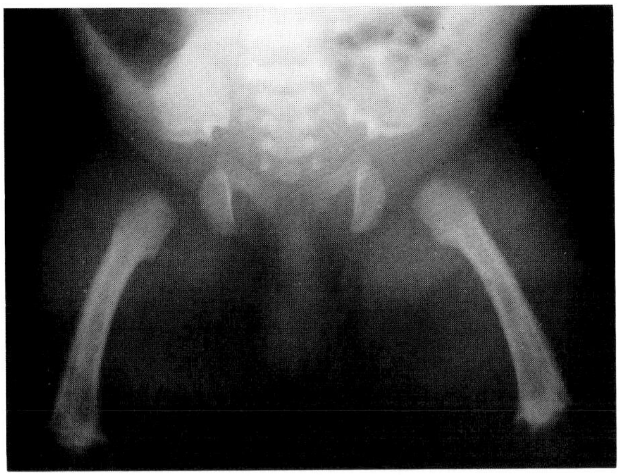

Fig. 8–17 Achondroplasia in a newborn. Note the characteristic short, broad femurs with flared metaphyses and the squared, hypoplastic iliac wings.

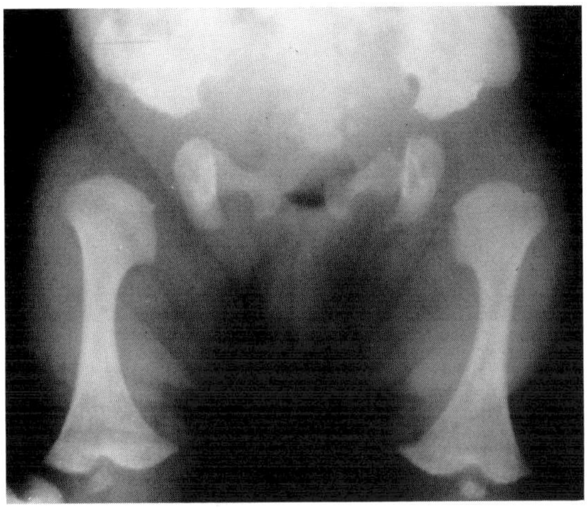

Fig. 8–18 Metatropic dwarfism. Prominence of the metaphyses of the femurs gives a dumbbell appearance.

used to help distinguish many of these conditions (Fig. 8–84). Nevertheless, certain long bone configurations are peculiar to some of these conditions.

Enlargement of the metaphyseal regions of the shortened long bones results in a dumb-bell appearance. This characteristic shape is most commonly seen in metatropic dwarfism (Fig. 8–18), Kneist syndrome, and severe pseudoachondroplasia.

Some conditions are characterized by long bone shortening that is more prominent in the middle segment of the extremities. This middle segment (mesomelic) shortening can be seen with mesomelic dwarfism (Fig. 8–19), dyschondrosteosis (Madelung's deformity), nail-patella syndrome, Ellis-van Creveld syndrome, Robinow's syndrome, and the ulnofibular dysplasias.

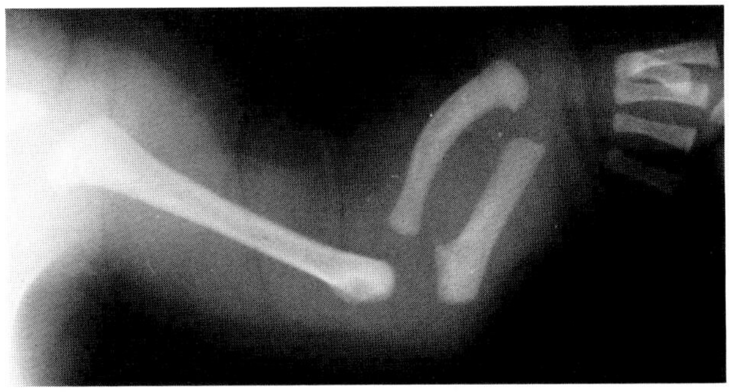

Fig. 8–19 Mesomelic dwarfism. The shortened and bowed bones of the forearm are typical of the middle segment shortening in this syndrome.

LONG THIN BONES

Congenital/developmental
- Osteogenesis imperfecta
- Arthrogryposis
- Marfan's syndrome
- Contractural arachnodactyly
- Cockayne syndrome
- Winchester syndrome
- Progeria
- Kenny-Caffey syndrome
- Stickler syndrome
- Hallermann-Streiff syndrome
- Werdnig-Hoffman disease

Systemic/metabolic
- Homocystinuria
- Rheumatoid arthritis

Miscellaneous
- Neurologic or neuromuscular disease
- Prolonged immobilization

Long Thin Bones

The most common cause of gracile bones is disuse of the extremity because of the hypotonia or paralysis

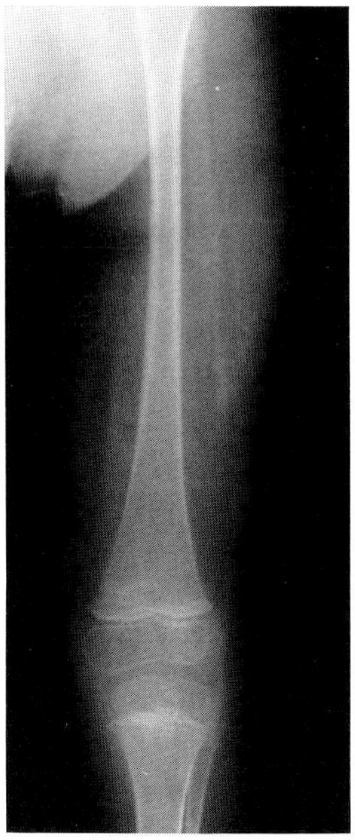

Fig. 8–20 Neurologic disease. Note the thin, gracile long bones with marked muscular atrophy.

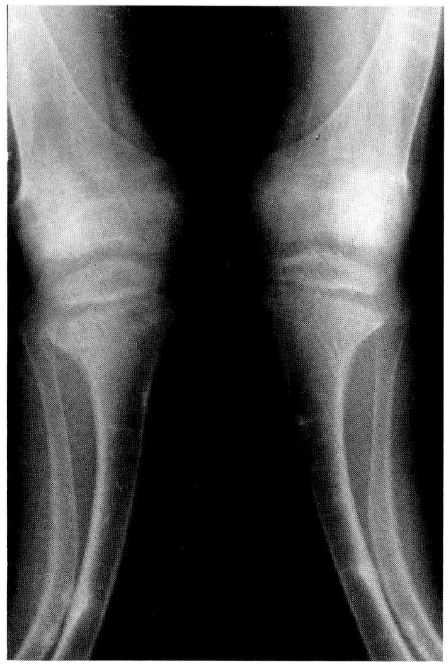

Fig. 8–21 Fanconi rickets secondary to glycogen storage disease. The long bones of the lower extremities are bowed with multiple pseudofractures, widened growth plates, and indistinct and irregular metaphyses.

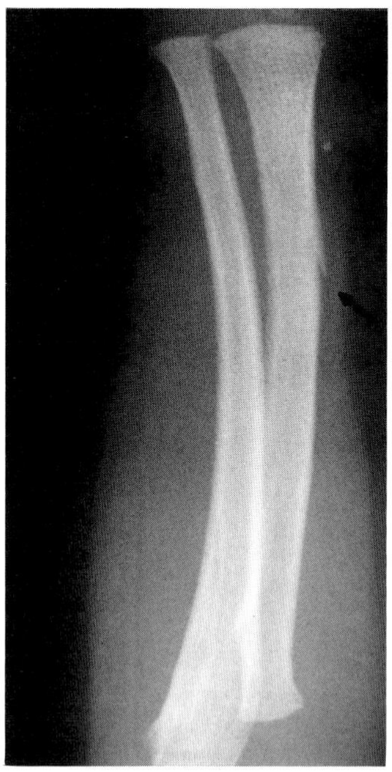

Fig. 8–22 Bending fracture. Note the exaggerated bending of the ulna associated with a greenstick fracture of the radius (*arrow*).

that accompanies many types of neurologic or neuromuscular disease (Fig. 8–20). Arthrogryposis describes a heterogenous group of conditions with an abnormal muscle-to-fat ratio and multiple congenital joint contractures. Other conditions that would lead to chronically decreased mobility, such as rheumatoid arthritis or severe trauma, can also result in long thin bones.

A number of bone dysplasias are also characterized by thin, gracile bones (see list). In the Kenny-Caffey syndrome, although the bones are thinned, the cortex is thickened resulting in stenosis of the medullary cavity. Lengthening of the long bones is more prominent in congenital contractural arachnodactyly, Marfan's syndrome, and homocystinuria.

Bowed Bones

Generalized bowing of the long bones is most often caused by either metabolic abnormalities leading to osteomalacia or to one of a variety of bone dysplasias. The list of bone dysplasias characterized by bowed long bones is rather extensive, and other features of these syndromes must be used for differentiation (see *Syndromes and Dysplasias*); achondroplasia is the most common dwarfing syndrome to exhibit bowed bones.

Rickets is the most common metabolic abnormality leading to softened, bowed bones. Weight bearing causes the bowing in these patients to be more prominent in the lower extremities (Fig. 8–21). In the neonate, bowed bones may be due to softened bones in utero, as occurs in such conditions as hypophosphatasia and osteogenesis imperfecta congenita. These conditions must be differentiated from the bowing that can occur as a result of abnormal intrauterine positioning or oligohydramnios.

Often, the bowing deformity that is caused by osteomalacic bones or abnormal intrauterine positioning will be quite asymmetrical or even focal. Focal bowing deformity also suggests bending fractures, which are common in childhood. Comparison views of the extremities are extremely helpful in identifying these injuries, which can be quite subtle (Fig. 8–22). Focal bowing of long bones may also occur following infection or trauma. Bowing of the tibia and fibula can be seen in patients with neurofibromatosis prior to the development of a congenital pseudoarthrosis. Nevertheless, this is also a common site for bowing due to abnormal intrauterine positioning. It is important to note that the curvature of congenital pseudoarthrosis of the tibia and fibula is anterolateral (Fig.

BOWED BONES

Congenital/developmental
- Achondroplasia
- Osteogenesis imperfecta congenita
- Metaphyseal dysplasia
- Madelung's deformity
- Diastrophic dwarfism
- Hypochondroplasia
- Thanatophoric dwarfism
- Campomelic dwarfism
- Larsen's syndrome
- Pseudoachondroplasia
- Asphyxiating thoracic dystrophy
- Melnick-Needles syndrome
- Ellis-van Creveld syndrome
- Parastremmatic dwarfism
- Contractural arachnodactyly
- Achondrogenesis
- Short rib-polydactyly syndromes
- Mesomelic dwarfism
- Robinow's syndrome

Systemic/metabolic
- Rickets
- Hyperparathyroidism
- Hypophosphatasia
- Hyperphosphatemia
- Mucopolysaccharidoses
- Mucolipidoses

Miscellaneous
- Intrauterine positional deformity
- Oligohydramnios

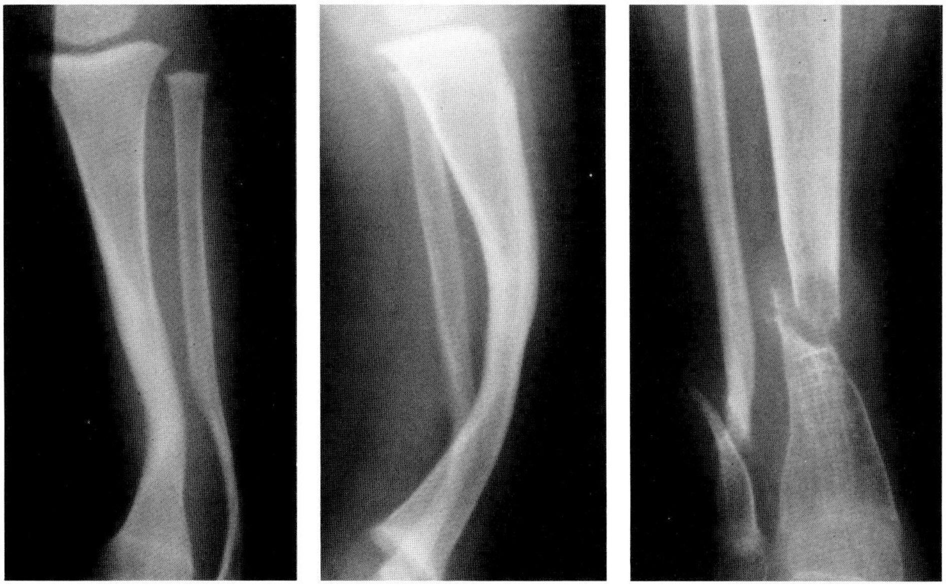

Fig. 8–23 Congenital pseudoarthrosis of the tibia and fibula in a patient with neurofibromatosis. **(A)** Anterioposterior and **(B)** lateral radiographs taken when the child was young, demonstrated characteristic anterolateral bowing and thinning of the shaft of the tibia and fibula. **(C)** The same patient later developed typical pseudoarthroses at the previous sites of bowing.

8–23), as opposed to the characteristic posteromedial bending associated with faulty intrauterine positioning. The pseudoarthroses associated with neurofibromatosis also demonstrate dysplastic bone changes, including thinning and cortical irregularity.

Focal Hypoplasia or Aplasia

Focal bone hypoplasia more commonly involves the upper extremities. Hypoplasia or aplasia often involves the radius and the first and second digits of the hand and is referred to as a radial ray deficiency (Fig. 8–24). This abnormality is a part of a number of syndromes and anomalies; the most well known include the Holt-Oram syndrome, Poland's syndrome, Fanconi's anemia, and the TAR (thrombocytopenia-absent radius) syndrome. The Holt-Oram syndrome is characterized by congenital heart disease and variable anomalies of the upper extremity, clavicle, and chest wall. Poland's syndrome combines partial or complete absence of the pectoralis muscles and anomalies of the ipsilateral upper extremity. In the TAR syndrome, the radii are absent bilaterally, but the thumbs are always present. In Fanconi's ane-

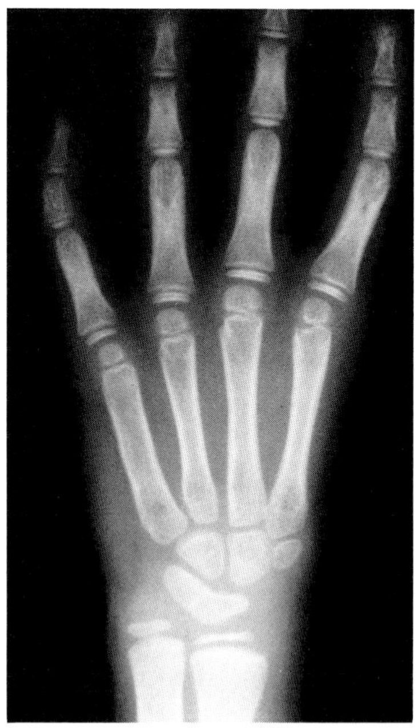

Fig. 8–24 Radial ray deficiency. Hypoplasia of the radius and absence of the thumb in a patient with Holt-Oram syndrome.

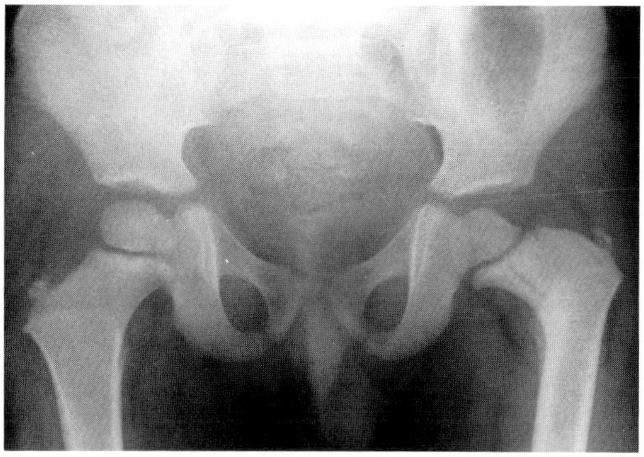

Fig. 8–25 Congenital coxa vara. The angle between the femoral shaft and neck is decreased and the growth plate lies at an oblique angle.

mia, radial ray deformity accompanies hematologic disorders, renal anomalies, and increased incidence of malignancies. The radial ray deformity is also a component of the VATER association.

Congenital underdevelopment of the femur is known as the proximal focal femoral deficiency syndrome. In its mildest form, the femoral dysgenesis is manifest as a decreased angle between the femoral neck and shaft and is referred to as congenital coxa vara (Fig. 8–25). More severe forms of this condition result in a variable degree of hypoplasia of the proximal femur, with resultant dysplasia of the ipsilateral acetabulum (Fig. 8–26). Various forms of hypoplasia or absence of the tibia with an intact fibula also occur.

Synostoses and Pseudoarthroses

Synostosis of bones is usually a congenital abnormality and is frequently associated with sex chromosome abnormalities such as Klinefelter's syndrome and the XXXY syndrome. The proximal radius and ulna is the most common site of the fusion and is associated with congenital dislocation of the radial head (Fig. 8–27). Radioulnar synostosis may also be seen with a number of other syndromes (Ehlers-Danlos syndrome, fetal alcohol syndrome, Holt-Oram syn-

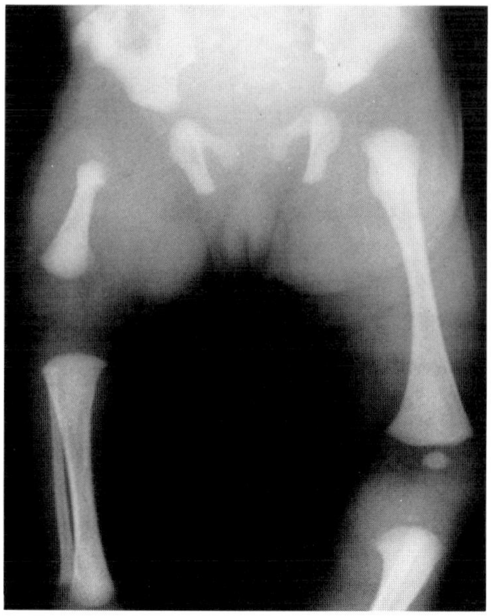

Fig. 8–26 Proximal focal femoral deficiency. The right femur is markedly hypoplastic and tapered.

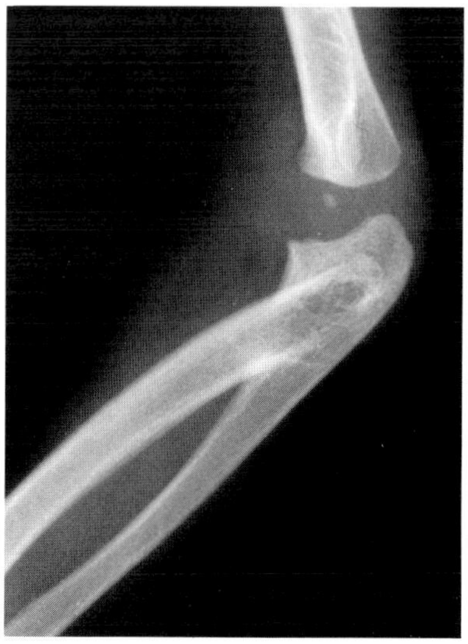

Fig. 8–27 Radioulnar synostosis associated with congential dislocation of the radial head. The proximal radius is tapered, rounded, and fused to the proximal ulna.

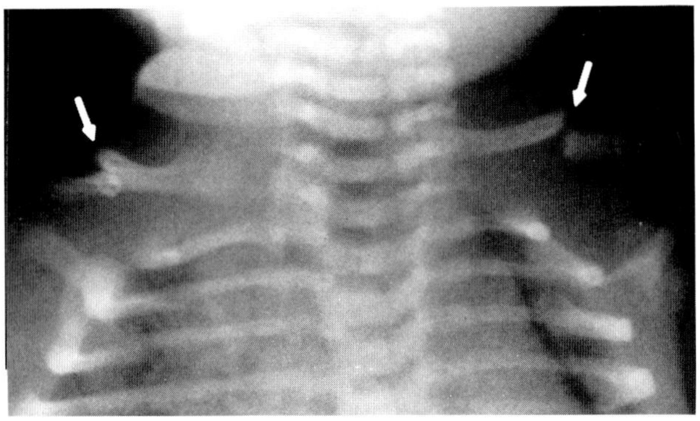

Fig. 8–28 Bilateral congenital pseudoarthroses of the clavicles. Note the rounded and slightly expanded ends of the bones at the sites of the pseudoarthroses (*arrows*).

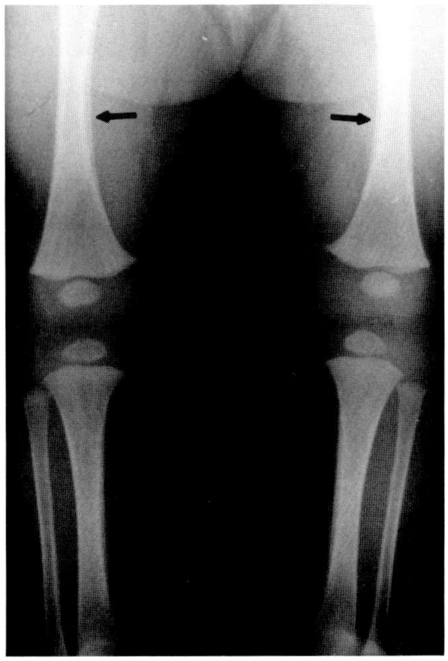

Fig. 8–29 Physiological periosteal new bone in a 3-month old. A thin layer of diaphyseal periosteal new bone is present along the medial aspects of the femurs and tibias (*arrows*).

drome) or it may be an isolated anomaly. Acquired synostoses may also occur, usually following a severe inflammatory process of the bone. This is a well known phenomenon in infantile cortical hyperostosis (Caffey's disease). Post-traumatic synostoses also occur.

Pseudoarthroses are more likely to be acquired than congenital. These pseudoarthroses are usually the sequela of fracture nonunion and are somewhat more frequent in patients with focal or generalized increased bone fragility (osteogenesis imperfecta, osteoporosis, osteomyelitis, bone cysts).

Congenital pseudoarthroses occur most commonly in the clavicle and the lower extremity. Pseudoarthrosis of the clavicle is usually an isolated anomaly and must be differentiated from the more common clavicular fracture. A clavicular pseudoarthrosis will show no evidence of healing and the ends of the bone adjacent to the disruption are rounded and bulbous (Fig. 8–28). The tibia and fibula are the other common sites for pseudoarthrosis and are most often seen in patients with neurofibromatosis (Fig. 8–23). Pseudoarthrosis of the femur occurs in conjunction with the proximal focal femoral deficiency syndrome. Other less common sites include the radius and ulna.

Periosteal New Bone

Periosteal new bone deposition in children is most often a reaction to irritation of the periosteum by a disease process arising from within the bone or in the adjacent soft tissues or joints. The presence of a periosteal reaction always indicates pathology, except in young infants (aged 2 to 6 months). In some infants, commonly premature infants, a thin layer of diaphyseal periosteal new bone may appear transiently. This reaction is most commonly seen in the femurs, tibia, and humeri, tends to be more prominent along the medial aspect of the diaphysis (Fig. 8–29), and probably reflects unusually vigorous bone growth in these normal infants.

A wide variety of disease processes can result in periosteal new bone formation in children (see list). The list of possible etiologies can be shortened by classifying the periosteal new bone as one of four configurations: (1) solid, (2) lamellar, (3) spiculated, and (4) ballooned.

PERIOSTEAL NEW BONE

Congenital/developmental
- Pachydermoperiostosis
- Macrodystrophia lipomatosa
- Neurofibromatosis

Inflammation
- Congenital syphilis
- Osteomyelitis
- Juvenile rheumatoid arthritis
- Caffey's disease

Neoplasm
- Leukemia/lymphoma
- Metastatic neoplasm
- Infantile hamartomatosis

Trauma/surgery
- Fractures

Systemic/metabolic
- Hypervitaminosis A, D
- Scurvy
- Copper deficiency
- Prostaglandin E therapy
- Healing rickets
- Thyroid acropachy
- Gangliosidosis
- Mucolipidosis II
- Hyperphosphatemia
- Gaucher's disease

Miscellaneous
- Hypertrophic osteoarthropathy
- Bone infarction
- Cellulitis
- Normal infants
- Mastocytosis

Solid periosteal reactions may be straight or lumpy, but usually the layer of periosteal new bone is rather thick. This type of periosteal reaction indicates an indolent disease process such as a healing fracture or a chronic soft tissue infection. Infantile cortical hyperostosis (Caffey's disease) is an uncommon condition that presents with soft tissue swelling and exuberant periosteal reaction that is often solid in appearance. The precise etiology is unknown, although it is probably an inflammatory condition, very likely caused by a virus. The most commonly involved bones include the mandible (80 to 90 percent), clavicle, ribs, and long bones. Flat bones such as the calvaria and the scapula can also occasionally be involved

A

B

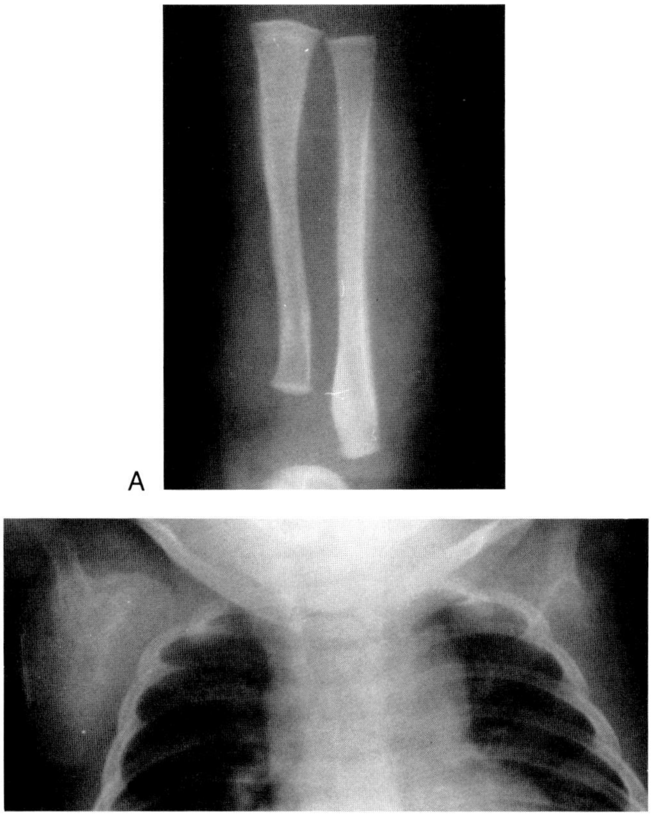

Fig. 8–30 Infantile cortical hyperostosis (Caffey disease). Soft tissue swelling and solid periosteal reaction involving **(A)** the ulna and **(B)** the right scapula.

A

B

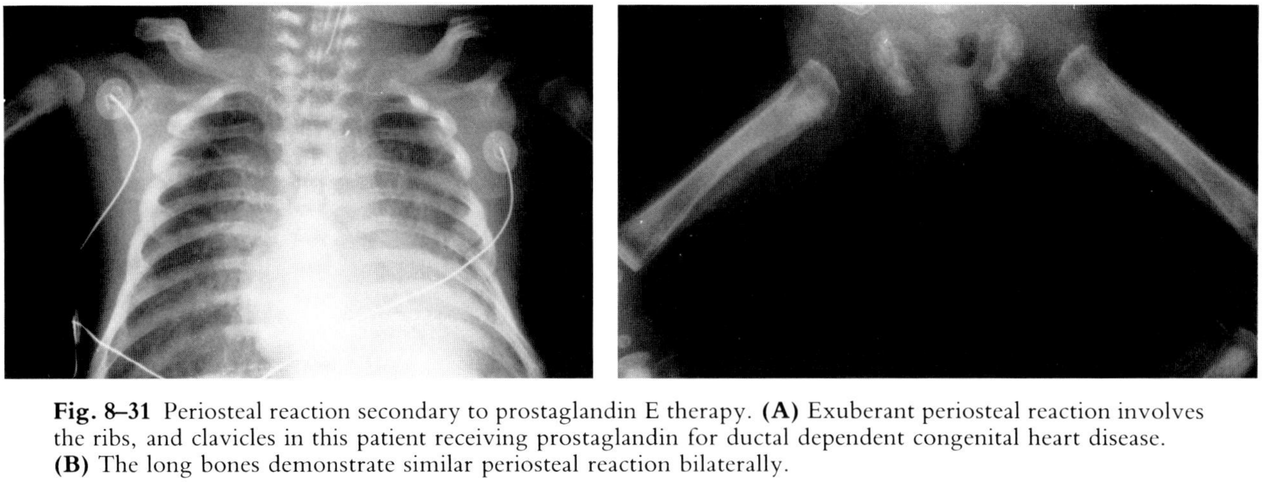

Fig. 8–31 Periosteal reaction secondary to prostaglandin E therapy. **(A)** Exuberant periosteal reaction involves the ribs, and clavicles in this patient receiving prostaglandin for ductal dependent congenital heart disease. **(B)** The long bones demonstrate similar periosteal reaction bilaterally.

(Fig. 8–30). The periosteal reaction is confined to the diaphysis and tends to spare the metaphysis. Although this is a self-limiting condition that gradually resolves, residual synostoses and bowing deformity may remain. Other conditions exhibiting this type of periosteal reaction include histiocytosis X, hypertrophic osteoarthropathy, pachydermoperiostosis, prostaglandin E therapy (Fig. 8–31), venous stasis, and thyroid acropachy (unusual in childhood).

A thin, single, solid layer of periosteal new bone characteristically occurs in more active disease processes such as osteomyelitis, bone infarction, healing rickets, hypervitaminosis A and D, neonatal infection (syphilis, rubella), and even malignant tumors (primary and secondary) (Fig. 8–32). As these diseases

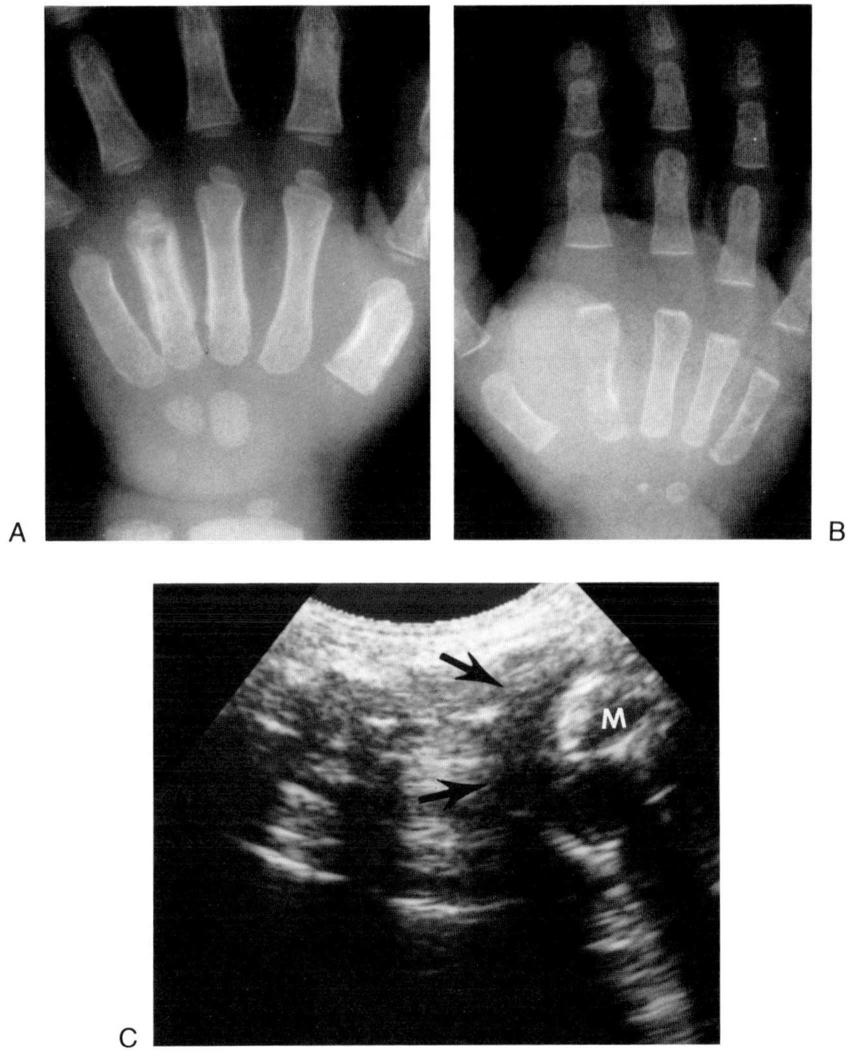

Fig. 8–32 Solid periosteal reaction. **(A)** Bone infarction involving the first and fourth metacarpals in this patient with sickle cell disease is manifest by bone destruction and periosteal reaction. **(B)** Osteomyelitis of the second metacarpal in a patient with chronic granulomatous disease. **(C)** A transverse sonogram of the hand reveals a cloak of hypoechoic edema or abscess (*arrows*) surrounding the involved metacarpal (*M*).

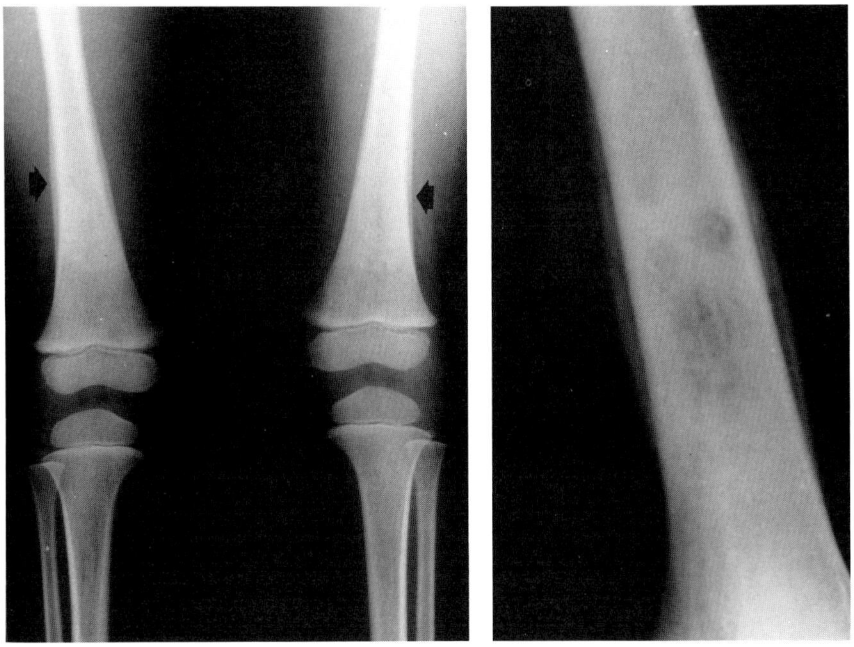

A B

Fig. 8–33 Thin periosteal reaction. **(A)** Thin layers of periosteal new bone in the femurs of a patient with leukemia (*arrows*). Note the transverse bands of decreased bone density in the metaphysis. **(B)** Bone destruction and lamellar periosteal new bone due to osteomyelitis of the femur.

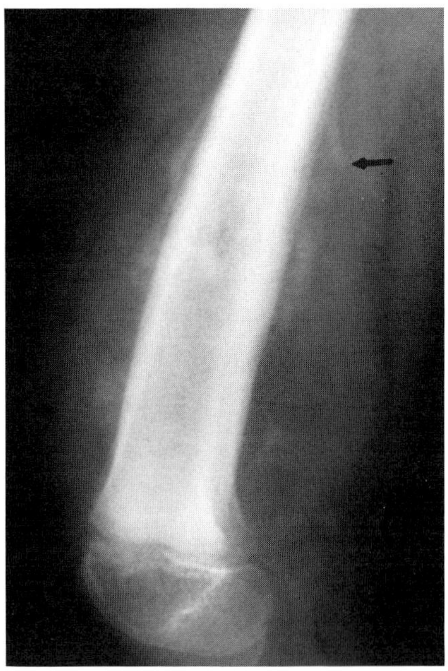

Fig. 8–34 Osteosarcoma of the distal femur. Interruption of the periosteal reaction (*arrow*), spiculated periosteal reaction, and a large soft tissue mass are common in this aggressive tumor.

progress or become more aggressive, multiple layers may be deposited giving an "onion-skin" or lamellar appearance (Fig. 8–33). Highly aggressive lesions, such as malignant bone tumors, break through the cortex and elevate the periosteum so rapidly that an interrupted periosteal reaction occurs. The resulting Codman's triangle is highly characteristic (Fig. 8–34).

A spiculated pattern of periosteal reaction is the result of new bone growth perpendicular to the long axis of the bone along Sharpey's fibers, which extend from the bone cortex to the elevated periosteum (Fig. 8–35). This pattern is only seen with highly aggressive lesions and is virtually pathognomonic of bone malignancy. The most common malignancies involving the bone in childhood include osteosarcoma, Ewing's sarcoma, metastatic neuroblastoma, leukemia, lymphoma, fibrosarcoma, and chondrosarcoma.

A single, thin but markedly elevated layer of periosteal new bone that cloaks the bone has been described as a ballooned periosteal reaction. This pattern is most commonly caused by the marked subperiosteal hemorrhage that occurs with fractures associated with child abuse and in neurologically impaired children (Fig. 8–36). The hemorrhage is probably the result of continued motion at the fracture site. Other causes of subperiosteal hemorrhage include neurofibromatosis, bleeding diathases, and scurvy. Mastocytosis and metabolic abnormalities such as gangliosidosis and hyperphosphatemia can occasionally cause ballooned periosteal new bone.

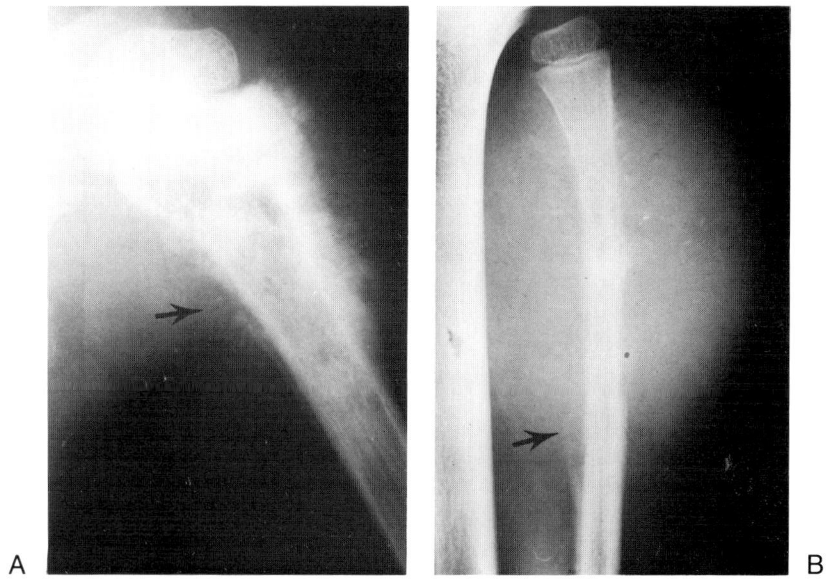

Fig. 8–35 Spiculated periosteal reaction. **(A)** Spiculated periosteal new bone (*arrow*) and dense tumor bone formation in osteosarcoma of the humerus. **(B)** Ewing's sarcoma of the fibula. Note the spiculations and Codman's triangle (*arrow*).

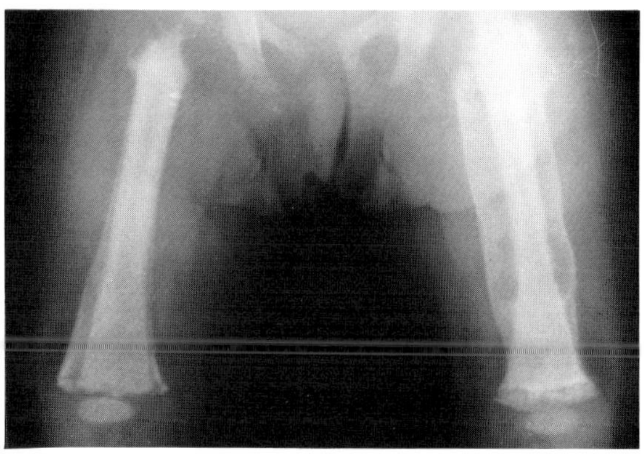

Fig. 8–36 Battered child syndrome. Multiple fractures and ballooned periosteal reaction due to physical abuse.

Focal Bone Sclerosis

The most common cause of an area of focal bone sclerosis in children is a healing stress fracture. These fractures most commonly occur in the proximal tibia and in older children (Fib. 8–37). Initially, healing stress fractures are not radiographically apparent; however as they begin to heal, a linear area of sclerosis in the region of the fracture develops, often accompanied by periosteal reaction. Before sclerosis development, scintigraphy is a sensitive method for detecting these often subtle fractures. Other common locations include the femoral neck, the fibula, and the metatarsals (Fig. 8–38).

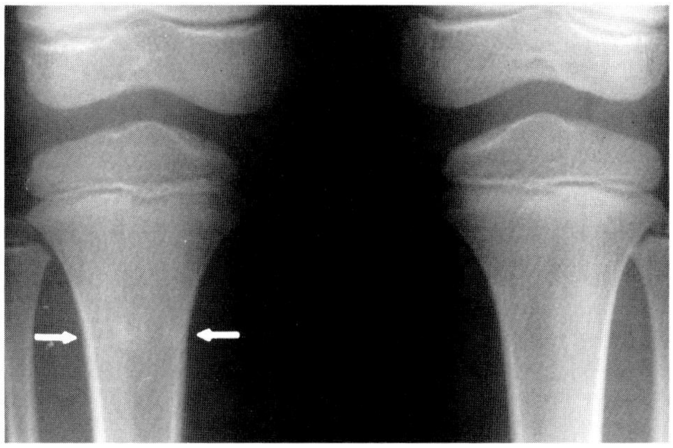

Fig. 8–37 Stress fracture of the proximal tibia. This healing stress fracture is manifest by periosteal reaction and a faint linear area of sclerosis (*arrows*) in the proximal tibia.

Developmental abnormalities such as healed fibrous cortical defects and fibrous dysplasia are moderately common causes of focal bone sclerosis. Healing bone infarction, healed histiocytosis X and, indeed, any healed lesion of bone can present as a sclerotic area. Patches of sclerotic bone occur in patients with tuberous sclerosis, particularly in the skull, long bones, vertebrae, and pelvis.

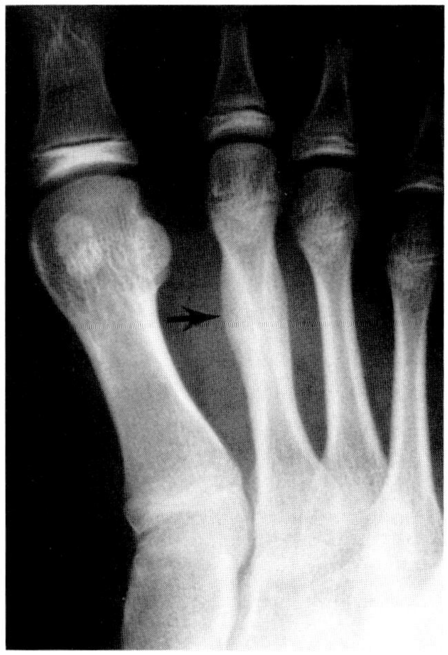

Fig. 8–38 Healing stress fracture of the metatarsal. Note the cortical thickening of the shaft of the second metatarsal (*arrow*) caused by a healing stress fracture.

FOCAL BONE SCLEROSIS

Congenital/developmental
- Fibrous dysplasia
- Healed fibrous cortical defect
- Bone island

Inflammatory
- Bone infarct
- Foreign body reaction
- Healing osteomyelitis

Neoplasm
- Osteoid osteoma
- Ewing's sarcoma
- Osteosarcoma
- Meningioma
- Osteoma
- Osteoblastic metastasis

Trauma/surgery
- Stress fracture

Systemic/metabolic
- Healed histiocytosis X
- Tuberous sclerosis

A number of bone tumors can cause a sclerotic appearance, although they are uncommon in children. The most common of these is the osteoid osteoma, a small, benign, highly vascular tumor that stimulates dense sclerosis in the surrounding bone (Fig. 8–39). These

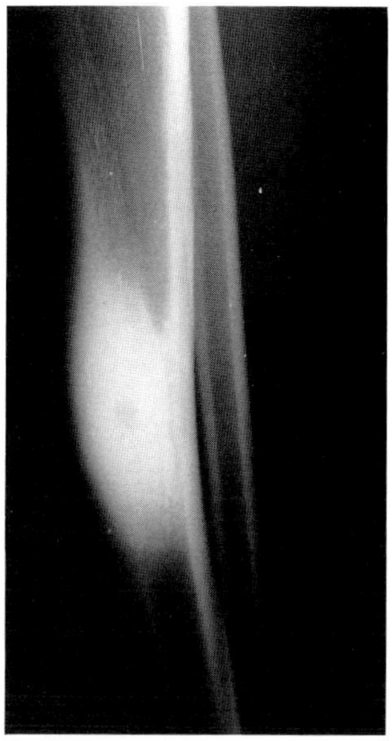

Fig. 8–39 Osteoid osteoma characteristically appears as a small radiolucent tumor nidus with prominent surrounding sclerosis. A cortical location is most common.

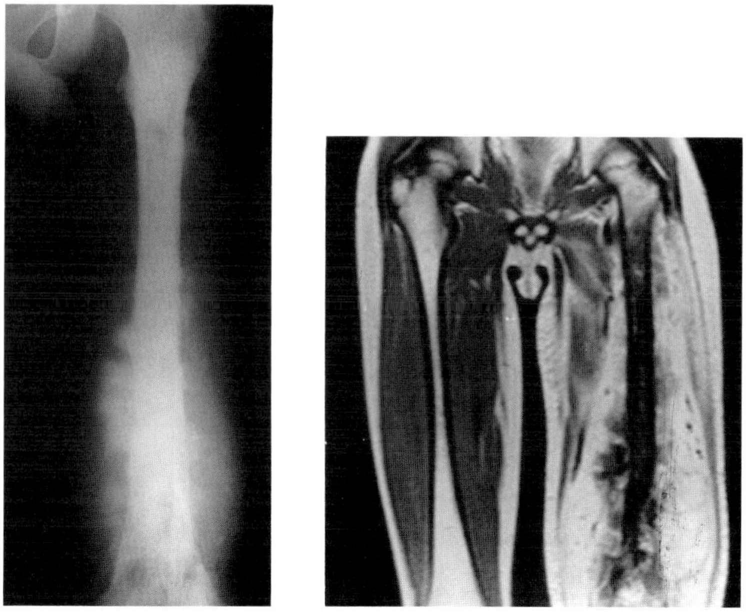

Fig. 8–40 Osteosarcoma. **(A)** Tumor bone formation in this large osteosarcoma of the femur resulted in sclerosis of the entire shaft of the involved bone. **(B)** A T_2-weighted coronal MRI provides better definition of the intraosseous and extraosseous extent.

lesions are quite painful and therefore require resection. Any bone may be affected, however the femur and tibia are the most common sites. The vertebrae and ribs can be involved, and this lesion should be considered whenever a painful scoliosis is encountered. It is imperative that the radiolucent tumor nidus be identified, as this lesion is prone to recur if the nidus is not completely excised. CT may be useful if plain radiographs fail to identify the nidus. The most common malignancies to present with sclerosis are Ewing's sarcoma and osteosarcoma (Fig. 8–40). Osteoblastic metastases are rare in childhood.

Focal Osteolytic Lesions

Focal areas of bone destruction can be the result of a wide variety of conditions. To facilitate the analysis of these lesions, certain features should be systematically evaluated, including the number of lesions; the location of the lesion within the bone; the pattern of bone destruction; the appearance of the margins of the lesion; the presence of calcification, ossification, or periosteal new bone; and the presence or absence of a soft tissue mass. Using these findings, one can usually offer a reasonable differential diagnosis.

Multiple osteolytic lesions are usually due to a widespread disease process, including metastatic malignancy, leukemia or lymphoma, and tumors associated with syndromes or skeletal dysplasias (e.g., Ollier's disease, multiple osteochondromatosis). Osteomyelitis in children commonly presents as multiple osteolytic lesions as it is more commonly caused by hematogenous spread of infection rather than local extension. Histiocytosis X is a relatively common cause of multiple osteolytic lesions (Fig. 8–41). Benign fibrous cortical defects can also be multiple.

FOCAL OSTEOLYTIC LESIONS

Congenital/developmental
- Fibrous cortical defect
- Nonossifying fibroma

Inflammation
- Osteomyelitis
- Bone infarction
- Neonatal infection (e.g., syphilis)
- Rheumatoid arthritis
- Tuberculous or fungal arthritis

Neoplasm/cyst
- Unicameral bone cyst
- Fibrous dysplasia
- Enchondroma
- Chondroblastoma
- Osteosarcoma
- Ewing's sarcoma
- Leukemia/lymphoma
- Metastatic malignancy
- Malignant fibrous histiocytoma
- Chondrosarcoma
- Fibrosarcoma
- Congenital fibromatosis
- Hemangioma
- Lymphangioma
- Chondromyxoid fibroma
- Aneurysmal bone cyst
- Giant cell tumor

Systemic/metabolic
- Brown tumor (hyperparathyroidism)
- Histiocytosis X
- Hemophilia (intraosseous hemorrhage)
- Intraosseous lipoma
- Foreign body granuloma

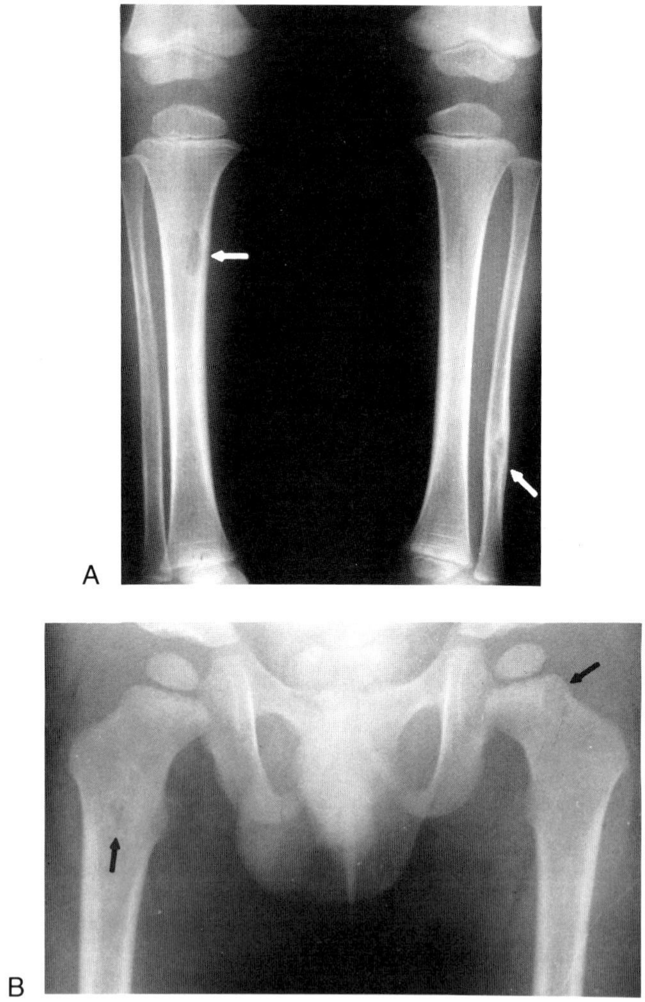

Fig. 8–41 Histiocytosis X. Multiple well defined osteolytic lesions involve **(A)** the right tibia, the left fibula (*arrows*), and **(B)** the proximal femurs bilaterally (*arrows*).

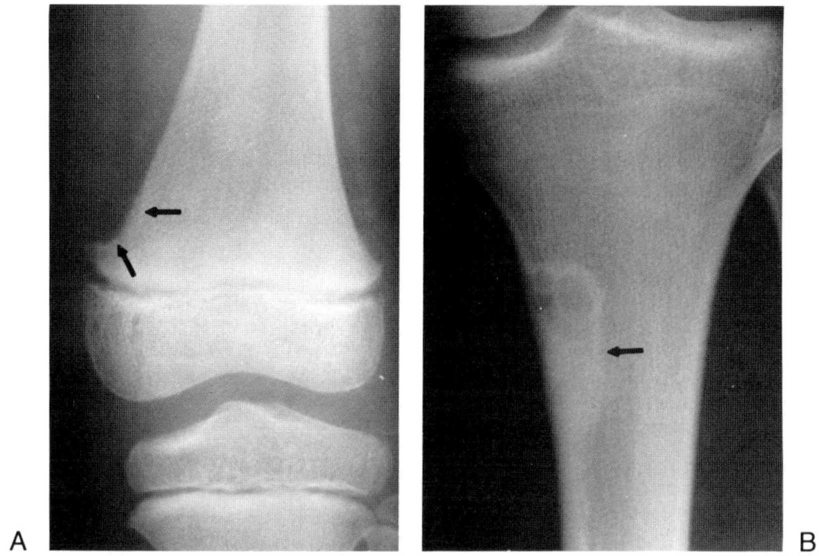

Fig. 8–42 Benign fibrous cortical defects. **(A)** A typical well defined osteolytic cortical defect in the metaphysis of the distal femur (*arrows*). **(B)** A larger lesion in the proximal tibia shows evidence of healing (*arrow*).

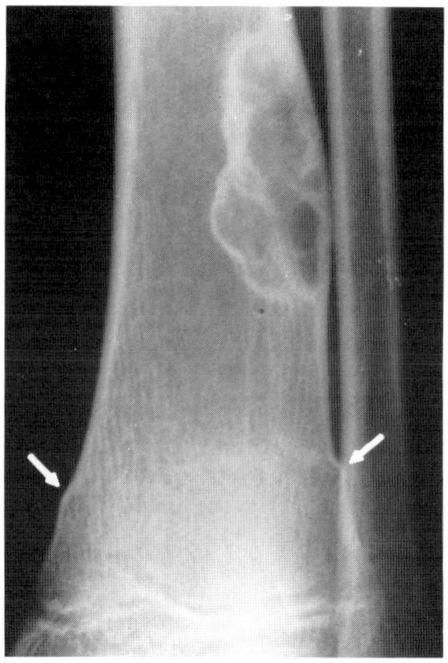

Fig. 8–43 Nonossifying fibroma. These benign lesions typically are eccentric with a sclerotic border and commonly have a bubbly appearance. Note the buckle fracture through the distal tibia (*arrows*), which led to the discovery of this asymptomatic lesion.

Lesions that occupy an eccentric position in the bone very often arise in the cortex. A common example is the benign fibrous cortical defect. These small, well-defined lesions most commonly occur in the metaphyses around the knees and are more common medially than laterally (Fig. 8–42). These defects are of no clinical importance and eventually heal completely. Nonossifying fibroma is a similar, although larger lesion involving the cortex (Fig. 8–43). Occasionally, low grade osteomyelitis will produce a similar appearance.

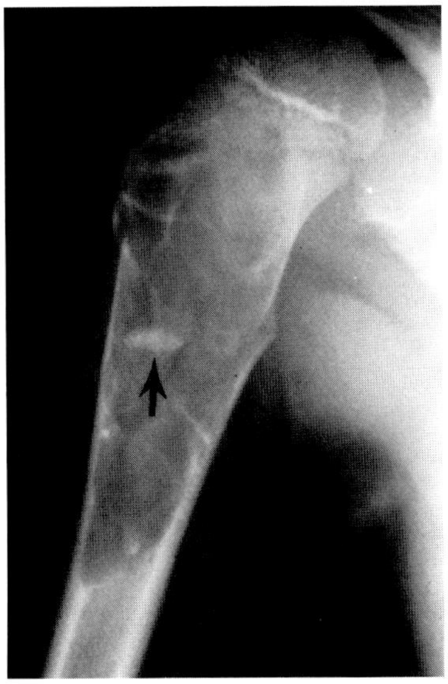

Fig. 8–44 Solitary bone cyst with pathologic fracture. This large, well defined, cyst of the proximal humerus has resulted in a pathologic fracture. Note the fallen fragment (*arrow*).

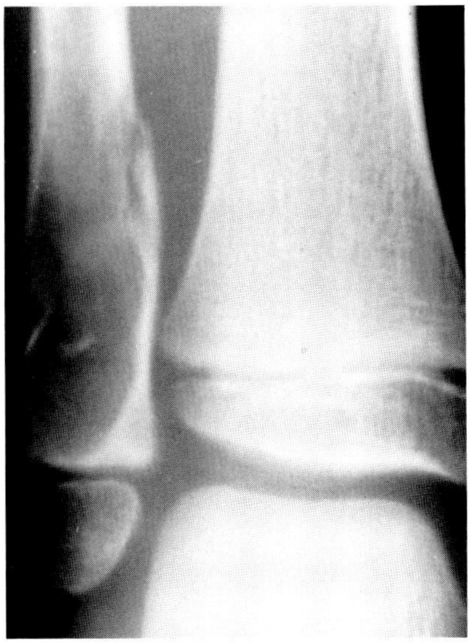

Fig. 8–45 A fractured bone cyst of the distal fibula similar to that pictured in Figure 8–44.

Lesions that arise within the medullary bone occupy a central location. A typical example of this type of lesion is the solitary or unicameral bone cyst. These fluid-filled cysts appear as radiolucent, thin-walled metaphyseal lesions that can expand the bone and thin the cortex (Fig. 8–44). The presence of a solitary cyst weakens the bone making it susceptible to fracture. When a fracture occurs, a small bone fragment may fall into the cyst cavity, creating the characteristic "fallen fragment sign" (Fig. 8–45). These lesions will slowly heal, especially following repeated fractures; however, intervention is often desirable to hasten the healing process. Most bone tumors are central within the bone, except for the osteotoid osteoma and nonossifying fibroma, which are more commonly cortical. Osteolysis due to osteomyelitis can involve both the medullary cavity and the cortex.

In lesions affecting the long bones, the portion of the bone involved can be a useful discriminator. The metaphysis is the most common location for lesions such as osteomyelitis, metastatic disease, bone cysts, many bone tumors, and bone infarction. Diaphyseal lesions are less common, and include Ewing's sarcoma, histiocytosis X, and fibrous dysplasia. Epiphyseal lesions are rather uncommon. Osteolytic defects of the epiphysis may be caused by osteomyelitis, rheumatoid arthritis, tuberculous or fungal arthritis, osteochondritis dissecans, or rarely, histiocytosis X or bone cysts. Chondroblastoma and giant cell tumors are the only tumors that commonly affect the epiphysis.

The rate of bone destruction can be inferred from the appearance of the margins of an osteolytic lesion. Benign or slowly progressive lesions are usually sharply defined, with clear differentiation between the lesion and the surrounding normal bone. Sclerotic margins may be present, particularly in such lesions as bone cysts, Brodie's abscess, fibrous dysplasia hemangioma, lymphangioma, giant cell tumor, aneurysmal bone cyst, and occasionally enchondroma. Sharply defined lesions without a sclerotic border include histiocytosis X, osteomyelitis, fibrous dysplasia, osteitis fibrosa cystica, and intraosseous hemorrhage (Fig. 8–46).

Aggressive lesions causing rapid bone destruction are characterized by ill-defined and irregular margins that are difficult to distinguish from surrounding normal bone. Often the lesion will cause a "moth-eaten" or permeative appearance rather than a discrete area

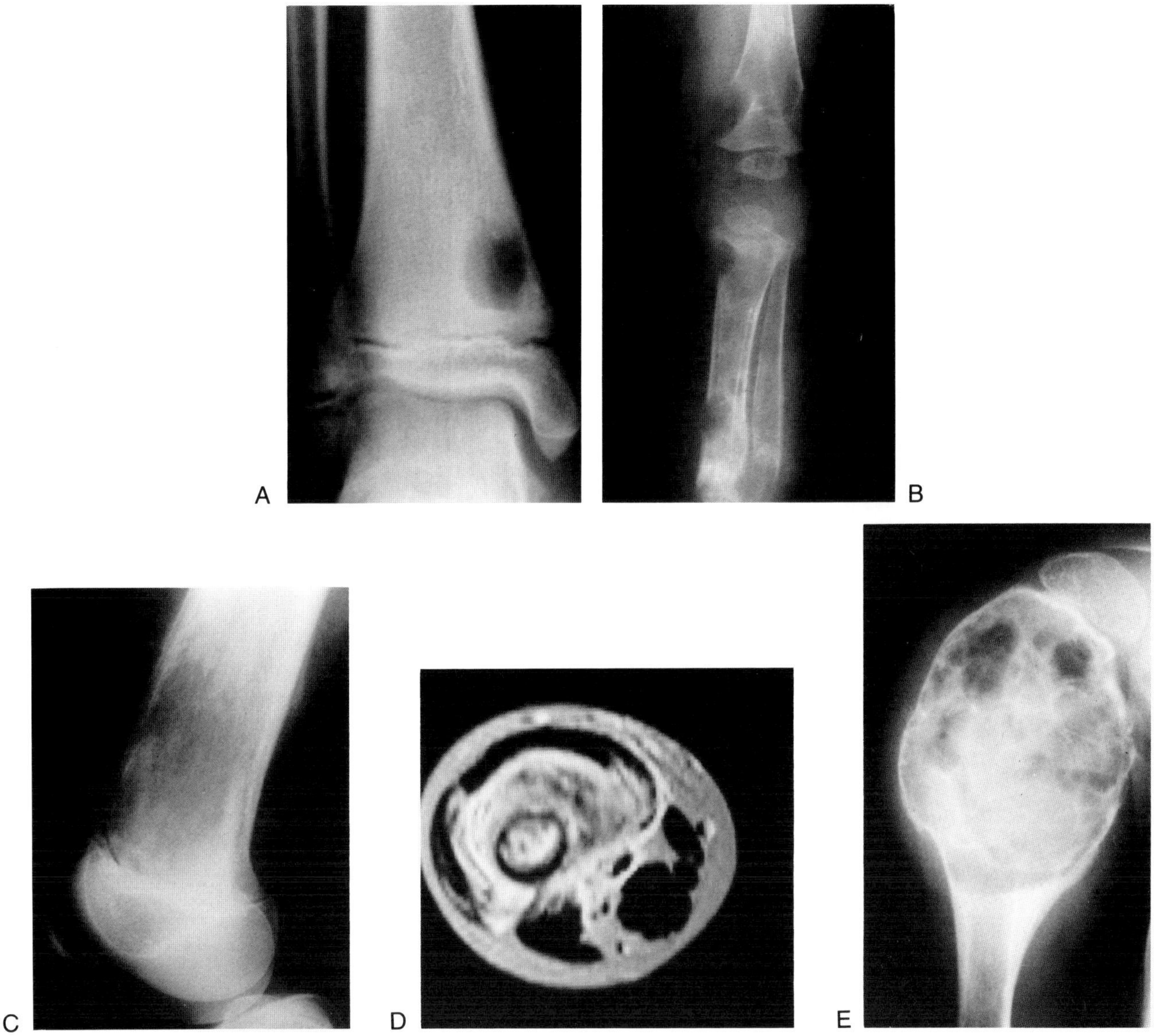

Fig. 8–46 Metaphyseal defects. **(A)** This Brodie's abscess of the distal tibia appears as a well-defined osteolytic lesion with little or no surrounding sclerosis. **(B)** Multiple osteolytic lesions and periosteal reaction in an infant with generalized hamartomatosis. **(C)** This osteolytic osteosarcoma of the femur has poorly defined margins. **(D)** T_2-weighted axial MRI better defines both the intraosseous and extraosseous extent of the lesion. **(E)** The markedly expansile, bubbly appearance of this well defined lesion is characteristic of aneurysmal bone cyst.

of osteolysis, particularly in diseases such as acute osteomyelitis, malignant bone tumors, leukemia, lymphoma, metastatic disease, and bone infarction. The presence of ossification or calcification within the lesion may help to characterize the matrix type. Cartilaginous lesions have an amorphous and sometimes circular pattern of calcification. Dense ossification is often seen in bone producing lesions such as osteosarcoma (Fig. 8–40). The presence and type of periosteal reaction can also be helpful in determining the etiology of an osteolytic lesion (see pp. 388–393).

The appearance of the soft tissues should not be neglected when examining bone lesions. Edema of the deep soft tissues adjacent to the bone can be an early clue to the presence of osteomyelitis. A soft tissue mass adjacent to an osteolytic lesion usually indicates that it is an aggressive lesion that has broken through the cortex (e.g., malignant bone tumors).

Exostoses

Bony or cartilaginous outgrowths from bones occur with primary bone tumors or as a result of trauma. Osteochondroma, one of the most common bone tumors of childhood, is a benign osteocartilaginous tumor that usually occurs in the metaphysis of a long bone near a joint. Although most of these lesions occur in the long bones of the lower extremities, almost any bone can be involved (Fig. 8–47). They appear as sessile or pedunculated lesions that tend to point away from the adjacent joint and cause widening of the metaphysis because of abnormal modeling (Fig. 8–48). A cartilaginous cap serves as the site of growth of these lesions, which continues until fusion of the epiphyses. Solitary osteochondromas are usually of little clinical significance; however when large, they may cause deformity, pain, or limitation of joint motion. Malignant degeneration is very uncommon, occurring in less than 1 percent of cases. The syndrome of multiple osteochondromatosis, in which multiple bilateral osteochondromas are present, is associated with a slightly higher rate of malignant transformation, however the incidence remains well below 10 percent.

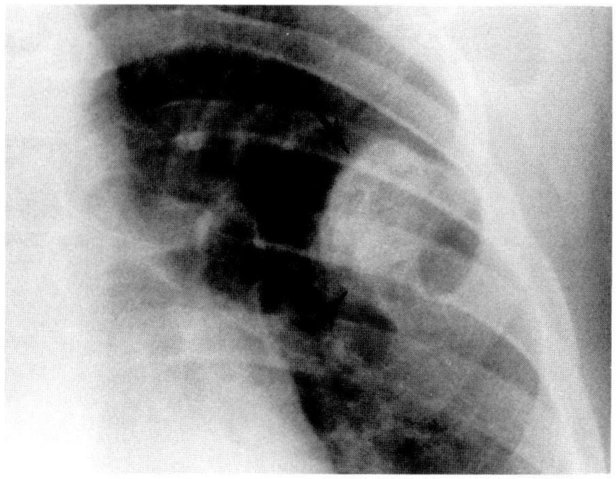

Fig. 8–47 Osteochondroma of the rib. This lesion (*arrows*) was initially mistaken for a lung nodule.

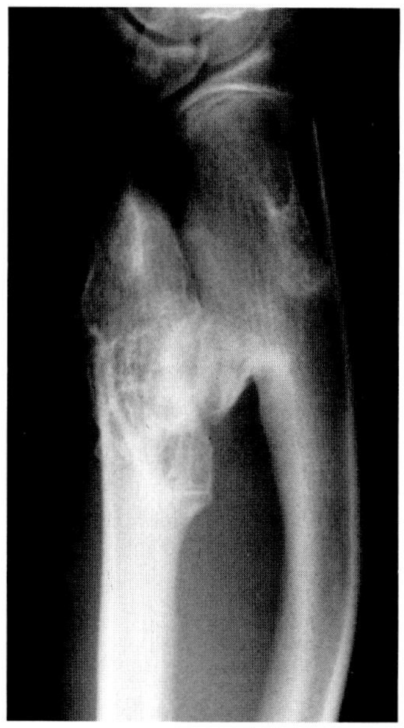

Fig. 8–48 Multiple osteochondromatosis. These large osteochondromas involving the distal radius and ulna resulted in significant widening and deformity of the bones.

Epiphyseal osteochondromas are unusual, however a sessile unilateral epiphyseal osteochondroma is the cause of epiphyseal dysplasia hemimelica (Trevor's disease) (Fig. 8–49). This condition most commonly involves the ankle or the knee and results in a varus or valgus deformity.

The supracondylar process of the humerus is a relatively common anomaly consisting of a vestigial bony spur extending medially from the anterior surface of the distal humeral shaft, pointing toward the elbow (Fig. 8–50). Usually this lesion is insignificant, however it can occasionally be fractured or cause nerve compression. Calcaneal spurs are occasionally seen in normal infants and in campomelic dwarfs. Bony spurs extending from the outer surface of the iliac wing, called iliac horns (Fig. 8–51), are associated with the nail-patella syndrome (osteo-onychodysplasia).

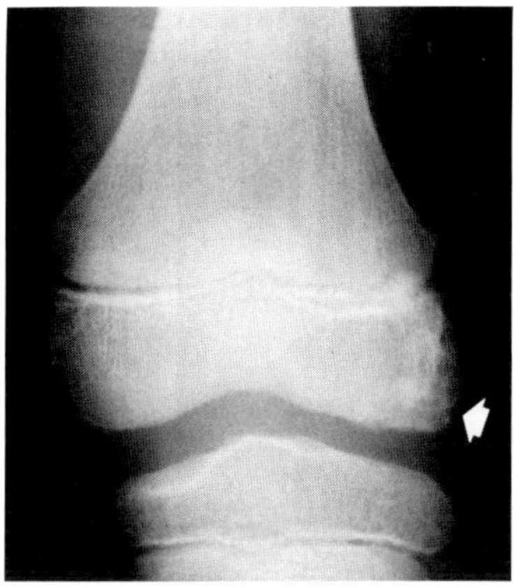

Fig. 8–49 Epiphyseal dysplasis hemimelica (Trevor disease). The lateral portion of the distal femoral epiphysis is enlarged by a sessile osteochondroma (*arrow*).

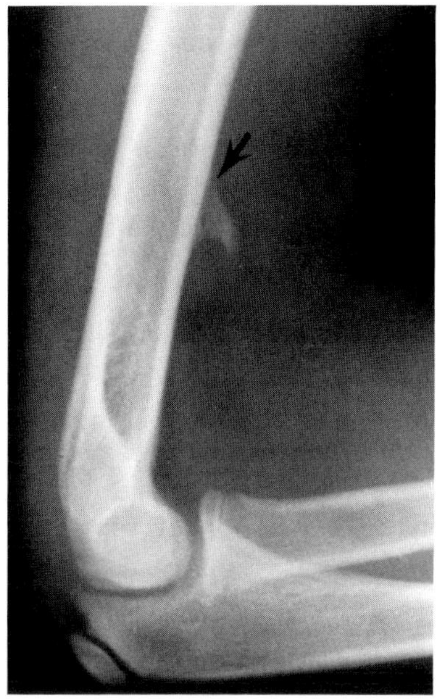

Fig. 8–50 Supracondylar process of the humerus. Note the presence of a fracture at the base of the spur (*arrow*).

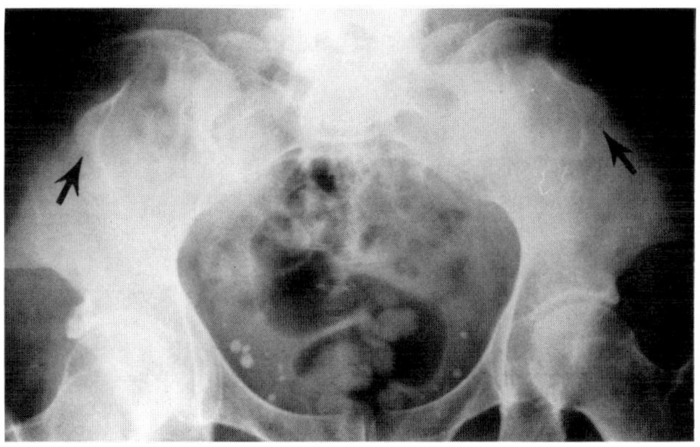

Fig. 8–51 Iliac horns. Bilateral exostoses extend from the outer surface of the iliac wings bilaterally (*arrows*).

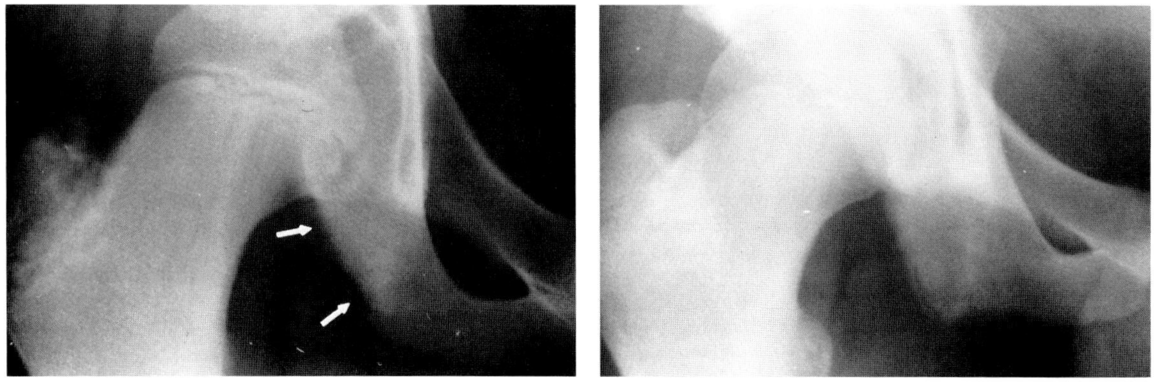

A B

Fig. 8–52 Ischial apophysis avulsion. **(A)** Acute avulsion of the ischial apophysis can appear as an area of cortical erosion along the lateral aspect of the ischium (*arrows*). **(B)** As the fracture heals, exuberant callus formation may create an exostosis, which is occasionally mistaken for a bone tumor.

Acquired exostoses are usually the result of healed avulsion fractures or myositis ossificans in children. Avulsion of the ischial apophysis frequently results in a bony exostosis (Fig. 8–52). Degenerative exostoses are rare in childhood, however they most commonly occur as a result of chronic hyperflexion injuries of the foot.

EPIPHYSEAL ABNORMALITIES

Enlarged Epiphyses

The epiphyses may appear relatively enlarged in conditions in which the long bones are short or thin (e.g., many dwarfing syndromes and neurologic diseases). True enlargement of the epiphyses is most often caused by the hyperemia associated with chronic joint inflammation. This hyperemia also results in osteoporosis of the epiphysis, causing it to appear demineralized and coarsely trabeculated. This appearance is most often seen in patients with rheumatoid arthritis and hemophilic arthropathy (Fig. 8–53). Chronic infections of the joint, particularly tuberculosis and fungal infections, can give the same appearance. In hemophilia, chronic synovial hypertrophy leads to erosions of the epiphyseal margins, causing them to be irregular. Characteristically, the intracondylar notch of the distal femoral epiphysis becomes widened (Fig. 8–54), a feature that helps to distinguish hemophilia from juvenile rheumatoid arthritis. Occasionally this finding occurs with tuberculous arthritis.

Epiphyseal neoplasms can cause the epiphysis to be enlarged, often in a nonuniform manner. A well-known example of this is epiphyseal dysplasia hemimelica, which is caused by an osteochondroma of the epiphysis (Fig. 8–49). Fibrous dysplasia of the epiphysis is a rare occurrence. Healed Legg-Perthes disease results in a proximal femoral epiphysis that is both enlarged and flattened.

ENLARGED EPIPHYSES

Congenital/developmental
- Winchester syndrome

Inflammation
- Rheumatoid arthritis
- Hemophilic arthropathy
- Tuberculous arthritis
- Fungal arthritis
- Chronic pyogenic arthritis

Neoplasm
- Epiphyseal dysplasia hemimelica
- Fibrous dysplasia

Miscellaneous
- Legg-Perthes disease (healed)

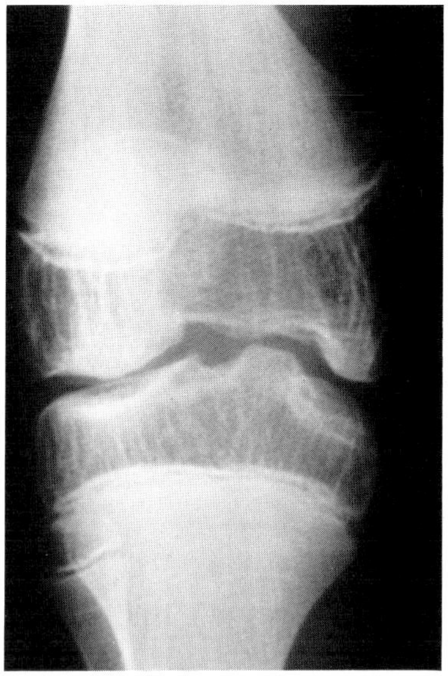

Fig. 8–53 Hemophilia. Chronic hyperemia caused by recurrent hemarthrosis results in enlargement, demineralization, and coarse trabeculation of the epiphyses about the knees of this patient with hemophilia.

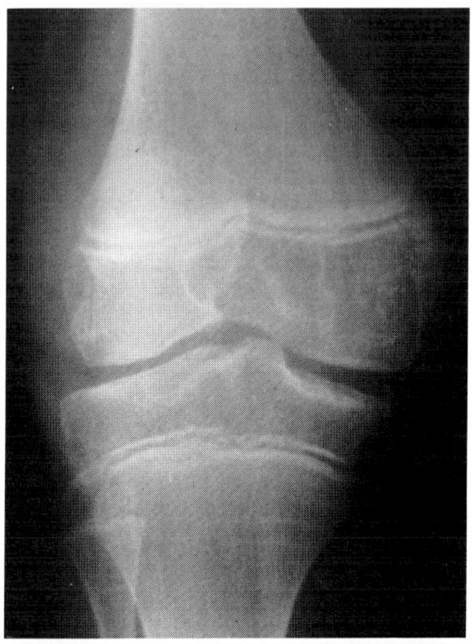

Fig. 8–54 Hemophilic arthropathy. Note the epiphyseal enlargement and widening of the intercondylar notch.

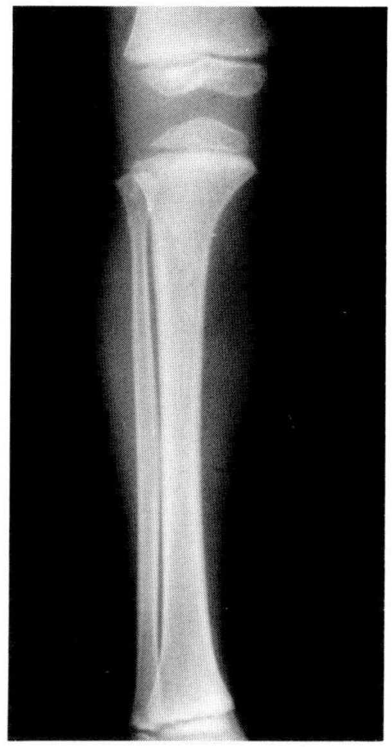

Fig. 8–55 Spondyloepiphyseal dysplasia. Generalized smallness and irregularity of the epiphyses is present.

Small Epiphyses

When a generalized pattern of small epiphyses is encountered, congenital dysplasia or dysgenesis of the epiphysis is the most likely cause. This pattern most commonly occurs in multiple epiphyseal dysplasia, spondyloepiphyseal dysplasia, and congenital hypothyroidism (Fig. 8–55). In all of these conditions, the epiphyses are small, irregular, and often frag-

> SMALL EPIPHYSES
>
> Congenital/developmental
> - Multiple epiphyseal dysplasia
> - Spondyloepiphyseal dysplasia
> - Congenital dislocating hip
> - Delayed bone age
>
> Inflammation
> - Following osteomyelitis, septic arthritis, or other injury
>
> Systemic/metabolic
> - Hypothyroidism
> - Morquio's disease
>
> Miscellaneous
> - Legg-Perthes disease (early)

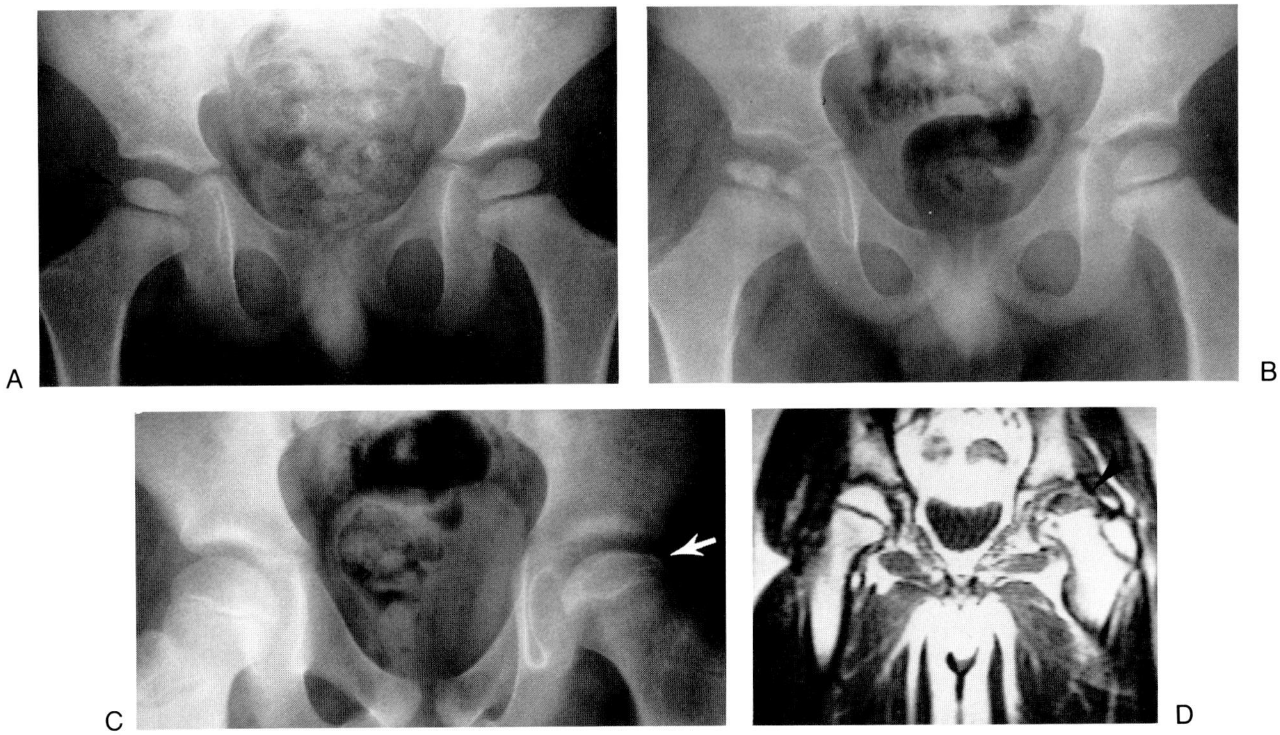

Fig. 8–56 Legg-Perthes disease. **(A)** This 5-year-old presented with a 2-week history of limping on the right lower extremity. Early radiographs of the hips showed only a small and slightly sclerotic right femoral head epiphysis (*arrow*). **(B)** Nine months later, marked flattening and fragmentation of the right epiphysis is evident. **(C)** An older patient with Perthes disease on the left. Note demineralization at the left femur except for the small femoral head (*arrow*). **(D)** T_1-weighted coronal MRI demonstrates the loss of normal signal intensity in the necrotic left femoral head (*arrowhead*).

mented. Infants with Morquio's disease often present with bone changes that are very similar to spondyloepiphyseal dysplasia congenita, including small epiphyses.

Isolated smallness of an epiphysis is usually due to some type of insult involving the joint or the epiphysis. A small and sometimes sclerotic proximal femoral epiphysis is one of the earliest findings of Legg-Perthes disease (idiopathic avascular necrosis of the femoral head) (Fig. 8–56). Often the epiphysis appears small before any apparent irregularity or fragmentation of the epiphysis occurs, making it an extremely useful finding for early diagnosis. A small femoral head epiphysis can also be seen in patients with a congenital dislocating hip. Early therapy of this condition, however, can allow the femoral head to return to a normal size.

Irregular or Fragmented Epiphyses

Epiphyseal fragmentation (or severe irregularity) may be seen, involving a single epiphysis or many epiphyses and may be congenital or acquired. If the fragmentation is due to a bone dysplasia, usually multiple epiphyses will be involved. These conditions include multiple epiphyseal dysplasia, spondyloepiphyseal dysplasia and the Dyggve-Melchior-Clausen syndrome (Fig. 8–57). Morquio's disease, a mucopolysaccharidosis, is accompanied by bony changes very similar to spondyloepiphyseal dysplasia including fragmented epiphyses. Meyer's dysplasia is a condition in which the development of the femoral head epiphyses is markedly delayed. As the femoral heads ossify, they have a very irregular, fragmented appearance; nevertheless, the heads continue to slowly develop and eventually have a normal appearance in

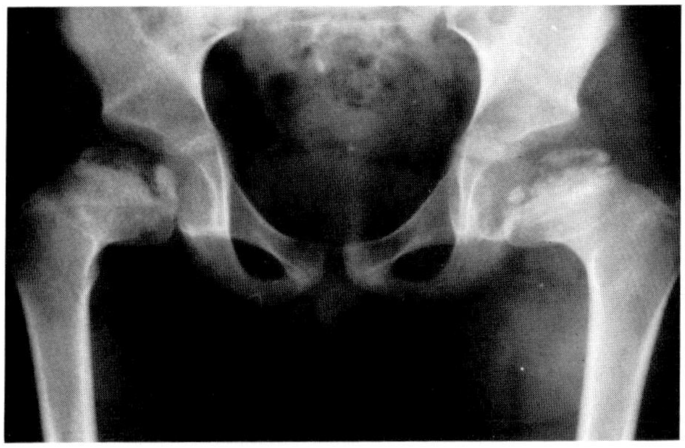

Fig. 8–57 Multiple epiphyseal dysplasia. Small fragmented femoral head epiphyses in a patient with multiple epiphyseal dysplasia.

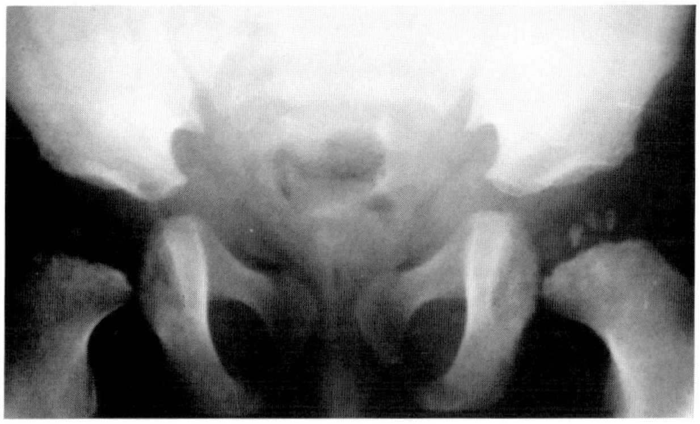

Fig. 8–58 Hypothyroidism. Epiphyseal dysgenesis results in very small fragmented epiphyses.

FRAGMENTED EPIPHYSES

Congenital/developmental
- Multiple epiphyseal dysplasia
- Spondyloepiphyseal dysplasia
- Meyer's dysplasia (femoral head)
- Thiemann's disease (middle and proximal phalanges)
- Tricho-rhino-phalangeal syndrome (femoral head)
- Dyggve-Melchior-Clausen syndrome

Inflammation
- Osteomyelitis/septic arthritis
- Rheumatoid arthritis

Neoplasm
- Epiphyseal dysplasia hemimelica

Trauma/surgery
- Frostbite (hands, feet)

Systemic/metabolic
- Conditions causing avascular necrosis
  - Sickle cell disease
  - Steroid therapy
  - Gaucher's disease
  - Collagen vascular disease
- Hypothyroidism (epiphyseal dysgenesis)
- Morquio's disease

Miscellaneous
- Legg-Perthes disease
- Other causes of avascular necrosis (e.g., following treatment of congenital hip dislocation)

most cases. Epiphyseal dysgenesis, the result of infantile hypothyroidism, appears as small, irregular or fragmented epiphyses, which then return to normal after therapy (Fig. 8–58). Isolated femoral head and phalangeal epiphyseal irregularity are seen with tricho-rhino-phalangeal syndrome and Thiemann's disease, respectively.

Acquired forms of epiphyseal irregularity and fragmentation are more common and are more likely to be isolated rather than diffuse abnormalities. Avascular necrosis is the most common cause of epiphyseal fragmentation, and can be caused by a number of conditions and diseases that lead to compromised vascularity to the epiphyses, especially the femoral head epiphyses. When avascular necrosis of the femoral heads is bilateral, it is often caused by a generalized disease process such as sickle cell disease, Gaucher's disease, or collagen vascular disease. Steroid therapy is also a common cause of avascular necrosis of the femoral head.

More commonly unilateral aseptic necrosis of the femoral head occurs, and is most often an idiopathic condition known as Legg-Perthes disease. Once fragmentation of the femoral head is seen the condition is in an advanced stage; therefore, it is desireable to detect Legg-Perthes disease before fragmentation oc-

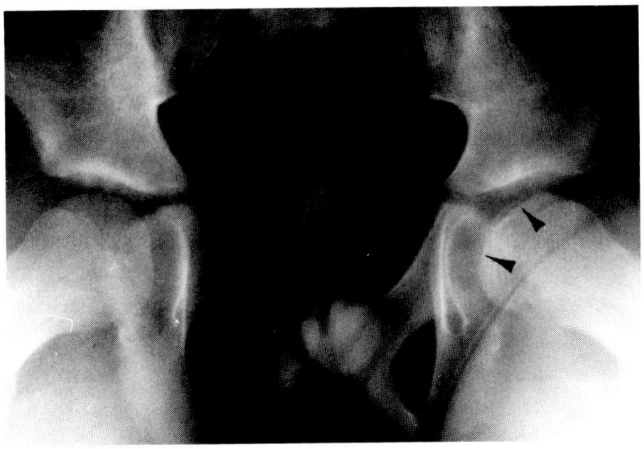

Fig. 8–59 Legg-Perthes disease. The radiolucent subchondral crescent (*arrowheads*) is a highly specific early finding in avascular necrosis of the left femoral head.

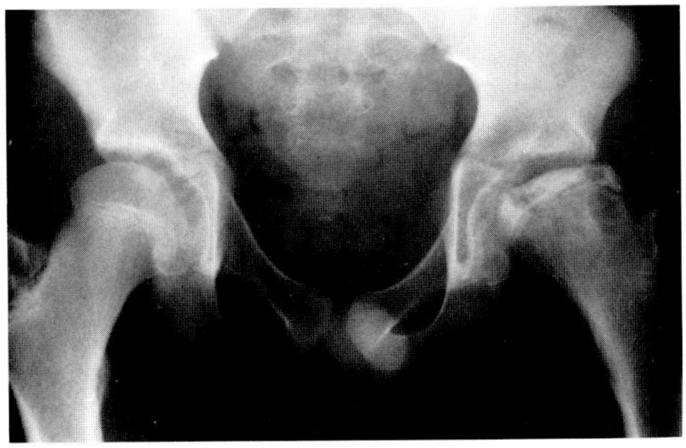

Fig. 8–60 Advanced Perthes disease. Advanced changes in this condition include marked flattening, sclerosis, and fragmentation of the left femoral head, widening of the femoral neck, and metaphyseal cystic lesions.

curs. The earliest findings of Legg-Perthes disease consist of smallness and sclerosis of the femoral head, occasionally accompanied by a subchondral lucent crescent representing an early fracture (Fig. 8–59). Demineralization of the bones and soft tissue atrophy about the affected hip serve as useful adjunctive findings in the condition. Gradually the necrotic femoral head becomes flattened, fragmented, and resorbed. Eventually the epiphysis reconstitutes; however in those cases in which treatment is delayed, the head can be quite deformed, flattened, and enlarged. The femoral neck appears shortened and widened and cystic changes may occur in the metaphysis (Fig. 8–60).

Inflammatory conditions such as osteomyelitis, septic arthritis, and rheumatoid arthritis can also cause isolated fragmented epiphyses. Avascular necrosis occasionally complicates surgical and nonsurgical treatment of certain hip disorders such as congenitally dislocating hip.

Stippled Epiphyses

A peculiar form of epiphyseal fragmentation consists of a dense punctate pattern involving not only the epiphyses but also the carpal and tarsal bones and the cartilaginous junctions in the spine and pelvis. Stippled epiphyses are most often seen in infants with

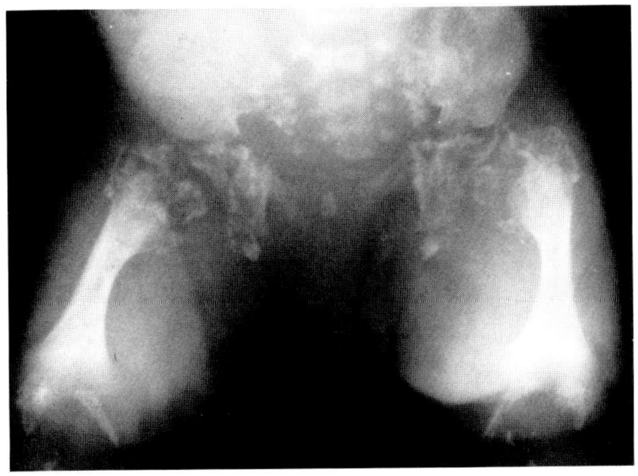

Fig. 8–61 Chondrodystrophia calcificans congenita. Note the characteristic stippling of the epiphyses and the cartilaginous junctions of the pelvis.

chondrodystrophia calcificans congenita or punctate epiphyseal displasia (Fig. 8–61). Two forms of this condition have been identified: a severe, autosomal recessive, lethal rhizomelic form and a less severe, autosomal dominant Conradi-Hünermann type. Less common hereditary syndromes associated with stippled epiphyses include the Zellweger (cerebrohepatorenal) syndrome, trisomy 18, trisomy 21, and GM_1-gangliosidosis. Congenitally acquired conditions such as warfarin embryopathy and fetal alcohol syndrome have also been associated with stippled epiphyses.

Cone-Shaped Epiphyses

Cone-shaped epiphyses with the apex pointing towards a V-shaped metaphysis are usually seen in the hands and feet (Fig. 8–62). This epiphyseal configuration is not uncommon in normal children. Nevertheless, such epiphyses can also be a part of a number of syndromes and bone dysplasias. The tricho-rhino-phalangeal dysplasia type I is characteristically associated with cone-shaped epiphyses, short metacarpals and metatarsals, irregularity and fragmentation of the femoral heads, sparse hair, and an abnormally shaped nose. Similar phalangeal cone-shaped epiphyses are seen in association with chronic renal disease in the conorenal syndromes. This type of epiphysis can occur in many other syndromes, such as achondroplasia, Ellis-van Crevald syndrome, cleidocranial dysostosis, the orodigitofacial syndromes, otopalatodigital syndrome, the acrocephalosyndactyly syndromes, asphyxiating thoracic dystrophy, epiphyseal dysplasias, metaphyseal dysostosis, Seckel's syndrome, and pseudo or pseudopseudohypoparathyroidism.

Any epiphysis may acquire a cone shape as a result of various types of insults at the epiphyseal-metaphyseal junction. Common causes include epiphyseal-metaphyseal fractures, osteomyelitis, bone infarction, frostbite, or radiation injury. Cone-shaped epiphyses have also been described in association with focal growth arrest due to vitamin A intoxication.

Epiphyseal Defects

Marginal defects of the epiphyses are most commonly caused by either traumatic injury or inflammatory

---

EPIPHYSEAL DEFECTS

Congenital/developmental
- Normal defects in femoral head (fovea centralis) and posterior femoral condyle
- Histiocytosis X

Inflammation
- Rheumatoid arthritis
- Tuberculous arthritis
- Fungal arthritis
- Osteomyelitis

Neoplasm
- Synovial tumors
- Fibrous defect

Trauma/surgery
- Osteochondritis dissecans
- Avulsion injuries

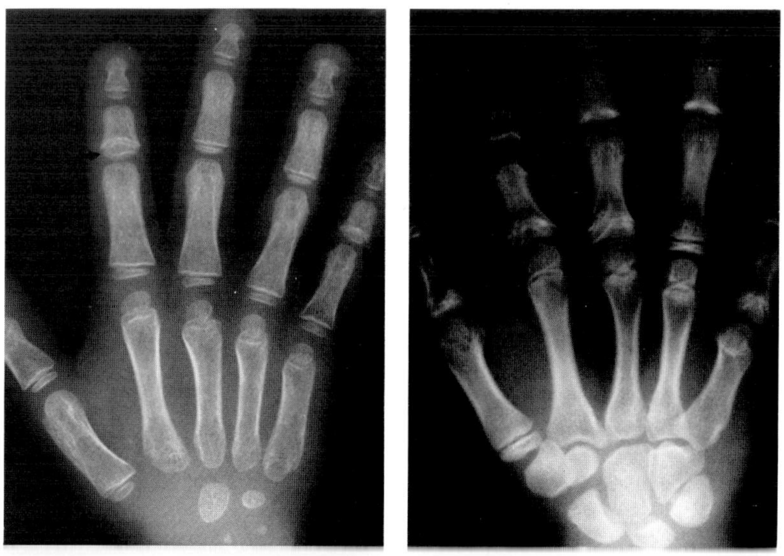

A B

Fig. 8–62 Cone-shaped epiphyses in the hands. **(A)** Note the coned epiphyses (*arrows*) and short phalanges in this patient with brachydactyly. **(B)** Typical cone-shaped epiphyses in trichorhinophalangeal syndrome.

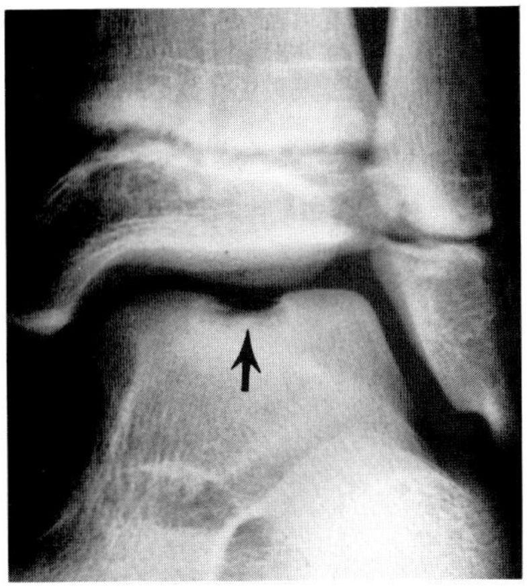

Fig. 8–63 Osteochondritis dissecans of the talus. A characteristic defect (*arrow*) along the articular surface of the talus.

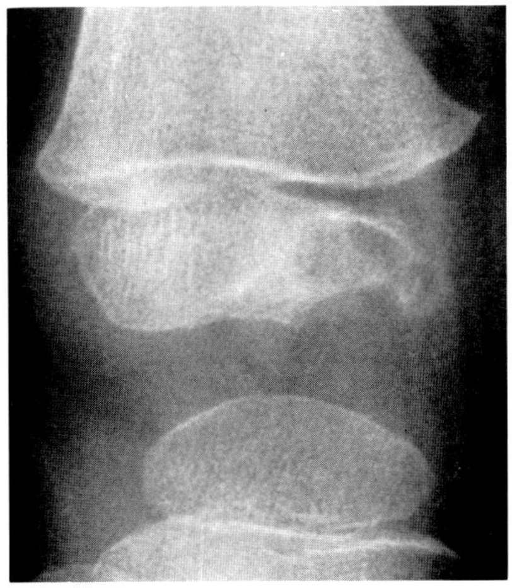

Fig. 8–64 Epiphyseal osteomyelitis. This destructive lesion with sclerotic borders involving the distal femoral epiphysis resulted from low-grade osteomyelitis.

processes involving the joint. Avulsion fractures involving the epiphysis are particularly common in the knee. Trauma is probably one of the principal causes of osteochronditis dissecans, leading to avascular necrosis of a portion of articular cartilage and its underlying subchondral bone. As the necrotic fragment of bone separates from the parent bone, it leaves a depression in the epiphysis at its site of previous location, usually in the lateral surface of the medial femoral condyle. Other less commonly affected sites include the talus (Fig. 8–63), capitellum, femoral head, and patella. Familial incidence is not an uncommon occurrence and multiple epiphyses may be involved in a single patient; thus, hereditary and constitutional predisposition to this condition may contribute to its occurrence.

Synovial hypertrophy can lead to erosion-type defects in the epiphyses, most often caused by chronic arthritides such as rheumatoid arthritis. Chronic infectious arthritis can also cause synovial hypertrophy, most commonly tuberculous or fungal arthritis. Occasionally, osteomyelitis may originate in the epiphysis (Fig. 8–64). Synovial tumors and tumorlike conditions, such as pigmented villonodular synovitis, are rare in childhood. Other rare causes of epiphyseal defects include histiocytosis X and benign fibrous defects.

METAPHYSEAL ABNORMALITIES

Transverse Bands

The metaphyses of the long bones in children frequently display early signs of illnesses resulting in poor enchondral bone growth. This evidence usually consists of bands of increased or decreased density extending transversely across the metaphysis. In some cases, both types of bands can occur. Although alone these bands are nonspecific, in the appropriate clinical setting they can be suggestive of a number of specific diagnoses.

Multiple, thin dense transverse metaphyseal bands, sometimes interposed between radiolucent bands, are rather common in children. These bands usually represent trophic changes resulting from variable rates of bone growth in children with multiple episodes of illness, trauma, or other insults (Fig. 8–65). Multiple growth arrest lines, or perhaps more appropriately growth recovery lines, associated with clinical signs of hypopituitarism are the hallmark of psychosocial dwarfism (Fig. 8–66). These patients suffer from a transient and reversible form of growth hormone deficiency due to an undesireable home environment.

TRANSVERSE METAPHYSEAL BANDS

- Dense
  - Congenital/developmental
    - Osteopetrosis
  - Inflammation
    - Healing neonatal infections
  - Systemic/metabolic
    - Chronic heavy metal intoxication (lead)
    - Severe illness or trauma
    - Healing rickets
    - Chronic illness
    - Hypervitaminosis D
    - Hypercalcemia
    - Scurvy
  - Miscellaneous
    - Psychosocial dwarfism
    - Chemotherapy
- Lucent
  - Inflammation
    - Neonatal infections (syphilis, rubella)
  - Neoplasms
    - Leukemia
    - Lymphoma
    - Metastasis
  - Systemic/metabolic
    - Severe illness or trauma
    - Scurvy

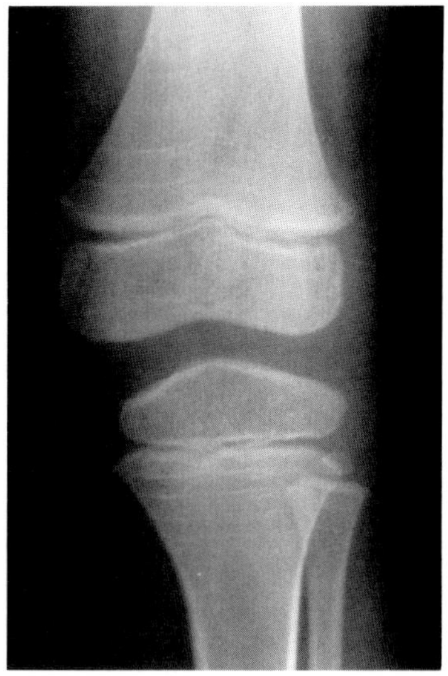

Fig. 8–65 Growth resumption lines. Multiple transverse bands of increased density in the metaphyses of a child with leukemia. The evenly spaced transverse lines mark the regular periodic chemotherapy treatments.

When removed from this environment, normal growth resumes rapidly, often so rapidly that exuberant brain growth leads to spreading of the cranial sutures. Alternating bands of radiodensity and radiolucency are also sometimes seen in osteopetrosis, but in these patients the characteristic extreme density of all of the bones suggests the diagnosis (Fig. 8–12).

A single radiodense band in the region of the zone of provisional calcification is not an uncommon finding in normal children, especially during the summer months when they are exposed to extended periods of sunlight. In other patients, however, these bands are abnormal and are most characteristic of chronic

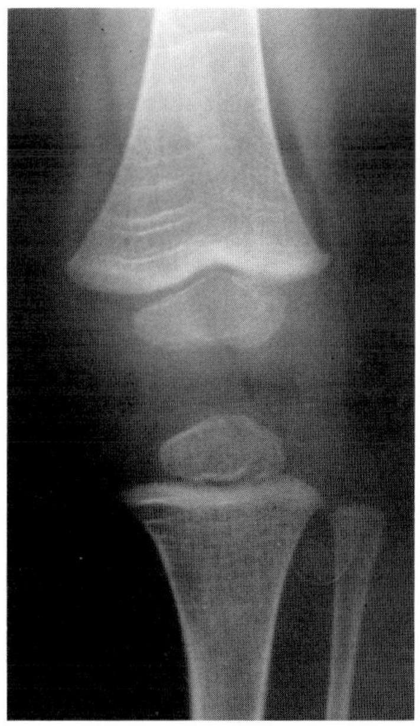

Fig. 8–66 Psychosocial dwarfism. Multiple dense, thin transverse bands across the metaphyses are a characteristic finding in this condition.

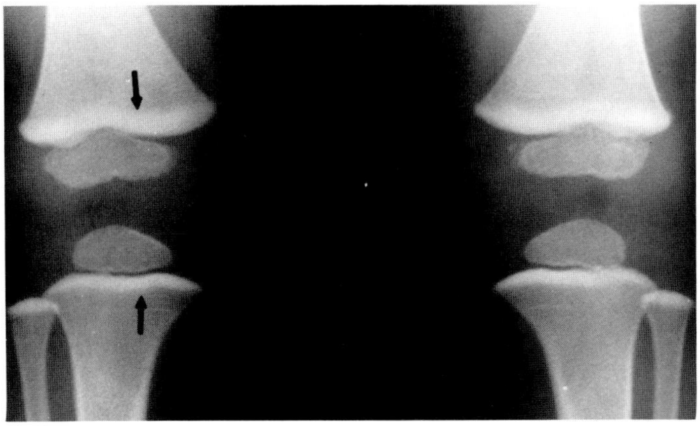

Fig. 8–67 Lead intoxication. Note the markedly thickened and dense zones of provisional calcification (*arrows*). These lines are the result of a combination of abnormal bone formation and lead deposition in the growing metaphysis.

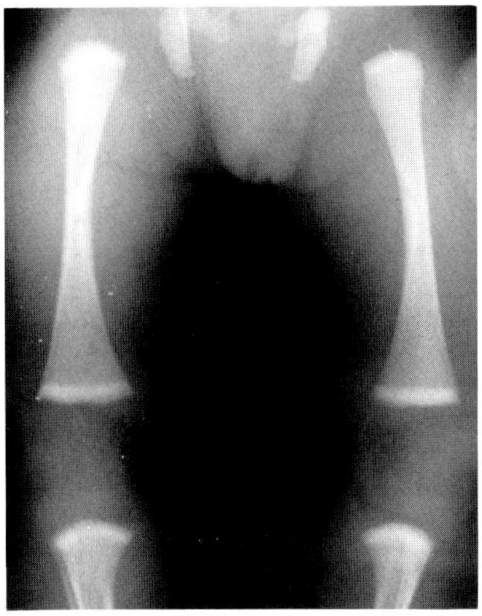

Fig. 8–68 Congenital syphilis. Metaphyseal bands of increased density in these infants represent altered enchondral bone formation.

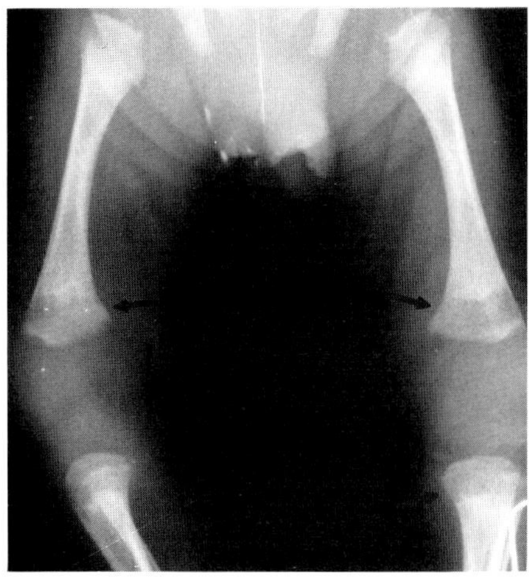

Fig. 8–69 Congenital syphilis. Trophic metaphyseal bands of decreased density (*arrows*) are a common finding in congenital syphilis.

heavy metal intoxication (Fig. 8–67). Lead is the most common culprit; however, arsenic, bismuth, fluoride, mercury, lithium, phosphorus, and radium poisoning can cause similar dense metaphyseal bands. Multiple episodes of lead intoxication can sometimes occur, resulting in multiple radiodense bands and widening of the metaphyses (Erlenmeyer flask deformity). Dense metaphyseal bands are sometimes seen in newborn infants with congenital syphilis (Fig. 8–68). Hypercalcemia and hypervitaminosis D are less common causes of a single radiodense metaphyseal band.

Solitary radiolucent transverse metaphyseal bands also occur and most often represent a nonspecific trophic change secondary to some form of severe illness or trauma. In neonates, such bands suggest a neonatal infection, most commonly syphilis (Fig. 8–69). Nevertheless, radiolucent bands may also be an early sign of malignancy in children, particularly leukemia, lymphoma, or metastatic disease (Fig. 8–70). These lines are especially well seen at both ends of the femurs, the proximal humeri, and the proximal tibias. Scurvy is an uncommon cause of a similar

A 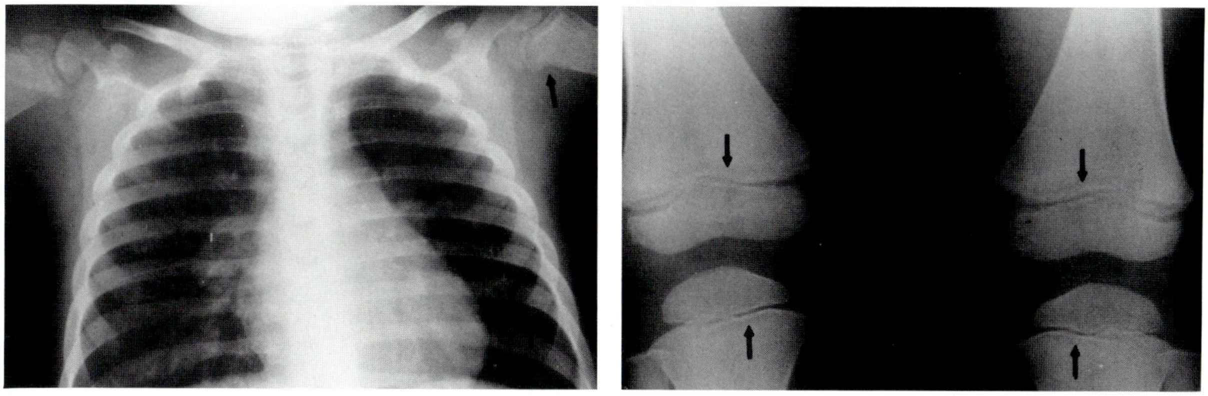 B

Fig. 8–70 Leukemia. **(A)** Radiolucent transverse bands in metaphyses such as these in the proximal humerus are often the initial radiographic finding of leukemia. Erosion of the medial metaphyseal cortex of the proximal humerus (*arrow*) is a suggestive, but nonspecific, finding in leukemia. Right hilar lymphadenopathy was also present in this patient. **(B)** Bands of decreased density at the knees in early leukemia (*arrows*).

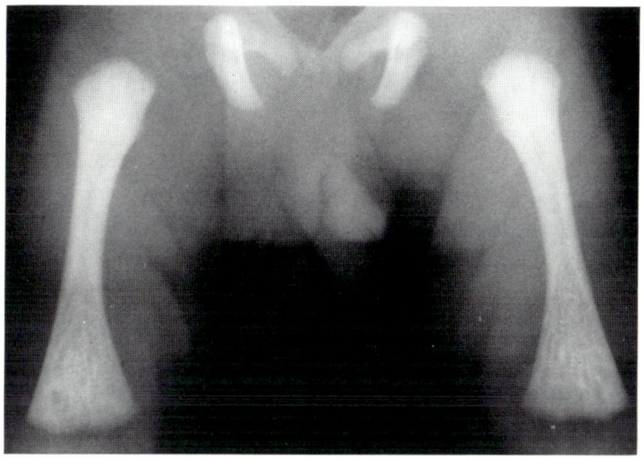

Fig. 8–71 Congenital rubella. The femoral metaphyses demonstrate the typical "celery stalk" appearance of congenital rubella infection in this newborn infant.

radiolucent transverse metaphyseal band. In any of these conditions, the metaphysis is weakened, which may lead to pathologic fracture.

Congenital rubella infection may result in metaphyseal abnormalities in up to 50 percent of cases. Multiple longitudinally oriented metaphyseal radiolucencies are typically seen, giving a "celery stalk" appearance (Fig. 8–71). These changes may occur in all of the long bones but are more prominent around the knees. The bone changes of rubella may be present at birth or develop in the first few weeks of life. In most cases complete healing has occurred by 3 to 6 months of age. Occasionally progression occurs, resulting in irregular or destroyed metaphyses. Congenital cytomegalovirus infection may result in similar bony changes, however epiphyseal maturation tends to be normal. Delayed epiphyseal maturation is seen in congenital rubella syndrome.

Splayed and Cupped Metaphyses

Splaying and cupping of the metaphysis may be due to a number of congenital or acquired conditions that result in disturbed enchondral bone growth (see list). Similar changes may occur at the rib ends in

SPLAYED AND CUPPED METAPHYSES

Congenital/developmental
- Metaphyseal dysostosis
- Achondroplasia
- Hypochondroplasia
- Pseudoachondroplasia
- Hypophosphatasia
- Thanatophoric dwarfism
- Metatropic dwarfism
- Kniest syndrome
- Ellis-van Creveld syndrome
- Mesomelic dwarfism
- Short-rib polydactyly syndrome
- Diastrophic dwarfism
- Chondrodystrophia calcificans congenita
- Spondylometaphyseal dysplasia
- Cephaloskeletal dysplasia (Taybi-Linder syndrome)
- Melnick-Needles syndrome

Inflammation
- Osteomyelitis/infarction (healed)

Trauma/surgery
- Epiphyseal-metaphyseal injury (healed)

Systemic/metabolic
- Rickets
- Hypervitaminosis A
- Phenylketonuria

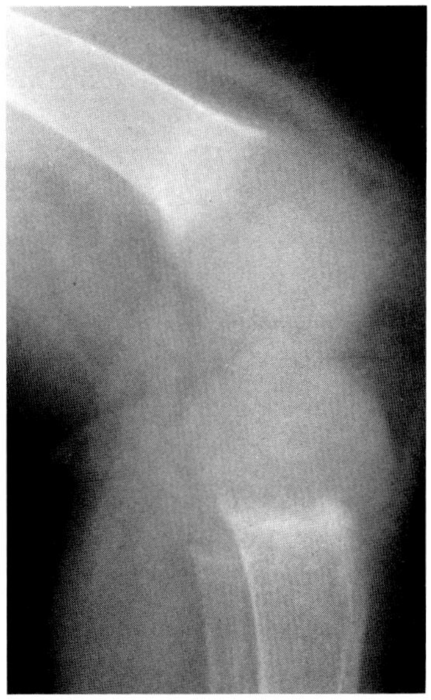

Fig. 8–72 Eight-month-old patient with rickets secondary to biliary atresia. Typical cupping, flaring, and fraying of the metaphyses is seen in the long bones of the lower extremity.

these conditions. This is a common finding in many bone dysplasias, the most common of which are achondroplasia and metaphyseal dysostosis.

The most common cause of acquired metaphyseal cupping and flaring is rickets. The metaphyses in this condition also appear indistinct and frayed, reflecting the lack of normal bone mineralization (Fig. 8–72). Similar metaphyseal changes can occur in hypophosphatasia and in some cases of metaphyseal dysostosis. In the healing phases of rickets, the cupping can become even more pronounced, but improved density appears in the zones of provisional calcification. Focal metaphyseal cupping and splaying is most often caused by some insult to the growth plate, generally infection, trauma, or infarction. Hypervitaminosis A occasionally results in focal growth plate damage with resultant cupping and splaying of the metaphysis.

Metaphyseal Fragments or Spurs

Spurs extending from the medial edge of the distal femoral and proximal tibial metaphyses are a common finding in children with "physiologic" bowing due to tibial torsion (Fig. 8–73). This is usually a self-limiting condition in young children. More severe beaking with ventral fragmentation involving the proximal medial tibial metaphysis is characteristic of Blount's disease (Fig. 8–74). This condition is a developmental abnormality resulting from a growth disturbance of the medial portion of the proximal tibial epiphysis. The deformity results in a marked genu varum and requires surgical correction by osteotomy in most cases. Bilateral symmetrical metaphyseal spurs have also been noted in infants with Menkes' (kinky hair) syndrome, a rare condition caused by abnormal copper metabolism.

Actual fragmentation at the margins of the metaphysis most often indicates the presence of an epiphyseal-

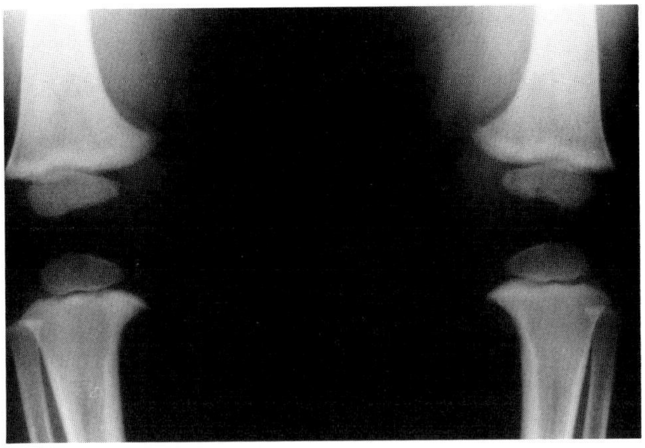

Fig. 8–73 Tibial torsion. Metaphyseal beaking and bowing at the knees usually spontaneously corrects as the child matures.

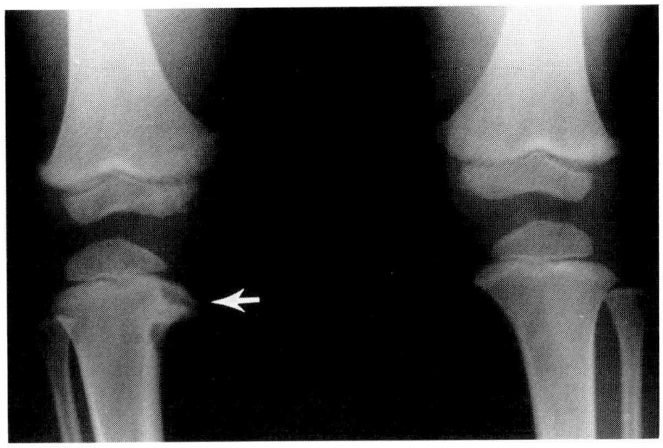

Fig. 8–74 Blount's disease. Prominent beaking of the medial tibial metaphysis on the right is accompanied by irregularity and metaphyseal sloping (*arrow*).

METAPHYSEAL FRAGMENTS OR SPURS

- Congenital/developmental
  - Menkes' (kinky-hair) syndrome
  - Blount's disease
- Trauma
  - Epiphyseal-metaphyseal fractures
    - Routine trauma
    - Breech delivery
    - Battered child syndrome
    - Rickets
    - Scurvy
    - Hyperparathyroidism
    - Neurogenic
    - Leukemia/lymphoma
    - Metastases
    - Osteomyelitis
    - Congenital infections

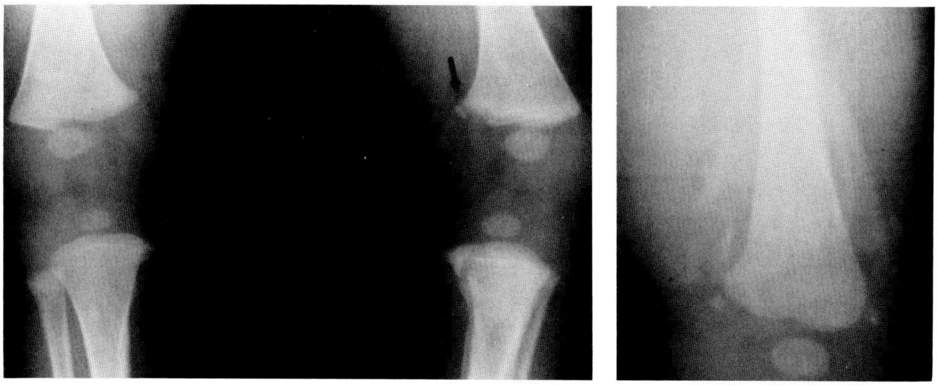

A B

Fig. 8–75 Battered child syndrome. **(A)** Typical corner and ring metaphyseal avulsion fractures in a battered infant (*arrows*). **(B)** Similar metaphyseal avulsion fractures with ballooned periosteal reaction is a result of trauma during a breech delivery.

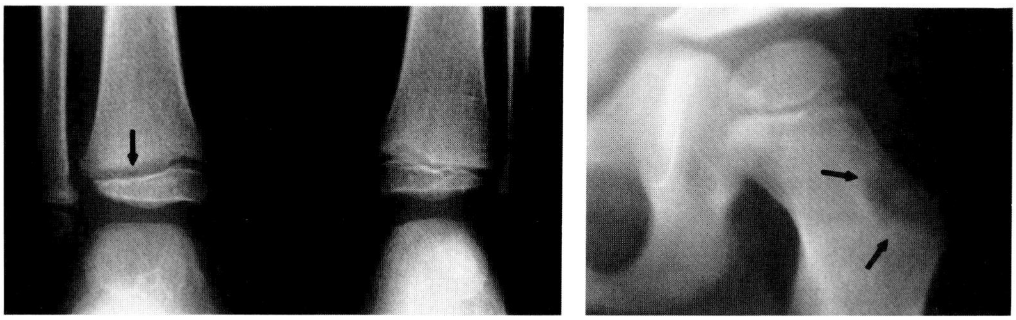

A B

Fig. 8–76 Osteomyelitis. **(A)** Early metaphyseal destruction by osteomyelitis of the distal right tibia (*arrow*). **(B)** Homogeneous destruction in the metaphyseal-equivalent region of the greater trochanter caused by osteomyelitis (*arrows*).

metaphyeal fracture. This type of fracture can occur with routine trauma, however it is also characteristically seen in neonates who deliver in a breech position and in the battered child syndrome (Fig. 8–75). Whenever the metaphyses are weakened by metabolic disease, malignancy, or infection similar fractures can occur.

Metaphyseal Destruction

The metaphysis of the long bones in children is often the first site to reflect bone involvement by generalized disease processes (see list, p. 415). Homogeneous destruction of the metaphysis is seen in many conditions, but is most suggestive of osteomyelitis, infarction, or the trophic changes that accompany congenital infections such as syphilis and rubella (Fig. 8–76). A similar appearance may occur with histiocytosis X or with advanced neoplasms.

An inhomogeneous or moth-eaten pattern of metaphyseal destruction is more commonly seen with malignancies that involve bone. Leukemia, lymphoma, and metastatic neuroblastoma are the most common causes of a moth-eaten metaphysis in children, although osteomyelitis can have a similar appearance (Fig. 8–77). Primary bone tumors such as osteosarcoma, fibrosarcoma, and Ewing's sarcoma are less common but can have the same appearance. Early metaphyseal destruction in malignancies such

METAPHYSEAL DESTRUCTION

Congenital/developmental
- Histiocytosis X

Inflammation
- Osteomyelitis
- Congenital infections

Neoplasm/cyst
- Leukemia
- Lymphoma
- Metastases (neuroblastoma)
- Ewing's sarcoma (other sarcomas)
- Primary bone tumor
- Fibrous cortical defect
- Solitary bone cyst

Miscellaneous
- Bone infarction

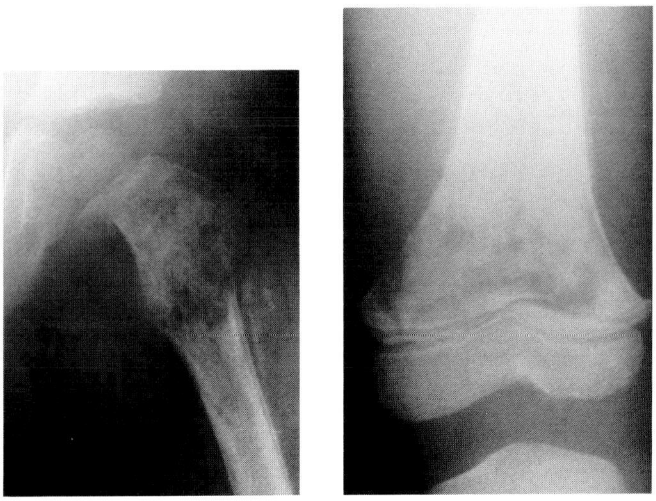

A B

Fig. 8–77 Moth-eaten metaphyseal destruction. **(A)** Irregular, patchy destruction of the proximal left femur caused by metastatic neuroblastoma. **(B)** Moth-eaten destruction of the distal femoral metaphysis with periosteal reaction and deep, soft tissue edema due to osteomyelitis.

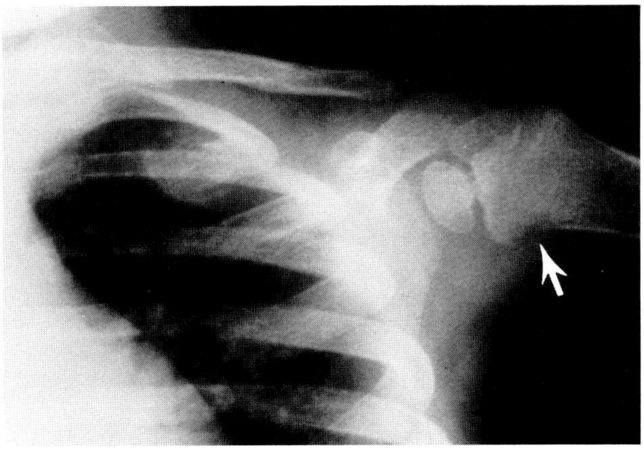

Fig. 8–78 Leukemia. Note the erosion of the medial cortex of the proximal humeral metaphysis (*arrow*) and destruction of the anterior portion of the first rib.

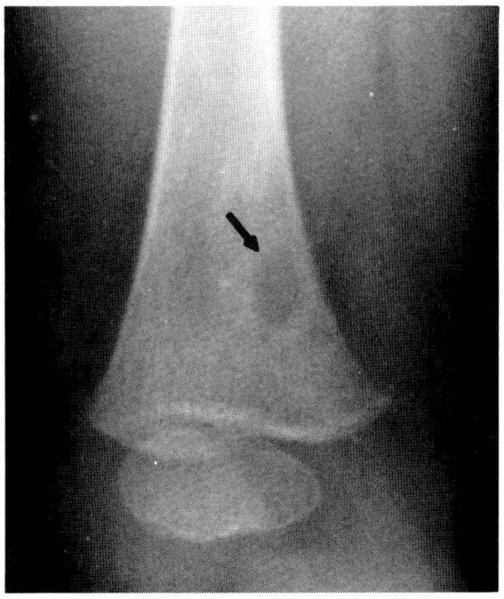

Fig. 8–80 Leukemia. A focal area of bone destruction (*arrow*) in the metaphysis of a patient with leukemia.

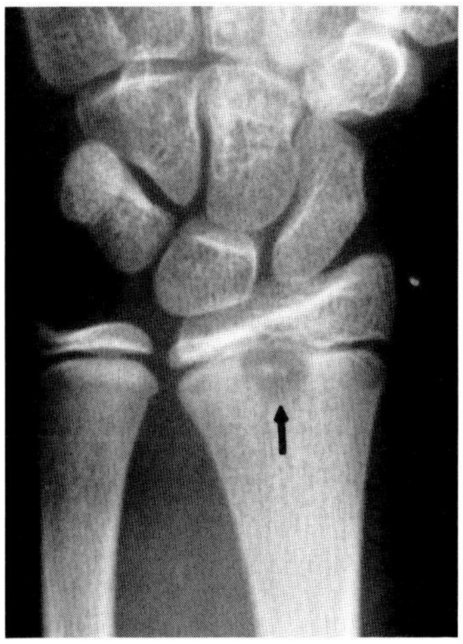

Fig. 8–79 Osteomyelitis of the distal radius. Note the focal area of metaphyseal destruction (*arrows*).

as leukemia may take the form of erosion of the medial cortex of the metaphyses, seen best in the proximal humerus or tibia (Fig. 8–78).

A focal osteolytic defect in the metaphysis of a child is usually due to osteomyelitis (Fig. 8–79). If the infection is low grade and chronic, the lesion may have sclerotic margins (Brodie's abscess). A solitary bone cyst appears as a central, focal osteolytic lesion with a thin, sharply defined margin. A small, well-defined osteolytic defect involving the metaphyseal cortex usually represents a fibrous cortical defect. These lesions are benign and very common and should not be mistaken for osteomyelitis or other destructive metaphyseal processes. Occasionally malignancies such as leukemia or metastatic neuroblastoma present as a focal osteolytic metaphyseal defect (Fig. 8–80).

Growth Plate Widening

The physis, or growth plate, is a relatively weak area in the bones of children; therefore, injuries to the extremities commonly result in a fracture at this site. These fractures range from simple separation of the epiphysis from the metaphysis to more complex injuries involving fractures of the epiphysis and metaphysis. In such injuries the growth plate appears widened, but this finding can be subtle if no associated bony fragment is detectable. Comparison views of the normal contralateral extremity are often extremely useful for detecting subtle epiphyseal-metaphyseal fractures (Fig. 8–81).

Generalized widening of the physes is most often caused by metabolic abnormalities, resulting in faulty enchondral bone growth (see list). A common example is rickets, which presents with growth plate widening and a frayed, splayed, and cupped metaphysis (Fig. 8–82). Hyperparathyroidism may also result in a widened growth plate. In children, hyperparathyroidism due to renal disease (renal osteodystrophy)

GROWTH PLATE WIDENING

Congenital/developmental
- Metaphyseal chondrodysplasias

Trauma/surgery
- Epiphyseal-metaphyseal fractures
- Slipped capital femoral epiphysis

Systemic/metabolic
- Rickets
- Hyperparathyroidism
- Hypophosphatasia
- Gangliosidosis
- Mucolipidosis II
- Hypothyroidism (severe)

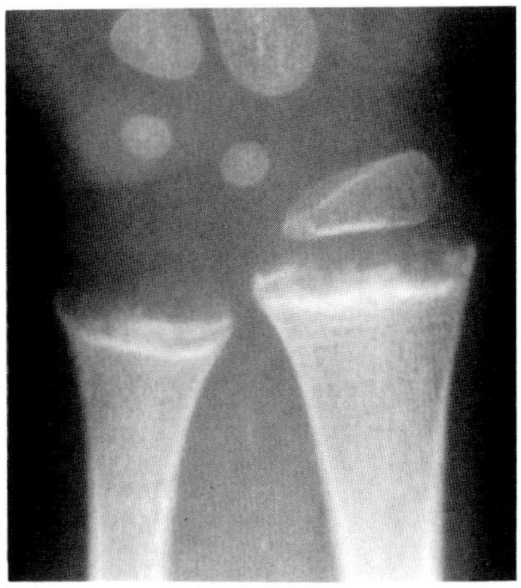

Fig. 8–82 Rickets. Note the apparent widening of the epiphyseal-metaphyseal junction with cupping and fraying of the metaphysis in this patient with rickets caused by renal tubular acidosis.

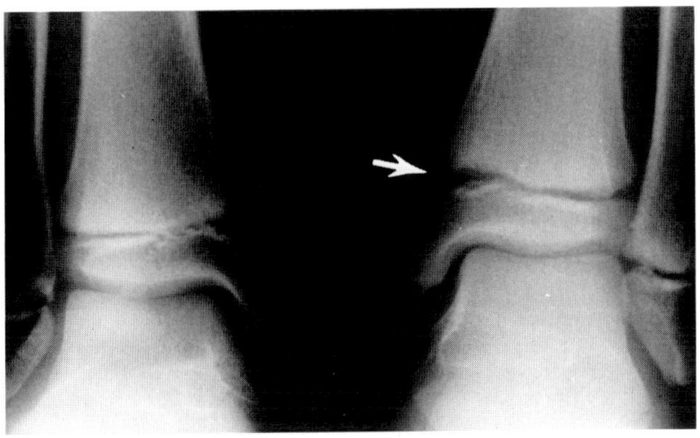

Fig. 8–81 Epiphyseal-metaphyseal fracture of the distal tibia. Detection of a subtle Salter-Harris I fracture (*arrow*) is facilitated by comparison with the contralateral normal ankle.

is the most common cause; primary hyperparathyroidism is rare in childhood. Generalized gangliosidosis, mucolipidosis type II, and the Jansen type of metaphyseal chondrodysplasia can all mimic hyperparathyroidism in infants. The other forms of metaphyseal chondrodysplasia may also demonstrate a widened growth plate, however the metaphyseal edges tend to be sclerotic and irregular. Hypophosphatasia and severe hypothyroidism may also result in generalized growth plate widening.

Widening of the proximal femoral growth plate is an early finding of slipped capital femoral epiphysis (Fig. 8–83). This condition occurs in early adolescence

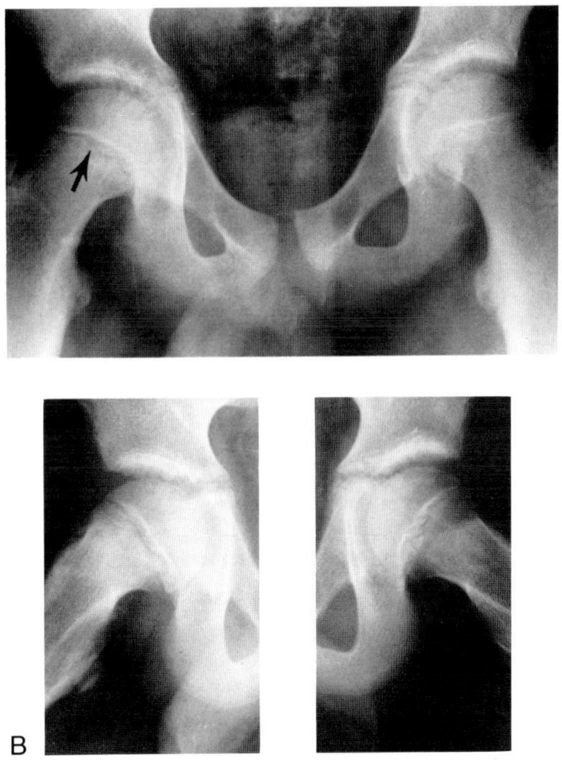

A

B

Fig. 8–83 Slipped capital femoral epiphysis. **(A)** The right proximal femoral physis is widened as compared with the normal left hip (*arrow*). **(B)** Lateral views demonstrate mild posterior slippage of the right femoral head on the metaphysis.

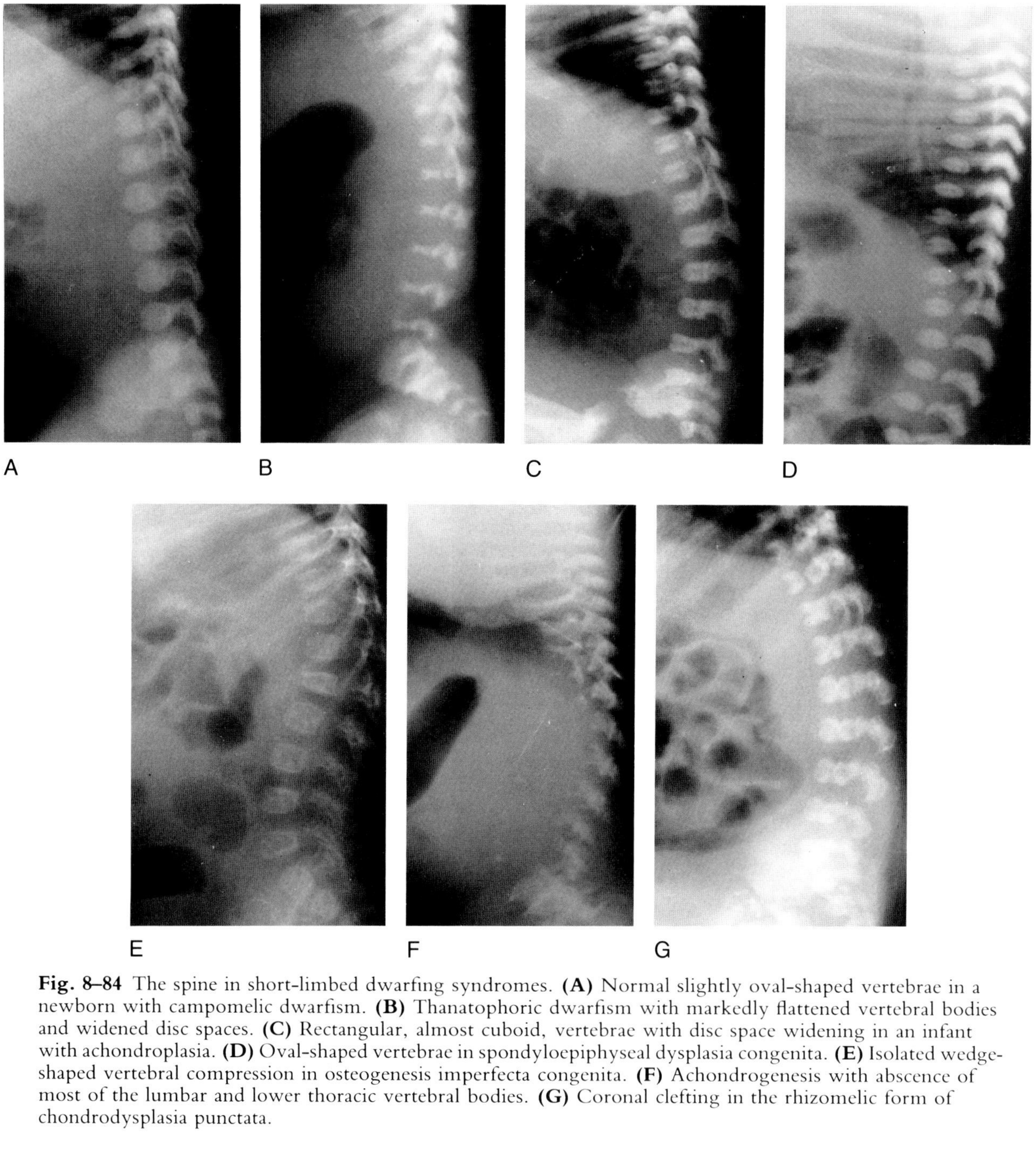

Fig. 8–84 The spine in short-limbed dwarfing syndromes. **(A)** Normal slightly oval-shaped vertebrae in a newborn with campomelic dwarfism. **(B)** Thanatophoric dwarfism with markedly flattened vertebral bodies and widened disc spaces. **(C)** Rectangular, almost cuboid, vertebrae with disc space widening in an infant with achondroplasia. **(D)** Oval-shaped vertebrae in spondyloepiphyseal dysplasia congenita. **(E)** Isolated wedge-shaped vertebral compression in osteogenesis imperfecta congenita. **(F)** Achondrogenesis with abscence of most of the lumbar and lower thoracic vertebral bodies. **(G)** Coronal clefting in the rhizomelic form of chondrodysplasia punctata.

and is most likely caused by chronic subclinical trauma to the physis. Eventually, the capital femoral epiphysis slips posteriorly and medially and is usually best visualized on a frogleg view. Bilateral, but often metachronous, slippage occurs in approximately 10 percent of cases.

Syndromes and Dysplasias

The classification of a patient's illness as one of the many congenital syndromes or skeletal dysplasias can be an intimidating task because of the enormous number and variety of abnormalities that characterize these conditions. This task is usually relegated to the pediatric radiologist or geneticist who has more frequent exposure to such patients and several excellent reference texts are available. Nevertheless, familiarity with some of the bone abnormalities that are common to many of these conditions can aid in the initial evaluation of such patients. Extensive lists of differential diagnoses are beyond the scope of this text, however the following points may be used to develop a systematic approach to the problem.

The spine is often helpful in the initial evaluation of a patient with a suspected syndrome or dysplasia. Certain characteristic vertebral body shapes are particularly useful for categorizing the various types of short-limbed dwarfs in the neonatal period (Fig. 8–84). Very flat, waferlike vertebrae are characteristic of thanatophoric dwarfism, metatropic dwarfism, and some of the Kneist-like dysplasias. In the Kneist syndrome, the vertebral bodies are less flattened and coronal clefts may be seen in both the Kneist syndrome and Kneist-like dysplasias. In spondyloepiphyseal dysplasia and hypochondrogenesis, the vertebrae are underdeveloped with a flat and rather oval shape. Wedge-shaped flattening due to compression occurs in osteogenesis imperfecta, especially the tarda form. Total absence of some or all of the vertebral bodies occurs in achondrogenesis, hypophosphatasia, and osteogenesis imperfecta congenita. Achondroplasia, hypochondroplasia, the short rib polydactyly syndromes, and the rhizomelic form of chrondrodystrophia punctata all demonstrate vertebral bodies with a cuboid or rectangular shape. The latter condition also shows coronal clefting of the vertebral bodies. Various types of segmentation anomalies occur with spondylothoracic dysplasia, dyssegmental dwarfism, and the dominant form of chondrodystrophia calcificans congenita. Other short-limbed dwarfing syndromes such as asphyxiating thoracic dystrophy, Ellis-van Creveld syndrome, campomelic dwarfism, diastrophic dwarfism and mesomelic dwarfism demonstrate normal spines. A narrowed spinal canal is also a useful finding in the diagnosis of achondroplasia and a number of other chondrodystrophies. Anterior and posterior scalloping in older children may result in a spool-shaped vertebra. This appearance is characteristic of conditions such as Melnick-Needles syndrome, neurofibromatosis, trisomy 21, and some of the chondrodystrophies and storage diseases.

Anomalies in the atlantoaxial region commonly accompany various syndromes and dysplasias. Hypoplasia or absence of the dens of C2 may occur as an isolated anomaly or may accompany such conditions as achondroplasia, trisomy 21, spondyloepiphyseal dysplasia congenita, and the mucopolysaccharidoses such as Morquio's disease. In many of these conditions, this anomaly is accompanied by instability at C1-C2. In some cases, the widening of the C1-dens distance can be quite dramatic (Fig. 8–85).

The most commonly encountered long bone abnormality in syndromes and dysplasias involves shorten-

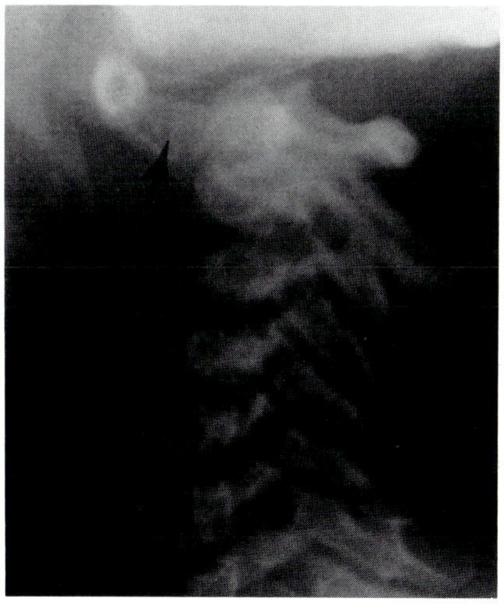

Fig. 8–85 Spondyloepiphyseal dysplasia. Mild hypoplasia of the dens is accompanied by instability at C1-C2, as evidenced by the widened C1-dens distance (*arrow*).

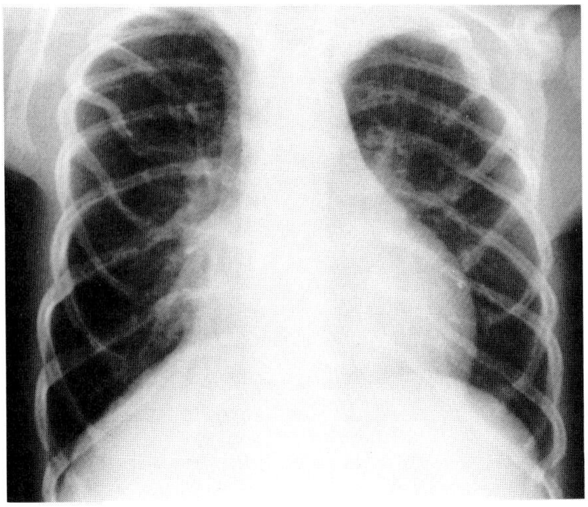

Fig. 8–86 Melnick-Needles osteodysplasty. Note the thin, twisted ribs.

ing of some or all of the long bones. This shortening may be categorized as proximal (rhizomelic), middle (mesomelic), or distal (acromelic). The long bones may be thin (overtubulation) or thick (undertubulation) (see lists, pp. 383 and 382). The epiphyses are small in dysplasias such as multiple epiphyseal dysplasia and spondyloepiphyseal dysplasia, sometimes with epiphyseal fragmentation (see lists, pp. 403 and 405). Splayed and cupped metaphyses characterize a number of syndromes and dysplasias (see list, p. 412). Twisted bones are an unusual finding that is most often seen in Melnick-Needles syndrome (Fig. 8–86), although it occasionally occurs with neurofibromatosis.

Pelvic bone abnormalities can be helpful in diagnosing a number of syndromes and dysplasias, particularly the chondrodystrophies, storage diseases, and chromosomal abnormalities. These abnormalities often involve either an increase or decrease in the acetabular angle (Fig. 8–87). When the angle is decreased (flattened acetabular roof), the iliac wings are often small and appear square-shaped. In some cases the acetabular roof will be irregular with deep sciatic notches, which is typical of many of the disproportionate dwarfing syndromes such as achondroplasia, asphyxiating thoracic dystrophy, Ellis-van Creveld syndrome, short rib polydactyly syndrome, metatropic dwarfism, spondyloepiphyseal dysplasia congenita, and thanatophoric dwarfism. Morquio's disease also demonstrates a similar appearance. Hypoplastic iliac wings with decreased acetabular angles but normal sciatic notches are characteristic of trisomy 21, tri somy 13, Morquio's disease, acrocephalosyndactyly syndromes, Cornelia de Lange syndrome, nail patella

A

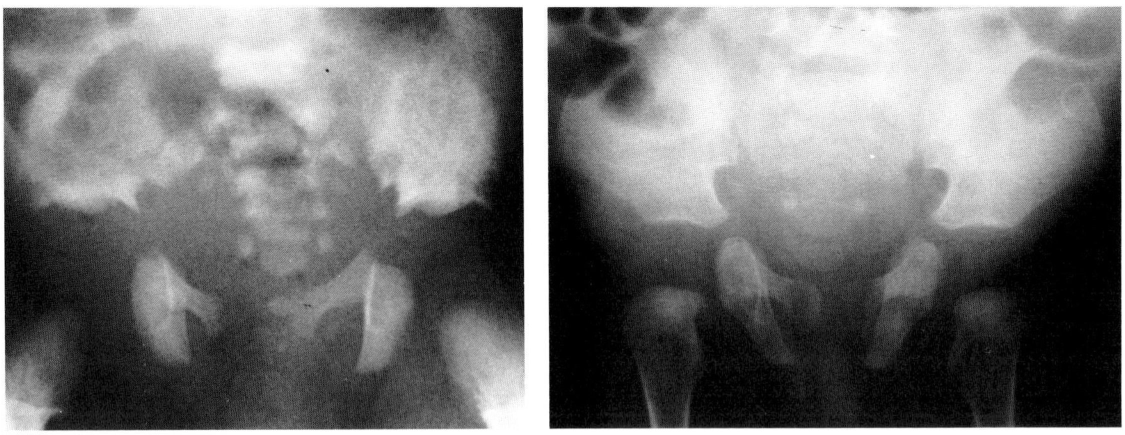

B

Fig. 8–87 Abnormal acetabular angles. **(A)** Characteristic small square iliac wings with decreased acetabular angles in a patient with achondroplasia. **(B)** Decreased acetabular angles and underossified pubic bones in trisomy 21.

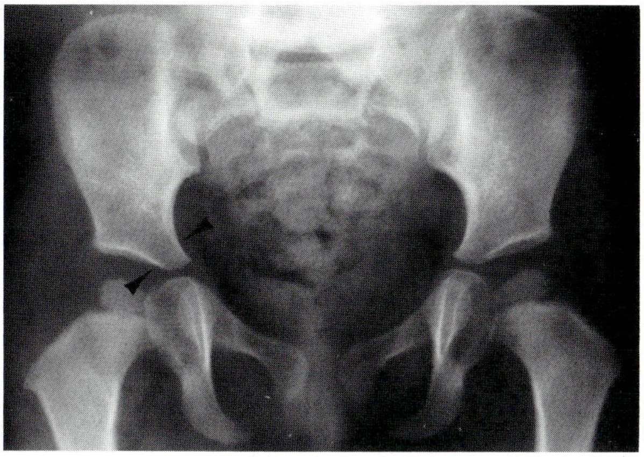

Fig. 8–88 Trisomy 18. The acetabular angles are increased with characteristic constriction of the lower iliac wing (*arrowheads*).

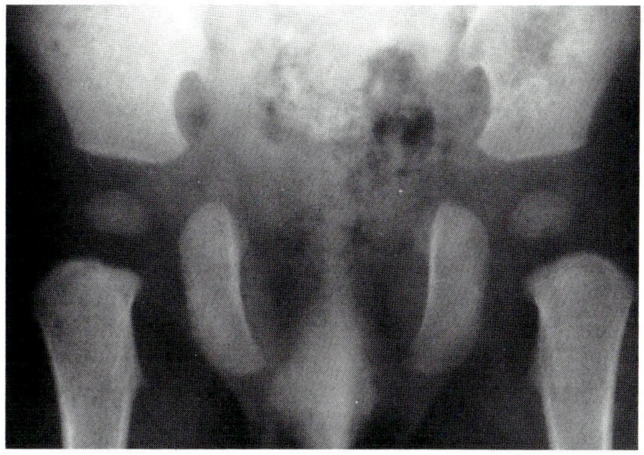

Fig. 8–89 Cleidocranial dysostosis. Note the absence of the pubic bones.

syndrome, Rubinstein-Taybi syndrome and Weissenbacher-Zweymuller syndrome. Increased acetabular angles with constriction of the lower portion of the iliac wing are typical of trisomy 18, Melnick-Needles syndrome, and many of the storage diseases other than Morquio's disease (Fig. 8–88). Steep acetabular angles are also seen with congenital hip dislocation. Hypoplastic or unossified pubic bones are characteristic of cleidocranial dysostosis, chondrodystrophia calcificans congenita, spondyloepiphyseal dysplasia congenita, the Taybi-Lindner syndrome, and many of the chondrodystrophies (Fig. 8–89).

Bony abnormalities in the hands and feet are common components of many congenital syndromes and dysplasias. Hand changes are especially prevalent and include shortening of the metacarpals or phalanges, triphalangeal thumb, clinodactyly, syndactyly, polydactyly, and carpal coalition (Fig. 8–90). Similar abnormalities may be present in the feet.

Segmentation abnormalities of the sternum can occasionally provide helpful information regarding the possible syndrome. Hypersegmentation of the sternum occurs in trisomy 21, whereas hyposegmentation is associated with trisomy 18, campomelic

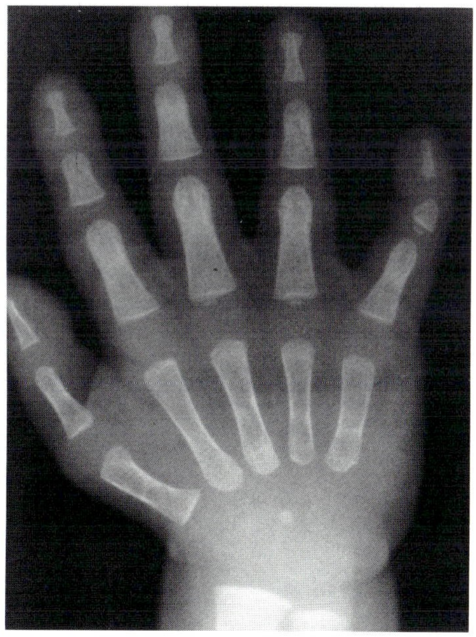

Fig. 8–90 Cornelia de Lange syndrome. Note the hypoplasia and curving in of the fifth digit.

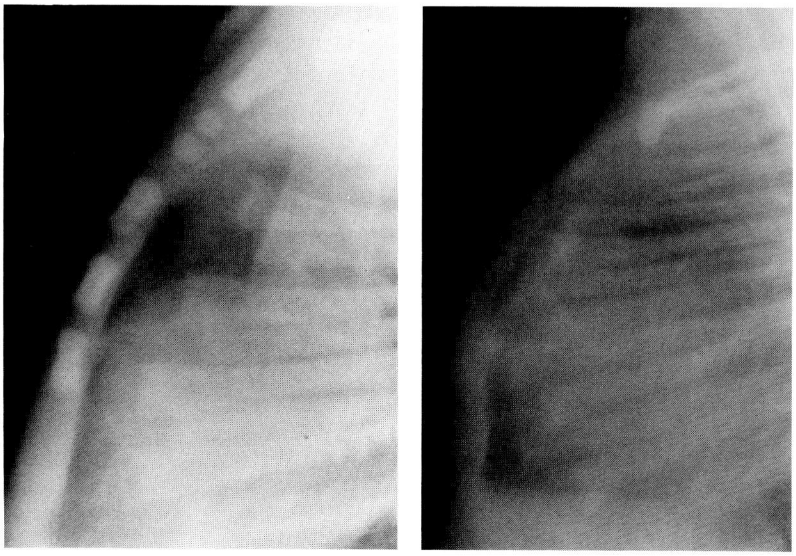

Fig. 8–91 Segmentation abnormalities of the sternum. **(A)** Hypersegmentation of the sternum in a patient with trisomy 21. **(B)** Sternal hyposegmentation associated with trisomy 18.

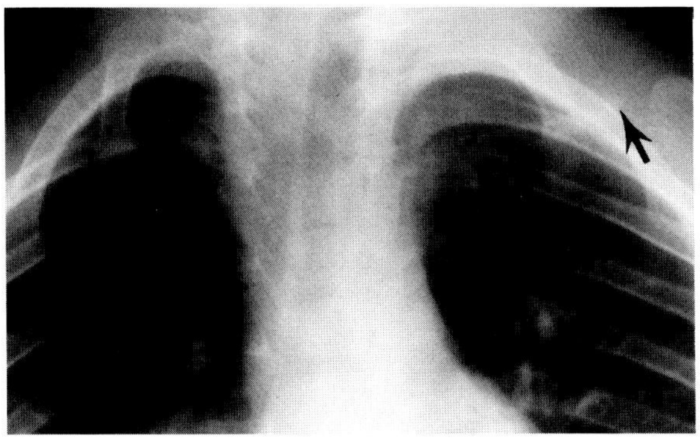

Fig. 8–92 Cleidocranial dysostosis. The clavicles are markedly hypoplastic (*arrows*).

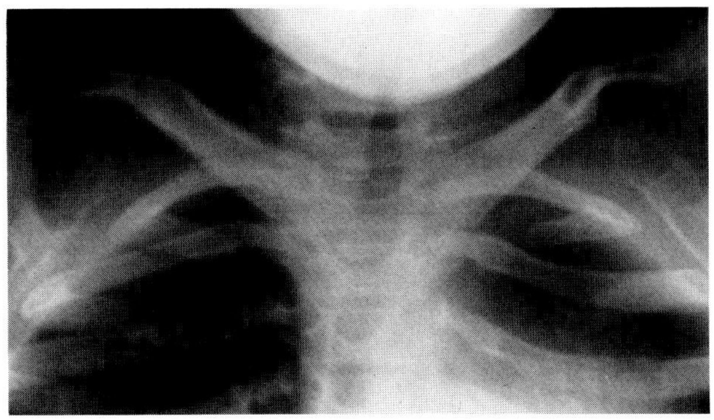

Fig. 8–93 Holt-Oram syndrome. A handlebar configuration of the clavicles is common in this condition.

dwarfism, Noonan syndrome, and Cornelia de Lange syndrome (Fig. 8–91). Hypoplasia of the clavicles occurs in cleidocranial dysostosis, Holt-Oram syndrome, Goltz syndrome, progeria, trisomy 13, and trisomy 18 (Fig. 8–92). Clavicles with a lateral hook ("handlebar") are characteristic of the Holt-Oram syndrome and can also be seen in campomelic dysplasia, diastrophic dysplasia, thrombocytopenia-absent radius (TAR) syndrome, and trisomy 18 (Fig. 8–93). In the storage diseases the clavicles may be very short and broad. Miscellaneous bone abnormalities such as abnormal bone density, synostosis, pseudoarthroses, and exostoses have been covered in previous sections.

SOFT TISSUES

Extremity Enlargement

Enlargement of the extremities may be due to enlargement of the bone, muscle, fat, or all of these. Unilateral enlargement of both the bony and soft tissue components of an extremity is referred to as hemihypertrophy and usually involves all of the structures on one side of the body. However, it tends to be more prominent in the lower extremities (Fig. 8–94). The etiology of hemihypertrophy is uncertain and sometimes it is an isolated abnormality. On the other hand, hemihypertrophy is frequently associated with intra-abdominal tumors, the most well known of which is Wilms' tumor of the kidney. Hemihypertrophy can also occur with benign cystic kidney disease and in the Beckwith-Weidemann syndrome.

Localized enlargement of an extremity or a portion of an extremity often occurs as a response to hyperemia associated with an arteriovenous fistula, hemangioma, or lymphangioma of the involved extremity. Abnormalities of the lymphatic system such as congenital absence or hypoplasia, surgical disruption, or compression by a mass may result in lymphedema causing localized soft tissue enlargement. Focal soft tissue enlargement caused by a mesenchymal abnormality of unknown etiology occurs in both neurofibromatosis and macrodystrophia lipomatosa. Focal enlargement of the soft tissues because of deep soft tissue edema can be an important early finding in osteomyelitis in children (Fig. 8–95).

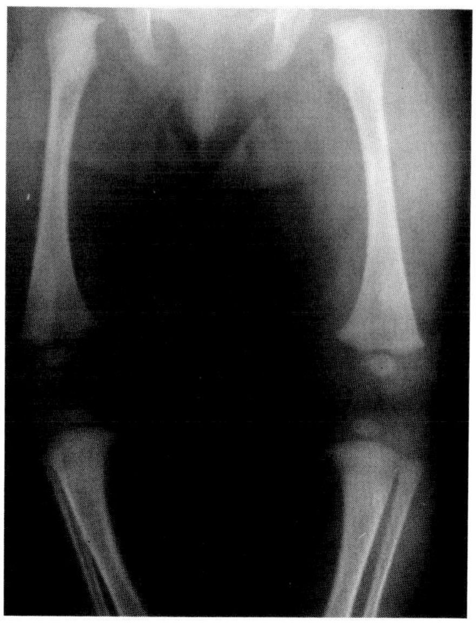

Fig. 8–94 Hemihypertrophy. The enlargement of the soft tissues and long bones on the left was idiopathic in this infant.

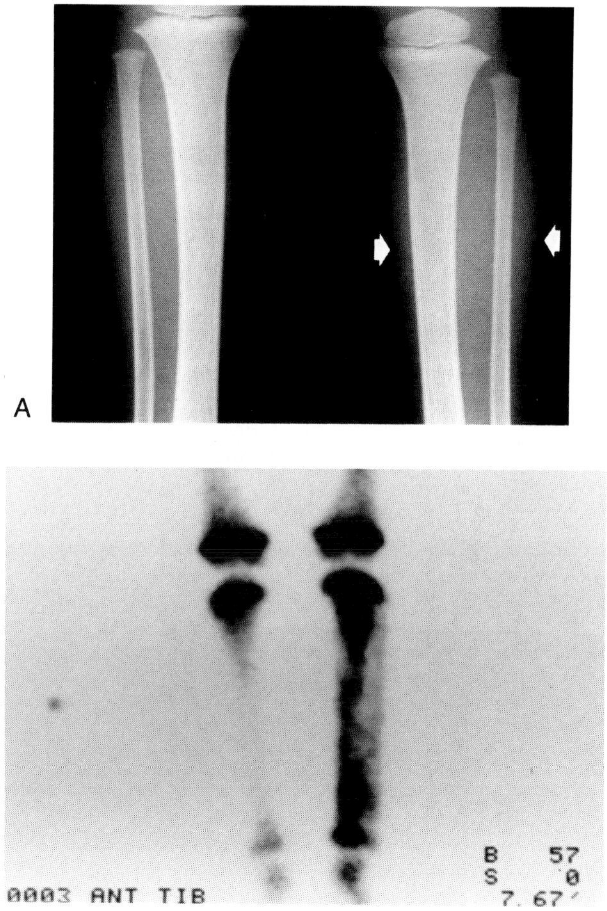

Fig. 8–95 Osteomyelitis of the left tibia. **(A)** Thickening of the deep soft tissues of the left leg (*arrows*) suggested the presence of deep edema due to osteomyelitis, even though no bony destruction could be identified. **(B)** The diagnosis was confirmed by a technetium bone scan, which showed diffusely increased tracer uptake in the left tibia.

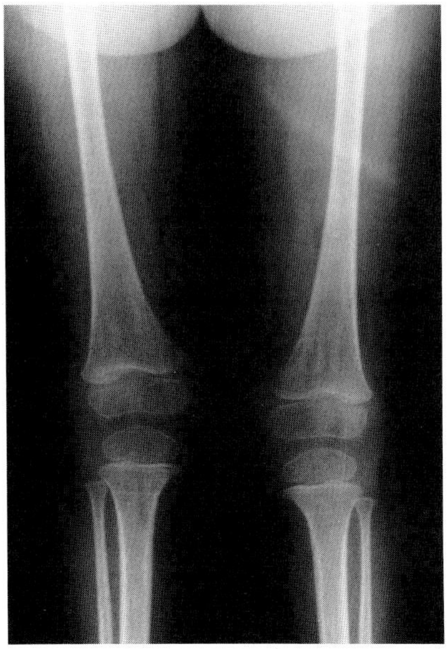

Fig. 8–96 Neurologic disease. The bones are gracile and the muscle bulk is markedly diminished.

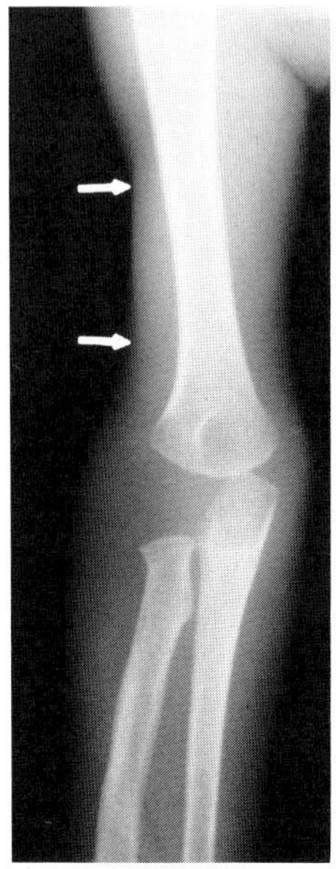

Fig. 8–98 Diencephalic syndrome. Note the marked decrease in subcutaneous fat (*arrows*).

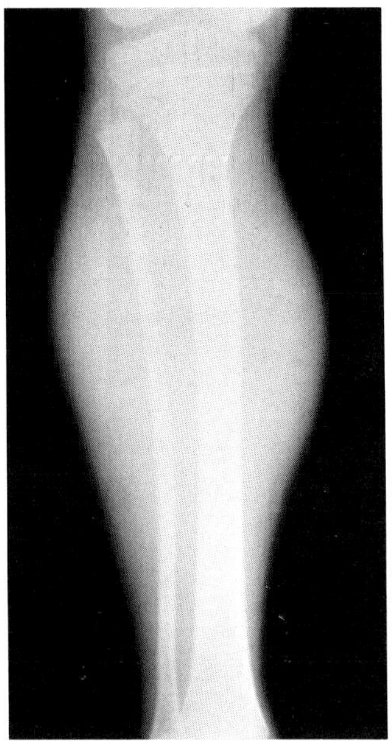

Fig. 8–97 Hypertrophic muscular dystrophy. Enlargement of the soft tissues was caused entirely by increased muscle bulk.

A

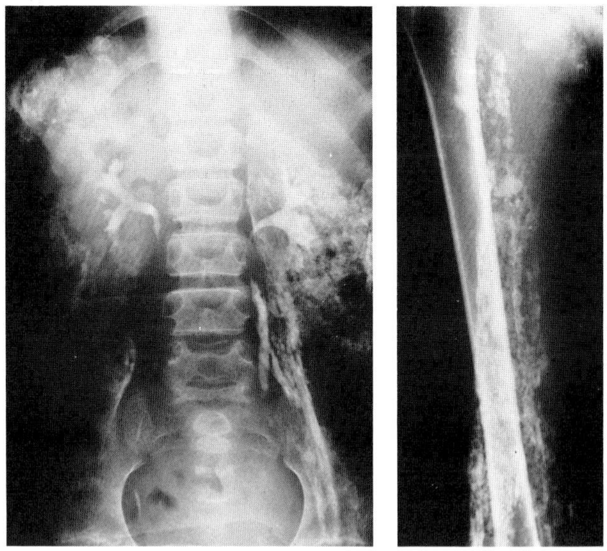

B

Fig. 8–99 Dermatomyositis. Extensive calcification was present in the soft tissues of the **(A)** body wall and **(B)** extremities.

Generalized soft tissue enlargement because of a disproportionate increase in subcutaneous fat is rather common and may be caused by simple obesity, increased exogenous or endogenous steroids, Prader-Willi syndrome, and Lawrence-Moon-Beidl syndrome. If the excessive fat is associated with a decrease in the muscle bulk, some form of neuromuscular disease is usually responsible (Fig. 8–96). Soft tissue enlargement due to increased muscle bulk is uncommon but can occur in some forms of muscular dystrophy, congenital muscular hypertrophy, and occasionally in normal exercise hypertrophy (Fig. 8–97).

Atrophy of the Extremity

Atrophy of the soft tissues of an extremity is most commonly secondary to some form of neurologic disease. Small extremities on one side of the body can be seen in the Russell-Silver syndrome, however the smallness is caused by abnormal growth of the extremities as reflected by a discrepancy of the bone age of each side of the body. Decreased soft tissues because of a decrease in the amount of subcutaneous fat may result from severe malnutrition. The diencephalic syndrome is an unusual condition in which a tumor in the region of the anterior hypothalamus results in abnormal fat metabolism; patients often show a complete absence of subcutaneous fat (Fig. 8–98). Congenital lipodystrophy is also characterized by a severe loss in subcutaneous fat which may be generalized or localized.

Soft Tissue Calcifications

Calcification within the soft tissues in infants and children is uncommon and may take one of several forms (see list). Irregular, amorphous calcifications may occur in the soft tissues after the resolution of muscular abscesses and hematomas. Sheets of amorphous calcifications occur with collagen vascular diseases, especially dermatomyositis and systemic lupus erythmatosis (Fig. 8–99). Early, focal post-traumatic myositis ossificans may appear as a focal area of amorphous calcification; later, these calcifications may take

SOFT TISSUE CALCIFICATIONS

Congenital/developmental
- Nevoid basal cell carcinoma syndrome*
- Ehlers-Danlos syndrome†
- Myositis ossificans progressiva‡
- Tumoral calcinosis*
- Calcinosis universalis*

Inflammatory
- After soft tissue abscess*
- Thrombophlebitis‡

Neoplasm
- Hemangioma†
- Lymphangioma†
- Generalized infantile fibromatosis*
- Calcifying epithelioma*

Trauma/surgery
- Myositis ossifications‡
- Posthemorrhage (hemophilia)*
- Foreign bodies*,†,‡
- Extravasation of calcium salt injections*

Systemic/metabolic
- Immobilization*,†
- Burns*,‡
- Collagen vascular diseases*
- Hyperparathyroidism*
- Hypervitaminosis D*
- Arteriosclerosis (e.g., progeria)‡

Miscellaneous
- Fat necrosis (infants)*
- Idiopathic vascular calcification‡
- Postsubcutaneous emphysema (neonate)*
- Varicose veins†

* Amorphous.
† Stonelike.
‡ Formed.

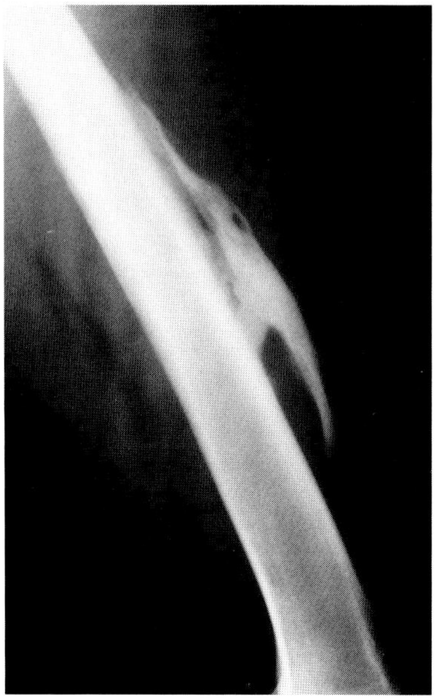

Fig. 8–100 Myositis ossificans. Masslike calcification of the soft tissues of the anterior thigh secondary to trauma.

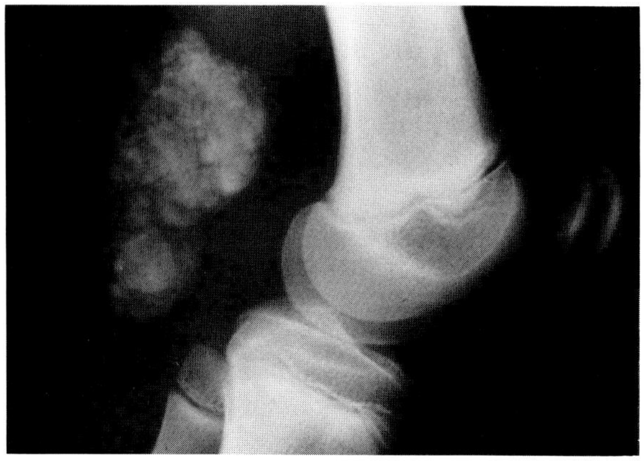

Fig. 8–101 Tumoral calcinosis. Note the large, flocculant mass of calcification posterior to the knee joint.

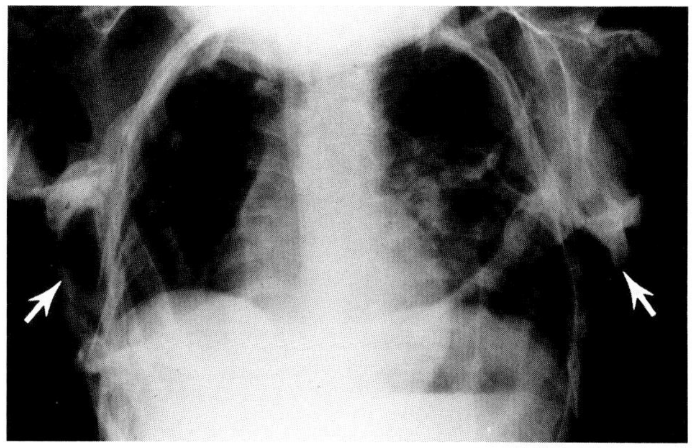

Fig. 8–102 Myositis ossificans progressiva. Massive, diffuse ossification of the soft tissues (*arrows*) in a 6-year-old patient.

on a more formed, masslike appearance (Fig. 8–100). Soft tissue calcifications may also follow severe burns, trauma, or other causes of prolonged immobilization such as neurologic disease. Hypercalcemia due to hyperparathyroidism or hypervitaminosis D can occasionally result in irregular soft tissue calcifications. In infants, rather extensive soft tissue calcification may result from fat necrosis. This condition is generally believed to result from local ischemia due to trauma or, occasionally, hypothermia. Foreign bodies within the soft tissues may mimic calcifications. Other causes of amorphous calcifications include the nevoid basal cell carcinoma syndrome, calcinosis universalis, generalized infantile fibromatosis, and extravasation of calcium salt injections. Tumoral calcinosis is a rare condition in which large masses of flocculent calcifications occur in the periarticular regions (Fig. 8–101). Occasionally these lesions are cystic, filled with a milk of calcium-type fluid.

Formed masses of calcification are characteristic of myositis ossificans progressiva, an inherited mesodermal disorder characterized by progressive inflammation and ossification of fascia, ligaments, tendons, and connective tissue. This ossification appears as sheets of dense bone that generally begin near joints and in the posterior spinal ligament and eventually extend into the muscles and subcutaneous tissues (Fig. 8–102). Microdactyly of the thumbs and great toes can be a helpful associated finding in the early stages of the disease before extensive ossification develops. Linear or tubular vascular calcifications are rare in children, but are occasionally seen in children who

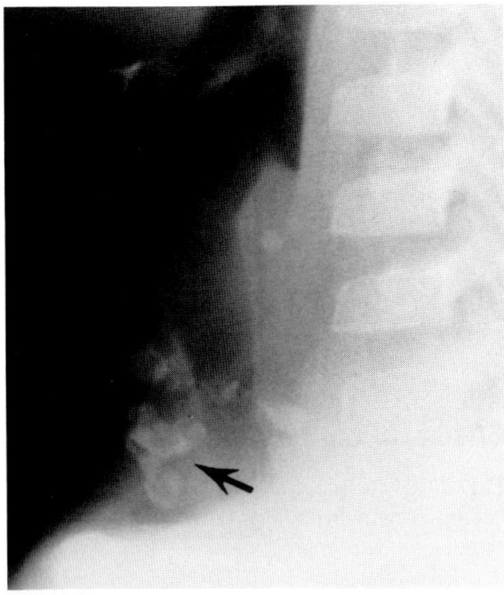

Fig. 8–103 Hemangioma of the neck. Characteristic phleboliths within this tumor were evident on the plain radiograph (*arrow*).

have early arteriosclerosis such as that which occurs with progeria. In infancy, idiopathic vascular calcifications have been reported.

Stonelike calcifications within the soft tissues are most commonly seen in angiomatous tumors such as hemangioma or lymphangioma (Fig. 8–103). Phleboliths may also develop in venous varicosities. Peculiar calcifed nodules, which have a stonelike appearance, have been reported in several cases of Ehler-Danlos syndrome.

SKULL

Enlarged Skull

The most common cause of cranial enlargement in young children before cranial suture closure is hydrocephalus. Hydrocephalus may be caused by congenital causes such as aqueductal stenosis or Arnold-Chiari malformation, or may be acquired. Acquired hydrocephalus is most often a communicating type of hydrocephalus caused by adhesions secondary to meningitis or subarachnoid hemorrhage. Noncommunicating hydrocephalus caused by intraventricular hemorrhage in premature infants is also quite common. Intracranial masses (tumors, cysts) may cause obstruction of the cerebral spinal fluid pathways leading to hydrocephalus. Hydranencephaly is an uncommon developmental condition in which the cerebral hemispheres are virtually absent, most likely because of some form of vascular or infectious insult. The enlarged skull is filled with cerebrospinal fluid, which may mimic massive hydrocephalus (Fig. 8–104). The

LARGE SKULL

Congenital/developmental
- Hydrocephalus (aqueductal stenosis, Arnold-Chiari malformation, Dandy-Walker cyst)
- Chondrodystrophies
- Cleidocranial dysostosis
- Sotos syndrome
- Craniometaphyseal dysplasia
- Russell-Silver syndrome
- Neurofibromatosis
- Familial megalencephaly
- Zellweger syndrome
- Riley-Smith syndrome

Inflammation
- Postmeningitis hydrocephalus

Neoplasm/cyst
- Large brain tumor or cyst
- Multiple hemangiomatosis syndrome

Trauma/surgery
- Subdural hematoma
- Hydrocephalus caused by posthemorrhagic adhesions

Systemic/metabolic
- Storage diseases

Miscellaneous
- Any cause of skull thickening
- Subdural effusions
- Hydranencephaly

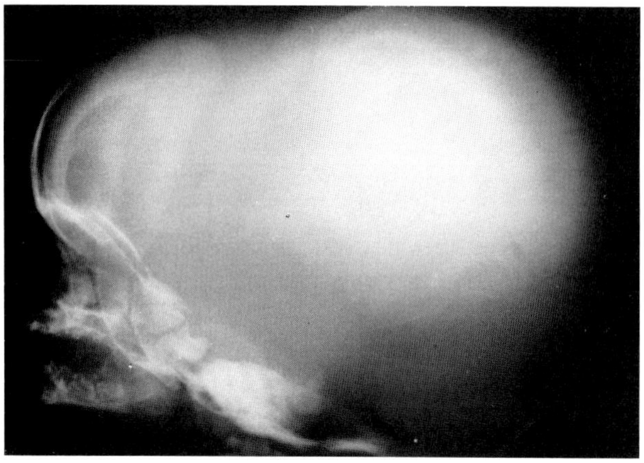

Fig. 8–104 Hydranencephaly. The skull is markedly enlarged and thinned.

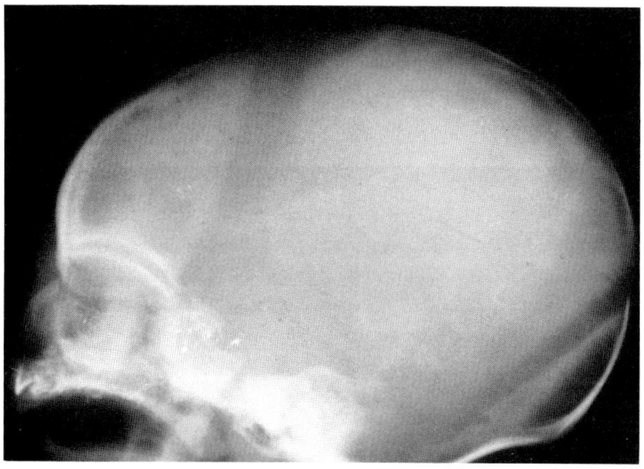

Fig. 8–105 Intracranial hemorrhage. Post-traumatic subdural hematoma resulted in cranial enlargement and spreading of the sutures in this child.

common carotid artery is small in these patients, a finding that helps to differentiate it from severe hydrocephalus.

Cranial enlargement with widening of the cranial sutures may also be the result of trauma resulting in intracranial hematoma (Fig. 8–105). This is an important finding, particularly in cases of suspected child abuse. Nonspecific subdural effusions may also occasionally lead to cranial enlargement.

Cranial enlargement is a common component of a number of congenital and developmental syndromes. Any cause of thickening of the skull will also lead to cranial enlargement. Enlargement of the brain is a less common cause of skull enlargement. This occurs in some of the mucolipidoses and mucopolysaccharidoses. A benign familial form of megalencephaly has also been described.

Small Skull

A small skull (microcephaly) is most often a reflection of an absent or atrophic brain. Anencephaly is the most severe form of maldevelopment of the brain, with only a small remnant of midbrain and brain stem present. Numerous syndromes are associated with poor brain development and resultant microcephaly (Fig. 8–106). Congenitally acquired infections such as rubella, cytomegalovirus, toxoplasmosis, and herpes often result in a poorly developed brain and a small skull. Microcephaly also occurs with fetal alcohol syndrome.

SMALL SKULL

Congenital/developmental
- Anencephaly
- Cephaloskeletal dysplasia
- Chromosomal abnormalities (e.g., trisomy 21, trisomy 18)
- Cockayne's syndrome
- Universal craniosynostosis
- Cornelia de Lange syndrome
- Dyggve-Melchior-Clausen syndrome
- Fanconi's anemia
- Holoprosencephaly
- Lissencephaly
- Meckel's syndrome
- Other syndromes associated with brain atrophy or mental retardation

Systemic/metabolic
- Homocystinuria
- Lesch-Nyhan syndrome
- Pyruvate dehydrogenase complex deficiency

Miscellaneous
- Congenital infections (TORCH syndrome)
- Psychosocial dwarfism
- Fetal alcohol syndrome
- Brain atrophy due to other causes

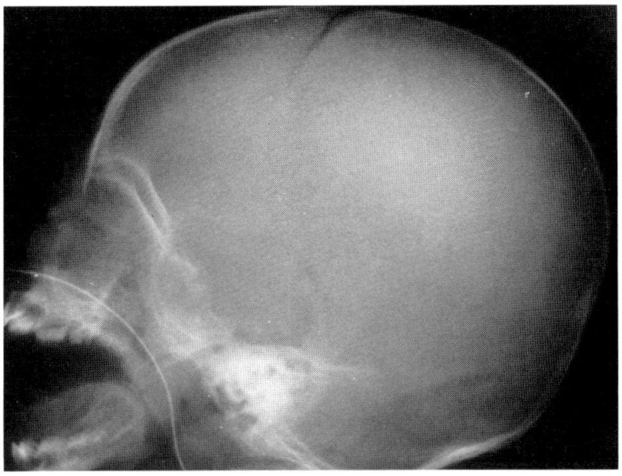

Fig. 8–106 Failure to thrive. A small skull with narrow sutures resulted from poor brain growth in this 3-month-old infant.

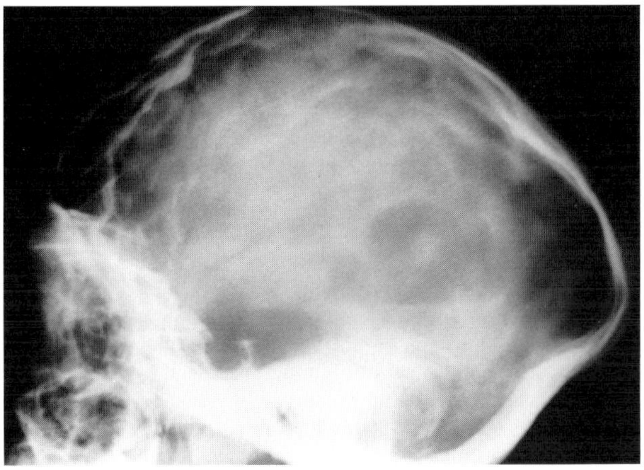

Fig. 8–107 Universal craniosynostosis. Early closure of all of the sutures resulted in microcephaly and chronically increased intracranial pressure. Note the prominent inner table convolutional markings and enlargement of the sella turcica.

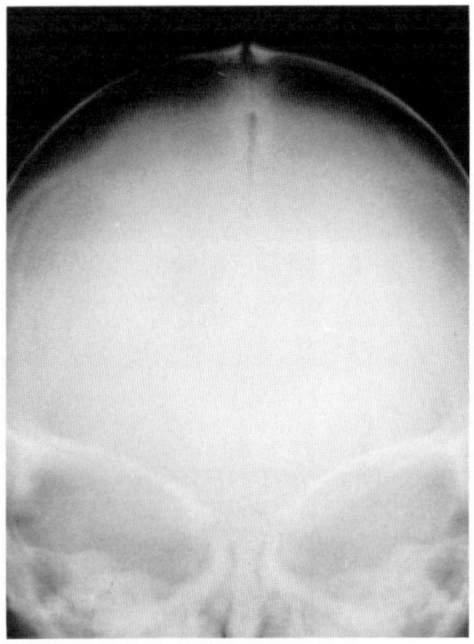

Fig. 8–108 Sagittal craniosynostosis. The abnormal sagittal suture demonstrates the characteristic narrowing with sharp edges and bony bridging seen with primary craniosynostosis.

Poor brain growth results in a lack of stimulation of skull growth and can lead to premature closure of the cranial sutures. This must be differentiated from the primary forms of craniosynostosis in which chronically increased intracranial pressure leads to the development of increased cranial convolutional markings and demineralization and enlargement of the sella turcica (Fig. 8–107). When the primary form of premature synostosis of the sutures occurs, the bone growth along the edges of the suture is impaired, resulting in a narrowed suture with knife-sharp edges and with sclerosis and ridging along the margins of the suture (Fig. 8–108). Eventually actual bony bridging will be seen. Universal craniosynostosis produces the most severe microcephaly, but more commonly some of the sutures will remain open. In such cases

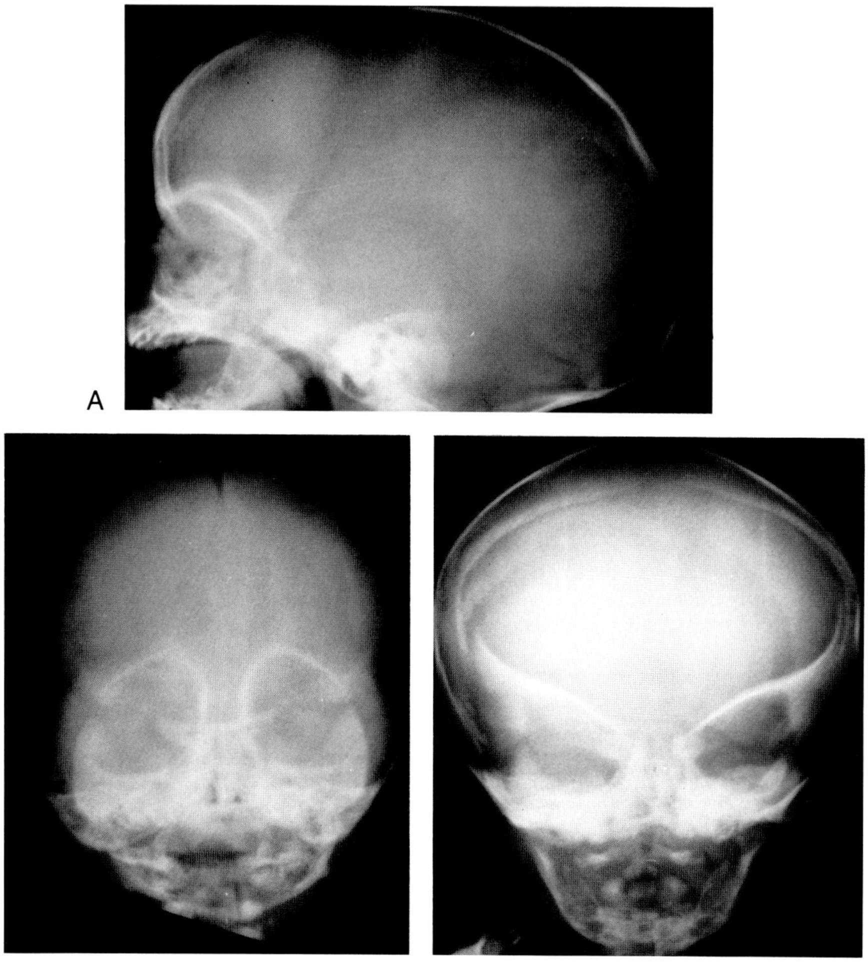

Fig. 8–109 Craniosynostosis. **(A)** Early closure of the sagittal suture results in an elongated (dolicocephalic) skull. **(B)** Medial slanting of the orbits because of premature closure of the metopic suture. **(C)** "Harlequin eye" deformity caused by coronal craniosynostosis.

the head circumference may not be particularly small, but the head shape will always be abnormal. The sutures involved in the synostosis determine the configuration of the skull. For example, sagittal synostosis results in a narrow elongated head (dolichocephaly), whereas bilateral coronal synostosis results in a short, wide skull with elevated sphenoid wings, hypertelorism, and "harlequin" type orbits (Fig. 8–109). Any combination of sutural involvement may occur and very bizarre configurations may result. Unilateral smallness of the calvaria may occur when only a portion of the brain is atrophic, such as in the Dyke-Davidoff-Masson syndrome or the Russell-Silver syndrome.

Thickened Skull

Generalized thickening of the calvaria usually results in increased density of the skull that may be homogeneous or inhomogeneous. The most common cause of a homogeneously dense thickened skull is longstanding decreased intracranial pressure, usually re-

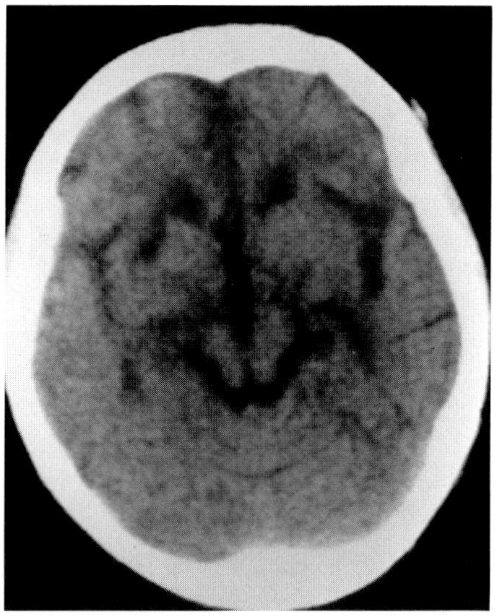

Fig. 8–110 Skull thickening secondary to brain atrophy. Axial CT scan demonstrates the thickened skull associated with enlargement of the intracranial cerebrospinal fluid spaces consistent with atrophy.

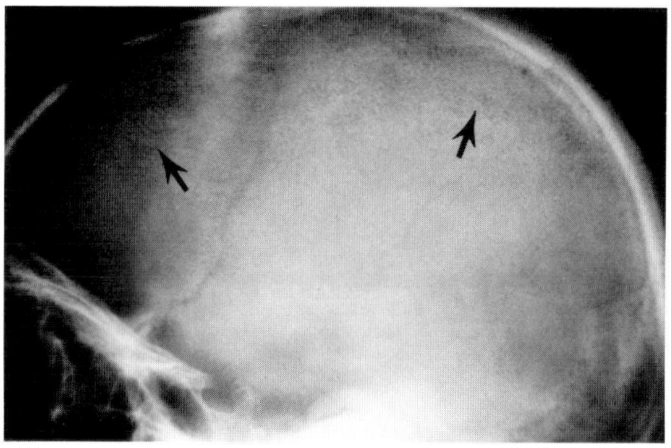

Fig. 8–111 Secondary hyperparathyroidism. Note the salt and pepper pattern of the skull (*arrows*).

GENERALIZED SKULL THICKENING

Congenital/developmental
- Osteopetrosis
- Acrodysostosis
- Cockayne's syndrome
- Craniometaphyseal dysplasia
- Congenital total lipodystrophy
- Osteopathia striata
- Pyknodyostosis
- Endosteal hyperostosis (van-Buchem)
- Melorheostosis
- Myotonic dystrophy

Neoplasm/cyst
- Leukemia/lymphoma
- Metastases

Systemic/metabolic
- Chronic anemia
- Hypoparathyroidism/pseudohypoparathyroidism
- Hyperparathyroidism
- Rickets (healing)
- Dilantin therapy
- Hypervitaminosis D
- Idiopathic hypercalcemia
- Storage diseases
- Polycythemia
- Hyperphosphatasia
- Fluorosis

Miscellaneous
- Brain atrophy
- After shunt placement for hydrocephalus

sulting from brain atrophy or after successful shunting of hydrocephalus (Fig. 8–110). A similar appearance occurs in a number of bone dysplasias and occasionally in the healing stages of renal osteodystrophy.

Metabolic abnormalities lead to skull thickening with a pattern of patchy sclerosis. These conditions include hyperparathyroidism, hyperphosphatemia, hypophosphatasia, and healing rickets. In hyperparathyroidism, the skull often exhibits a granular, "salt and pepper" pattern (Fig. 8–111). Lamellated thickening has been seen with hyperphosphatemia and sickle cell anemia.

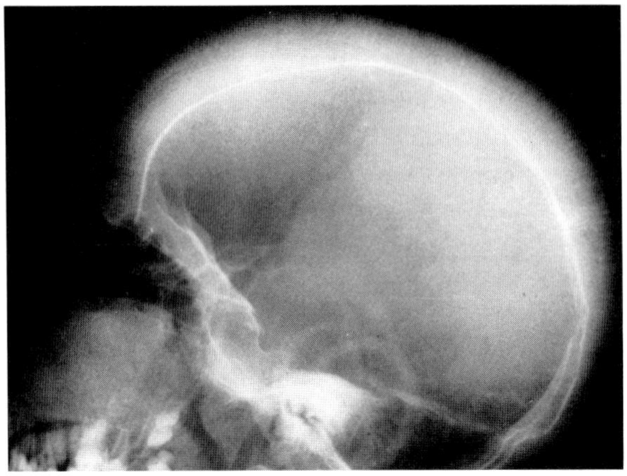

Fig. 8–112 Thalassemia. Marked thickening of the skull and facial bones is caused by marrow proliferation in this hemoglobinopathy.

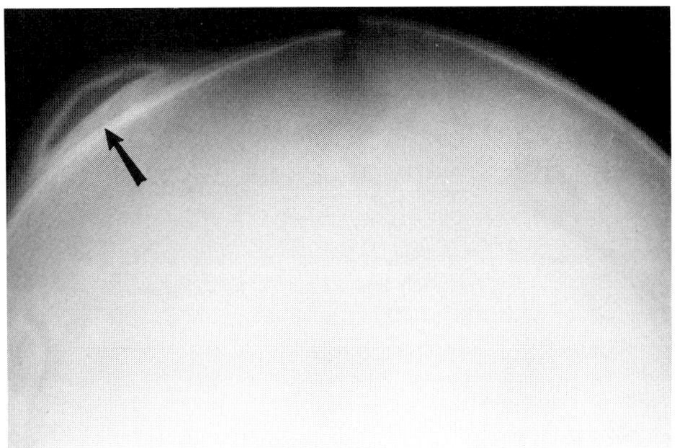

Fig. 8–113 Calcified cephalohematoma. In the healing stages, such hematomas appear as focal thickening of the skull with a radiolucent center (*arrow*). The defect in the left skull represents a surgical burr hole.

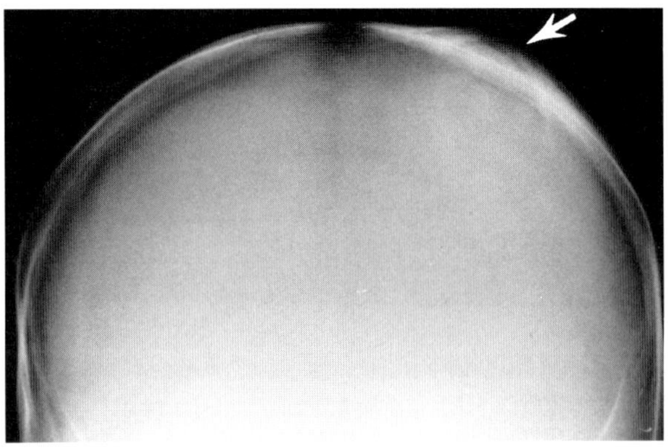

Fig. 8–114 Cephalohematoma. Focal thickening of the skull because of a healed calcified cephalohematoma (*arrow*).

Hematologic conditions thicken the skull by enlarging the diploic layer of the calvaria (Fig. 8–112). Often multiple vertical striation are also present. The most common cause of this pattern are the chronic anemias such as sickle cell disease, thalassemia, iron deficiency anemia, hereditary spherocytosis, and polycythemia. Leukemia, lymphoma, and metastatic disease can occasionally produce a similar appearance, however these conditions are more likely to result in a focal thickening of the skull.

Localized thickening of the calvaria may involve focal areas of the cranial vault or isolated thickening of the skull base. Localized areas of thickening and sclerosis of the skull may occur due to chronic osteomyelitis or adjacent cellulitis, healing histiocytosis X, tuberous sclerosis, sickle cell disease, iron deficiency anemia, leukemia, or metastatic neuroblastoma. Cephalohematomas are a common occurrence in the postnatal period. During the healing phase, they may appear as a focal area of skull thickening with a central radiolucency (Fig. 8–113). Once the healing is complete, a focal, homogeneously thickened area involving both the inner and outer table often persists, sometimes for years (Fig. 8–114). Neoplasms such as hemangioma, meningioma, osteoma, and osteogenic sarcoma, are unusual causes of focal skull thickening in childhood.

Large focal areas of skull thickening and sclerosis are most often due to fibrous dysplasia (Fig. 8–115). The frontal and basal regions of the skull are most commonly involved. These lesions are composed of varying amounts of fibrous tissue, cartilage, and immature bone and may exhibit varying amounts of radiolucency and sclerosis. Unilateral thickening of the skull can be associated with ipsilateral cerebral hemiatrophy in the Dyke-Davidoff-Masson syndrome.

A number of bone dysplasias result in skull thickening that is isolated to the skull base. Skull base thickening commonly occurs with fibrous dysplasia. Clivus chordoma is the most common neoplasm to cause skull base thickening. These tumors arise from primitive notochord remnants and appear as destructive lesions, often with irregular calcifications. Meningioma is a rare cause of basal skull thickening in children.

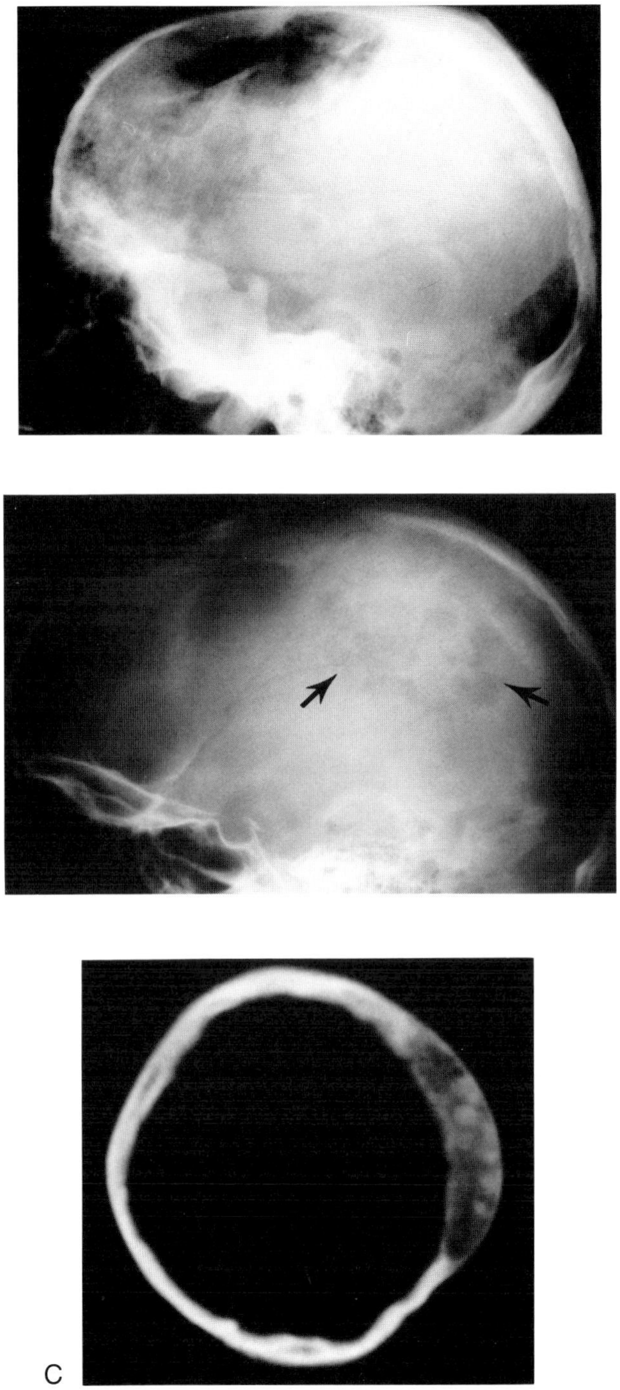

Fig. 8–115 Fibrous dysplasia. **(A)** Multiple areas of skull thickening are common in this condition. **(B)** This mixed lytic and sclerotic lesion of the parietal bone was caused by fibrous dysplasia (*arrows*). **(C)** Axial CT scan at bone window settings demonstrates the focal thickening and mixed attenuation of the lesion.

FOCAL SKULL THICKENING

Congenital/developmental
- Osteopetrosis*
- Craniometaphyseal dysplasia*
- Diaphyseal dysplasia*
- Melnick-Needles osteodysplasty*
- Metaphyseal chondrodysplasia (Jansen)*
- Cleidocranial dysostosis*
- Otopalatodigital syndrome*
- Melorheostosis*
- Fibrous dysplasia

Inflammatory
- Chronic infection

Neoplasm
- Meningioma
- Hemangioma
- Clivus chordoma*
- Other primary bone tumors
- Leukemia
- Metastatic neuroblastoma

Trauma/surgery
- Cephalohematoma (healed)

Systemic/metabolic
- Chronic anemias
- Histiocytosis X (healing)

Miscellaneous
- Cerebral hemiatrophy (Dyke-Davidoff-Masson syndrome)

* Base of skull only.

Thin Skull

Generalized thinning of the calvaria is a common finding in the normal premature infant. Otherwise, a thin calvaria is most often associated with some type of syndrome or bone dysplasia (see list). Generalized skull thinning is characteristic of osteogenesis imperfecta, cleidocranial dysostosis, Melnick-Needles syndrome, progeria, and aminopterin fetopathy (the use of aminopterin during the first trimester of pregnancy) (Fig. 8–116). Metabolic abnormalities such as rickets and hypophosphatasia also result in a thin skull. Increased intracranial pressure caused by chronic and untreated hydrocephalus can also result in generalized thinning of the cranium.

Chronically increased intracranial pressure more commonly results in prominent convolutional markings because of pressure from the gyri upon the inner table of the skull (Fig. 8–117). These markings are most often seen with slowly progressive space-occupying lesions of the brain such as hydrocephalus, neoplasms, and cysts. In such patients, other signs of increased intracranial pressure are usually seen, such as widened cranial sutures and enlargement and demineralization of the sella turcica. The various forms of primary craniosynostosis also lead to prominent convolutional markings of the skull. The mark-

THINNING OF THE SKULL

Congenital/developmental
- Osteogenesis imperfecta
- Craniolacuna
- Chromosomal abnormalities (trisomy)
- Cleidocranial dysostosis
- Melnick-Needles syndrome (osteodysplasty)
- Progeria
- Aminopterin fetopathy
- Craniosynostosis

Neoplasm/cyst
- Intracranial neoplasm or cyst*

Trauma/surgery
- Chronic subdural hematoma*

Systemic/metabolic
- Rickets
- Hypophosphatasia
- Neurofibromatosis*

Miscellaneous
- Hydrocephalus (untreated)
- Prematurity

* Focal.

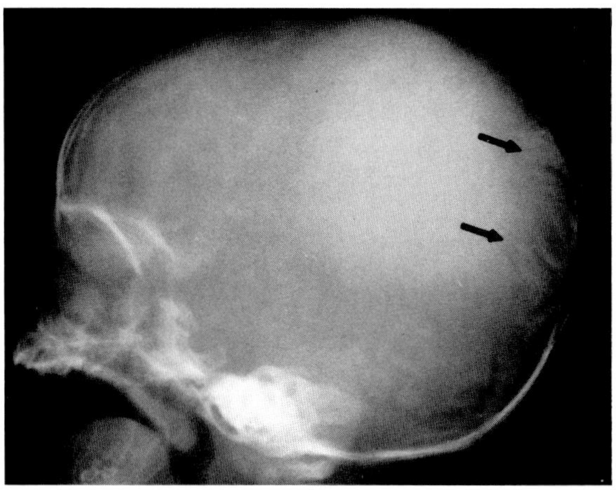

Fig. 8–116 Osteogenesis imperfecta congenita. The skull is thin with multiple Wormian bones (*arrows*).

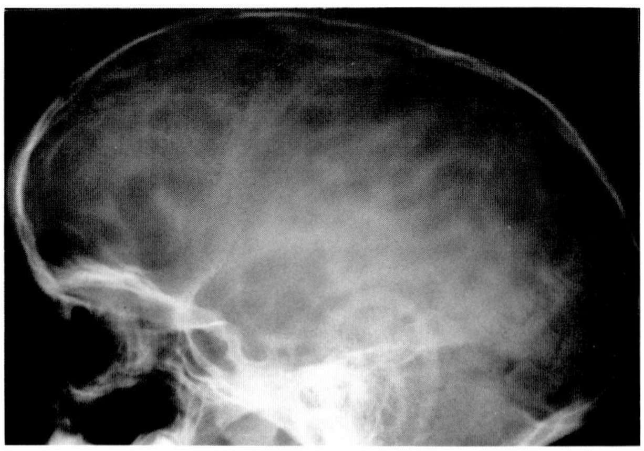

Fig. 8–117 Sagittal craniosynostosis. Increased convolutional markings on the inner table of the skull are caused by chronically increased intracranial pressure.

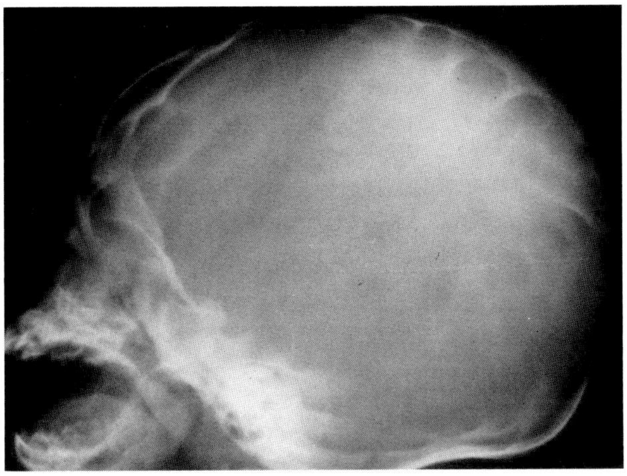

Fig. 8–118 Lacunar skull (Lückenschädel). Note the characteristic dysplastic changes involving the inner table of the skull in this newborn infant.

ings are most prominent with universal craniosynostosis, however locally increased markings can occur along the margins of any suture that closes prematurely. Secondary craniosynostosis caused by abnormalities such as healing rickets, hypophosphatasia, and hypercalcemia can also result in prominent convolutional markings.

Lacunar skull (Lückenschadel) is an abnormality of inner table bone formation associated with focal defects in the dura. This results in a pattern that is often mistaken for increased convolutional markings (Fig. 8–118). Lacunar skull is seen almost exclusively in newborns with meningoceles, meningomyeloceles, or encephaloceles. Although hydrocephalus is often present, the lacunar pattern is not due to increased intracranial pressure in such cases. The pattern resolves by 6 to 8 months of age.

Focal areas of calvarial thinning are most often caused by an underlying, slowly expanding lesion such as a neoplasm or some type of cyst. A chronic subdural hematoma may also result in a focal area of thinning. Dysplastic skull changes associated with neurofibromatosis also present as localized areas of calvarial thinning.

Widened Cranial Sutures

True widening of the cranial sutures is the result of increased intracranial pressure due to a variety of causes. This pressure may be caused by mass lesions such as neoplasms, cysts, or enlarged ventricles; intracranial hemorrhage or infection; cerebral edema; pseudotumor cerebri; or various encephalopathies (e.g., lead, hypervitaminosis A). An interesting form of increased intracranial pressure occurs in the recovery phase of psychosocial dwarfism. These children suffer from growth retardation because of some form

WIDENED CRANIAL SUTURES

Congenital/developmental
- Cleidocranial dysostosis
- Osteogenesis imperfecta
- Pachydermoperiostosis
- Progeria
- Pyknodysostosis
- Metaphyseal dysplasia (Jansen)
- Aminopterin fetopathy
- Megalencephaly
- Hydranencephaly
- Intrauterine infections

Inflammation
- Intracranial infection (meningitis, cerebritis, abscess)
- Encephalopathy (lead, vitamin A intoxication)

Neoplasm/cyst
- Intracranial tumor or cyst

Trauma/surgery
- Intracranial bleeding
- Brain edema

Systemic/metabolic
- Rickets
- Prematurity
- Psychosocial dwarfism (recovery phase)
- Hypothyroidism
- Hyperparathyroidism
- Hypophosphatasia

Miscellaneous
- Pseudotumor cerebri
- Hydrocephalus
- Subdural hygroma

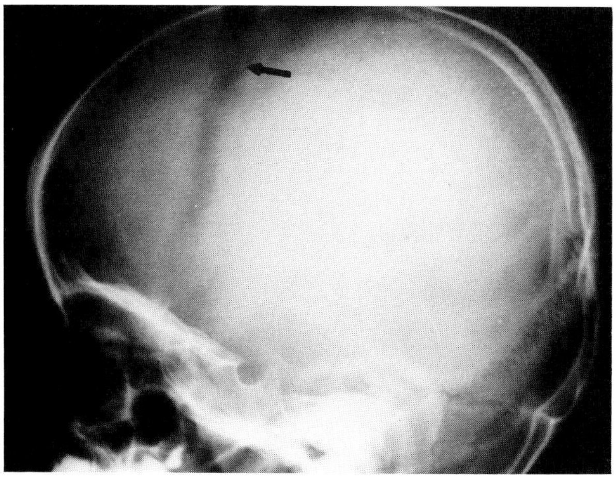

Fig. 8–119 Psychosocial dwarfism. In the healing stages of this condition, rebound brain growth can result in transient increased intracranial pressure and widening of the sutures (*arrow*).

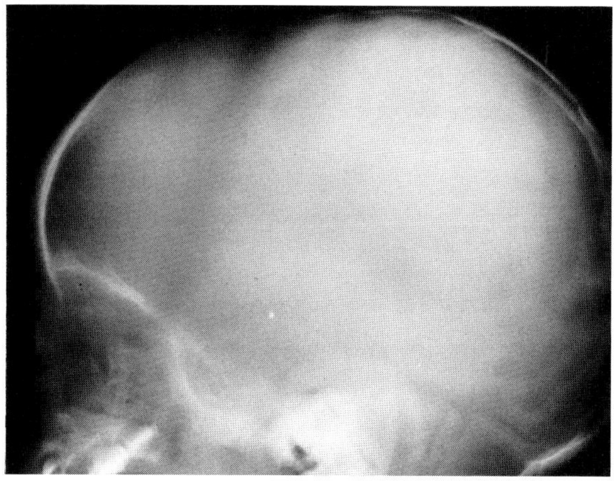

Fig. 8–120 Rickets. Abnormal mineralization of the skull causes the cranial sutures to appear widened.

of psychosocial deprivation. When removed from this undesireable environment, these children undergo rapid recovery with remarkable rebound growth. This rapid brain growth can result in temporary cranial sutural widening that, at times, can be quite alarming (Fig. 8–119). A similar phenomenon can occur following the treatment of hypothyroidism and other conditions that cause generalized growth retardation.

Apparent cranial suture widening is the result of generalized demineralization of the skull or impaired membranous bone formation. Demineralizing metabolic bone disease such as rickets or hypophosphatasia commonly results in wide-appearing sutures (Fig. 8–120). A number of bone dysplasias are associated with poor membranous bone formation. Delayed ossification of the skull with apparently widened sutures is a common occurrence in premature infants.

Wormian Bones

Intrasutural, or wormian bones, commonly occur as a normal variant in infants. They are generally located in the lambdoid sutures (Fig. 8–121). Wormian bones have been associated with a number of congenital and developmental syndromes. They may also be seen with metabolic abnormalities such as hypothyroidism or hypophosphatasia.

WORMIAN BONES

Congenital/developmental
- Osteogenesis imperfecta
- Cleidocranial dysostosis
- Pyknodysostosis
- Pachydermoperiostosis
- Chromosomal abnormalities (trisomies)
- Progeria
- Hallermann-Streiff syndrome
- Aminopterin fetopathy
- Menkes' syndrome
- Prader-Willi syndrome

Systemic/metabolic
- Hypophosphatasia
- Hypothyroidism

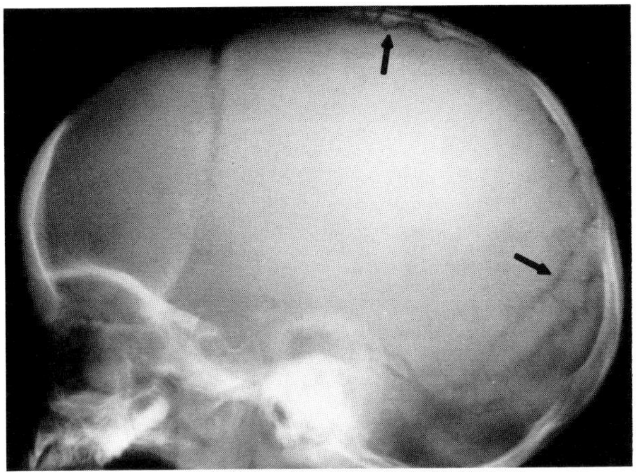

Fig. 8–121 Cleidocranial dysostosis. Wormian bones are seen in the lambdoid and sagittal sutures (*arrows*).

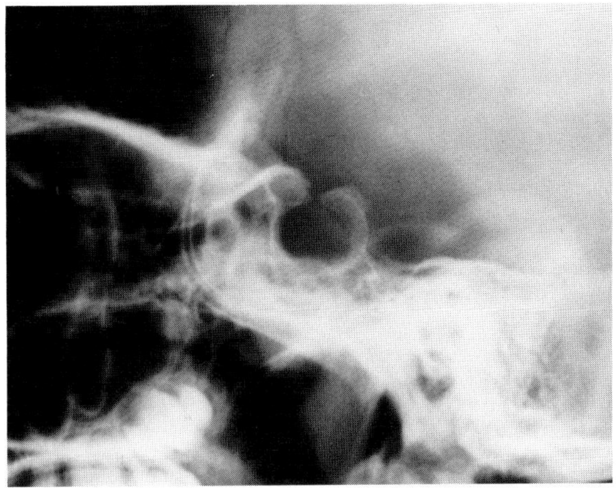

Fig. 8–122 Pituitary adenoma. Enlargement of the sella turcica in a child with a chromophobe adenoma of the pituitary gland.

Sella Turcica Abnormalities

Enlargement of the sella turcica in children is most commonly caused by a neoplasm that either originates within the pituitary gland or in the parasellar region (see list, p. 438). Enlargement of the pituitary gland itself is usually caused by a pituitary adenoma (chromophobe or eosinophilic) (Fig. 8–122). The pituitary gland may also become enlarged because of the rebound hypertrophy that may occur in hypothyroidism and after the total adrenalectomy for Cushing's syndrome with adrenal hyperplasia. The latter is referred to as Nelson syndrome and the enlargement is because of formation of a pituitary adenoma. Pituitary hypertrophy tends to cause a rounded enlargement of the sella, which has been described as a "cherry" sella.

The most common childhood tumor to extend from the suprasellar region into the sella is the craniopharyngioma. These tumors often contain curvilinear or amorphous calcifications, which may be visible on a skull radiograph (Fig. 8–123). Arachnoid cysts may also extend into the sella turcica causing enlargement. The cyst may be congenital or may arise following intracranial hemorrhage or infection. Other parasellar masses, such as meningiomas, hypothalamic tumors, or internal carotid artery aneurysms, are quite rare.

Enlargement of the sella can be a late finding in any condition that causes chronically elevated intracranial pressure. The dysplasia of the sphenoid bone that sometimes occurs with neurofibromatosis can also lead to deformity and enlargement of the sella. In some children, the sella has a shallow and elongated configuration; it may occur in normal children. This "stretched" sella appearance may occur in conjunction with generalized cranial enlargement. Similar con-

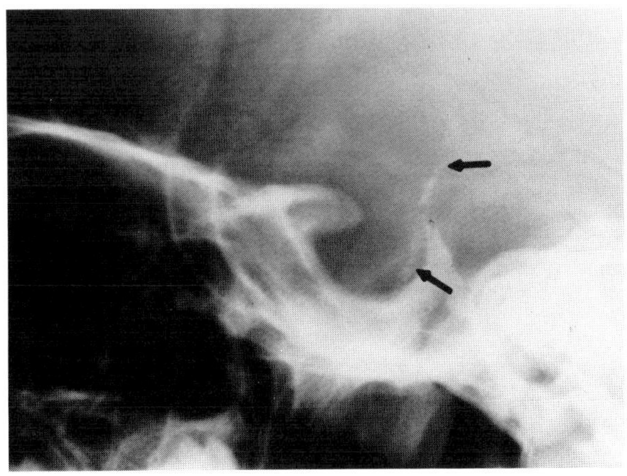

Fig. 8–123 Craniopharyngioma. Curvilinear calcifications (*arrows*) and sellar enlargement are characteristic of this childhood tumor.

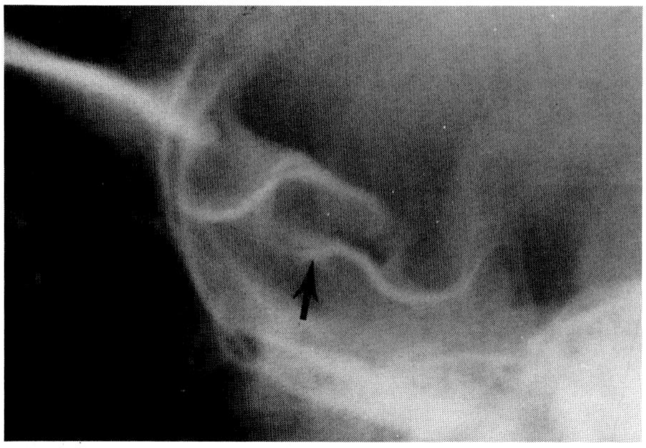

Fig. 8–124 Optic glioma. Erosion of the tuberculum sella by this tumor involving the optic chiasm has created a scooped sella configuration (*arrow*).

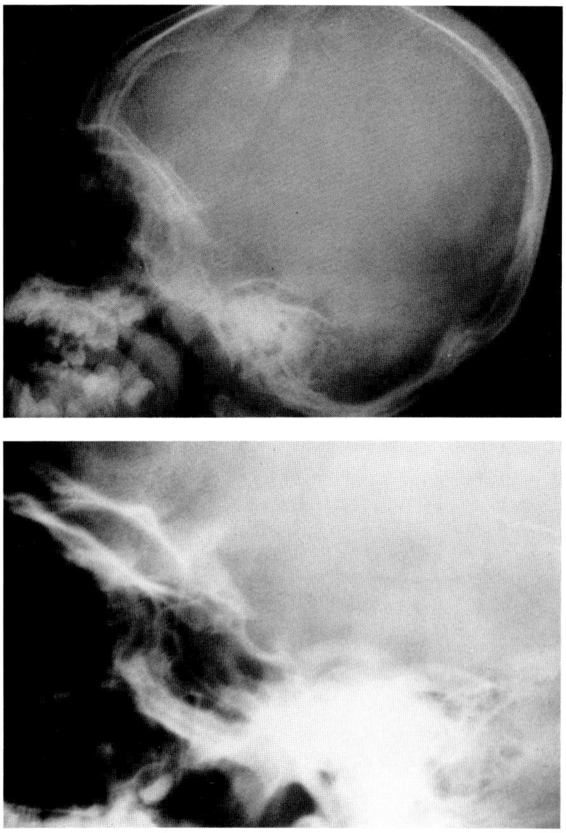

A

B

Fig. 8–125 Small sella turcica. **(A)** Chronically decreased intracranial pressure due to atrophy of the brain has resulted in a small, thickened skull and a small sella turcica. **(B)** A small sella in a patient with hypopituitarism.

LARGE SELLA TURCICA

Congenital/developmental
- Neurofibromatosis (dysplastic sella)
- Universal craniosynostosis
- Empty sella syndrome

Neoplasm/cyst
- Craniopharyngioma
- Pituitary adenoma
- Optic chiasm glioma (scooped sella, J-shaped sella)
- Parasellar meningioma
- Hypothalamic tumor
- Clivus chordoma
- Arachnoid cyst

Systemic/metabolic
- Hypothyroidism
- Nelson's syndrome
- Storage diseases (J-shaped sella)

Miscellaneous
- Chronically elevated intracranial pressure (hydrocephalus, mass)
- Aneurysm of internal carotid artery

figurations such as the scooped (omega) sella or the J (boat) sella are most commonly seen with tumors involving the optic chiasm (Fig. 8–124). The J-shaped sella is also associated with some of the mucolipidoses and mucopolysaccharidoses.

A small sella is most often a normal variant. However, just as increased intracranial pressure can lead to enlargement of the sella, a small sella turcica may result from chronically decreased intracranial pressure, most often caused by brain atrophy or the successful shunting of hydrocephalus (Fig. 8–125). Hypopituitarism is an uncommon cause of a small sella turcica.

Destructive Skull Lesions

Bone destruction involving the skull occurs in two general patterns: (1) discrete lytic lesions that may be single or multiple, and (2) more diffuse areas of permeative osteolysis. A wide variety of conditions may

A

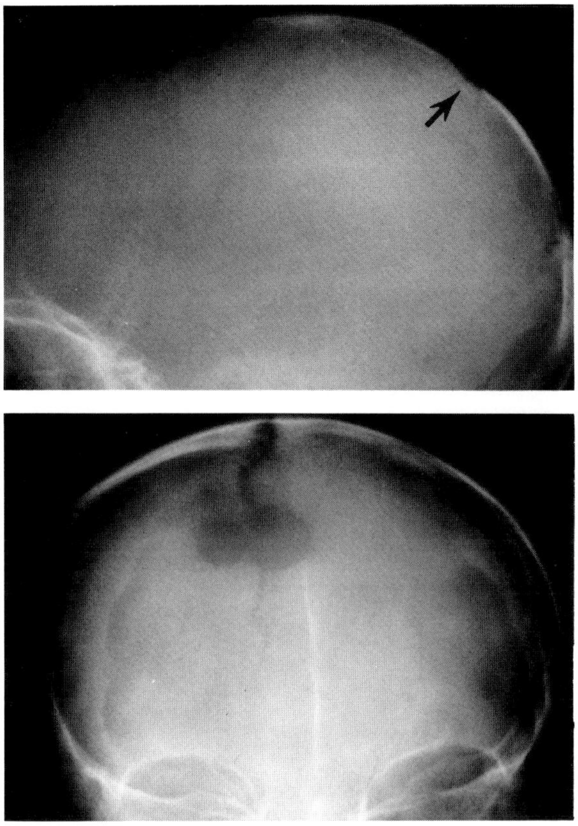

B

Fig. 8–126 Normal variants in the skull. **(A)** Accessory parietal fontanelle can be seen along the sagittal suture between the anterior and posterior fontanelles (*arrow*). **(B)** Typical bilateral parietal foramina.

A

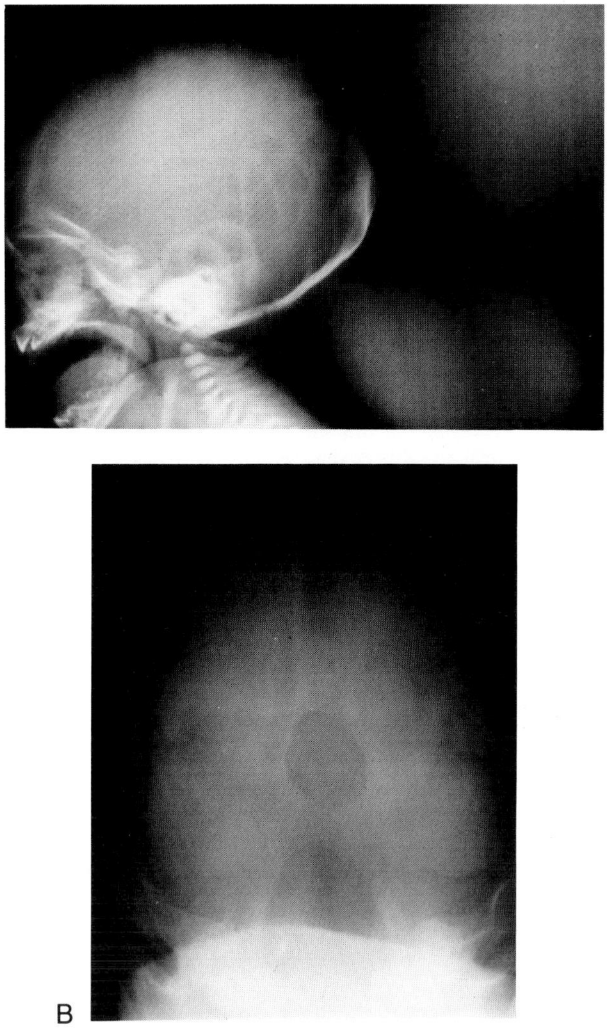

B

Fig. 8–127 Posterior encephalocele. **(A)** Note the lacunar skull and the large soft tissue mass extending from the posterior skull in this newborn infant. **(B)** The occipital skull defect can be clearly identified on this Towne view.

lead to discrete lytic skull lesions (see list, p. 440). Common nonpathologic causes of apparent skull destruction include areas of skull thinning caused by venous lakes and pacchionian granulations. Developmental variants such as parietal foramina or the inioindinial canal in the region of the torcula may also be mistaken for areas of osteolysis. Several types of accessory fontanelles may also occur, giving an appearance of a lytic skull lesion. These may occur along the sagittal suture anterior to the posterior fontanelle (accessory parietal fontanelle) (Fig. 8–126); in the midline, anterior to the anterior fontanelle (metopic fontanelle); and laterally at the junction of the posterior fossa sutures. Pathologic developmental anomalies include the encephalocele and the congenital dermal sinus. Both of these lesions are more common in the occipital region (Fig. 8–127), although they may also occur in the frontal or lateral regions. An encephalocele is a defect of the skull with a variable amount of brain tissue bulging through the defect. A congenital dermal sinus is a persistent midline sinus extending from the skin surface to the brain or meninges that predisposes the patient to intracranial infections. CT and MRI are the most useful methods for delineating the anatomy in such conditions.

LYTIC SKULL LESIONS

Congenital/developmental
- Fibrous dysplasia
- Encephalocele
- Neurofibromatosis
- Congenital dermal sinus
- Intradiploic ectopic neural tissue
- Parietal foramina
- Venous lakes
- Pacchionnian granulations
- Inioindinial canal

Inflammatory
- Osteomyelitis
- Congenital syphilis
- Caffey disease

Neoplasm/cyst
- Metastatic disease
- Epidermoid
- Leukemia/lymphoma
- Scalp tumor
- Aneurysmal bone cyst
- Hemangioma
- Dermoid
- Primary bone tumor

Trauma/surgery
- Leptomeningeal cyst
- Burr hole
- Radiation necrosis
- Intraosseous hematoma
- Cephalohematoma (healing)

Systemic/metabolic
- Histiocytosis X

The presence or absence of sclerosis of the margins of a lytic skull lesion may be a helpful differentiating feature. Epidermoids and aneurysmal bone cysts of the skull usually have markedly sclerotic borders (Fig. 8–128). Other lesions that may show a variable amount of sclerosis include fibrous dysplasia, encephaloceles, osteomyelitis, leptomeningeal cysts, healing cephalohematomas, and calvarial hemangiomas and dermoids (Fig. 8–129). Lytic skull lesions that usually show no sclerosis of their margins include metastases, histiocytosis X, and areas of radiation or postoperative necrosis. Multiple osteolytic skull

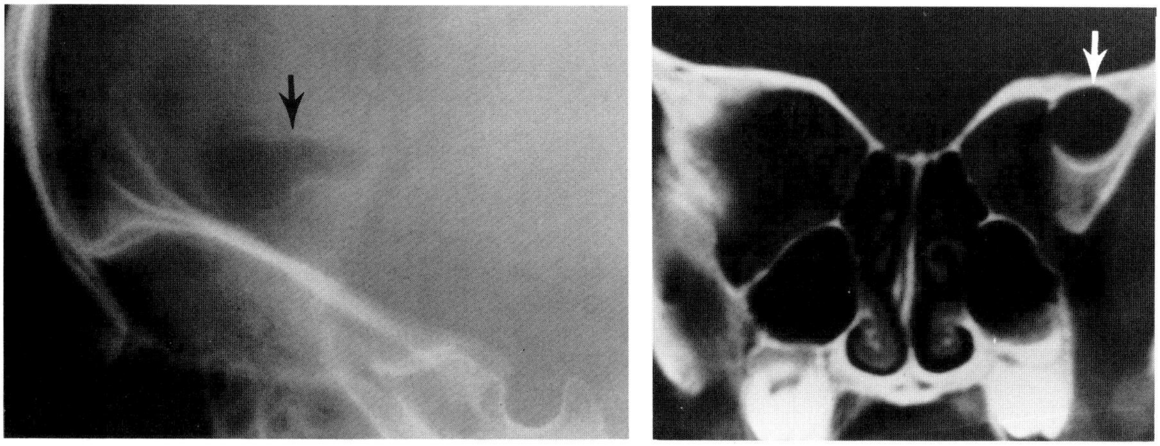

Fig. 8–128 Epidermoid of the skull. **(A)** These tumors characteristically appear as a radiolucent defect with sclerotic borders (*arrow*). **(B)** Coronal CT scan at bone window settings demonstrates an epidermoid of the sphenoid bone (*arrow*).

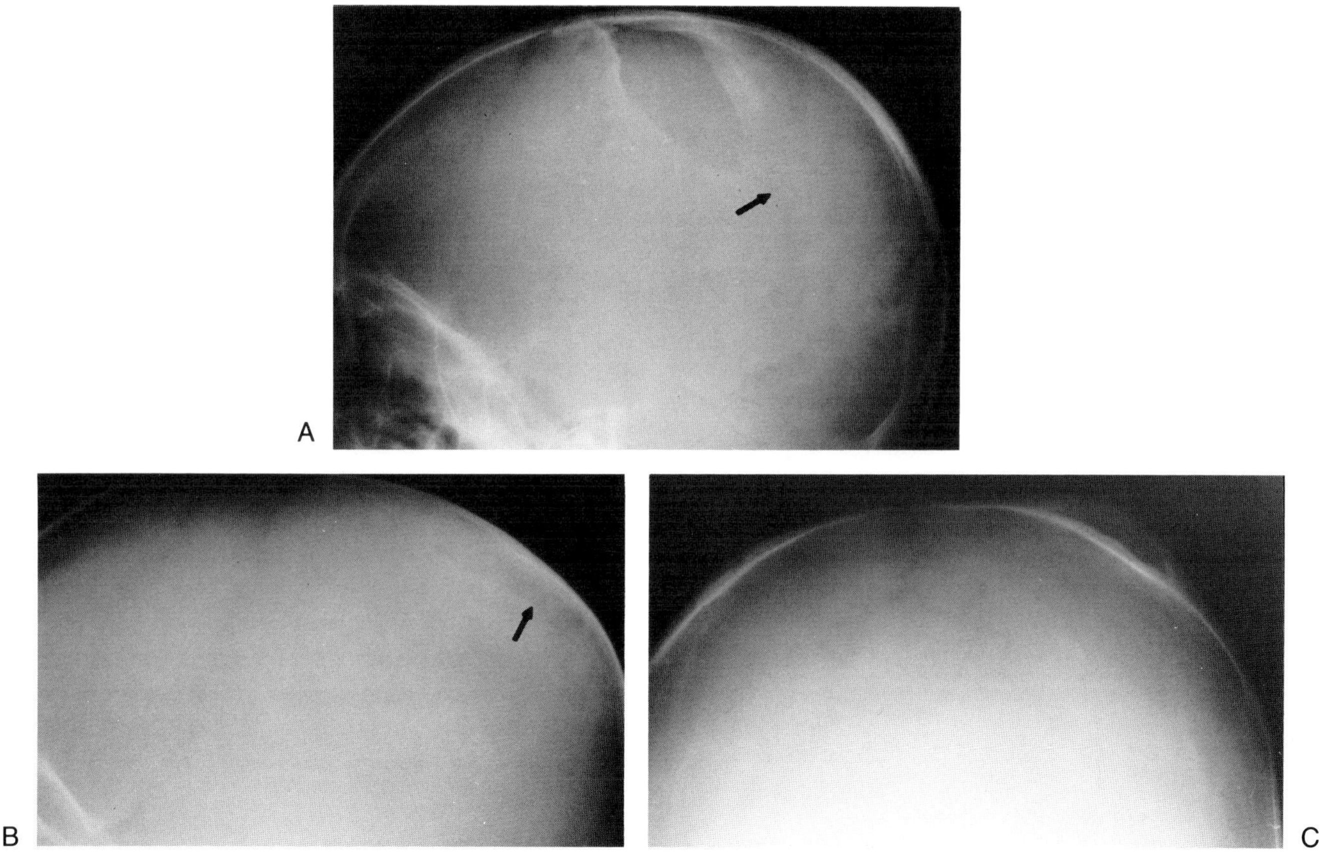

Fig. 8–129 Lytic skull lesions with variable sclerosis. **(A)** Leptomeningeal cyst. This lesion is a late complication of a skull fracture associated with a dural tear. Herniation of the meninges through the fracture results in a pulsatile mass, which enlarges the fracture at this site. The typical appearance is an elliptical, scalloped, sharply defined radiolucent skull defect. Occasionally the fracture line can be identified extending from the edge of the defect (*arrow*). **(B)** In the healing stages, when early calcification is occurring, a cephalohematoma may appear as a radiolucent skull defect (*arrow*), unless **(C)** a tangential view is obtained.

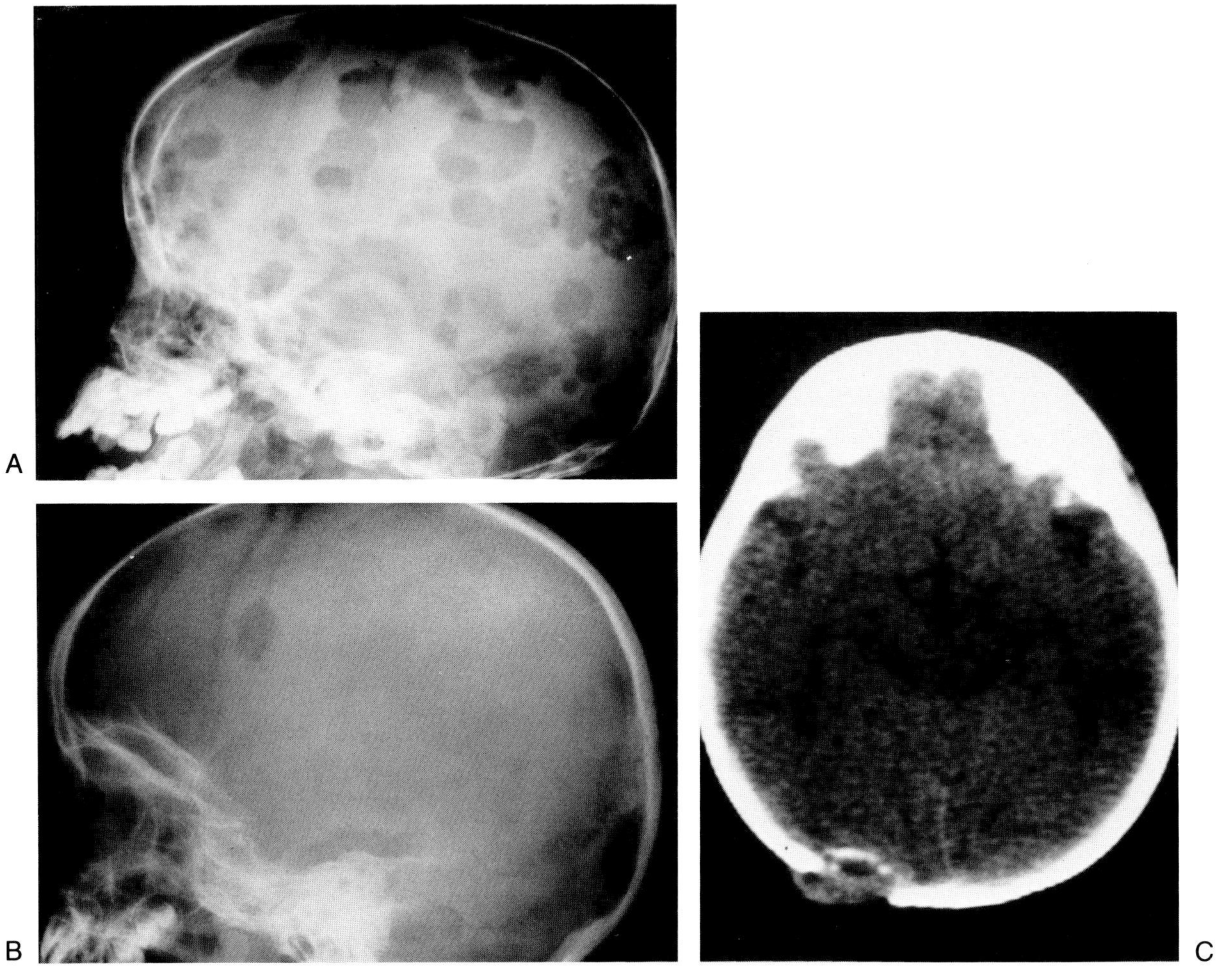

Fig. 8–130 Histiocytosis X. **(A)** Multiple lytic skull lesions in a patient with Letterer-Siwe disease. **(B)** Two osteolytic defects caused by eosinophilic granuloma. **(C)** The soft tissue component of the defect is demonstrated by axial CT scan.

lesions are most often caused by histiocytosis X, leukemia, lymphoma, or metastatic malignancy (Fig. 8–130).

Areas of indistinct, permeative bone destruction in the skull are most commonly caused by malignant neoplasms such as metastatic disease, leukemia, and lymphoma (Fig. 8–131). Less commonly, osteomyelitis may cause multiple areas of bone destruction, giving a permeative appearance. The patchy demineralization that occurs with hyperparathyroidism (salt and pepper skull) sometimes resembles permeative bone destruction.

PERMEATIVE SKULL DESTRUCTION

Inflammatory
- Osteomyelitis

Neoplasm
- Metastatic disease
- Leukemia/lymphoma
- Primary bone tumors

Systemic/metabolic
- Hyperparathyroidism

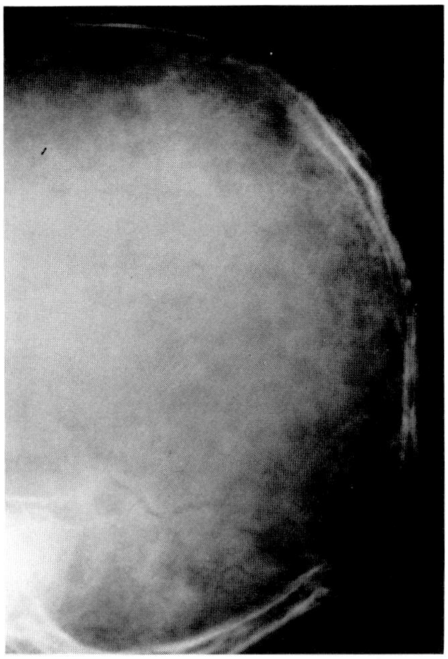

Fig. 8–131 Leukemia. Multiple small osteolytic defects result in a permeative pattern of destruction in this patient with skull involvement by leukemia.

SPINE

Focal Sclerosis

Focal areas of sclerosis in a vertebra may involve the vertebral body or the posterior elements, however all such lesions are uncommon in children. Neoplasms are probably the most common cause of focal vertebral sclerosis, and a large percentage will be osteoid osteomas (Fig. 8–132). These benign but painful lesions most commonly occur in the neural arches and

FOCAL SCLEROSIS OF VERTEBRAE

Congenital/developmental
- Congenital abnormalities of apophyseal joint
- Bone island
- Tuberous sclerosis
- Healed histiocytosis X

Inflammation
- Healed osteomyelitis

Neoplasm/cyst
- Osteoid osteoma
- Ewing's sarcoma
- Osteosarcoma
- Hodgkin's lymphoma
- Osteoblastic metastases

Trauma/surgery
- Healed fracture

Miscellaneous
- Idiopathic solitary sclerotic pedicle

A

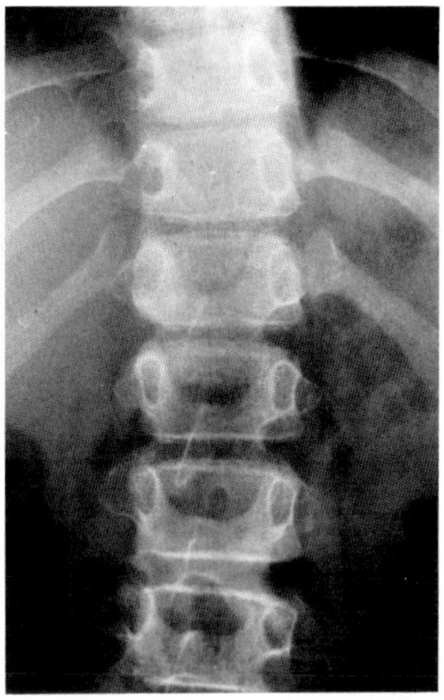

B

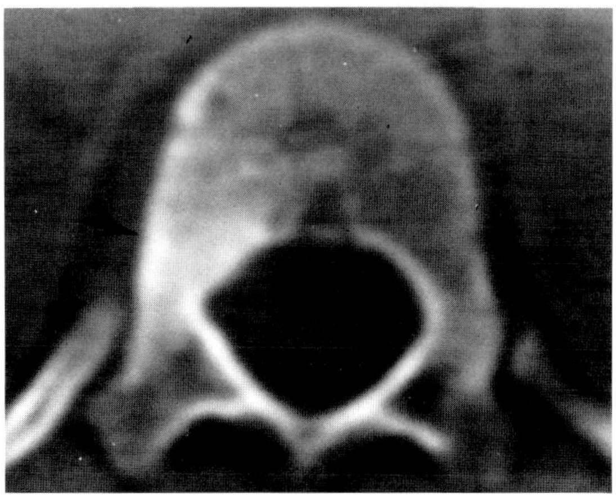

Fig. 8–132 Osteoid osteoma of the spine. **(A)** Sclerosis of the right pedicle of T12 was seen in this patient with painful scoliosis. **(B)** Axial CT scan permitted more precise localization of the tumor (*arrow*).

spinous process and are sometimes difficult to detect on the plain radiograph. CT and nuclear scintigraphy may aid in the detection of lesions with little sclerosis. Ewing's sarcoma, Hodgkin's lymphoma, and osteosarcoma are other neoplasms that rarely can cause focal areas of sclerosis in the spine. Osteoblastic metastases are extremely rare in childhood.

Congenital abnormalities of the apophyseal joint can lead to abnormal stresses, which may lead to sclerosis around the joint. This most often occurs in the lumbar spine. Bone islands and the sclerotic lesions of tuberous sclerosis are very unusual in the vertebrae. Any healed lesion of the spine (e.g., osteomyelitis, fracture, histiocytosis X) will appear as an area of focal sclerosis involving the spine. Occasionally an idiopathic, isolated sclerotic pedicle can occur in a normal patient.

Abnormalities of the Pedicles

When evaluating the pediatric spine, one should always take note of both the size and shape of the pedicles (see list, pp. 444 and 445). Pedicle enlargement is uncommon, but can occur when the pedicle is involved by a variety of neoplasms. The osteoid osteoma causes a sclerotic and sometimes enlarged pedicle. Giant osteoblastoma is pathologically similar to the osteoid osteoma, however it causes an enlarged radiolucent pedicle. Other tumors such as hemangioma, lymphangioma, or osteochrondroma are even less common. Congenital or acquired unilateral arch deficiency has been shown to result in compensatory hypertrophy of the contralateral pedicle.

A pedicle may be small or deformed on a congenital basis and is usually associated with other vertebral anomalies. Congenital absence of a pedicle is rare and most commonly occurs in the cervical spine. Small pedicles have also been known to occur because of previous radiation therapy. Dysplastic pedicles are occasionally seen in patients with neurofibromatosis. Pedicle destruction is usually due to tumor involvement, most often metastatic neuroblastoma, leukemia, or lymphoma (Fig. 8–133). Histiocystosis X and primary bone tumors are rare causes of pedicle destruction.

Flattened pedicles occasionally occur as normal variants in the lumbar spine. Pathologic pedicle flattening is almost always because of some type of intraspinal tumor (Fig. 8–134), although large intraspinal cysts occasionally cause the same appearance.

ENLARGED PEDICLE

Congenital/developmental
- Contralateral arch deficiency (single)
- Unilateral hypertrophy (multiple)

Neoplasm/cyst
- Osteoblastoma
- Hemangioma
- Lymphangioma
- Osteoid osteoma
- Osteochondroma
- Other tumors

Platyspondyly

When flattened vertebral bodies are encountered, it is important to note whether one, several, or all of the vertebrae are involved (see list, p. 445). Flattening of all the vertebrae is referred to as universal platyspondyly, which is most often caused by a congenital bone dysplasia (e.g., osteogenesis imperfecta, spondyloepiphyseal dysplasia, and thanatophoric or metatropic dwarfism) or metabolic abnormality (Morquio's disease) (Fig. 8–135). The flattening in these

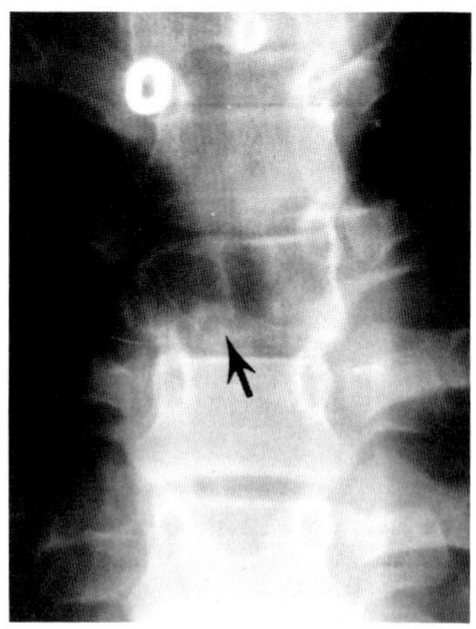

Fig. 8–133 Aneurysmal bone cyst. Pedicle destruction in this child was caused by an aneurysmal bone cyst (*arrow*).

SMALL, FLATTENED, OR ABSENT PEDICLE

Congenital/developmental
- Normal variant*
- Vertebral anomalies*
- Congenital absence†
- Neurofibromatosis*

Neoplasm
- Intraspinal tumor or cyst‡
- Metastatic disease†
- Leukemia/lymphoma†
- Primary bone tumor†

Trauma/surgery
- Postradiation therapy*

Systemic/metabolic
- Histiocytosis X†
- Neurofibromatosis*

* Small; dysplastic.
† Destroyed; absent.
‡ Flattened.

PLATYSPONDYLY

Congenital/developmental
- Osteogenesis imperfecta*,†
- Spondyloepiphyseal dysplasia*
- Thanatophoric dwarfism*
- Metatropic dwarfism*
- Achondrogenesis*
- Kniest syndrome*
- Dygvve-Melchior-Clausen syndrome*

Inflammation
- Osteomyelitis

Neoplasm/cyst
- Metastatic disease†
- Leukemia/lymphoma†
- Hemangioma

Trauma/surgery
- Fracture†

Systemic/metabolic
- Osteoporosis/osteomalacia†
- Histiocytosis X†
- Sickle cell disease*
- Morquio's disease
- Hypothyroidism

* Universal.
† Isolated (may be multiple).

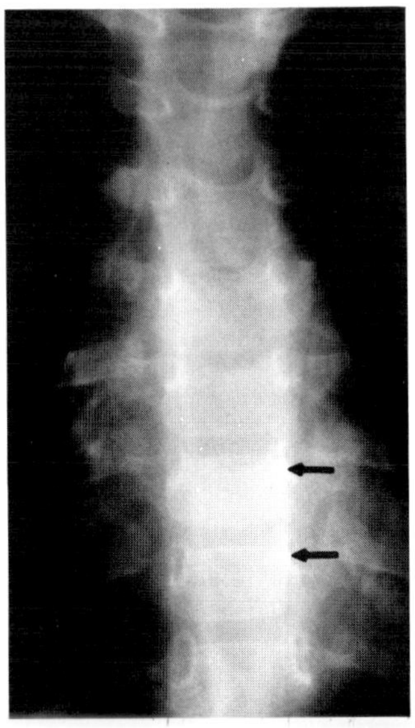

Fig. 8–134 Intraspinal mass. Angular scoliosis of the spine with flattening of the pedicles (*arrows*) as a result of an intraspinal tumor.

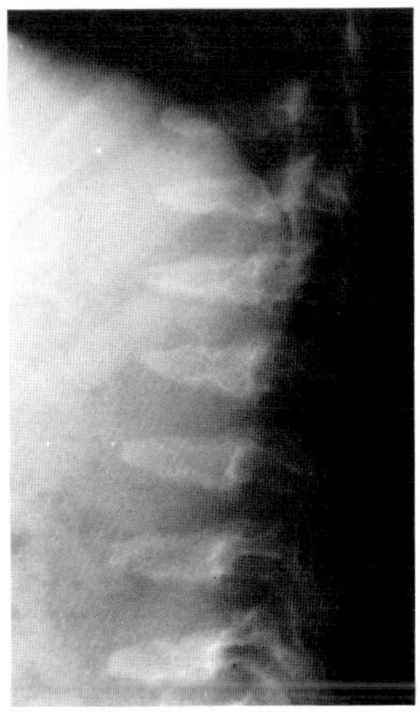

Fig. 8–135 Morquio's disease. Universal platyspondyly is common in patients with this mucopolysacchardiosis.

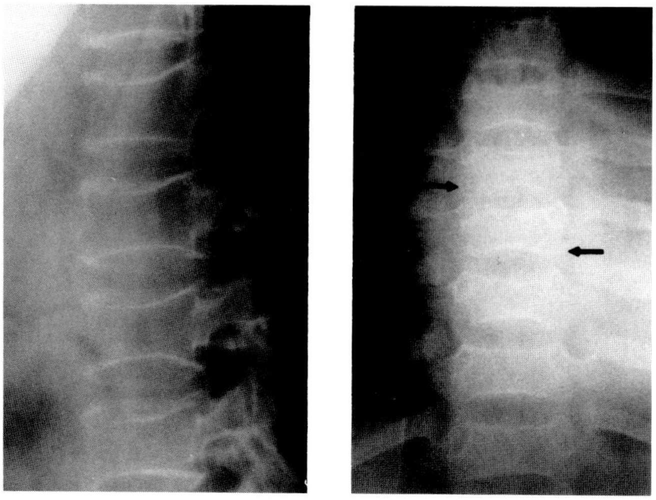

Fig. 8–136 Flattened vertebrae. **(A)** Biconcave deformity of the vertebrae is caused by osteoporosis in this child receiving steroids. **(B)** In this child with sickle cell disease, the spine shows characteristic biconcave deformity of the vertebrae. In some vertebrae, the characteristic central step-off pattern can be seen (*arrows*).

conditions is usually generalized, but is not necessarily uniform throughout the spine. In sickle cell disease, the vertebrae characteristically develop a biconcave configuration, often with an acute central step-off (Fig. 8–136). Occasionally, severe osteoporosis or osteomalacia may result in compression fractures involving all the vertebrae.

Platyspondyly isolated to one or several vertebrae is most commonly due to a fracture, either pathologic or traumatic. Vertebral trauma generally produces greater compression anteriorly (wedge-shaped vertebrae) (Fig. 8–137). The vertebrae of patients with osteogenesis imperfecta are prone to this type of compression fracture as well.

Any cause of vertebral destruction can lead to compression and flattening of the vertebral body. Infection is the commonest cause of vertebral destruction and most often results in a uniform or irregular flattening of the vertebrae with narrowing of the disc space (Fig. 8–138). Fungal infections of the spine lead to vertebral destruction, however the disc spaces tend to be preserved. Vertebral destruction by neoplasms such as leukemia, lymphoma, and metastatic neuroblastoma or sarcoma is not uncommon. Primary bone neoplasms are rather rare in children.

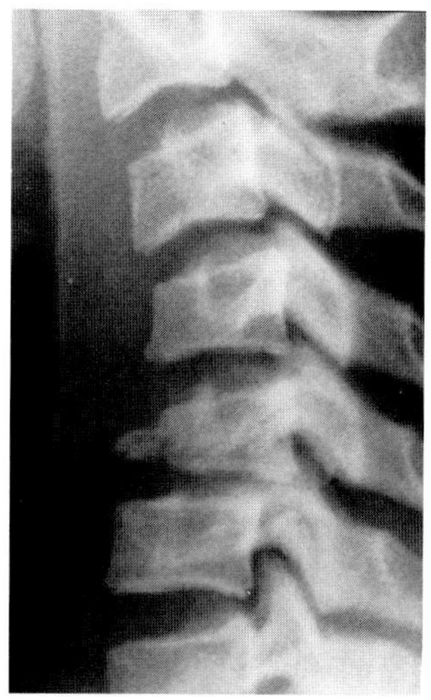

Fig. 8–137 Vertebral compression fracture. A hyperflexion injury as a result of a motor vehicle accident resulted in this compression fracture of C5 with posterior subluxation of C5 on C6.

Histiocytosis X should also be considered when destruction of one or several vertebral bodies is encountered. Profound vertebral body flattening (vertebra plana) is a typical manifestation of this disease. The adjacent disc spaces are maintained despite the presence of marked vertebral flattening (Fig. 8–139).

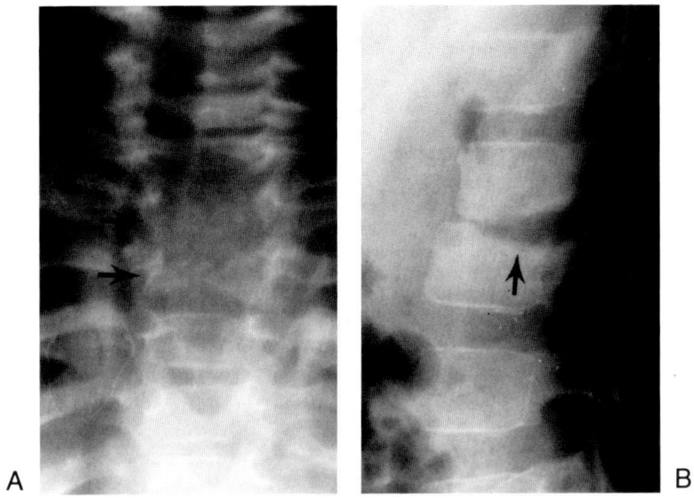

Fig. 8–138 Infectious spondylitis. **(A)** Flattening and destruction of upper thoracic vertebrae because of infection with tuberculosis (*arrows*). **(B)** Disc space infection can later lead to destruction of the adjacent vertebral bodies (*arrow*).

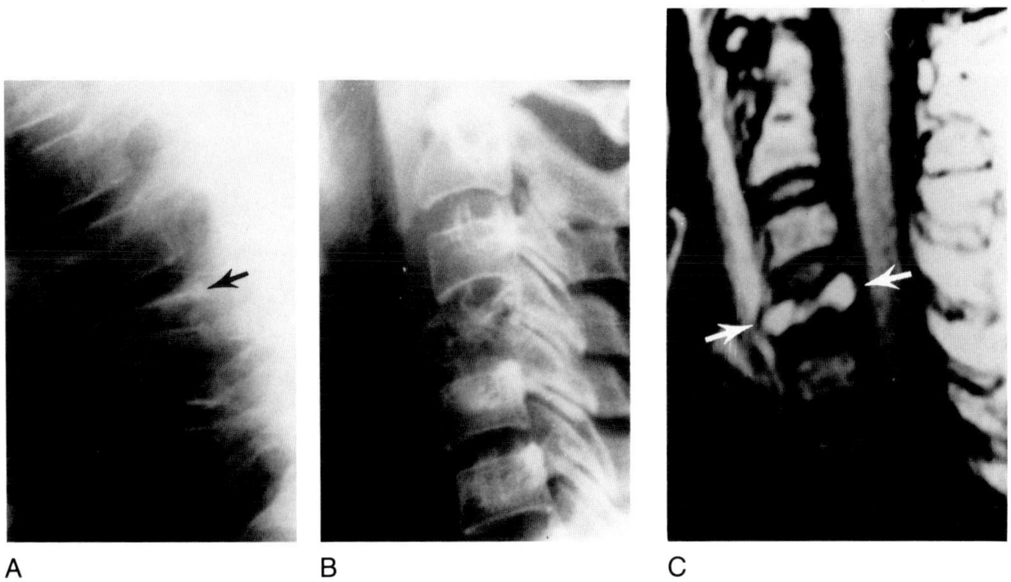

Fig. 8–139 Histiocystosis X. **(A)** Characteristic vertebra plana deformity (*arrow*). **(B)** Eosinophilic granuloma involving C4 caused the flattening and decreased density of this vertebral body on the plain radiograph. **(C)** On T_1-weighted sagittal MRI, the involved vertebra displays increased signal intensity, and marked flattening and widening (*arrows*). Note preservation of the discs adjacent to C5.

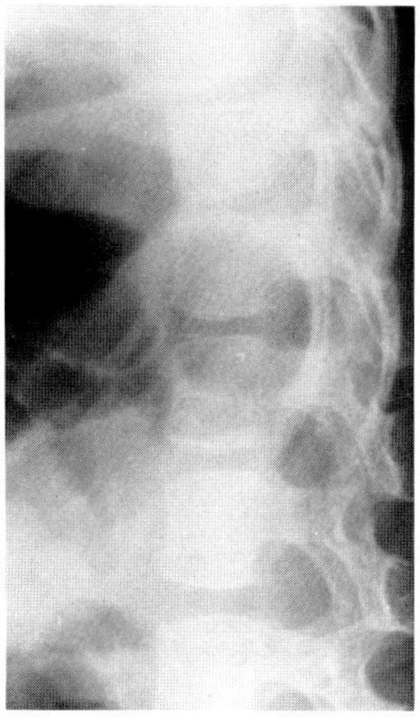

Fig. 8–140 Tall vertebrae. Note the increased height of the vertebrae in the spine of this child with neurologic damage caused by congenital rubella infection.

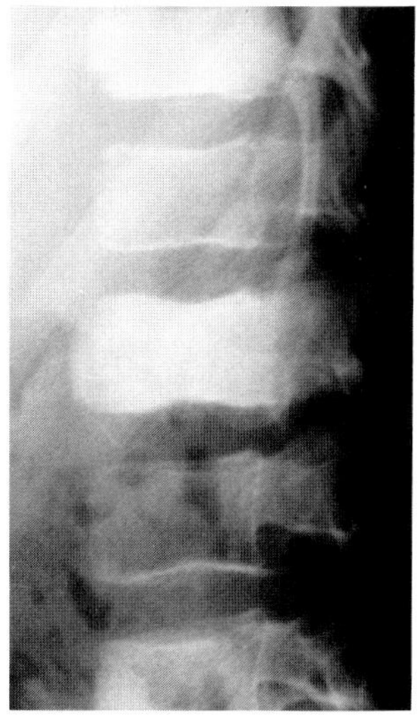

Fig. 8–142 Ewing's sarcoma. Following treatment, Ewing's sarcoma of the spine appears as an enlarged, but sclerotic, vertebral body.

A

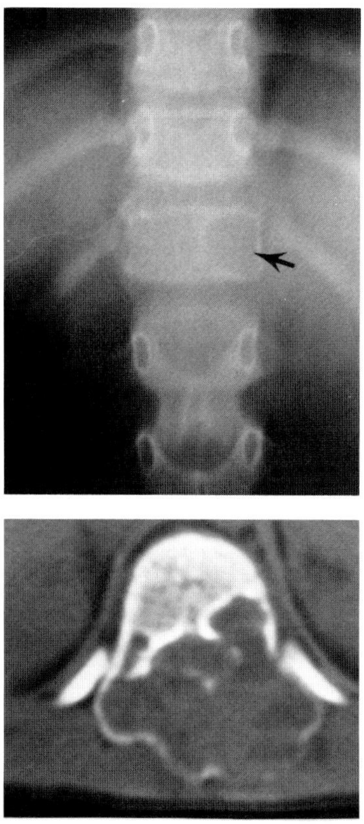

B

Fig. 8–141 Aneurysmal bone cyst. **(A)** Note the enlarged pedicles of T12 (*arrow*). **(B)** Axial CT scan demonstrates the lobulated, expansile nature of this lesion.

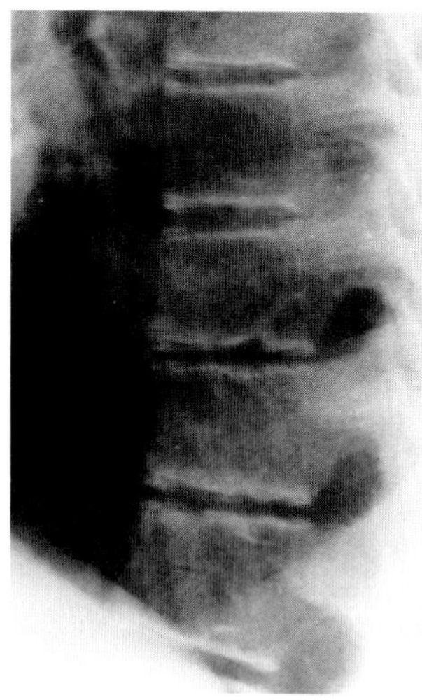

Fig. 8–143 Scheuermann's disease. Mild wedge deformity and end plate irregularity in the lower thoracic spine are typical findings in this condition.

Other Vertebral Shapes

In the normal neonate, the vertebral bodies often have a round or oval configuration, particularly at the thoracolumbar junction. Prominent central vein grooves are often present along the anterior and sometimes the posterior aspect of the vertebral body. Increased prominence or persistence of the central vein grooves can be seen in hypothyroidism, osteopetrosis, thalassemia, sickle cell disease, Gaucher's disease, leukemia, lymphoma, and metastatic malignancy. As the infant matures, the vertebrae becomes more rectangular. With the appearance of the ring epiphyses, a normal squared appearance occurs. Underdevelopment of the vertebrae, which occurs in some of the bony dysplasias, results in oval-shaped vertebral bodies.

Increased height of the vertebral bodies is most often associated with hypotonia and the absence of vertical stress (Fig. 8–140). Tall vertebrae may be seen with a variety of congenital abnormalities that result in mental or physical retardation (e.g., trisomy 21, rubella syndrome) and with other crippling neuromuscular disorders. Isolated enlargement of a vertebral body is usually caused by bone cysts or neoplasms. Aneurysmal bone cysts are the most common cysts to involve a child's spine, giving an expanded, radiolucent, and bubbly appearance (Fig. 8–141). Neoplasms such as hemangioma, lymphangioma, and osteoblastoma may also have a rather cystic appearance. Treated Ewing's sarcoma of the spine often results in an enlarged but sclerotic vertebra (Fig. 8–142).

Mild anterior wedging of the vertebral bodies is a common normal finding in the thoracic and upper cervical spine. When wedging occurs in other areas or is more pronounced, the wedging should be considered pathologic. Scheuermann's disease (juvenile kyphosis) is characterized by kyphosis that is secondary to the anterior wedging (greater than 5 degrees) of at least three adjacent vertebrae (Fig. 8–143). This condition usually develops around puberty, and although the etiology is unknown, chronic mechanical injury due to hyperflexion has been postulated. When anterior wedging caused by any condition is marked, a pronounced localized kyphosis or gibbus deformity may occur. Gibbus deformity is typically seen with Scheuermann's disease, healed infection such as tuberculosis, and conditions with chronic anterior flexion such as neurofibromatosis and some of the chondystrophies (Fig. 8–144).

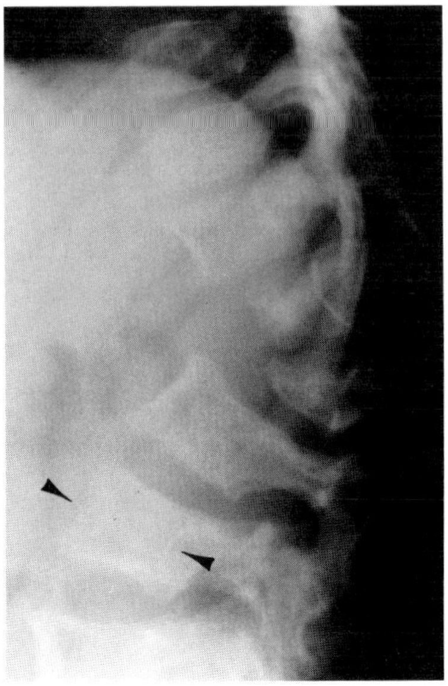

Fig. 8–144 Neurofibromatosis. Dysplastic vertebral bodies at the thoracolumbar junction caused a marked gibbus deformity in this patient with neurofibromatosis. Note the anterior and posterior scalloping of the vertebral bodies (*arrowheads*).

Scalloped Vertebrae

Mild posterior and anterior scalloping may occur in normal patients, particularly in the lumbar spine. When posterior scalloping becomes more prominent, pathologic erosion caused by an expansile intraspinal process should be considered. Lesions such as intraspinal tumors or cysts, syringomyelia or hydromyelia, uncontrolled communicating hydrocephalus, and dural ectasia may all result in posterior scalloping of the vertebrae (Fig. 8–145). Dural ectasia most commonly occurs in patients with neurofibromatosis and is caused by a mesenchymal developmental abnormality. Dural ectasia can also be idiopathic, or may be associated with Marfan's or Ehlers-Danlos syndromes. Posterior scalloping in patients with achondroplasia and other chondrodystrophies is usually accompanied by a narrow spinal canal; crowding in the spinal canal often leads to cord and nerve compression later in life.

Anterior scalloping is much less common than posterior scalloping, and occurs most often in patients

SCALLOPED VERTEBRAE

Congenital/developmental
- Neurofibromatosis*,†
- Achondroplasia†
- Ehlers-Danlos syndrome†
- Marfan's syndrome†

Neoplasm/cyst
- Intraspinal tumor, cyst†
- Leukemia/lymphoma*
- Metastatic disease*
- Intra-abdominal tumors*

Systemic/metabolic
- Storage diseases†

Miscellaneous
- Syringomyelia†
- Communicating hydrocephalus (long-standing)†

* Anterior.
† Posterior.

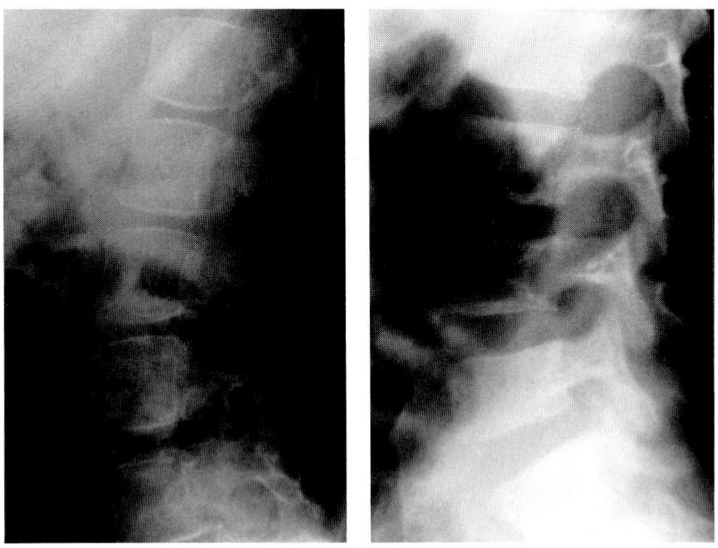

Fig. 8–145 Posterior scalloping. **(A)** A large intraspinal dermoid resulted in expansion of the spinal canal and posterior scalloping of the vertebral bodies. **(B)** Posterior scalloping of the lumbar vertebrae in a patient with neurofibromatosis.

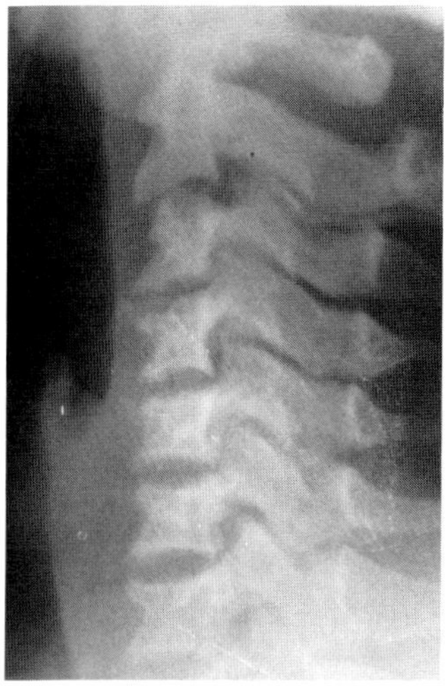

Fig. 8–146 Neurofibromatosis. Prominent anterior and posterior scalloping of the cervical vertebra result in a spool-shaped appearance of the vertebrae in this patient with neurofibromatosis.

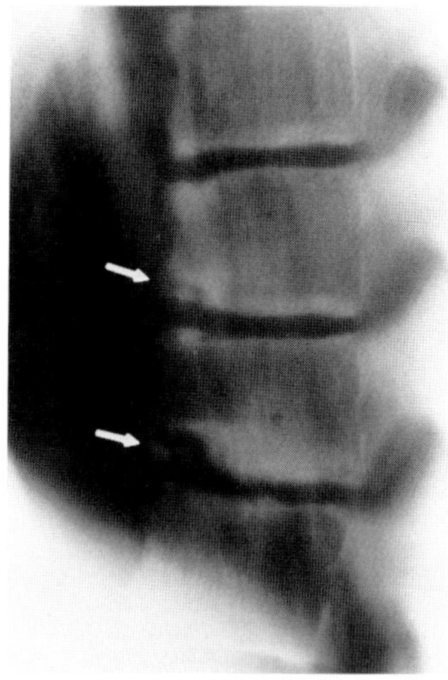

Fig. 8–147 Scheuermann's disease. Note the fragmented beak along the anterior and inferior margin of several of the vertebral bodies (*arrows*).

with neurofibromatosis. Erosion due to intra-abdominal tumors is less common and abdominal aneurysms are very rare in children. Vertebral destruction due to leukemia, lymphoma, or metastasis may create a scalloped appearance to the anterior vertebral body. When prominent anterior and posterior scalloping occur together, the vertebra takes on a spool shape. This appearance is most pronounced in trisomy 21, Melnick-Needles syndrome, and neurofibromatosis (Fig. 8–146).

Beaked Vertebrae

A beak or hook along the anterior aspect of the vertebral body is not an uncommon finding in the thoracolumbar region. This beaking is nearly always associated with some degree of kyphosis and is probably caused by acute or chronic hyperflexion in this region. Smooth beaks at the thoracolumbar junction can occasionally be seen in normal infants and are most likely secondary to exaggeration of the normal kyphosis present in young infants. As the infant matures, the vertebrae return to a normal shape.

More pronounced beaking can occur from an acute hyperflexion injury of the spine. The beak is usually rather irregular or fragmented in acute injuries. A similar irregular beaking occurs in Scheuermann's disease, in which mechanical stresses due to chronic hyperflexion probably play an important part (Fig. 8–147). Any condition characterized by hypotonia may result in vertebral beaking due to chronic hyperflexion. Often in these conditions the beak will appear smooth rather than fragmented. This appearance is commonly seen in conditions such as the mucopolysaccharidoses, mucolipidoses, gangliosidosis, Mor-

BEAKED VERTEBRAE

Congenital/developmental
- Achondroplasia
- Neurofibromatosis

Trauma/surgery
- Acute flexion injury
- Scheuermann's disease

Systemic/metabolic
- Storage diseases
- Hypothyroidism

Miscellaneous
- Hypotonia due to neuromuscular disease

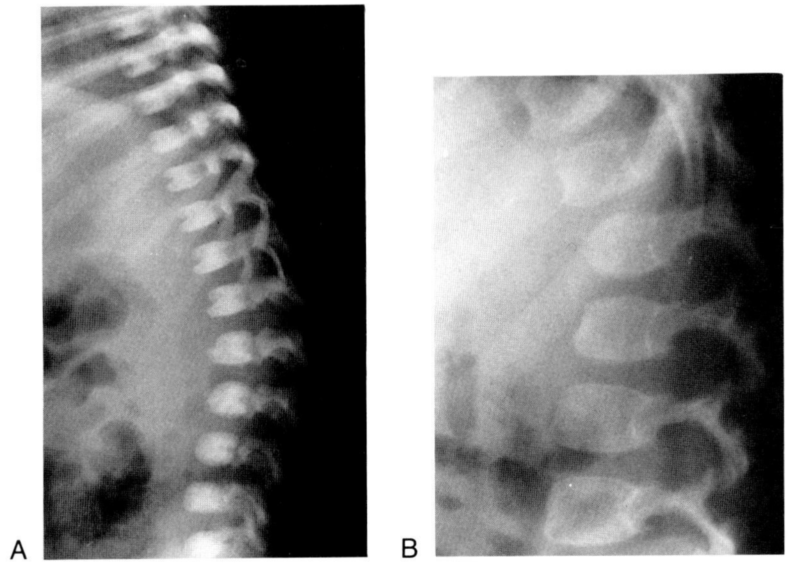

Fig. 8–148 Inferior beaking. **(A)** Smooth inferior beaks at and around the thoracolumbar junction are commonly seen in hypotonic patients such as this newborn with neonatal hypothyroidism. **(B)** Similar beaking is present in this older patient with Hurler's disease.

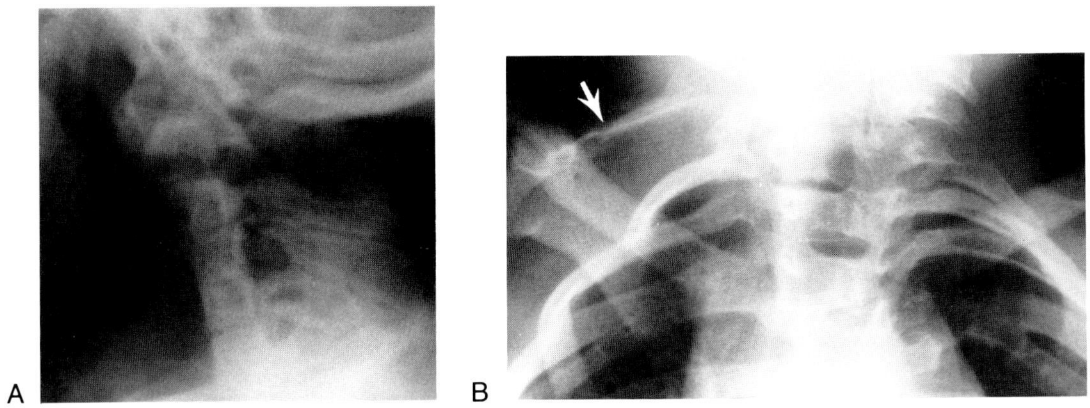

Fig. 8–149 Klippel-Feil syndrome. **(A)** The neck is shortened as a result of fusion of several of the cervical vertebrae. **(B)** Sprengel's deformity (*arrow*) commonly accompanies this syndrome.

quio's disease, hypothyroidism, and neuromuscular disease (Fig. 8–148). Immaturity of the spine also plays a role in some of the storage diseases and hypothyroidism. Associated disc space narrowing and eventual posterior herniation of the nucleus pulposus can occur in some cases.

Fused Vertebrae

Fusion of the vertebral bodies commonly occurs on a congenital basis. Such fusion often occurs at C2–C3, and can be isolated or associated with the Klippel-Feil syndrome. In this syndrome, congenital fusion of at least two vertebrae results in a short neck with limited motion and varying degrees of torticollis (Fig. 8–149). Other associated deformities include Sprengel's deformity (elevation and rotation of the scapula), cervical ribs, scoliosis, kyphosis, congenital deafness, renal or ovarian agenesis, and congenital heart disease.

Acquired fusion of the vertebral bodies can occur following the healing of any process that destroys

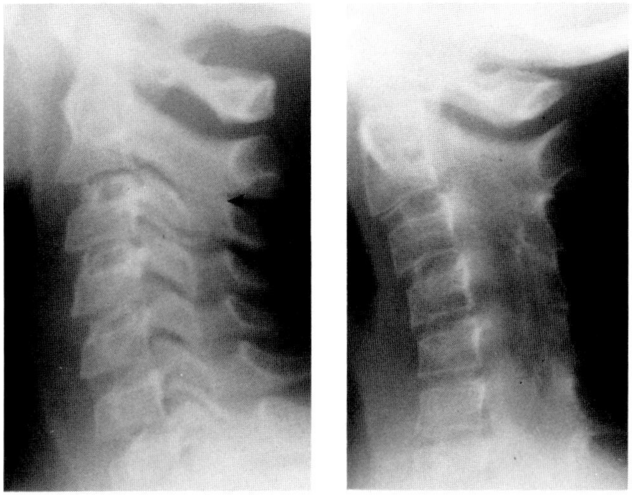

Fig. 8–150 Juvenile rheumatoid arthritis. **(A)** Early spinal involvement consists of fusion at C2-C3 (*arrow*). **(B)** Two years later, complete fusion of the cervical spine has occurred.

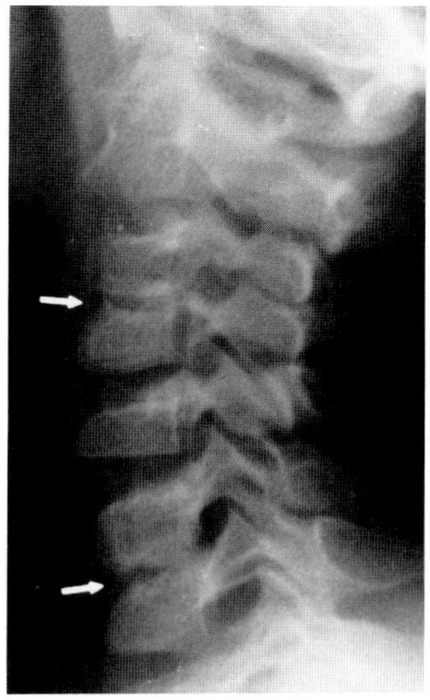

Fig. 8–151 Block vertebrae. Multiple partially fused vertebral bodies with rudimentary intervening discs (*arrows*) occurred on a congenital basis in this patient.

the intervertebral disc. Nonspecific discitis or spinal osteomyelitis are the most common causes of disc destruction, although severe trauma can have a similar result. In the late stages of Scheuermann's disease, the involved vertebral bodies may fuse in a fixed gibbus deformity. Vertebral fusion due to ankylosing spondylitis rarely occurs during childhood.

Fusion of the apophyseal joints is most commonly associated with juvenile rheumatoid arthritis. Apophyseal joint narrowing usually begins at the C2-C3 and C5-C7 levels. Late in the disease, complete fusion of the spine can occur (Fig. 8–150). Healed trauma or infection involving the apophyseal joints may also result in fusion.

Disc Space Narrowing

Causes of disc space narrowing may be either congenital or acquired. Narrowing is sometimes due to congenital underdevelopment of the disc, which in its most severe form results in block vertebra (Fig. 8–151). Congenital narrowing may occur anywhere in the spine and sometimes involves multiple vertebrae. The vertebrae adjacent to the narrowed disc space may be slightly small but otherwise tend to appear normal.

DISC SPACE NARROWING

Congenital/developmental
- Congenital narrowing (block vertebra)
- Spondyloepiphyseal dysplasia
- Cockayne's syndrome
- Ruvalcaba syndrome
- Kniest syndrome

Inflammation
- Discitis/spondyloarthritis
- Osteomyelitis
- Ankylosing spondylitis

Trauma/surgery
- Acute flexion injuries
- Scheuermann's disease

Systemic/metabolic
- Morquio's disease

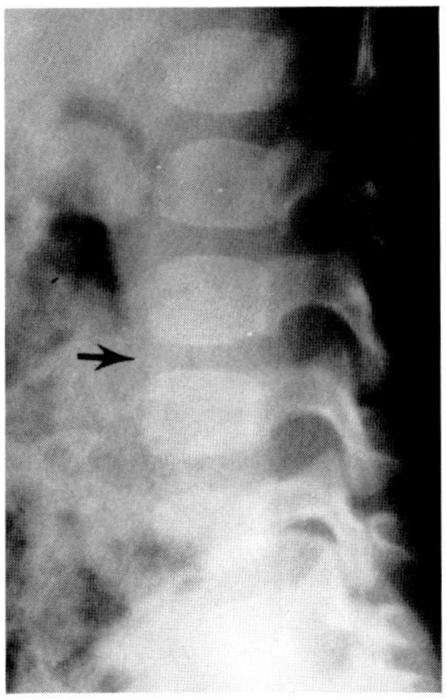

Fig. 8–152 Nonspecific discitis. The initial plain radiographs showed only minimal narrowing of the disc space (*arrow*).

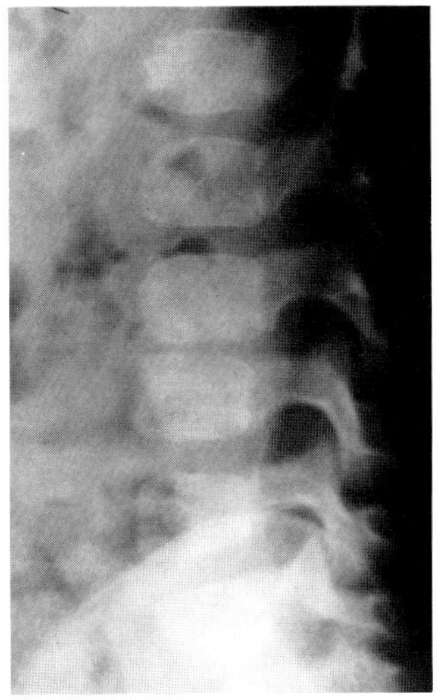

Fig. 8–153 A later radiograph of the area shown in Figure 8–152 shows significant disc space narrowing with destruction and sclerosis of the adjacent vertebral end plates.

Acquired disc space narrowing is most commonly a result of infectious or inflammatory disc destruction. In children, disc space narrowing constitutes the earliest radiographic finding in nonspecific discitis (Fig. 8–152). This condition has been variably attributed to infection or trauma, although most favor an infectious etiology. Very early in the disease when the disc narrowing is quite subtle, radioisotope bone scans are helpful. Later in the disease process, some degree of destruction of the adjacent vertebral bodies can occur resulting in an appearance indistinguishable from osteomyelitis (Fig. 8–153). Disc narrowing due to ankylosing spondylitis is rare in childhood.

Both acute and chronic trauma may result in disc destruction and resultant disc space narrowing. Most commonly these injuries are due to hyperflexion, sometimes with a rotational component. Scheuermann's disease is probably caused by chronic, subclinical hyperflexion trauma, resulting in disc space narrowing, end plate irregularity, and anterior wedging of at least three adjacent vertebral bodies. A portion of the disc commonly herniates into the weakened end plate causing Schmorl's nodes or a fragmented beak along the anterior aspect of the vertebral body (Fig. 8–147). Similar changes have been noted in several congenital syndromes and dysplasias.

Disc Calcification

The usual forms of calcification of the intervertebral discs that occur in adults, associated with such conditions as degenerative disc disease, ochronosis, ankylosing spondylitis, CPPD (calcium pyrophosphate dihydrate) arthropathy, hypervitaminosis D, or hemochromatosis, are very rare in children. Occasionally idiopathic calcification of the disc occurs in older children (Fig. 8–154), usually affecting the cervical and upper thoracic spine. Often the calcifications are accompanied by neck pain, muscle spasm, and fever. The involved discs tend to be slightly thickened; occasionally herniation of the disc occurs. The symptoms usually resolve spontaneously with only symptomatic therapy, and the calcifications gradually disappear.

Dislocation of the Spine

Vertebral body dislocation most commonly results from flexion-rotation injuries involving the cervical spine. The radiographic findings in such traumatic injuries in children are the same as those encountered in adults. Nevertheless, a few differences should be noted. The C1-dens distance is wider in children than in adults, commonly measuring 2 to 3 millimeters and even 4 to 5 millimeters in a small percentage of normal patients. In addition, this distance can occa-

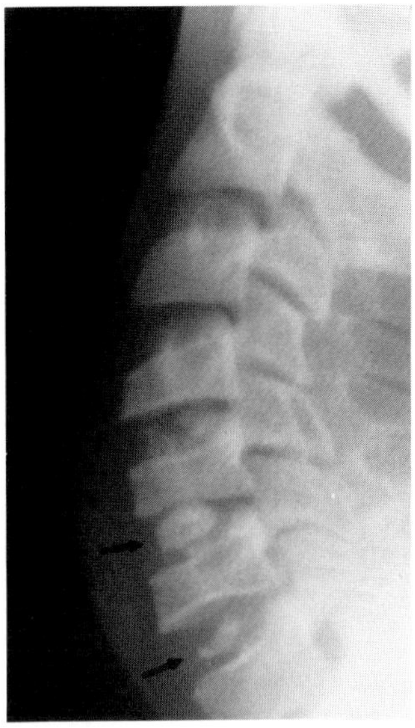

Fig. 8–154 Idiopathic disc calcification. Multiple calcified discs were seen in the lower cervical and upper thoracic spine of this 12-year-old patient (*arrows*).

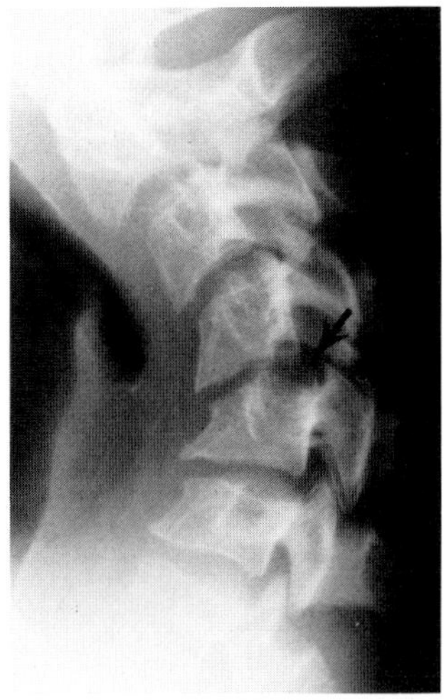

Fig. 8–155 Post-traumatic cervical subluxation. Note the subluxation of the cervical vertebrae following a motor vehicle accident (*arrow*). This hyperflexion injury also resulted in anterior compression of several of the vertebrae.

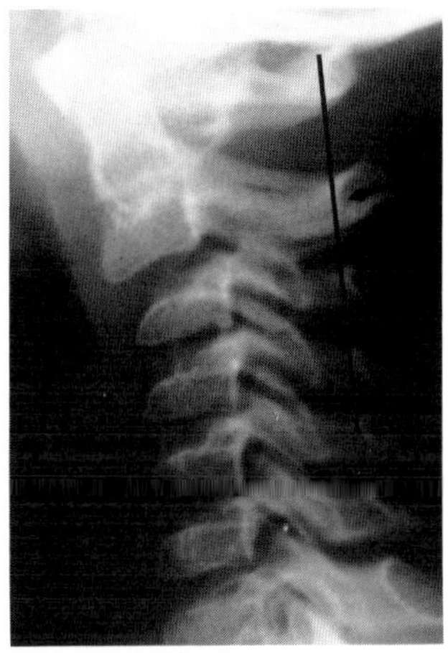

Fig. 8–156 Physiologic subluxation at C2-C3. Although C2 is mildly anteriorly subluxed on C3, the anterior cortex of the C2 spinous process lies within 1.5 mm of the posterior cervical line (*arrow*).

sionally increase by 1 to 2 millimeters with flexion even in the absence of a true dislocation. Nevertheless, dislocation of C1 on C2 can occur after trauma and any hypermobility on flexion and extension views should be viewed with caution. A common cause of pathologic widening of the C1-dens distance is the congenital ligamentous laxity associated with hypoplasia of the dens and the first cervical vertebra. This abnormality is most often seen in syndromes such as trisomy 21, Morquio's disease, chondrodystrophia punctata, and some storage diseases (Fig. 8–85). The hypermobility in these patients can be quite alarming; in some cases cord compression can result. Laxity of the ligaments in the absence of dens hypoplasia may occur in patients with rheumatoid arthritis.

Dislocation of the vertebral bodies most often consists of an anterior dislocation involving the cervical spine. Lateral dislocation less commonly occurs and is caused by severe rotation and flexion or extension injuries. Most dislocations in children are post-traumatic (Fig. 8–155), although rarely infections or congenital anomalies of the spine may result in dislocation. In children, a mild degree of physiologic anterior subluxation is common in the upper cervical spine. Such subluxation may involve several vertebra or may be isolated to the C2-C3 level. This finding is usually noted on flexion radiographs and can suggest the pathologic dislocation that occurs with a hangman's fracture. A helpful differentiating feature is assessment of the posterior cervical line, a line drawn along the anterior cortex of the spinous processes of C1 and C3 (Fig. 8–156). In normal physiologic dislocation, this line should not lie more than 1.5 millimeters anterior to the anterior cortex of the spinous process of C2.

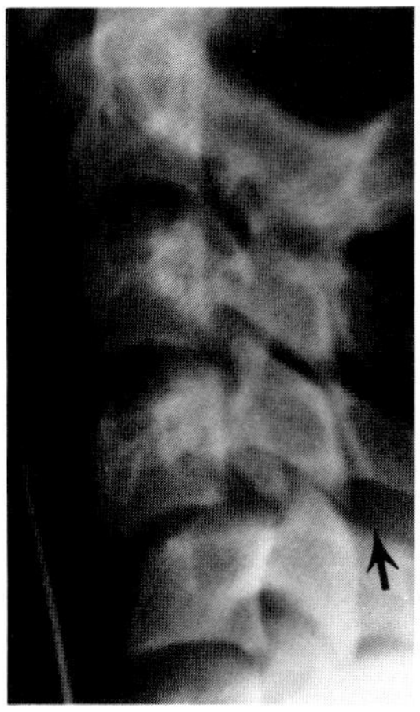

Fig. 8–157 Rotatory dislocation at C4-C5. Note the widened interspinous distance (*arrow*) and the asymmetery of the apophyseal joint at this level.

Rotatory dislocation of the cervical spine is often subtle and difficult to detect. Suggestive findings include malalignment of the spinous processes on the anteroposterior view, narrowing or nonuniform visualization of the apophyseal joints on the lateral view, and increased interspinous distance (Fig. 8–157). Occasionally, congenital anomalies of the posterior elements may mimic these findings.

Scoliosis

Scoliosis is a common condition in childhood, defined as lateral curvature and rotation of a portion of the spine. Scoliosis may be classified as one of two basic types: structural and functional (nonstructural). Structural scoliosis often has a rotatory component and consists of a primary and secondary (compensatory) curve. Usually the curve with the least flexibility on lateral bending is considered the primary curve. Nonstructural scoliosis is not associated with a compensatory curve and little rotation is present. The patient usually can voluntarily correct the curvature and stand erect. Nonstructural scoliosis is often due to poor posture or a leg length discrepancy.

The more common types of scoliosis are structural in nature. Any condition that results in pronounced spasm of the paraspinal muscles, such as trauma or adjacent inflammatory processes, can result in a structural scoliosis. Lumbar scoliosis with concavity to the right is a common finding in patients with appendicitis (Fig. 8–158). In a large percentage of patients with structural scoliosis, the curvature is idiopathic in nature. Although the cause is unknown, some authors attribute it to asymmetrical growth of the vertebral epiphyses or to inherent muscle imbalance. Rotation is virtually always present and is usually towards the convex side of the curvature. In the adolescent form of idiopathic scoliosis, the female-to-male ratio is 5:1.

Other causes of structural scoliosis are much less common, however they must be excluded before the scoliosis can be considered idiopathic. Other forms of structural scoliosis may be caused by abnormalities

SCOLIOSIS

Congenital/developmental
- Vertebral anomalies (e.g., hemivertebra, unilateral bar)
- Osteogenesis imperfecta
- Chondrodystrophies
- Neurofibromatosis
- Arthrogryposis multiplex congenita
- Idiopathic

Inflammatory
- Rheumatoid arthritis
- Pyogenic or tuberculous spondylitis
- Postempyema
- Poliomyelitis

Neoplasm
- Osteoid osteoma
- Other bone tumors
- Intraspinal tumors

Trauma/surgery
- Spastic paralysis secondary to trauma, etc.
- Fracture/dislocation of spine
- Post-thoracoplasty
- Postirradiation

Miscellaneous
- Any cause of paraspinal muscle spasm
- Other neuromuscular disease (e.g., muscular dystrophy, cerebral palsy, syringomyelia, Friedreich's ataxia)
- Congenital heart disease
- Any cause of osteoporosis/osteomalacia
- Histiocytosis X

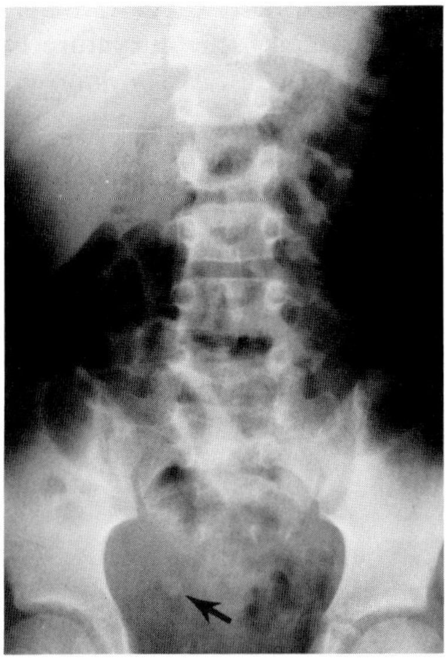

Fig. 8–158 Perforated appendicitis. Scoliosis with concavity to the right was associated with a soft tissue mass and fecalith (*arrow*) in the right lower quadrant (*arrow*).

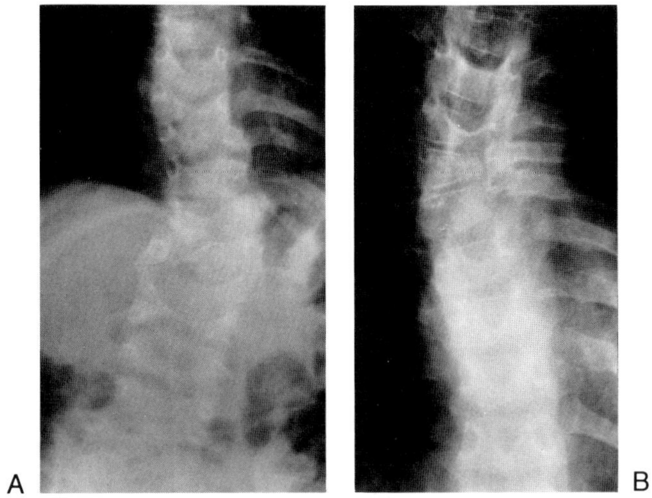

Fig. 8–159 Scoliosis. **(A)** Scoliosis was caused by multiple vertebral anomalies in this patient. **(B)** Thoracic scoliosis as a result of a unilateral bar on the left.

of the vertebrae (e.g., congenital anomalies, compression deformity, infections, tumors) (Fig. 8–159), neurologic disease (e.g., poliomyelitis, neurofibromatosis, intraspinal tumors, syringomyelia), or muscular disease (e.g., arthrogryposis syndromes, muscular dystrophy). In many of these conditions, the scoliosis is more angular with little evidence of rotation. An increased incidence of scoliosis occurs in patients with congenital heart disease, although the reason for the association is unclear.

Torticollis

Torticollis in children may be either congenital or acquired. Congenital torticollis is divided into two types. Postural congenital torticollis is thought to be caused by intrauterine malpositioning of the fetus; it is transient and resolves spontaneously. Muscular congenital torticollis results from a unilateral contracture of the sternocleidomastoid muscle and is usually associated with a fibrous mass within the sternocleidomastoid muscle (Fig. 8–160). The deformity may

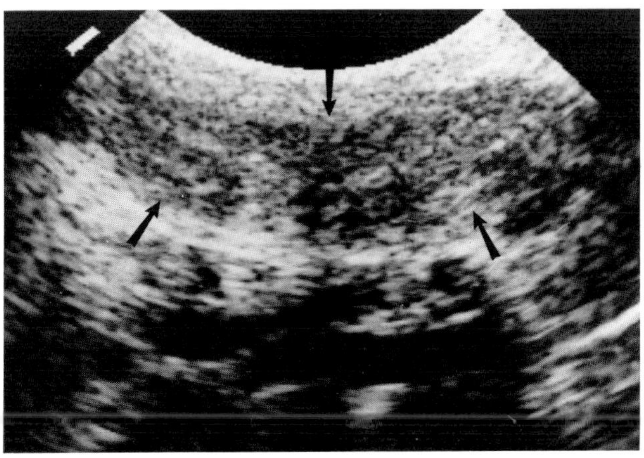

Fig. 8–160 Fibromatosis colli. Ultrasonography of the neck in this newborn with torticollis reveals a hypoechoic mass within the sternocleidomastoid muscle (*arrows*), a typical appearance of these fibromas.

be present at birth or may develop during the first 3 weeks of life. Treatment consisting of passive stretching exercises should be instituted to prevent development of secondary deformities of the face and head. The fibrous mass gradually disappears over the next 2 to 6 months. Acquired torticollis is most often the result of muscle spasm secondary to inflammation or trauma. Torticollis can also be a presenting symptom of tumors in the posterior fossa or upper cervical spine or spinal cord. Sandifer syndrome is a peculiar posturing of the neck associated with gastroesophageal reflux. When the reflux is corrected, the abnormal curvature disappears.

Because of the rotation involved in many cases of torticollis, the upper cervical spine appears rather disorganized radiographically. The C1-dens distance should always be noted, as it will be normal in patients with torticollis but increased in rotatory dislocation of C1-C2. In difficult cases, CT probably remains the most useful modality to demonstrate the anatomy.

Abnormalities of the Sacrum

A wide spectrum of congenital anomalies may affect the lower lumbar and sacral spine. Mild sacral hypoplasia may go unnoticed unless some form of motor dysfunction or bowel or bladder impairment occurs later in life. More severe forms of sacral hypoplasia or agenesis tend to present early in life with neurologic deficits, often associated with hypotonia and muscle wasting; club foot deformity; and incontinence. In the severe forms of sacral agenesis, portions of the lumbar spine may also be absent (Fig. 8–161). The lower extremities may be fused (mermaid deformity) and various gastrointestinal and genitourinary anomalies often are present. This entire constellation of anomalies has been referred to as the caudal regression syndrome, and are more common in infants of diabetic mothers.

A curved or crescent-shaped deformity of the sacrum with a unilateral concave defect is a typical appearance associated with an anterior or intrasacral meningocele (Fig. 8–162). Anterior sacral meningoceles are sometimes seen in patients with neurofibromatosis. Similar deformities occur in association with anorectal anomalies, presacral teratoma (Fig. 8–163), and tethered cord with or without a lipoma.

Erosion or destruction of the sacrum is most commonly caused by an adjacent neoplasm such as teratoma, sarcoma, or neuroblastoma. The teratoma or dermoid is the most common neoplasm in this region and may be intrapelvic, extrapelvic, or both. Up to 60 percent of these neoplasms contain calcifications that can be identified on plain radiographs. The pres-

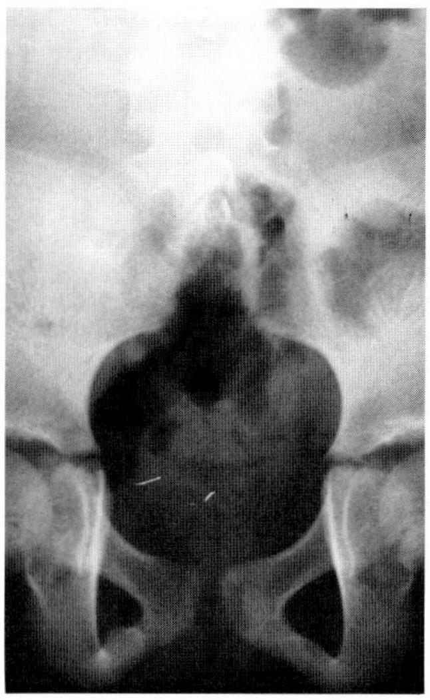

Fig. 8–161 Congenital absence of the sacrum. Absence of the sacrum and deformity of L5 were isolated congenital anomalies in this patient.

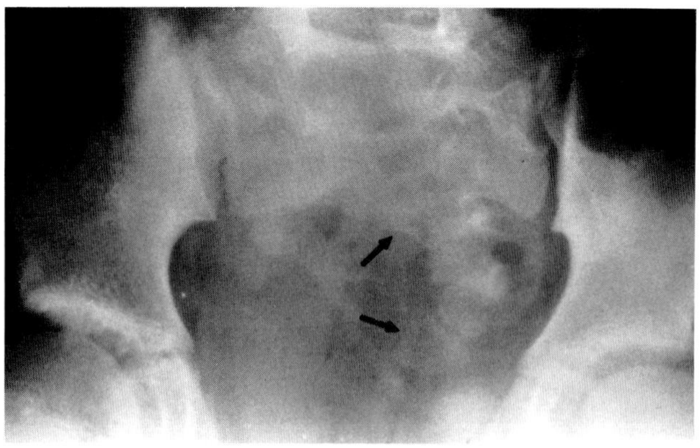

Fig. 8–162 Intrasacral meningocele. Note the crescent-shaped deformity of the sacrum (*arrows*), typical for this condition.

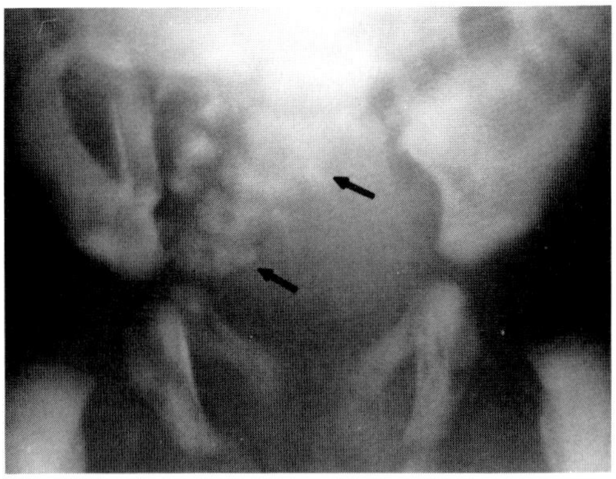

Fig. 8–163 Presacral teratoma. Curved deformity of the sacrum is similar to that seen with intrasacral meningocele.

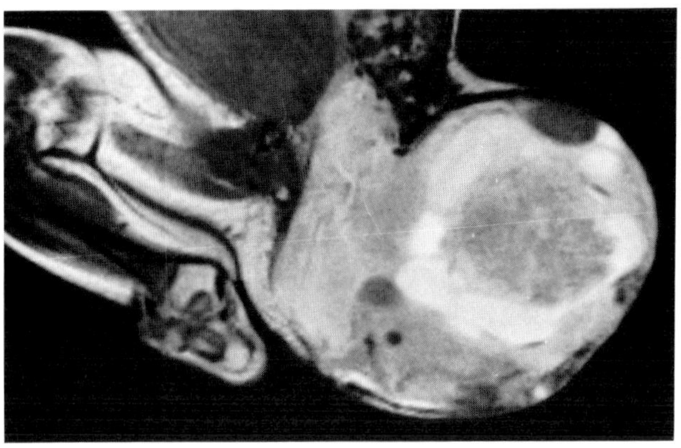

Fig. 8–164 Presacral teratoma. The varied tissue components and extent of this large teratoma were clearly identified on this T_1-weighted coronal MRI study.

ence of fat may also be detectable on plain radiographs, although ultrasonography, CT, and MRI are more sensitive for detecting the various tissue types within these complex neoplasms (Fig. 8–164). Although most teratomas are benign, all sacrococcygeal teratomas can be considered potentially malignant. Malignancy is somewhat more common in intrapelvic teratomas and in older infants. Sacral cordoma is a rare primary neoplasm of the sacrum. Destructive lesions such as metastases, infection, and histiocytosis X are much less common in the sacrum than in the remainder of the spine.

SUGGESTED READINGS

1. Alexander JE, Seibert JJ, Aronson J, et al: A protocol of plain radiographs, hip ultrasound, and triple phase bone scans in the evaluation of the painful pediatric hip. Clin Pediatr 27:175, 1988
2. Benz G, Brandeis WE, Willich E: Radiological aspects of leukemia in childhood. An analysis of 89 children. Pediatr Radiol 4:201, 1976
3. Caffey J: The early roentgenographic changes in essential coxa plana. AJR 103:620, 1968
4. Caffey J: The parent-infant traumatic stress syndrome (Caffey-Kempe syndrome) (battered babe syndrome). AJR 114:217, 1972
5. Ennis JT, Whitehouse G, Ross FGM, Middlemiss JH: The radiology of the bone changes in histiocytosis X. Clin Radiol 24:212, 1973
6. Gloebl HJ, Capitano MA, Kirkpatrick JA: Radiographic findings in children with psychosocial dwarfism. Pediatr Radiol 4:83, 1976
7. Graf R: The ultrasound examination of the hip. In Tonnis D (ed): Congenital dysplasia and dislocation of the hip in children and adults. Springer-Verlag, Berlin, 1984
8. Kozlowski K: Platyspondyly in childhood. Pediatr Radiol 2:81, 1974
9. Ozonoff MB: Pediatric Orthopedic Radiology. WB Saunders, Philadelphia, 1979
10. Swischuk LE: The beaked, notched, or hooked vertebra: its significance in infants and young children. Radiology 95:661, 1970
11. Swischuk LE, Hayden CK Jr: Rickets: a roentgenographic scheme for diagnosis. Pediatr Radiol 8:203, 1979
12. Tachdjian MO: Congenital Dislocation of the Hip. Churchill Livingstone, New York, 1982
13. Taybi H, Lachman RS: Radiology of Syndromes, Metabolic Disorders, and Skeletal Dysplasias. 3rd Ed. Yearbook Publishers, Chicago, 1990

Index

Page numbers followed by "f" designate figures; those followed by "t" designate tables.

D

H

M

N

P

R

U

V

W

X

Z